APPLIED NEUROPSYCHOLOGY OF CEREBROVASCULAR DISEASES

APPLIED NEUROPSYCHOLOGY OF CEREBROVASCULAR DISEASES

A PRACTICAL GUIDE TO BRAIN ARTERIES, LESION LOCALIZATION, AND REHABILITATION STRATEGIES

HELMUT HILDEBRANDT
Department of Neurology, Hospital Bremen-Ost, Bremen, Germany

NERGIZ TURGUT
Neuroscience Institute, Universidad San Francisco de Quito, Quito, Ecuador

MIRIAM HOLLAND-LETZ
Department of Neurology, Hospital Bremen-Ost, Bremen, Germany

ELSEVIER

ACADEMIC PRESS
An imprint of Elsevier

Academic Press is an imprint of Elsevier
125 London Wall, London EC2Y 5AS, United Kingdom
50 Hampshire Street, 5th Floor, Cambridge, MA 02139, United States

ISBN: 978-0-443-45450-9

For Information on all Academic Press publications
visit our website at https://www.elsevier.com/books-and-journals

Publisher: Megan Ball
Acquisitions Editor: Simonetta Harrison
Editorial Project Manager: Khyati Vat
Production Project Manager: Sathyavani Deiva Sigamani
Cover Designer: Raman Kumar

Typeset by MPS Limited, Chennai, India

Contents

Acknowledgments

This book reflects the collective efforts of colleagues, mentors, and supporting institutions.

We would like to express our gratitude to the patients of our early neurological rehabilitation unit, whose challenges and recovery journeys continuously shape our understanding of the healing brain. Working alongside them has not only informed the clinical insights presented in this book but has also furthered our commitment to improving their care and rehabilitation. We also thank our therapeutic and medical colleagues from the rehabilitation unit for decades of discussions on understanding patients' difficulties and identifying the most effective interventions to support them.

Some chapters reflect the intellectual and practical support of the Research Training Group (RTG) 2783, funded by the German Research Foundation (DFG)—Project ID 456732630. This is particularly the case for the chapters on transcranial direct current stimulation and visuospatial neglect.

We would like to thank Universidad San Francisco de Quito and its undergraduate program in psychology for their support. In particular, we thank the research assistants and students Joaquín Castro for the helpful organization of figures and licenses and Catalina Alvarez for the creation of several figures.

A book would not be possible without personal support. One of the authors (Nergiz Turgut) would like to express her personal gratitude to her family and friends, in particular her husband David and her daughter Lorin, as moments of distraction sometimes help to regain focus. She also thanks her mother as a role model and her father, himself an author, as an inspiration for cowriting this book. She is especially grateful to Prof. Dr. Helmut Hildebrandt for his mentorship and guidance over several years.

Introduction

The relevance of stroke for clinical neuropsychologists

Stroke, a sudden interruption of blood flow to the brain causing brain cells to die due to a lack of oxygen and nutrients, is now the third leading cause of death. In Germany, an incidence rate of 260,000 per year and a prevalence rate of more than one million strokes can be assumed. The incidence rate increases with age (doubling with each decade of age), which makes stroke a disease related to aging. With life expectancy increasing in most countries of the world, a consistent rise in stroke patients can be expected. In Germany, most patients (around two-thirds) in neurorehabilitation are stroke patients.

Knowledge of stroke patterns and their functional consequences, therefore, should be essential information for those working in the field of clinical neuropsychology. However, it is rarely an important part of textbooks (for an exception in German). While there are some excellent books on stroke and resulting neurological syndromes (one example is Bogousslavsky and Caplan), most of these textbooks focus on the *neurological* consequences of various stroke localizations, such as motor deficits and sensory loss, and are not written from the perspective of clinical neuropsychology. Even if neuropsychological studies are mentioned, cognition and emotions are not the structuring topics.

Another issue related to these books is the shift toward structural brain imaging for the diagnosis of acute stroke over the past two to three decades. Therefore the assessment of clinical syndromes, such as neglect (see Chapter 5) or aphasia (see Chapter 6) has lost much of its relevance for neurologists. In a similar vein, advances in acute stroke treatment mean that the earliest interventions can now decisively influence outcomes. The neurologist's primary role has shifted toward identifying the underlying cause of the symptoms and initiating treatment without delay. At the same time, hospital stays for stroke patients have become progressively shorter, with functional assessment and rehabilitation increasingly taking place outside acute care settings and beyond the main focus of neurological practice. It should be added that the *functional treatment* of the patients has never been a core task in neurology but the work of colleagues from physiotherapy, occupational therapy, speech therapy, and neuropsychology. Therefore specialized functional treatment is rarely discussed in existing textbooks on stroke syndromes.

Importantly, a similar gap exists in the training of nonmedical neurorehabilitation professionals. Medical knowledge related to stroke had received little attention in the training of the nonmedical neurorehabilitation professions. Here, the focus is often etiology-independent assessment of impairments and remaining abilities. Functional treatment approaches are often based on commonsense explanations of symptoms, on possible recovery pathways derived from ontogenetic development of functions (i.e., according to Bobath or Affolter), or on assuming existing tests as defining measures ("alertness" training). The available knowledge about crucial aspects, such as lesion localization, the impact of this localization, and the lesion size on prospect for recovery, is rarely considered in books on functional treatment of stroke patients. Even in domains with a strong research background, interventions are only rarely designed for patients with different lesions. For example, none of the developed neuropsychological treatments of memory disorder distinguish between those with and without involvement of the Papez circuit, and only a few studies on motor rehabilitation distinguish between those with and without destruction of the corticospinal tract inside the capsula interna.

Thus there is a reciprocal knowledge gap between the perspectives of medical and nonmedical professionals working with stroke patients treated in neurorehabilitation units. This gap hampers the work of clinical neuropsychologists, who are responsible for the functional assessment and treatment of these patients related to cognitive and affective impairments. This gap also hampers the development of stage- and severity-depending rehabilitation strategies that respond to the specific situation of single patients.

Effective assessment requires prioritization, because the brain retains many capacities. There is an urgent need to use available information on *individual* patients to restrict the assessment to the most critical domains. Such a reduction would increase the time for treatment. Something similar holds for the treatment of the patients. The severity of deficits may be due to the mere size of the lesion as a global effect but also to its specific localization (as a local effect). It may also depend on the acute overall state of the patient, irrespective of the stroke's lesion. Therefore treating patients raises questions like when to do what with which kind of patient. Again, any helpful information to decide on which approach should be taken is of immense importance, because face-to-face interventions are time-consuming and costly. Even more concerning than financial costs is the shortage of neuropsychologists available to treat the emerging number of patients. Therefore treatment should be focused and based on plausible and rational decisions.

As brain scans and their descriptions focus exclusively on questions of acute intervention, most neuroradiological reports are incomplete with regard to the information that could be inferred from the images concerning how to rehabilitate stroke patients. Even in the post-acute phase, brain scans are performed mainly to address acute medical concerns, such as detecting the development of hydrocephalus, evaluating the reduction of brain swelling after hemicraniectomy for bone flap reimplantation, or ruling out a second stroke in the event of a sudden clinical worsening. A direct interaction between neuroradiologists and neurorehabilitative professionals concerning neurorehabilitative questions is the very rare exception of what the dominant clinical routine is. Furthermore, in Germany, most of the rehabilitation units do not have access to clinical brain scanning devices at all, and the information about cerebrovascular events stems from scans that were done and reported on for the acute phase. Therefore the necessary information has to be derived by an independent inspection of the acute clinical scans from a neurorehabilitative perspective to gather information about size, localization of the stroke, already existing microangiopathy, and brain atrophy.

This book aims to address this knowledge gap and support clinical neuropsychologists in integrating medical information from the acute treatment phase into their work. The starting point will be a short introduction on what stroke is and how it is treated during the acute phase together with a description of the vessels of the brain. Afterward, the major brain arteries will be introduced, and typical cognitive and affective impairment patterns induced by a stroke to branches of one of them will be discussed. Information on the prognosis of deficits and their functional treatment will be added. This information will help clinical neuropsychologists to understand the medical reports of the patients and to formulate first and guiding hypotheses about the remaining deficits and possible treatments.

The second section of this book is focused on helping clinical neuropsychologists to understand clinical brain scans and to localize stroke lesions. To train orientation in clinical brain images, MRIcron, a free digital brain visualization software, is introduced. Moreover, clinical landmarks that are helpful to orient in cranial MRI and cranial CT scans are explained, and clinical example images of strokes and training tasks using MRIcron can be found in this section. The aim of this section is to teach clinical neuropsychologists to understand clinical brain scans and to use them for coming up with expectations of which functions might be impaired and what the prognosis might be.

The third and most extensive section of this book is focused on the treatment of stroke syndromes, such as neglect, hemianopia, aphasia, disorders of consciousness, and memory disorders. Each chapter distinguishes between phases of recovery and severity of impairment to propose different interventions, something we believe to be essential for neurorehabilitation. Another chapter introduces transcranial direct current stimulation (tDCS) as add-on treatment and the free SimNIBS software to enable the reader to perform a planning of positioning the electrodes according to lesion localization and phase of recovery.

The emphasis placed on *treatment* of cognitive and affective consequences of stroke expresses our conviction that treatment rather than assessment is the most important task of clinical neuropsychologists. Primarily, patients want to get help, not receive information on what they are unable to do at the current time. Still, helping patients to improve is impossible without insight into the consequences of stroke and profound knowledge of different treatment approaches that consider the state, severity, and prognosis of the impairment. It is also impossible without insight into the problems on the side of the patients, because any rehabilitation depends on the cooperation of both the neuropsychologist and the patient. And insight is based on rational and scientific-based information offered by the clinical neuropsychologist.

How to integrate diagnosing and treating the patients to achieve the best possible effects is proposed on a more theoretical level in the last chapter of the third part. Therefore, in the last chapter of this book, an integrated model will be proposed to put the different parts of the puzzle into one meaningful picture of neuropsychological work. This chapter will also cover fundamental aspects of virtual reality as a treatment option.

This book concludes with a brief appendix offering an overview of key tables, designed to serve as quick practical guidance. Reading this appendix can by no means replace the full reading of the chapters. Rather, it is designed to provide rapid orientation on which interventions should be initiated immediately upon first patient contact, with the relevant chapters serving for subsequent in-depth review. This approach parallels current trends in medical practice, and it may be advantageous for neurorehabilitation to adopt similar procedural structures.

However, there remains a substantial gap between acute neurological intervention and neurorehabilitation. This especially concerns the lack of well-designed studies encompassing the full spectrum of sensory, motor, cognitive, and affective disorders that compare different interventions across various stages of recovery. There is no immediate remedy for this lack of evidence, and the reader should be aware that most chapters on interventions are necessarily based on clinical experience rather than firm evidence-based knowledge. The perspectives presented in this book, therefore, inevitably reflect the authors' own clinical viewpoint—not out of any sense of grandiosity or megalomania, but with the aim of providing a starting point for future works on this topic that can be supported by more extensive empirical research.

Helmut Hildebrandt
Nergiz Turgut
Miriam Holland-Letz

CHAPTER

1

Brain arteries and related stroke syndromes

1.1 Cerebral blood flow and stroke

1.1.1 Cerebral blood flow

The predominant cause of vascular lesions is an interruption/occlusion of blood supply, not of venous blood outflow. Therefore cerebral blood supply plays a central role in understanding stroke and its consequences. Approximately 800 ml of blood is flowing through the brain each minute, about 1100 L a day [1,2]. Blood circulation is kept constant, regardless of the physical strain and differences in gravitational orientation. Impairments of this autoregulation induce vertigo during rapid postural changes, such as standing up quickly or turning the head. Constant blood supply is achieved by myogenetic autoregulation called the Bayliss effect: when the internal pressure of the vessel increases, the vessels constrict, while in the case of a drop in the internal pressure of the vessel, the vessel's diameter increases.

However, blood circulation is not only controlled on an automatic level. A cascade of central processes is involved in blood supply, too. This cascade involves the autonomic nervous system (ANS), especially the sympathetic branches of it. If specific organs of the body are highly active, they need more blood. Therefore blood flow to other inactive organs is suppressed by sympathetic innervation and vasoconstriction. Parasympathetic modulation of the vessels is important during the night. Vasodilatation increases blood flow and facilitates the drainage of metabolic waste products from the brain, which is important for normal cell function.

1.1.2 Disruption of cerebral blood supply

For the nervous system and especially for the brain cells, a loss of up to 50% of cerebral blood flow can be compensated, but a short drop below

Applied Neuropsychology of Cerebrovascular Diseases
DOI: https://doi.org/10.1016/B978-0-443-45450-9.00003-5

20 ml/100 g/min leads to reversible failures [2]. Such reversible failures are called transient ischemic attack (TIA). Patients enter the stroke unit with symptoms like hemiparesis or speech impairments that usually resolve within a couple of hours. However, at less than 15 ml/100 g/min, cell loss occurs. After 3–4 minutes of cardiac arrest, ganglion cells undergo necrosis, and after 9–10 minutes, brain death becomes inevitable. Physiological functioning of brain areas is thus given as long as more than 20% to 30% of the normal blood flow value is achieved. This means that the cells survive but are not performing the function they should perform because of a loss of blood supply. Once perfusion is restored, neuronal function can recover. This explains why the symptoms observed during TIAs are reversible.

In ischemia (another term for diminished blood supply to the brain), the vessels initially increase their diameter (vasodilation due to the Bayliss effect), although structural damage may already be present. As ischemia progresses vasoparalysis may develop: the vessels no longer respond with caliber changes. However, an increase in vessel diameter in the affected area is crucial for collateral blood flow. Connections between blood vessels, known as anastomoses, allow blood of adjacent arterial territories or of branches of the same artery not affected by the occlusion to reach the stroke territory. One important component of collateral circulation is formed by the leptomeningeal anastomoses. Blood from nearby arteries within the subarachnoid space is being redirected toward the stroke area. Fig. 1.1 illustrates this process. The left panel shows the anatomy of six different cerebral arteries (inferior view, brain tissue not shown, but the lateral ventricle as a gray structure). Immediately after occlusion of the right-sided artery shown in red, the clinical angiography demonstrates absent filling of the branches of this cerebral artery (center panel). Several minutes later, partial filling of these branches becomes visible (right panel), reflecting collateral blood flow through the leptomeningeal branches as indicated by the arrows [3].

1.1.3 Acute treatment of stroke

Filling through leptomeningeal anastomoses is important for the efficacy of contemporary treatment of stroke. Contemporary treatment is based on two interventions: first, pharmacological thrombolysis with the enzyme recombinant tissue plasminogen activator (rt-PA). The enzyme is infused and leads to thrombolysis as soon as the enriched blood reaches the occluded artery. Usually, the time since stroke onset should be less than 4.5 hours. Although studies now suggest that the treatment window might be longer, the effect of thrombolysis is higher if applied as early as possible. Second, thrombectomy is a mechanical interventional procedure by which a blood clot or thrombus is removed

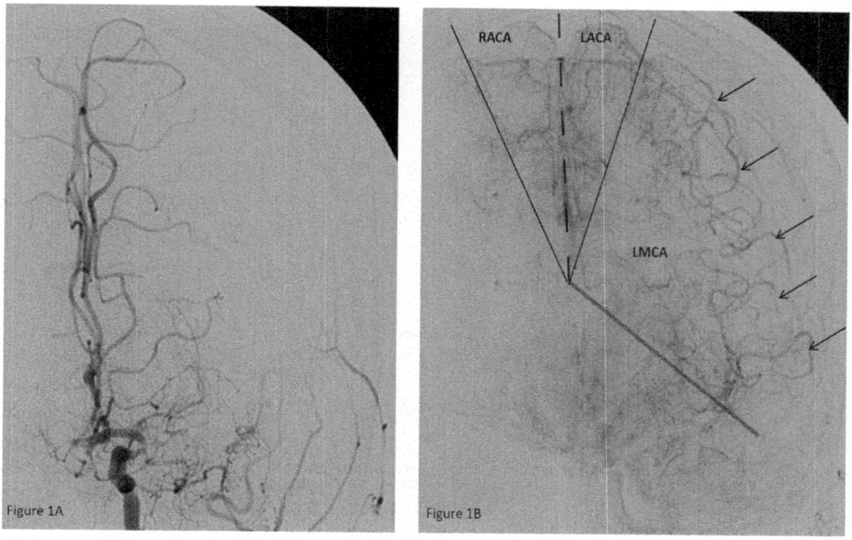

FIGURE 1.1 Stroke and the effect of leptomeningeal collaterals. *From Tariq N., Khatri R. Leptomeningeal collaterals in acute ischemic stroke. J Vasc Interv Neurol 2008;1(4):91–95.*

under image guidance using endovascular devices. The time window for thrombectomy is usually defined as less than 6 hours since stroke. Both interventions have an enormous effect on the outcome of strokes. But they depend on the existence of leptomeningeal anastomoses, strong enough to respond to the Bayliss mechanism to supply the brain tissue with enough blood for the physiological survival of the different cells.

Thrombolysis and thrombectomy not only have changed the survival rate after stroke, but they also have altered the typical lesion patterns observed on MRI scans (and therefore also the functional outcome). The left side of Fig. 1.2 shows how a complete acute stroke would look on a coronal image from the center of the brain reaching cortical areas. Depicted on the right side how the stroke would look like, if the leptomeningeal anastomoses are sufficient enough to enable the brain cells to survive until thrombolysis or thrombectomy re-opened the occluded artery. Therefore essential cortical brain areas could be rescued. In the subcortical parts of the brain, there are no leptomeningeal branches; these cells received no collateral blood supply and underwent cell death. However, a lack of leptomeningeal arteries might not be the only reason why subcortical structures cannot be rescued by thrombectomy as effectively as cortical areas. The use of endovascular tools may detach small arteriosclerotic plaques that travel through the arteries. Because subcortical arteries have a small caliber, even small plaques may lead to strokes. Still, the positive effect of thrombolysis and

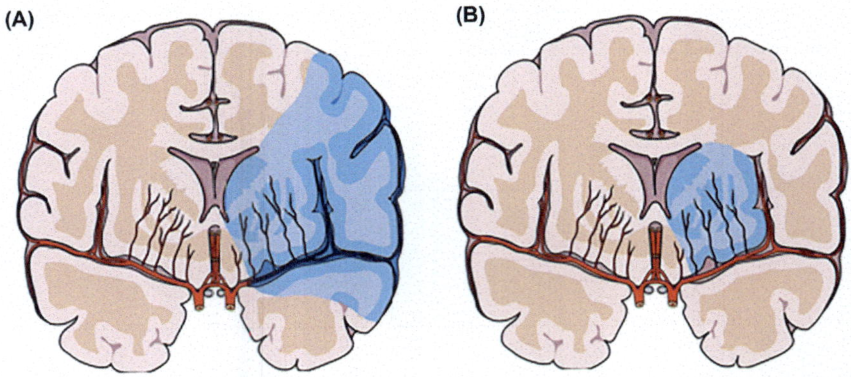

FIGURE 1.2 Coronal drawing of a combined cortical and subcortical stroke (A) versus a subcortical stroke (B). *From Guglielmi V., Quaranta D., Masone Iacobucci G. et al. Basal ganglia ischaemic infarction after thrombectomy: cognitive impairment at acute stage. Eur J Neurol 2023;30(12):3772–3779.*

thrombectomy on stroke outcome is enormous. This can be seen on MRI scans: many depict strokes restricted to subcortical structures and small cortical spots without collateral anastomoses, whereas in earlier decades, brain scans more often showed extended cortical and subcortical strokes [4].

1.2 Classification of strokes

In clinical routine practice, the terms global and focal hypoxia or ischemia are used, but only the latter refer to strokes. Before exemplifying the different terms of strokes and their relevance for neuropsychologists, global hypoxia should be explained.

1.2.1 Global hypoxia

Global hypoxia means that all cerebral arteries suffer from a loss of oxygen transport, for example, by pulmonary embolism, cardiac arrest, or strangulation trauma. Global hypoxia does not produce focal brain lesions, such as strokes, because by definition the whole brain is involved. However, usually some parts of the brain are more severely affected than others. This is due to the structure of vascularization and the dependence of specific neurons on oxygen. The first aspect will be discussed below in the context of low-flow stroke or strokes related to end arteries. The second aspect is important for neuropsychologists, because there are two types of neurons that require more oxygen supply than other neurons and are more sensitive to short-term blood supply loss. Specifically, magnocellular neurons of the dorsal visual pathway seem to need higher amounts of oxygen compared to parvocellular neurons [5,6], meaning that global hypoxia involves a risk of developing apperceptive and even form agnosia. The same holds for hippocampal neurons. Thus severe memory loss or amnesia is also a frequent consequence of hypoxia. Both conditions, agnosia and memory impairments, are core symptoms that are diagnosed and treated by a neuropsychologist.

1.2.2 Local hypoxia/stroke

Local hypoxia (strokes) is classified either according to the cause (embolic, atherothrombotic, hemodynamic), or by circumstance (hemorrhagic or not), by size (territorial, lacunar, microangiopathic), by the affected brain artery, or by location [2,7]. The first, causal classification is of lesser relevance to a neuropsychologist but highly important for physicians.

The second classification has an impact on the counseling of the patients and on coping with the illness. The existence of blood in the brain tissue leads to functional consequences, which may resolve after its resorption. Therefore the severe impairment the patients may experience may show a fast recovery as long as the blood is visible, for example, on cranial computer tomography (cCT) scans (i.e., has not been resolved, yet). However, after resorption, the recovery trajectory may be more prolonged compared to ischemic strokes. There is data that seems to indicate that recovery is slower (not necessarily smaller) in patients with intracerebral hemorhage (ICH) [8]. On top of that any kind of brain hemorrhage increases the risk of developing convulsions or symptomatic epilepsy. These different aspects should be discussed with the patients whenever they request such information or it is deemed necessary by the clinicians.

Stroke size is the third dimension used for classifying stroke. Fig. 1.3 depicts the different stroke patterns grouped by size.

On the right side (representing the left hemisphere), subcortical arteriosclerotic encephalopathy (SAE) is shown, which indicates many but very small strokes, which are not experienced by the patients as a single event. Some amount of SAE is quite common in elderly people and can be compensated for by cognitive reserve. However, if the SAE is severe enough, symptoms of cognitive and motor slowing, memory impairment, and urinary incontinence will become prominent.

In the middle column of Fig. 1.3, low-flow infarcts and watershed strokes are shown [9,10]. In both cases (low-flow and watershed strokes), the affected tissue is located at the distal end of the arterial supply and is therefore particularly vulnerable to reductions in cerebral perfusion.

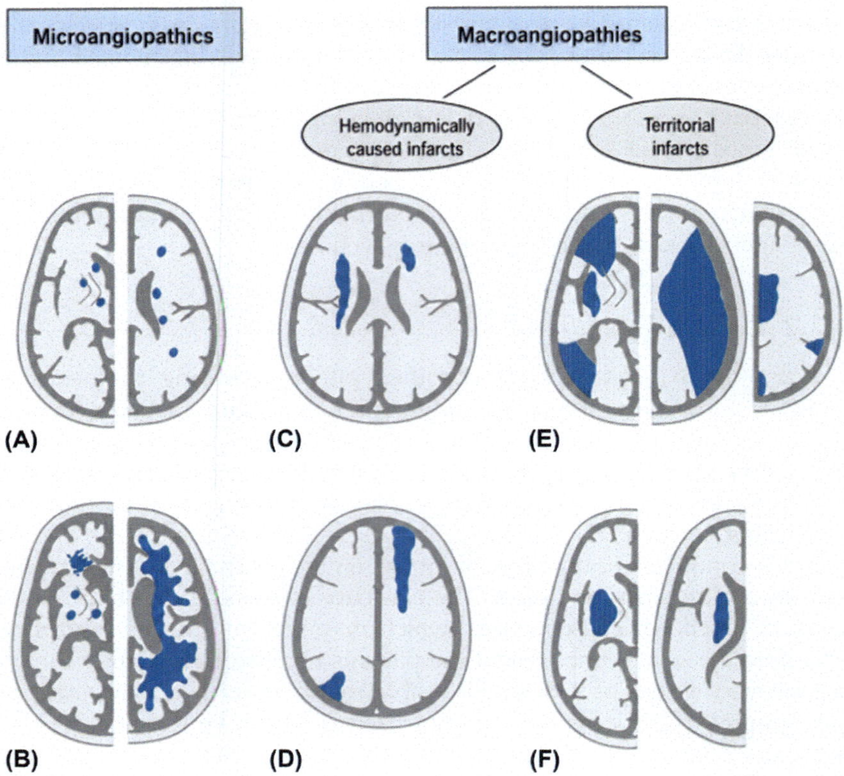

FIGURE 1.3 (A–F) Patterns of stroke. *From Poeck, K., & Hacke, W. (2006). Neurologie (12., aktualisierte und erweiterte Auflage). Springer. https://doi.org/10.1007/3-540-29998-X.*

Therefore any reduction in blood pressure will result in the consumption of most of the oxygen by the foregoing segments of the brain subserved by this artery. As a consequence, these distal territories become particularly vulnerable to ischemia. Watershed strokes often produce small arrow-shaped cortical lesions. This is because at this part of the brain, the branches of two different arteries end. Reduced blood flow therefore affects the tissue along the boundary between the two vascular territories. From a scientific point of view, such strokes are interesting because they mainly affect cortical structures of the frontal and dorsal premotor cortex (in the case of involvement of the middle cerebral artery (MCA) and anterior cerebral artery (ACA)).

Large stroke lesions are called "territorial" and are named by the artery involved. Most medical reports inform at least about the cause (e.g., embolic) of the stroke and the arteries involved ("MCA stroke"). Detailed neuroradiological reports also specify the branches or the localization of the stroke, such as right-sided middle cerebral stroke of the frontal branches or left-sided parietal middle cerebral stroke.

The localization of the infarct is highly important for the work of a neuropsychologist. It informs the selection of assessment tools, because of the expectation of which functions will be impaired. Additionally, it defines what kind of impairment would not be expected in the absence of atypical hemisphere dominance or earlier brain diseases. This knowledge helps to reduce the number of tests that need to be administered. However, if the patient deviates from what would be expected based on neuroimaging findings, further investigation is warranted. In such cases, one should consider whether additional brain regions are involved beyond those visible (e.g., due to the development of hydrocephalus in the days or weeks since the last brain scan was done, or by an ongoing independent neurodegenerative process). Alternatively, it should be examined whether psychogenic factors are part of the clinical picture the patient is presenting. Both considerations are important aspects of the neuropsychological investigation. For both reasons, an understanding of the anatomy of the cerebral arteries and the terminology used to describe different types of strokes is important to understand lesion localization, the expected functional consequences, and to guide the clinical work of neuropsychologists.

1.3 Non stroke cerebrovascular diseases

Before the different cerebral arteries are demonstrated in more detail, three nonstroke vascular diseases of the brain (or atypical causes of stroke) will be introduced shortly.

1.3.1 Spontaneous (non-traumatic) subarachnoid hemorrhage

The second most common vascular disease of the brain, although far less frequent than stroke, is subarachnoid hemorrhage (SAH) resulting from a ruptured aneurysm [2,7,11]. Aneurysms are protrusions of the arterial wall (Fig. 1.4). It is estimated that more than 10% of humans suffer from a small or large aneurysm, but only a few of these aneurysms rupture.

Cerebral vessels run outside the brain tissue within the subarachnoid space, that is, between the arachnoid and pia mater, before entering the cerebrum. Cerebral aneurysms within the subarachnoid space are often located proximal to the bifurcation of the internal carotid artery into the ACA and MCA, at the anterior communicating artery, and within the subarachnoid spaces surrounding the brainstem and cerebellum (see below). Because the walls of aneurysms are structurally weaker than those of normal arteries and may become progressively thinner as the

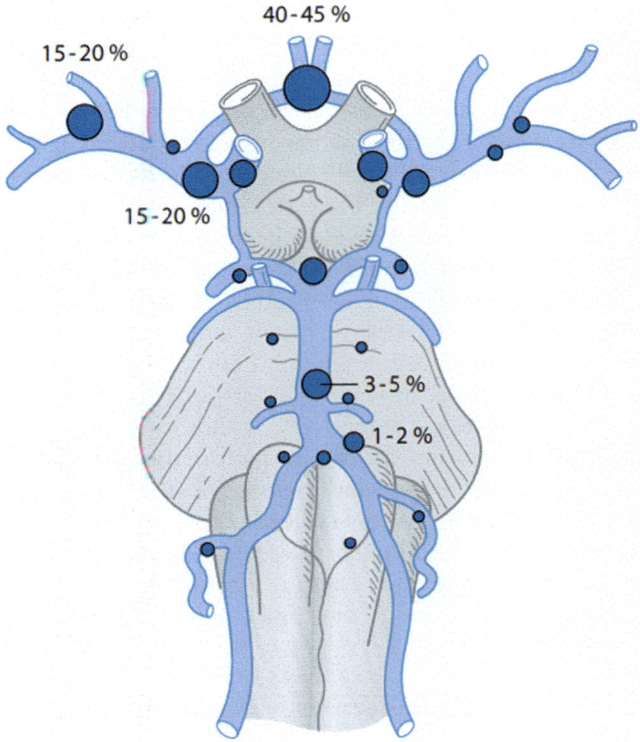

FIGURE 1.4 Schematic drawing of cerebral aneurysms. *From Poeck, K., & Hacke, W. (2006). Neurologie (12., aktualisierte und erweiterte Auflage). Springer. https://doi.org/10.1007/3-540-29998-X. Figure 9.1.*

aneurysm enlarges, fluctuations in blood pressure can cause rupture. In this case, blood is released into the subarachnoid space and, if the hemorrhage is sufficiently severe, may also extend into the brain tissue resulting in an intracerebral hemorrhage (ICH). This can cause cerebral ischemia through reduced blood flow following aneurysm rupture or through vasoconstriction triggered by blood affecting the neural mechanisms controlling the vessel caliber. Because the subarachnoid space is continuous over the surface of the brain, blood may spread to regions distant from the site of the rupture. This may further reduce cerebral blood flow through vasospasm and through increased intracranial pressure caused by the presence of blood within the subarachnoid space. Fig. 1.5 shows a clinical cCT, where the SAH was not produced by an aneurysm but by a traumatic brain injury.

When interpreting Fig. 1.5, it should be noted that acute blood appears hyperdense (white) in cCT scans. The SAH is evident from the hyperdense

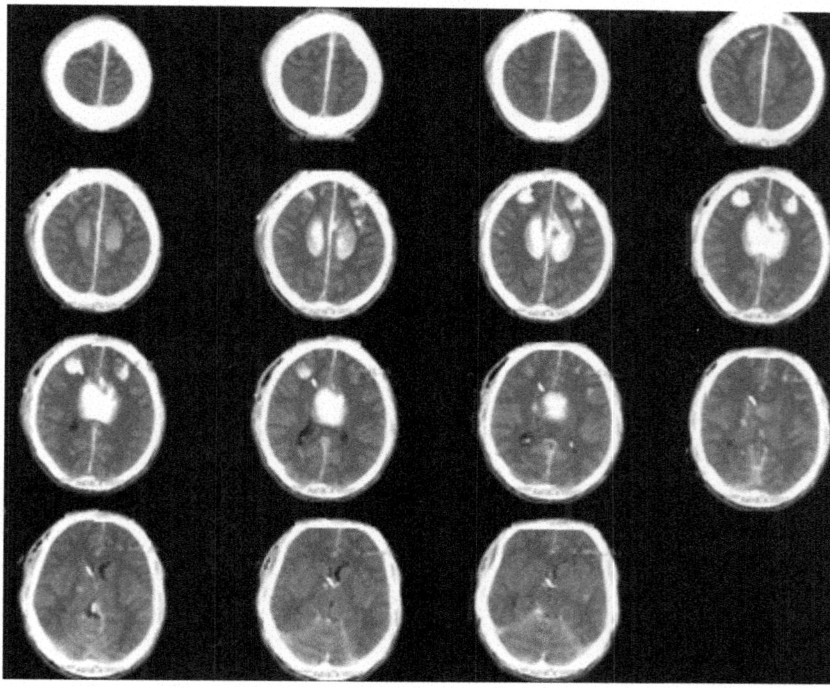

FIGURE 1.5 Clinical scan of subarachnoid hemorrhage.

appearance of the cerebral sulci. The scan also shows blood, visible as a white area, within the lateral ventricles (symmetrical structures in the center of the images) due to additional intraventricular hemorrhage as well as two symmetrical spots of blood in the frontal cortex (upper part of each image), indicating a bilateral shunting. Shunting was performed to reduce brain swelling.

1.3.2 Intracerebral hemorrhage

A second cerebrovascular disease is intracerebral hemorrhage (ICH) [2,7]. If such a hemorrhage is not a consequence or side effect of an ischemic stroke ("hemorrhagic transformation"), it is referred to as a spontaneous ICH. Causes of ICH are, among others, extremely high hypertension or a long history of hypertension, genetic coagulation disorders, or an arteriovenous malformation. Fig. 1.6A shows a schematic drawing of an ICH on the left and a reconstruction of an arteriovenous malformation on the right. Fig. 1.6B adds a clinical scan of an ICH (not of an arteriovenous malformation). As already mentioned, blood becomes

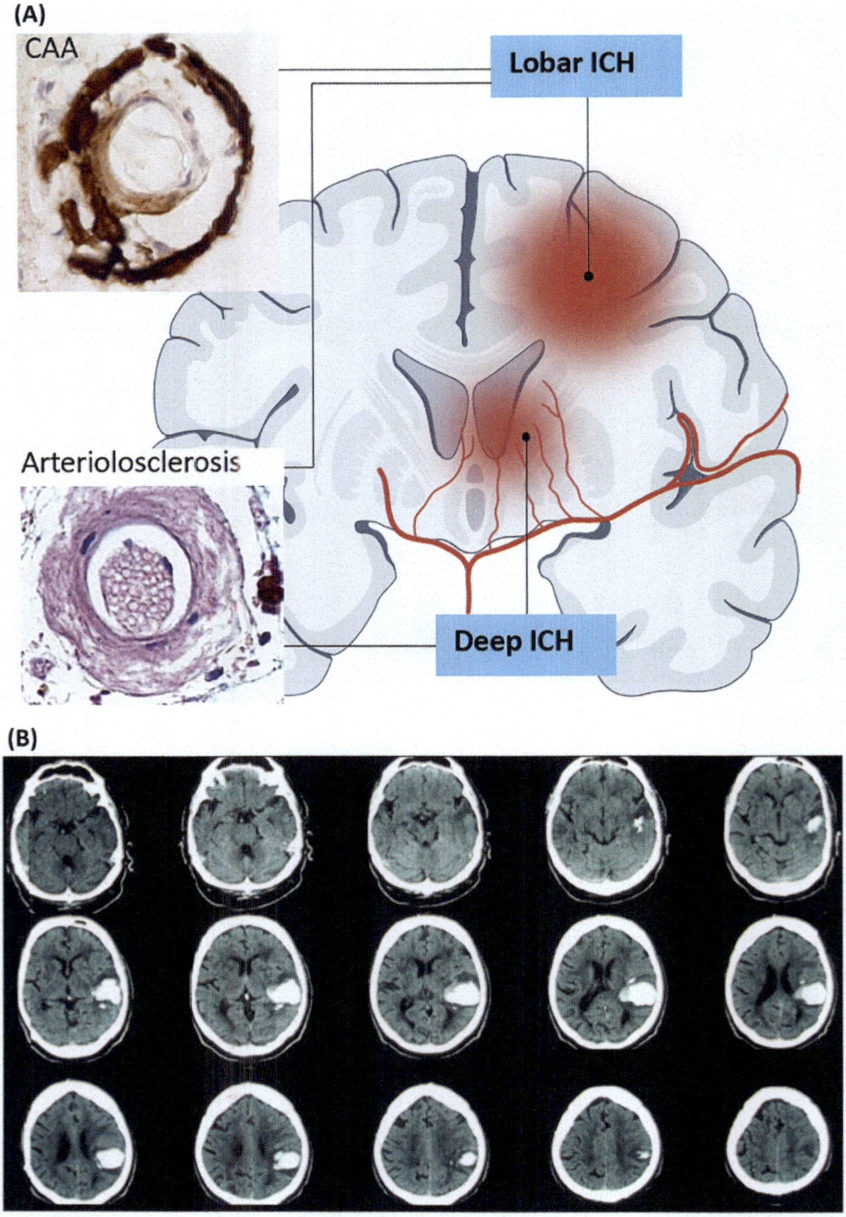

FIGURE 1.6 Arteriovenous malformation and clinical scan of intracerebral hemorrhage. *Source: (A) Seiffge, D. J., Fandler-Höfler, S., Du, Y., Goeldlin, B. M., Jolink, W. M. T., Klijn, C. J. M., & Werring, D. J. (2024). Intracerebral haemorrhage — mechanisms, diagnosis and prospects for treatment and prevention. Nature Reviews Neurology, 20(12), 723–736. https://doi.org/10.1038/s41582-024-01035-w.*

visible as a white area. Accordingly, there is a large white area on the right side of each transversal image (corresponding to the left hemisphere). The clinical scan illustrates several important features that should be considered when interpreting such scans. First, there are dark areas in the immediate neighborhood of the white area. These are called edema and reflect fluid accumulation associated with swelling and inflammatory processes. Second, the two black structures in the center of each section (the lateral ventricles) are not completely symmetrical. This indicates that the hemorrhage and associated swelling impact the width of these structures on the right side. Finally, a small line runs along the frontal cortex to the postcentral cortex. In images eight and nine, this line is shifted a little bit towards the left. Such a midline shift is also a sign of unilateral brain swelling. The shift is small in this clinical case. If it were more pronounced, decompressive surgery (removal of a portion of the skull to relieve intracranial pressure) may be necessary to rescue the patient's life.

1.3.3 Intracranial arterial dissection

The third nonstroke vascular disease is called arterial dissection, which involves a tear in the inner layers of the arterial wall [12]. In younger patients, a trauma caused by sharp movement is often the reason for an arterial dissection (e.g., while undergoing chiropractic treatment, which is a physiotherapeutic intervention, or certain sports with sudden head movements). In elderly patients, embolized atherosclerotic plaque fragments may also play a role.

If the inner layers of the arterial walls are dissected, blood will tend to enlarge the separation between its layers. In addition, thrombi may form at the site of the dissection and give rise to distal emboli (Fig. 1.7). This can lead to a complete occlusion of the artery. In many cases, lowering blood pressure allows the vessel wall to heal over time. The functional consequences depend on the duration of the dissection and the completeness of the occlusion. Dissections mainly occur in the vertebral artery but also the basilar artery. The vertebral arteries course through the transverse foramina of the cervical vertebrae before entering the skull. Their close relationship to the cervical spine may contribute to their vulnerability during sudden head and neck movements.

1.3.4 The vascular system of the brain: cortical branches of the middle cerebral artery and anterior cerebral artery

As already defined, stroke refers to the occlusion of the major cerebral arteries or their branches leading to structural brain damage [2,7,14–16].

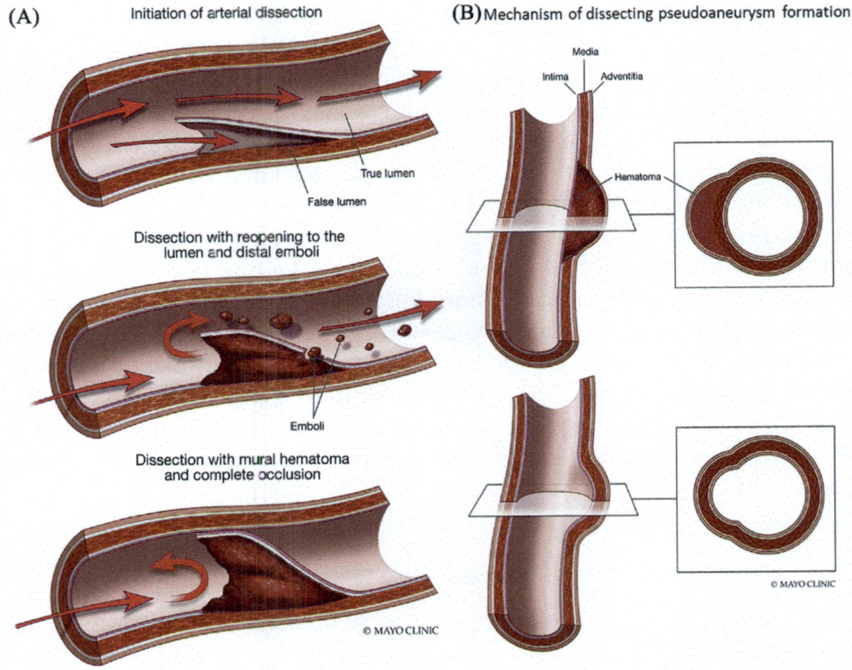

FIGURE 1.7 Intracranial artery dissection. Keser, Meschia [13].

To understand stroke from a neuropsychological perspective, knowledge about the cerebral vascular system is a prerequisite. To provide the necessary background several neuroanatomical terms will be introduced in the following sections.

The vascular supply of the brain is based on two major paired circuits (one anterior and one posterior for each hemisphere of the brain [14], for a more detailed description of the brain's blood supply, we refer to the book of Nieuwenhuys [17]). The anterior circulation originates from the common carotid artery and continues via the internal carotid artery, which reaches the subarachnoid space after entering the skull. The posterior circulation originates from the vertebral arteries, which arise extracranially from the subclavian arteries and unite to form the basilar artery. The basilar artery subsequently bifurcates into the paired posterior cerebral arteries. This is shown in Fig. 1.8 as a schematic drawing and as a clinical angiogram.

1.3.5 Circle of Willis

The two major supply circuits (anterior and posterior) are connected at the base of the brain by communicating arteries, creating a completely

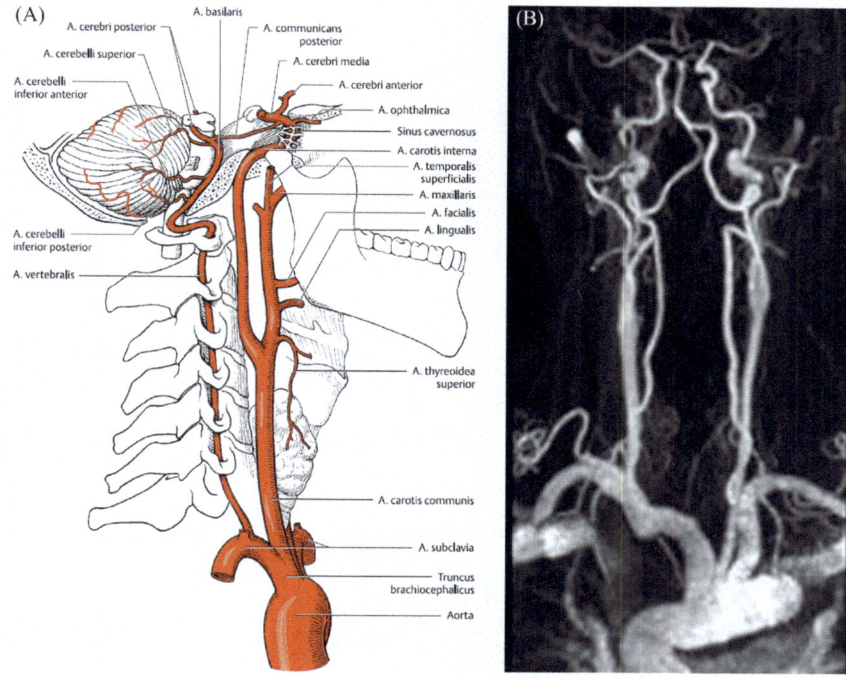

FIGURE 1.8 Schematic drawing and clinical scan of the brain's blood supply. *(A) From Bähr M., Bechmann I. Neurologisch-topische Diagnostik: Anatomie - Funktion - Klinik.* 11 überarbeitete Auflage Thieme *2021. Abb. 11.1.*

closed circuit called the Circle of Willis (Fig. 1.9) [7,17]. The exact configuration of these connections is interindividually variable. The arteries that close the circuit are the anterior communicating artery and the posterior communicating arteries. The Circle of Willis allows the brain to partially compensate for the occlusion of one of the three major arteries (the two internal carotid arteries and the basilar artery). However, the degree of compensation depends on the structure of the Circle of Willis: if the communicating arteries are small, compensation may be insufficient. Furthermore, because of the difference in caliber between the carotid arteries and the communicating arteries, the compensation is generally incomplete.

However, as discussed above, it may be complete enough to rescue brain tissue until thrombolysis or thrombectomy take place. The Circle of Willis is visible on clinical angiograms, but its inspection is possible only by rotating the view and following its course. A single sectional image is insufficient, because of the three-dimensional configuration of the circle. From a neuroanatomical point of view, it is important to

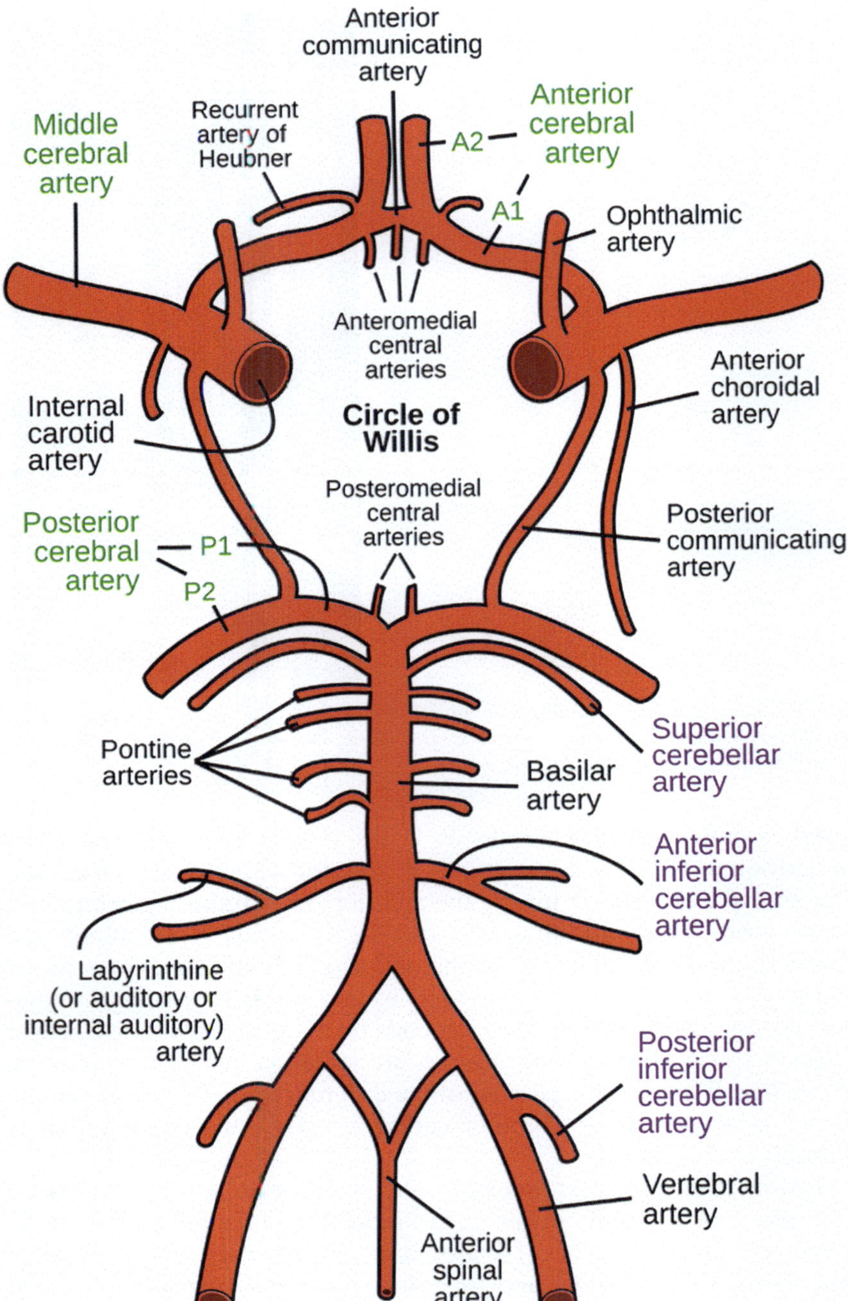

FIGURE 1.9 The Circle of Willis. *Wikimedia Commons. Author: McKay (own work). Licensed under Creative Commons Attribution-ShareAlike 4.0 International (CC BY-SA 4.0). https://commons.wikimedia.org/wiki/File:Circle_of_Willis_en.svg.*

mention that the two communicating arteries give rise to a series of small perforating arteries that provide essential subcortical structures (e.g., the thalamus and the ventral striatum). We will return to these vessels in a later section.

1.3.6 Major cerebral arteries and their vascular territories

The cerebral hemispheres are supplied by the three major cerebral arteries on each side (Fig. 1.10): the middle cerebral artery (MCA), anterior cerebral artery (ACA), and posterior cerebral artery (PCA) [14,17]. The MCA is by far the largest cerebral artery and supplies the lateral portion of the cortex. The ACA and PCA supply the medial portions (Fig. 1.11). The areas where the terminal branches of these arteries meet are called "watershed areas"—they also allow for inter-arterial anastomoses, complementing the intra-arterial anastomoses between different arterial branches.

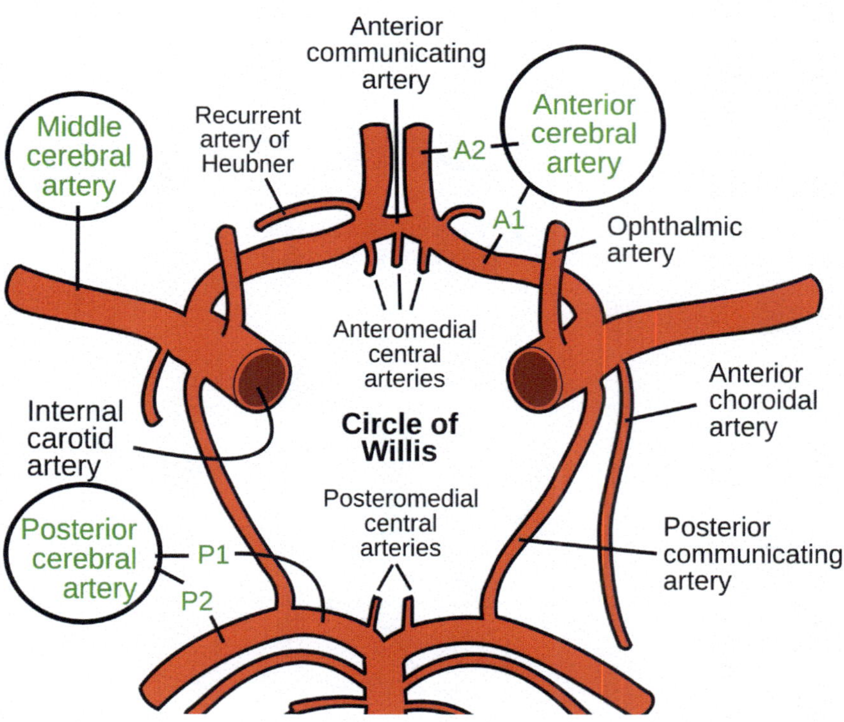

FIGURE 1.10 The three major cerebral arteries. *From The Circle of Willis. Wikimedia Commons. Author: McKay (own work). Licensed under Creative Commons Attribution-ShareAlike 4.0 International (CC BY-SA 4.0). https://commons.wikimedia.org/wiki/File:Circle_of_Willis_en.svg.*

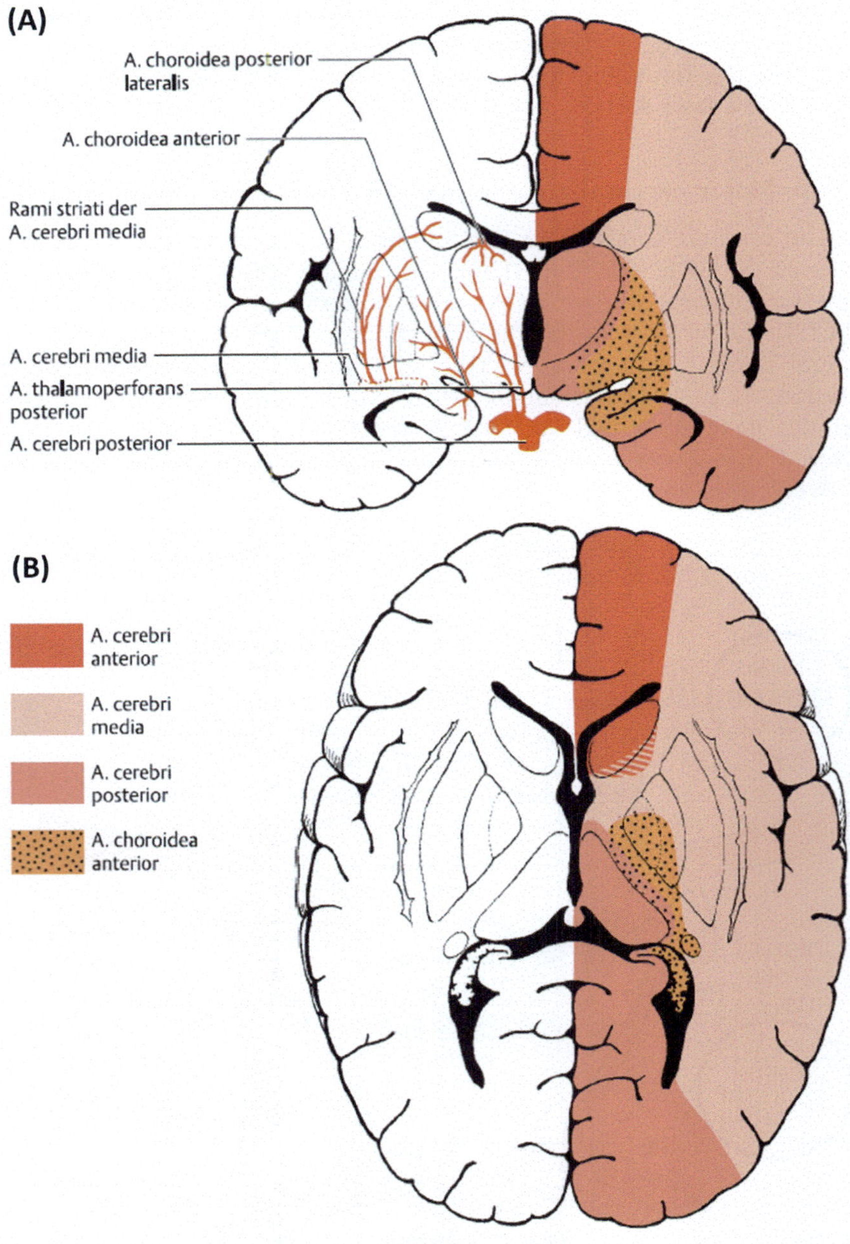

FIGURE 1.11 Schematic drawing of the cortex and its blood supply by the three major cerebral arteries in coronal (A) and axial (B) view. *From Bähr M., Bechmann I. Neurologisch-topische Diagnostik: Anatomie - Funktion - Klinik.* 11 überarbeitete Auflage Thieme *2021, Abb. 11.3.*

1.3.6.1 Middle cerebral artery

The MCA originates at the bifurcation of the internal carotid artery into middle and anterior cerebral arteries. Just before this bifurcation the ophthalmic artery arises from the internal carotid artery. Some patients experience transient monocular vision loss lasting from minutes to hours. This is called "amaurosis fugax" and represents a TIA in this territory [2,7]. Experiencing such events is associated with an increased risk of subsequent stroke, and warrants further medical evaluation. Before giving rise to the ophthalmic artery, the internal carotid artery follows a characteristic S-shaped course, which is called the carotid siphon, a region particularly prone to arteriosclerotic plaque formation [17].

After the internal carotid artery bifurcates into the MCA and ACA a distinction is made between the M1 segment, which is the part of the MCA before reaching the insular cistern, and the M2 segment. The perforating branches of the M1 segment (lenticulostriate arteries, often affected by strokes) supply the basal ganglia [14,17,19]. The anterior choroidal artery is one of these perforating arteries [20]. However, in some individuals, it arises from the internal carotid artery. The M2 segment begins at the insular cistern and courses within the subarachnoid space of the Sylvian fissure before dividing into branches that supply the lateral cerebral cortex [21]. The M2 segment supplies most of the lateral cerebral cortex as well as the U-fibers connecting adjacent gyri across the sulci. In contrast, the deep white matter tracts are mainly supplied by the perforating arteries. Stroke lesions therefore frequently involve both cortical regions and white matter pathways, making precise cognitive modeling of the resulting symptoms more difficult.

Fig. 1.12 shows the M2 segment of the MCA. The M2 segment is divided into three branches: the frontal trunk, the central-parietal trunk, and the inferior temporal trunk.

The branches of these trunks are named according to the sulci in which they course, and the same principle applies to the two other major cerebral arteries, the ACA and the PCA.

1.3.6.2 Anterior cerebral artery

For the ACA, an A1 and an A2 segment can be distinguished [17,22]. The A1 segment is the part before the anterior communicating artery and supplies parts of the orbitofrontal cortex. The anterior communicating artery connects the two branches of the ACA as part of the Circle of Willis. Perforating branches of the A1 segment (e.g., the recurrent artery of Heubner) and of the anterior communicating artery (e.g., the anteromedial central arteries) supply the basal forebrain and ventral basal ganglia. The A2 segment winds around the anterior corpus callosum, and supplies the corpus callosum, the cingulate gyrus, and the entire mesial (orbito-) frontal lobe (Fig. 1.13). Its terminal branches reach the precuneus

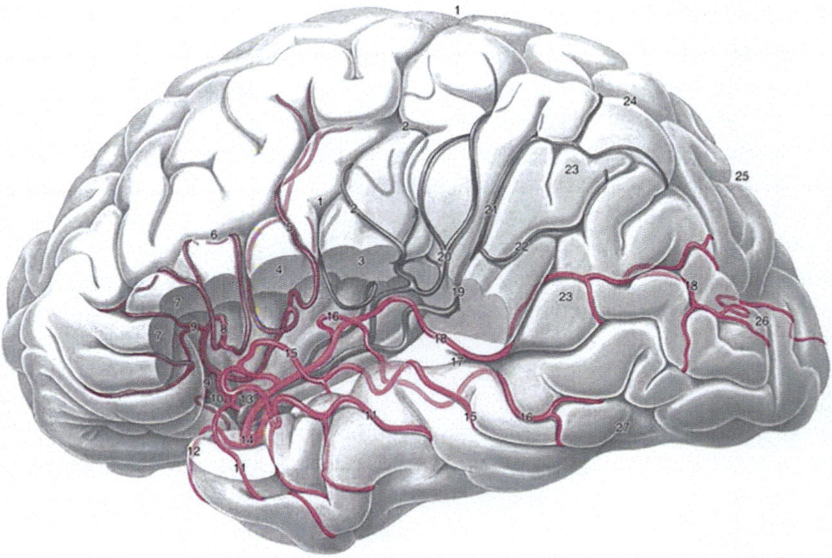

1 Central sulcus
2 Artery of the central sulcus (branches)
3 Postcentral gyrus
4 Precentral gyrus
5 Artery of the precentral sulcus
6 Inferior frontal sulcus
7 Inferior frontal gyrus, triangular part
8 Prefrontal artery (candelabrum artery)
9 Lateral frontobasal artery (branched)
10 Anterior trunk of the middle cerebral artery (ascending frontal artery)
11 Anterior temporal artery (branches)
12 Temporopolar artery
13 Middle trunk of the middle cerebral artery
14 Posterior trunk of the middle cerebral artery
15 Middle temporal artery
16 Posterior temporal artery
17 Superior temporal sulcus
18 Temporo-occipital artery
19 Lateral sulcus, posterior branch
20 Artery of the postcentral sulcus (anterior parietal artery)
21 Posterior parietal artery
22 Artery of the angular gyrus
23 Angular gyrus
24 Intraparietal sulcus
25 Parieto-occipital sulcus
26 Lunate sulcus
27 Anterior occipital sulcus

Alternative subdivision
11+15 Anterior temporal artery
16 Middle temporal artery
18 Posterior temporal artery
20 Parietal artery
21+22 Artery of the angular gyrus

FIGURE 1.12 Different branches of the M2 segment of the middle cerebral artery. *From Nieuwenhuys R., Voogd J., Huijzen C.van The Human Central Nervous System. 4th ed. Berlin: Springer-Verlag; 2008. Figure 4.4.*

and, in some individuals, the tip of the cuneus, that is, parts of the medial parietal cortex. In this region, the ACA forms anastomoses with the PCA.

1.3.6.3 Clinical consequences of middle and anterior cerebral artery strokes

Tables 1.1 and 1.2 summarize the different cortical branches of the MCA and the ACA and the expected neuropsychological and sensorimotor deficits. However, some of the listed deficits are not the result of a cortical stroke (and

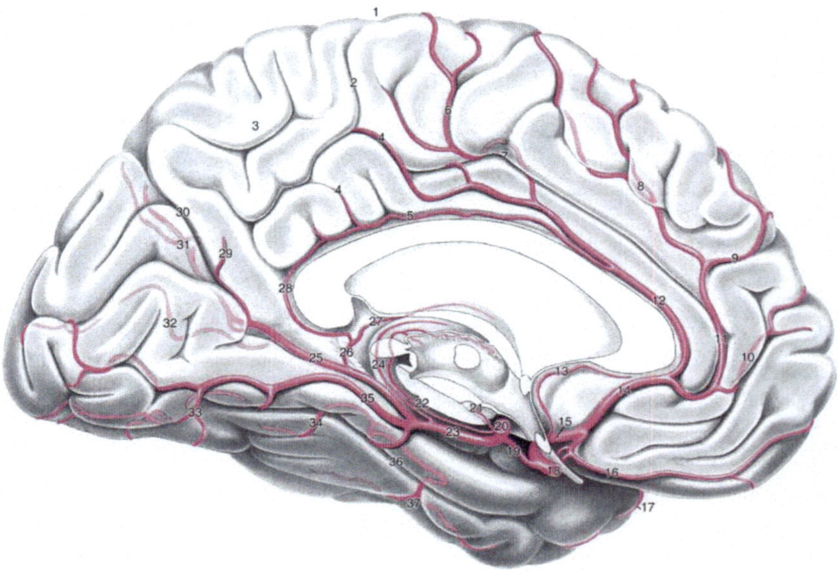

1 Central sulcus
2 Marginal branch of the cingulate sulcus
3 Precuneus
4 Artery of the precuneus
5 Pericallosal artery, posterior branch (anastomosis with 28)
6 Paracentral artery
7 Cingulate sulcus
8 Posteromedial frontal artery
9 Intermediomedial frontal artery
10 Anteromedial frontal artery
11 Callosomarginal artery
12 Pericallosal artery
13 Median artery of the corpus callosum
14 Anterior cerebral artery, postcommunicating part
15 Anterior communicating artery
16 Medial frontobasal artery
17 Temporopolar artery
18 Internal carotid artery
19 Posterior communicating artery
20 Posterior cerebral artery, precommunicating part
21 Posteromedial central arteries
22 Posterior medial choroidal branch
23 Posterior cerebral artery, postcommunicating branch
24 Posterior thalamic branches
25 Medial occipital artery
26 Cingulatethalamic artery
27 Superior thalamic branch
28 Dorsal branch of the corpus callosum (anastomosis with 5)
29 Parietal branch
30 Parieto-occipital sulcus
31 Parieto-occipital branch
32 Calcarine branch (in calcarine sulcus)
33 Posterior temporal branches
34 Medial intermediate temporal branch
35 Lateral occipital artery
36 Collateral sulcus
37 Anterior temporal branches

FIGURE 1.13 Schematic drawing of the anterior cerebral artery. *From Nieuwenhuys R., Voogd J., Huijzen C.van The Human Central Nervous System. 4th ed. Berlin: Springer-Verlag; 2008. Figure 4.2.*

not of a lesion of subcortical nuclei, which will be discussed below) but of a white matter lesion. MCA strokes may involve the optic radiation and therefore produce visual field defects. Such strokes may also impact the deep white matter and internal capsule, which will lead to hemiparesis or hemiplegia and sensory loss. Earlier explanations of ideomotor apraxia argued that the reason for this clinical syndrome is a disconnection between occipital and temporal cortical areas and the left premotor cortex caused by

TABLE 1.1 Cortical branches of the middle cerebral artery and resulting stroke syndromes.

Deficits related to the involved branch of the artery	Left middle cerebral artery	Right middle cerebral artery
Motor (frontal br.)	Distal-predominant paresis on the right; dysarthria.	Distal-predominant paresis on the left; dysarthria.
Action (frontal br.)	Apraxia (ideomotor and ideational). Apraxia of speech.	Apraxia affecting complex postures and visuoconstructional tasks.
Sensory (postcentral br.)	Impaired proprioception and tactile perception on the right.	Impaired proprioception and tactile perception on the left.
Language (frontal, parietal, and temporal br.)	Aphasia (e.g., Broca's aphasia). Central dyslexia, dysgraphia, and dyscalculia.	Impaired prosody and reduced comprehension of complex messages. Impaired mental rotation.
Memory (frontal, parietal, and temporal br.)	Impaired verbal learning and working memory abilities.	Impaired visuospatial learning and working memory abilities. Increased risk of confabulations.
Attention (frontal, parietal, and temporal br.)	Slowed information processing. Disinhibition. Impairment of the phonological loop.	Visuospatial neglect. Slowed information processing. Impaired feature binding.
Vision (parietal and temporal br.)	Impaired local visual attention. Right quadrantanopia or hemianopia. Optic ataxia affecting the right visual field.	Impaired global attention. Left quadrantanopia or hemianopia.
Emotional regulation (temporal br.)	Depression. Affective lability.	Depression. Reduced affective empathy.

damage to the superior longitudinal fasciculus or the arcuate fasciculus. Both fiber tracts receive their blood supply from the MCA.

We will return to the major syndromes associated with strokes of the major cerebral arteries in the following chapters. Their cognitive mechanisms will be discussed as far as necessary for clinical neuropsychological practice, and strategies for their diagnosis and, in particular, their treatment will be introduced.

TABLE 1.2 Cortical branches of the anterior cerebral artery and resulting stroke syndromes.

Deficits related to the involved branch of the artery	Left anterior cerebral artery	Right anterior cerebral artery
Motor (paracentral br.)	Monoparesis of the right leg	Monoparesis of the left leg
Action, executive function (pericallosal, callosomarginal br.)	Stimulus-bound behavior; severe impairment of planning.	Severe impairment of insight and delayed reward discounting. Pathological grasping and alien hand syndrome.
Language (pericallosal br.)	Akinetic mutism. Dynamic aphasia.	Slowing of speech.
Sensory (paracentral, precuneal br.)	Impaired proprioception of the right leg	Impaired proprioception of the left leg
Vision	None.	None.
Attention	Slowed information processing and reduced sustained attention.	Contralateral motor neglect. Profound slowed information processing.
Memory (A1 br., orbitofrontal br., perforating br.)	Memory impairments particularly affecting verbal information	Memory impairments particularly affecting visuospatial information
Emotional regulation	Reduced emotional expression. Impaired planning and goal representation.	Reduced emotional expression. Impaired future-oriented thinking and reward discounting.

1.4 Supply of subcortical structures—the perforating arteries

1.4.1 The basal ganglia

For a neuroanatomical description of the basal ganglia (consisting of the caudate nucleus, putamen, and globus pallidus), we refer to the book of Nieuwenhuys [17]. For the purpose of this chapter, it is sufficient to note that they are intimately involved in multiple loops that enable specific motor, cognitive, and affective functions. Moreover, the effects of basal ganglia lesions are typically lateralized: lesions or reduced activation of neurons involved in motor execution will cause deficits on the contralateral but not on the ipsilesional side [23,24]. This lateralization reflects the limited interhemispheric connectivity between the basal ganglia of the two hemispheres and the relatively sparse projections from the contralateral cortex to ipsilesional basal ganglia structures.

There is a topographic organization of the striatum (comprising the putamen and caudate nucleus) related to afferent and efferent connections. The dorsolateral putamen predominantly receives fibers from the primary motor cortex (Fig. 1.14). In contrast, the dorsomedial putamen primarily interacts with premotor areas, similar to the lateral portion of the caudate nucleus. The caudate nucleus is a long, curved structure that follows the lateral ventricle and shows a similar shape. The most anterior parts are called the head of the caudate, the central parts the body of the caudate nucleus, and the small and long part turning anteriorly and following the temporal horn of the lateral ventricle is called the tail of the caudate nucleus. The latter appears to be involved in visual learning; however, little is known about the clinical consequences of lesions affecting this region, and systematic studies are currently lacking. The body and the dorsal head of the caudate are connected with the frontal eye fields (Brodmann area 8), the prefrontal cortex (Brodmann areas 9 and 46), and the cingulate gyrus. The ventral head of the caudate nucleus (and the nucleus accumbens, a structure located medial to it) is predominantly connected with the limbic cortex.

To understand the consequences of stroke lesions in the basal ganglia, it is also important to mention that the globus pallidus has no direct fiber connections with the cortex but only with the striatum and different midbrain and thalamic structures [17]. The globus pallidus is thought to function as a relay station for a wide range of functions. Rather than being specialized for specific processes, it contributes to the inhibition of competing processes and facilitates processes that are relevant in a specific situation.

More recent models of the basal ganglia argue that one major function of the caudate nucleus may be the chunking and automatization of sequences of movements for the execution of complex actions [25,26]. When distinguishing between the learning, consolidation, and retrieval of such chunks, the basal ganglia appear to be particularly involved in their consolidation, i.e., the gradual automatization of action chains.

Bilateral damage to the basal ganglia therefore reduces the ability to automatize actions. There are also hints that even if learning movement patterns is possible after a basal ganglia stroke, there is an upper limit to the complexity of these chunks and that they function more rigidly than in healthy subjects. Fig. 1.15 shows impaired sequence learning in the basal ganglia, limited by the complexity of the rule, and Fig. 1.16 illustrates the relationship between the size of a basal ganglia stroke and motor learning impairment [27].

This recent model of basal ganglia function has not yet tested in larger clinical populations. However, it would predict that patients with basal

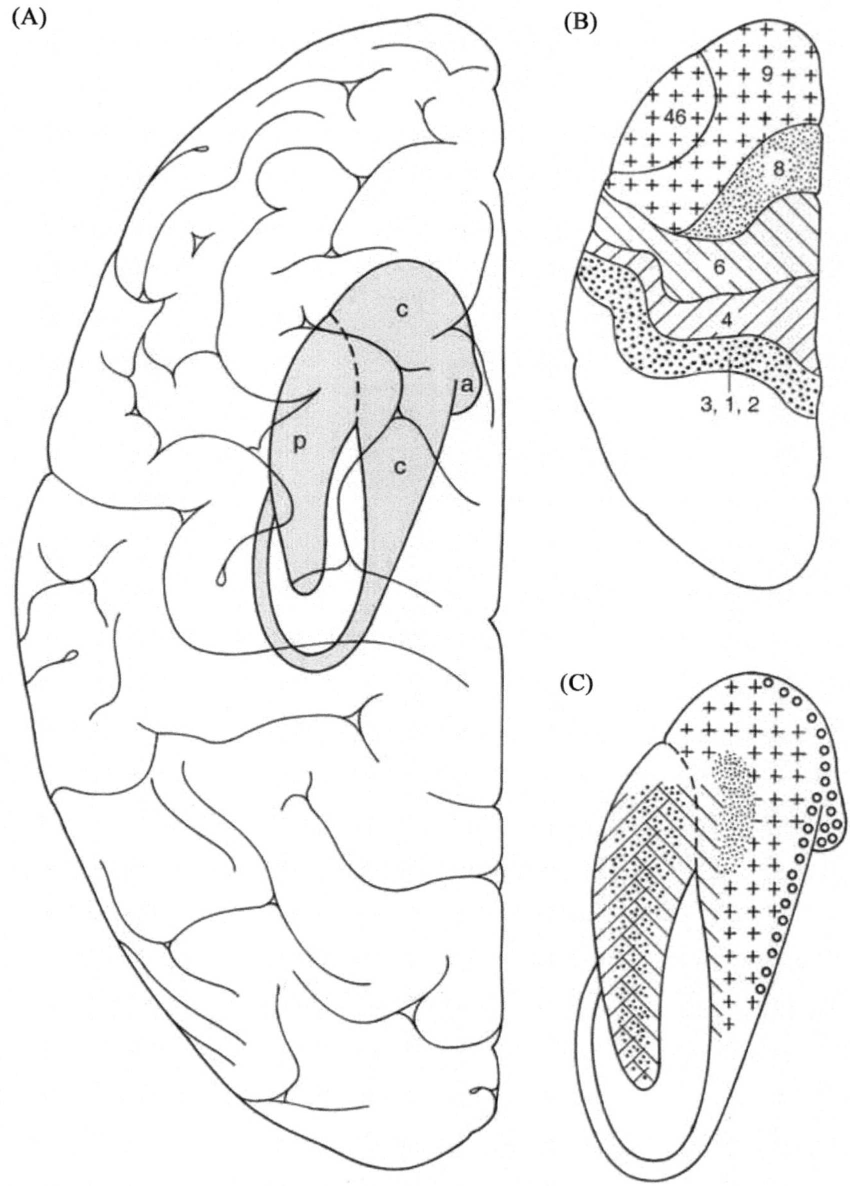

FIGURE 1.14 Schematic drawing of the basal ganglia and their cortical connections. (A) Superior view of the left hemisphere showing the location of the striatum (a, nucleus accumbens; c, caudate nucleus; p, putamen). (B) Brodmann areas on the right hemisphere. (C) Corresponding corticostriatal projection zones. The orbital and medial prefrontal cortices project to the ventral striatum, of which only a small portion is visible from above. *From Nieuwenhuys R., Voogd J., Huijzen C.van The Human Central Nervous System. 4th ed. Berlin: Springer-Verlag; 2008. Figure 14.1.*

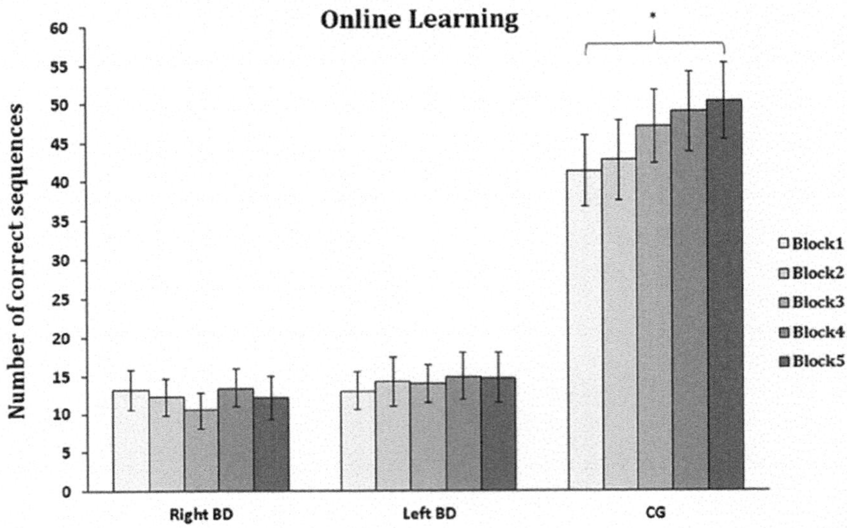

FIGURE 1.15 Loss of motor learning after basal ganglia stroke in patients with right brain damage (Right BD) or left brain damage (Left BD), and in healthy controls (CG). *From Russo C., Veronelli L., Casati C. et al. Explicit motor sequence learning after stroke: a neuropsychological study. Exp Brain Res 2021;239(7):2303–2316. Figure 3.*

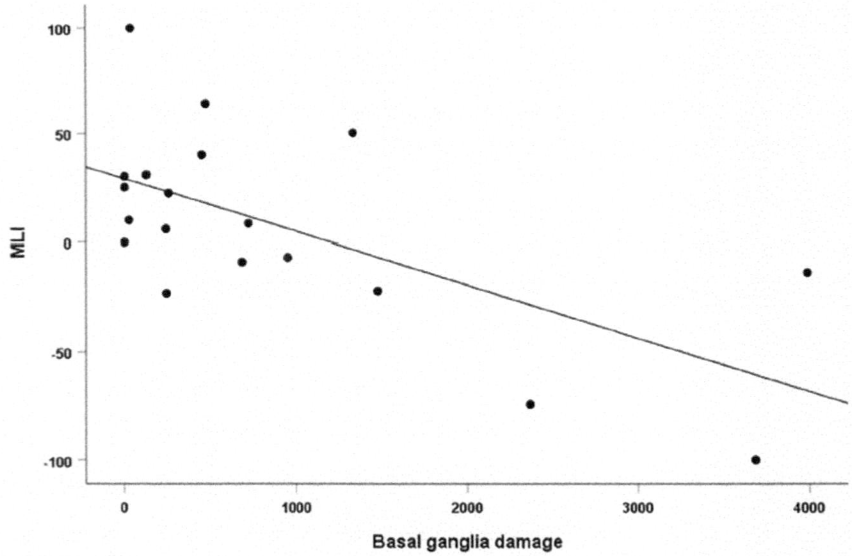

FIGURE 1.16 Relation between lesion size of basal ganglia stroke and motor learning. *From Russo C., Veronelli L., Casati C. et al. Explicit motor sequence learning after stroke: a neuropsychological study. Exp Brain Res 2021;239(7):2303–2316.*

ganglia lesions might improve only in simple motor functions but may have difficulties consolidating complex behavior. This would have an impact on functional outcome after stroke, for example, with regard to reintegration into a dynamic job environment. It might even have an impact on rehabilitation prospects if the consolidation deficit is severe, because rehabilitation is basically the relearning of skills.

1.4.1.1 *Blood supply of the basal ganglia by perforating arteries of the middle cerebral artery*

The brain's subcortical structures (basal ganglia, thalamus) are primarily supplied by perforating arteries, which branch off from the major arteries (MCA, ACA, PCA). The MCA supplies the largest parts of the basal ganglia, whereas the ACA and the anterior choroidal artery [20], supply the remaining regions (Fig. 1.17). The PCA and posterior choroidal arteries supply the hypothalamus and the thalamus with blood. We will come back to this topic below. Fig. 1.17 shows a schematic drawing of the perforating arteries of the MCA in a coronal view of the brain.

The M1 segment is the part of the MCA, where the perforating arteries originate [17,19]. They then travel through the brain tissue until they reach the dorsal and lateral parts of the basal ganglia. The ventral parts of the basal ganglia are supplied by the anterior choroidal artery (tail of the caudate nucleus, directly lateral to the temporal part of the lateral ventricle) or by perforating arteries of the ACA (ventral caudate nucleus, nucleus accumbens).

1.4.1.2 *Blood supply of the basal ganglia by perforating arteries of the anterior cerebral artery*

Fig. 1.18 shows the perforating arteries of the ACA [22]. These are called the anterolateral central arteries. The recurrent artery of Heubner is one of these perforating arteries, arising from the ACA in most individuals proximal to the anterior communicating artery. The vascular territory of the recurrent artery of Heubner includes the anteromedial part of the head of the caudate nucleus and the anteroinferior internal capsule, as well as parts of the putamen and the septal nuclei. Consequently, strokes affecting the recurrent artery of Heubner may lead to cognitive and emotional deficits [23]. The septum pellucidum is a small region in the mesial part of the frontal cortex accommodating cholinergic nuclei [17]. The basal forebrain is another part of the brain hosting cholinergic nuclei and is also supplied by perforating arteries of the anterior communicating artery. We will come back to this topic when discussing lesions resulting from a ruptured aneurysm of the anterior communicating artery below.

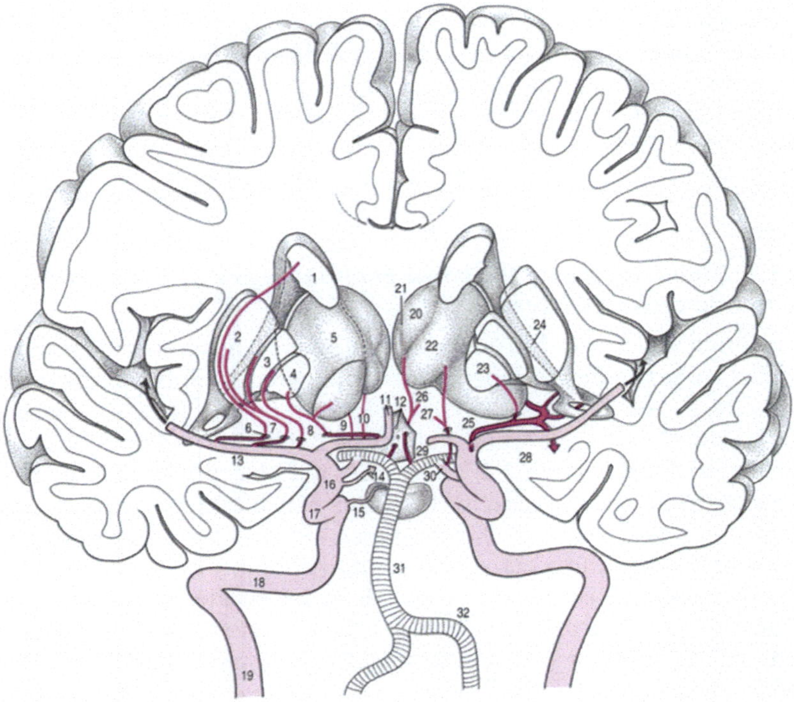

1 Caudate nucleus
2 Putamen
3 Globus pallidus, external segment
4 Globus pallidus, internal segment
5 Thalamus
6 Anterior perforated substance
7 Anterolateral central arteries, lateral branches
8 Anterolateral central arteries, medial branches
9 Long central artery (Heubner [16])
10 Anteromedial central arteries
11 Anterior cerebral artery
12 Posterior perforated substance
13 Middle cerebral artery, sphenoid part
14 Superior hypophyseal artery
15 Inferior hypophyseal artery
16 Internal carotid artery, cerebral part
17 Internal carotid artery, cavernous part
18 Internal carotid artery, petrous part
19 Internal carotid artery, cervical part
20 Medial nucleus of the thalamus
21 Midline nuclei of the thalamus
22 Anterior nucleus of the thalamus
23 Globus pallidus, internal segment
24 Tail of the caudate nucleus
25 Anterior choroidal artery
26 Subthalamus with posteromedial central arteries
27 Hypothalamus with hypothalamic branch
28 Amygdaloid nucleus
29 Posterior cerebral artery
30 Posterior communicating artery
31 Basilar artery
32 Vertebral artery

FIGURE 1.17 Perforating lenticulostriate arteries. *From Nieuwenhuys R., Voogd J., Huijzen C.van The Human Central Nervous System. 4th ed. Berlin: Springer-Verlag; 2008. Figure 4.8.*

1.4.2 Clinical consequences of basal ganglia strokes

1.4.2.1 Globus pallidus

Isolated lesions of the globus pallidus typically do not produce focal impairments. Clinical studies on such lesions suggest that apathy may be a consequence of pallidal strokes. Between 10% and 20% of patients with

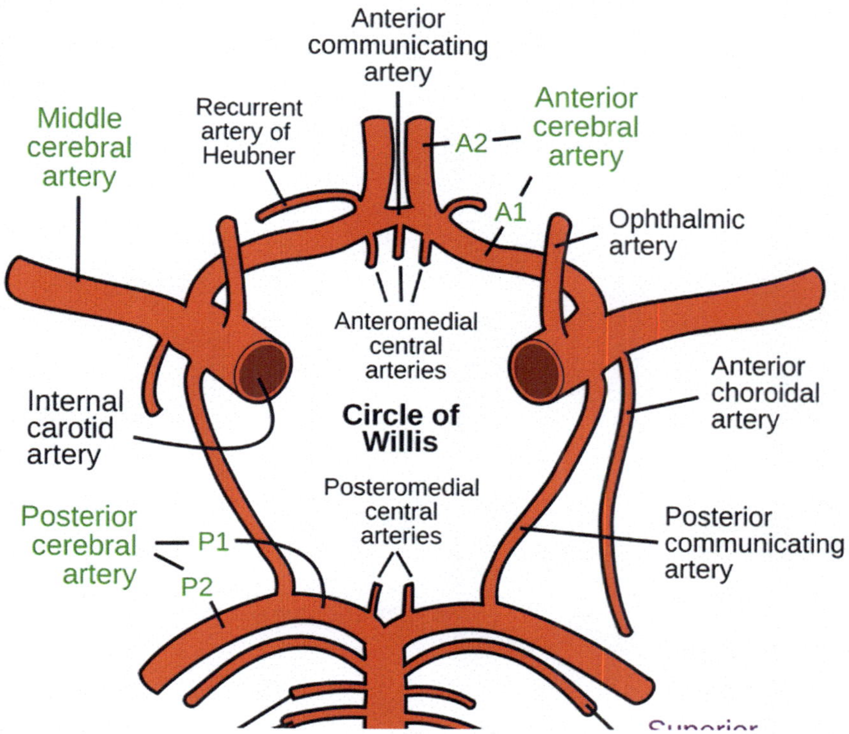

FIGURE 1.18 Origin of the perforating arteries from the Circle of Willis. *Author: McKay (own work). Licensed under Creative Commons Attribution-ShareAlike 4.0 International (CC BY-SA 4.0). https://commons.wikimedia.org/wiki/File:Circle_of_Willis_en.svg.*

pallidal lesions develop reduced drive. In some cases, isolated lesions of the putamen can cause mild aphasia and signs of neglect, depending on the lesion side (and handedness). If the lesions are small and truly restricted to the putamen, recovery is often rapid and largely complete [28]. Small lesions (lacunar strokes) of the lenticular nucleus impair memory performance, but only very mildly.

1.4.2.2 Striatum

Lesions of the striatum (i.e., the caudate nucleus and putamen) often produce motor, cognitive, and affective impairments [23,24]. Lesions of the body of the caudate nucleus are associated with motor weakness, dystonia, rarely hemichoreatic hyperkinesia, and only very rarely (if ever) classic parkinsonian symptoms such as unilateral tremor. The proportion of patients exhibiting motor deficits is high (up to 80%). However, it should be noted that the basal ganglia are surrounded by motor fiber tracts such as the corona radiata and the corticospinal tract (Fig. 1.19). Thus the likelihood

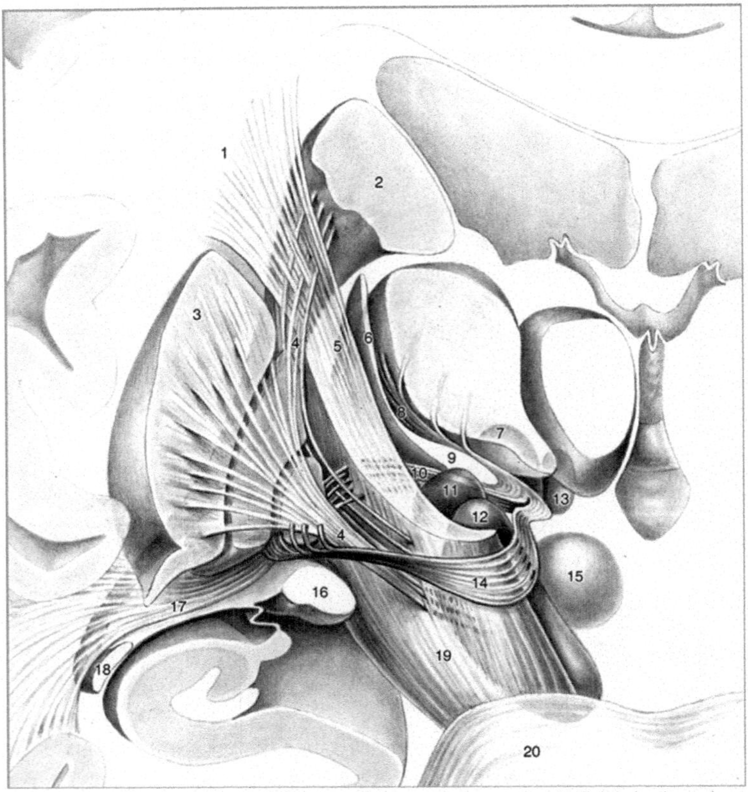

1 Corona radiata
2 Body of caudate nucleus
3 Putamen
4 Strionigral fibres
5 Internal capsule, posterior limb
6 Reticular thalamic nucleus
7 Centromedian thalamic nucleus
8 Thalamic fasciculus
9 Zona incerta
10 Lenticular fasciculus
11 Subthalamic nucleus
12 Substantia nigra
13 Parafascicular thalamic nucleus
14 Ansa lenticularis
15 Red nucleus
16 Optic tract
17 Internal capsule, sublentiform part
18 Tail of caudate nucleus
19 Cerebral peduncle
20 Pons

FIGURE 1.19 Coronal drawing of fiber tracts adjacent to the basal ganglia. *From Nieuwenhuys R., Voogd J., Huijzen C.van The Human Central Nervous System. 4th ed. Berlin: Springer-Verlag; 2008. Figure 14.6.*

that a stroke also involves fibers of these tracts is high, and this will lead to motor deficits. A clinical study reconstructing the involved perforating arteries showed that strokes of the anterolateral branches of the lenticulostriate arteries resulted much more often in motor deficits than those of the anteromedial branches. The anterolateral branches arise from the MCA M1 segment, whereas the anteromedial branches arise from the A1 segment, and only the anterolateral branches supply the internal capsule with blood.

In cases involving the head of the caudate nucleus, patients may present with aphasia (left hemisphere lesion) or neglect (right hemisphere lesion) [24]. The percentage of patients displaying these syndromes is between 40% and 50%, depending on the lesion's side. Dysarthria is a common consequence of lesions to the head of the caudate, if the lesion is located in the upper part and adjacent to the body of the caudate [19,23,24]. Lateral lesions of the head of the caudate can result in dysexecutive symptoms, and medial lesions may lead to akinetic mutism. Lesions in the ventral part of the caudate nucleus may lead to affective disorders such as apathy. Regardless of this fine-grained analysis of the head of the caudate, more than half of these patients suffer from apathy, which is more than twice as common as after pallidal strokes.

1.4.3 Prognosis of basal ganglia strokes

The prognosis of unilateral strokes limited to the basal ganglia is excellent. This is particularly true for strokes affecting the anteromedial branches of the perforating arteries, because patients are significantly less likely to experience motor impairments. However, this prognosis relates only to the ability to live independently. There are no studies looking more explicitly for neuropsychological deficits and for return to work. Moreover, if there are bilateral infarcts involving both basal ganglia structures, the prognosis is less favourable. Table 1.3 shows that about two-thirds of patients with striato-capsular strokes recover substantially. In this respect, it should be noted that by definition, strokes restricted to the basal ganglia are small lesions. Small cortical strokes also tend to have a good prognosis. The table also includes motor impairments and lesions within the internal capsule, a neighbouring structure, which contains the corticospinal fiber tracts responsible for hand movements. Consequently the recovery rate for isolated basal ganglia strokes alone is likely to be even higher.

1.5 The posterior cerebral artery

The cerebral cortex is supplied by three pairs of arteries, and the PCA has not yet been discussed [14,17,29]. The PCA is divided into four segments. The P1 segment (the part before the posterior communicating artery), supplies the hypothalamus, the corpora mammillaria, the medial thalamus, and parts of the midbrain. The P2 segment (located between

TABLE 1.3 Motor and cognitive deficits of basal ganglia strokes.

	Rascol et al. 1982	Santamarta et al. 1983	Bladin and Berkovic 1984	Levlne et al. 1988	Welller et al. 1990	Donnan et al. 19S1	Bolten and Lodder 1992	Welller et al. 1993	Nlcolal et al. 1996	Total (%)
Demographic data										
No. of patients	15	8	11	24	29	50	15	57	56	265(100)
M/F ratio		1/7	5/6	18/6	20/9	27/23	10/5	3/26	30/26	
Mean years (years)		48	53	59	55	63		53	68	
Age range (years)		34–65	50–84	26–88	22–86	24–88		16–89	35–89	
Clinical data										
Lacunar syndromes	15	1	2	5	6		:3	19	11	62/186(33)
Hemiparests	15	8	11	24	29	49	14	57	51	218/225(97)
Severe			9	18	13		10		29	79/135(59)
Moderate			0	4	12		4		0	20/135(15)
Mild			2	2	4		1		22	31/135(23)
Hemi-hypoesthesia	0	6	0	15	23	30	10	40	20	121/225(54)
Aphasta/neglect	0	4	8	17	8	35	11	26	3	127/225(56)

TABLE 1.3 (Continued)

	Rascol et al. 1982	Santamarta et al. 1983	Bladin and Berkovic 1984	Levlne et al. 1988	Welller et al. 1990	Donnan et al. 19S1	Bolten and Lodder 1992	Welller et al. 1993	Nlcolal et al. 1996	Total (%)
Prognosis										
No recovery	5/13	2	6	6	9	12		22		46/156(29)
Moderate recovery	0/13	4	3	4	4	23		12		44/156(28)
Complete recovery	8/13	2	2	14	11	15		I9		60/156(38)
Pathogenesis										
Cardiac source of embolism	2	8	5	5	14/24	7	7	25	29	83/225(37)
Internal carotid artery (ICA)	0/6	0	6/8	17	9	12/27	4	17	20	76/198(38)
Middle cerebral artery (MCA)	2/6	0	2/8	5	15	3/27	0	25	4	39/198(20)

From Pullicino P. Lenticulostriate arteries. In: Bogousslavsky J., Caplan L.R., editors. Stroke Syndromes 2 ed. Cambridge: Cambridge University Press; 2001. pp. 428–438.

the origin of the posterior communicating artery and the posterior choroidal artery) supplies the lateral thalamus, and strokes of the P2 segment and their consequences will be discussed below. The P3 segment (located distal to the origin of the posterior choroidal artery) supplies the mediobasal, inferior temporal lobe, and the medial parietal lobe (along the parieto-occipital sulcus). The P4 segment supplies the medial (e.g., the calcarine sulcus) and lateral occipital lobe.

The PCA forms anastomoses with the ACA at the level of the medial parietal cortex, more specifically within the subarachnoid space of the parieto-occipital sulcus and the posterior part of the cingulate cortex.

1.5.1 Posterior cerebral artery strokes

1.5.1.1 P4 segment strokes

Patients with strokes involving the P4 segment typically present with homonymous hemianopia or more restricted visual field loss in the contralesional visual field [29–31]. The retinotopic organization of the visual cortex follows two important gradients. The first one is a dorsal—ventral gradient: lesions superior to the calcarine sulcus result in defects in the lower half of the contralateral visual field. However, lesions inferior to the calcarine sulcus produce defects in the upper contralateral visual field. The second gradient follows the caudal-rostral axis. Lesions near the occipital pole produce defects surrounding the contralateral foveal visual field, whereas lesions more rostral within the occipital lobe affect the peripheral visual field. The reason for this retinotopic organization will be discussed in the chapter on visual field defects and their treatment (Chapter 4). It should also be noted that PCA strokes often do not impair the central (foveal or even macular) visual field. Most patients show foveal sparing. This is clinically important because preservation of approximately 4 degrees of foveal vision largely eliminates the risk of a hemianopic reading disorder. The most plausible explanation for this is that foveal vision is based on two independent blood circulations: one related to the PCA, the other related to the MCA. Because of this additional MCA supply, foveal vision often remains intact.

1.5.1.2 P3 segment strokes

The mediobasal temporal cortex is supplied by the P3 segment of the PCA [29,32]. There is some interindividual variation in this regard: in some individuals, the hippocampus is supplied by the PCA, whereas in others it is supplied by the anterior choroidal artery. Fig. 1.20 illustrates the vascular territories of the hippocampus and applies only when the hippocampus is exclusively supplied by the PCA.

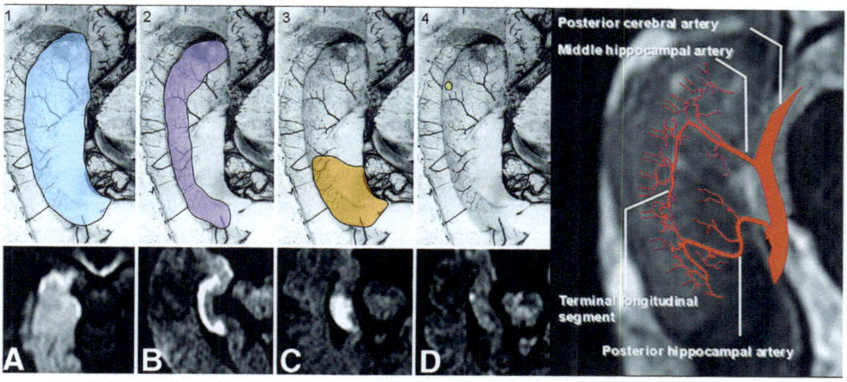

FIGURE 1.20 Blood supply of the hippocampus. *From Szabo K., Forster A., Jager T. et al. Hippocampal lesion patterns in acute posterior cerebral artery stroke: clinical and MRI findings. Stroke 2009;40(6):2042–2045.*

Even when the hippocampus itself is spared, P3 segment strokes may produce a hippocampal-like amnestic syndrome. This may occur because the P3 segment vascularizes the collateral sulcus, which contains cortical projections to and from the hippocampus. In fact, interaction between the hippocampus and the cortex is relayed through the collateral sulcus, including the entorhinal and transentorhinal cortices.

A stroke affecting the collateral isthmus may deafferent the hippocampus. This is of particular interest because the earliest neurodegenerative alterations in Alzheimer's disease occur here (Braak stage I and II) [34,35]. In a study by Cramon and Hebel [33], PCA strokes affecting the collateral isthmus of the left hemisphere led to severe deficits in verbal learning. In their study, only 11 of the participants showed hippocampal lesions, whereas 24 showed parahippocampal lesions and 21 showed lesions involving the collateral isthmus. Those patients with lesions affecting the left parahippocampus or the left collateral isthmus were all impaired in verbal word list learning and delayed recall. These patients were also impaired in verbal paired-associate learning, but not in verbal digit span forward, and only about 30% were impaired in a story recall task. The patients with homologous lesions in the right hemisphere were unimpaired in word-list learning and paired-associate learning, as were the patients with left PCA strokes sparing the hippocampus, parahippocampus, and collateral isthmus. These findings suggest a strong lateralization of word list learning and recall, and verbal paired-associate learning. Similar studies focusing on right hemisphere PCA strokes using spatial learning tasks revealed analogous findings for the Rey–Osterrieth Complex Figure (a test of visuospatial constructional ability and recall memory), although the effects were less pronounced than those observed for verbal learning [32,36,37]. One interpretation of this discrepancy between left and right PCA strokes could be that spatial learning and recall are less lateralized than verbal learning and recall. Another interpretation is that most clinical spatial learning and recall tasks allow for verbal encoding of the spatial information, which may help patients compensate for the impairment. Taken together, clinical impairment after right hemisphere P3 segment strokes is often mild to absent, whereas impairment after homologous left stroke is at least moderate.

The Fig. 1.21 shows a left hemisphere PCA stroke, sparing the occipital pole but involving the fusiform gyrus, parts of the optic radiation, the collateral sulcus, the parahippocampal region, and, in some sections, also the hippocampus. The expected clinical consequences include a right-sided visual field defect due to involvement of the optic radiation, possibly encompassing the entire upper quadrant and perhaps also parts of the lower quadrant. Severe verbal learning

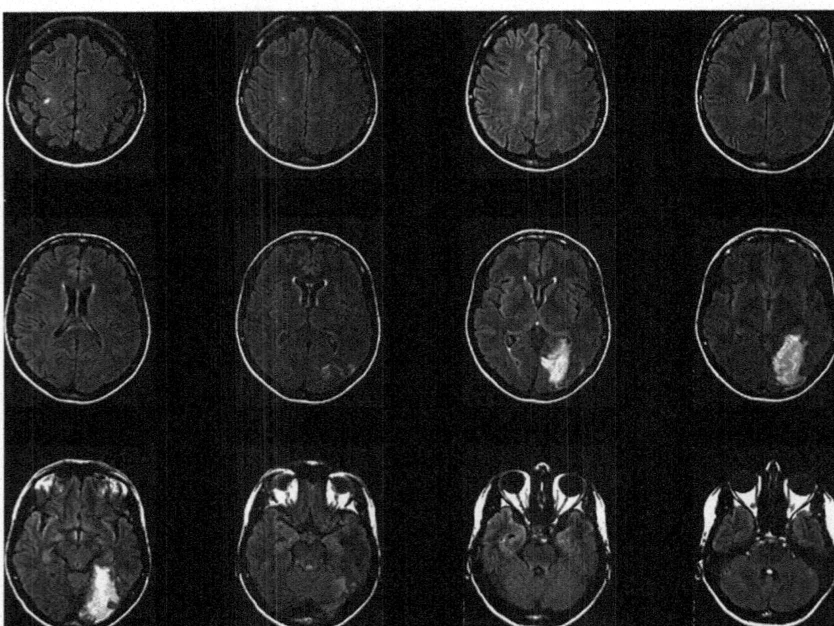

FIGURE 1.21 Clinical MRI scan of a posterior stroke.

and recall deficits would be expected because of the lesion's involvement of the parahippocampal region and extension into the hippocampus. Pure alexia is likely since the lesion affects the left ventral occipitotemporal cortex, including the fusiform gyrus, which plays a critical role in visual word recognition. Even though the most ventral images of the occipital and temporal lobes do not show a lesion, the lesion pattern also raises the possibility of associative agnosia because of the involvement of the fusiform gyrus and adjacent ventral visual association areas. We refer to Chapter 2 for guidance on the localization of brain lesions on clinical scans.

1.5.2 Clinical consequences of posterior cerebral artery strokes

Table 1.4 offers an overview of the impairments associated with PCA strokes depending on the affected hemisphere. Please note that the consequences of thalamic strokes will be discussed in the next chapter, because the thalamus is not only supplied by the PCA but also by

TABLE 1.4 Cortical branches of the posterior cerebral artery and associated stroke syndromes.

Possible consequences of PCA strokes	Posterior left	Posterior right
Motor	No paresis	No paresis
Somatosensory	Impaired right-sided proprioception and tactile perception (in case of thalamus involvement). Increased pain sensitivity for pain.	Impaired left-sided proprioception and tactile perception (in case of thalamus involvement). Increased pain sensitivity.
Language	Word finding difficulties	No change
Vision	Right homonymous hemianopia or quadrantanopia	Left homonymous hemianopia or quadrantanopia
Recognition	Visual associative agnosia. Hemianopic reading disorder. Pure alexia.	Neglect (with thalamus involvement). Hemianopic reading disorder. Prosopagnosia.
Memory	Severe verbal memory impairment	Mild visuospatial memory impairment
Affective	No change	No change
Behaviour	No change	No change

perforating arteries of the posterior communicating artery and the anterior choroidal artery.

1.6 Vascularization of the thalamus

The thalamus is a mesial brain structure that serves as a major relay station for most sensory information and plays an important role in motor execution, the modulation of cognitive functions (e.g., attention), and the regulation of arousal and wakefulness.

Like the cortex, functions related to motor control and cognition are localized in the anterior segments of the thalamus (Fig. 1.22). The sensory-perceptual nuclei are localized caudally, and the homeostatic nuclei are located medial to the sensory-perceptual nuclei. This can be easily illustrated for tactile and pain perception: tactile perception is relayed through the ventral posterolateral (VPL) and ventral posteromedial (VPM) nuclei. Pain perception, therefore, is represented more

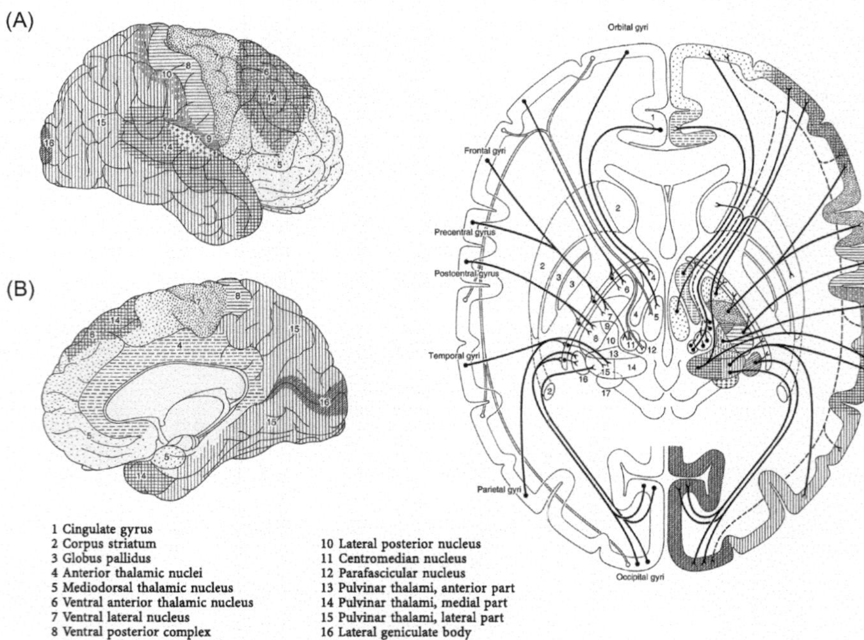

FIGURE 1.22 (A) and (B): Cortical efferences of different thalamic nuclei. *From Nieuwenhuys R, Voogd J., Huijzen C.van The human central nervous system. 4th ed. Berlin: Springer-Verlag; 2008. Figures 8.3 and 8.4.*

medially than tactile processing. The mesially located nuclei of the thalamus are related to attention and wakefulness. The thalamus has reciprocal connections with all cortical areas, and these connections are topographically organized. As a result, different thalamic nuclei are connected to different cortical regions and contribute to distinct sensory, motor, cognitive, and behavioural functions.

1.6.1 The thalamus as part of the Papez circuit

To understand the consequences of thalamic vascularization and stroke, it is important to consider the major thalamocortical loops involved in cognition. One of these loops is the Papez circuit (Fig. 1.23), which plays a major role in memory consolidation. The circuit originates in a hippocampal formation and projects via the fornical fimbria to the columns of the fornix to reach the mammillary bodies. From the mammillary bodies, the circuit continues via the mammillothalamic tract to the anterior nucleus of the thalamus and then via the medial and lateral longitudinal striae back to the hippocampus. Bilateral lesions of the Papez circuit typically lead to profound memory impairment, and may even result in anterograde amnesia [38]. Similar loops exist for functions such as motor execution, goal-directed behaviour, and mood regulation [17].

1.6.2 Thalamic blood supply

The vascularization of the thalamus resembles that of other subcortical structures and is provided by the perforating arteries arising from the PCA [20,29,39,40]. The following perforating arteries can be distinguished: the tuberothalamic artery, the paramedian thalamic arteries (thalamoperforating arteries), the thalamogeniculate arteries, and the anterior and the posterior choroidal arteries. They originate from the PCA, the posterior communicating artery, or the bifurcation of the basilar artery. Fig. 1.24 shows the different arteries supplying the thalamus and the vascular segments from which they arise.

Starting with the left side of Fig. 1.24, the paramedian artery supplies the central nuclei of the thalamus. A distinctive feature of this artery is that, in some individuals, it arises directly from the basilar artery before it divides into the left and right PCA. In this case, a stroke affecting the paramedian artery will produce bilateral thalamic lesions.

The next thalamic artery encountered when moving upstream is the tuberothalamic artery. The tuberothalamic artery does not arise directly from the PCA but from the posterior communicating artery. This artery supplies the anterior parts of the thalamus, including the anterior

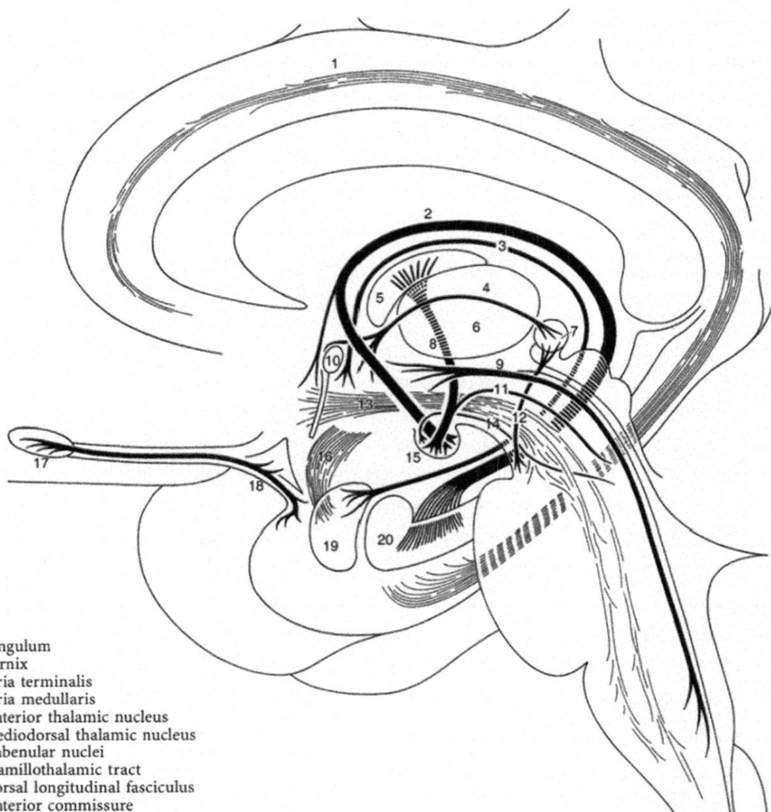

FIGURE 1.23 Schematic drawing of the Papez circuit. *From Nieuwenhuys R, Voogd J., Huijzen C.van The human central nervous system. 4th ed. Berlin: Springer-Verlag; 2008. Figure 23.2.*

thalamic nucleus, which is one of the major nuclei of the Papez circuit. Strokes affecting this artery may result in lateralized memory disorders, meaning that a left hemisphere stroke typically causes deficits in verbal learning and recall, whereas a right hemisphere stroke typically causes deficits in visuospatial learning and recall. In clinical routine practice, the lateralization of memory functions between the two anterior thalamic nuclei is a well-established finding. However, the question of

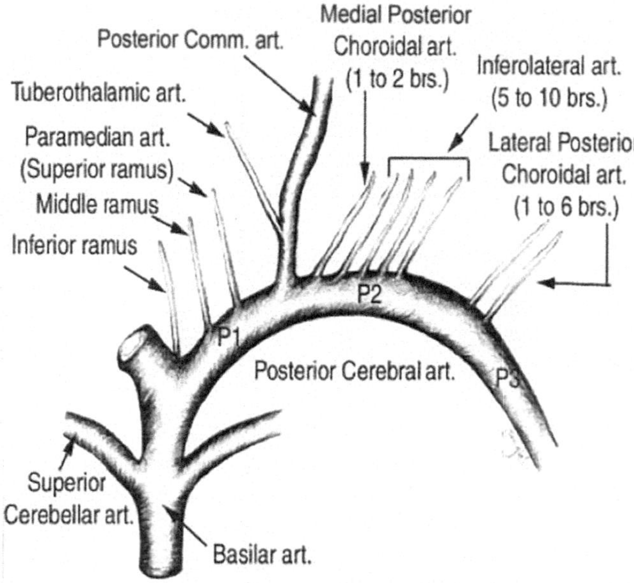

FIGURE 1.24 Perforating arteries of the posterior cerebral artery and thalamic blood supply. *From Schmahmann J.D. Vascular syndromes of the thalamus. Stroke 2003;34(9):2264–2278.*

whether this lateralization is as pronounced as that observed for the hippocampi remains unresolved. This may be because the fornix, which connects the hippocampus with the anterior thalamic nuclei, contains crossing fibers between the left and the right hemisphere at the level of the hippocampal fimbria and ventral to the anterior commissure. This would allow afferent and efferent projections to cross between the two hippocampi and the mammillary bodies of both hemispheres, potentially reducing the lateralization of functional deficits. However, the proportion of such crossing fibers remains unclear.

The next artery that arises from the PCA supplying the thalamus is the thalamogeniculate artery. This artery supplies the more lateral regions of the thalamus, whereas the anterolateral nuclei are often supplied by branches of the anterior choroidal artery (which does not arise from the PCA).

The last artery is the posterior lateral choroidal artery. It is involved in the vascularization of the posterior thalamus as well as the posterior parts of the internal capsule. Strokes affecting these arteries produce specific lesion patterns and should raise expectations about resulting deficits (Figs. 1.25 and 1.26) (Table 1.5) [41].

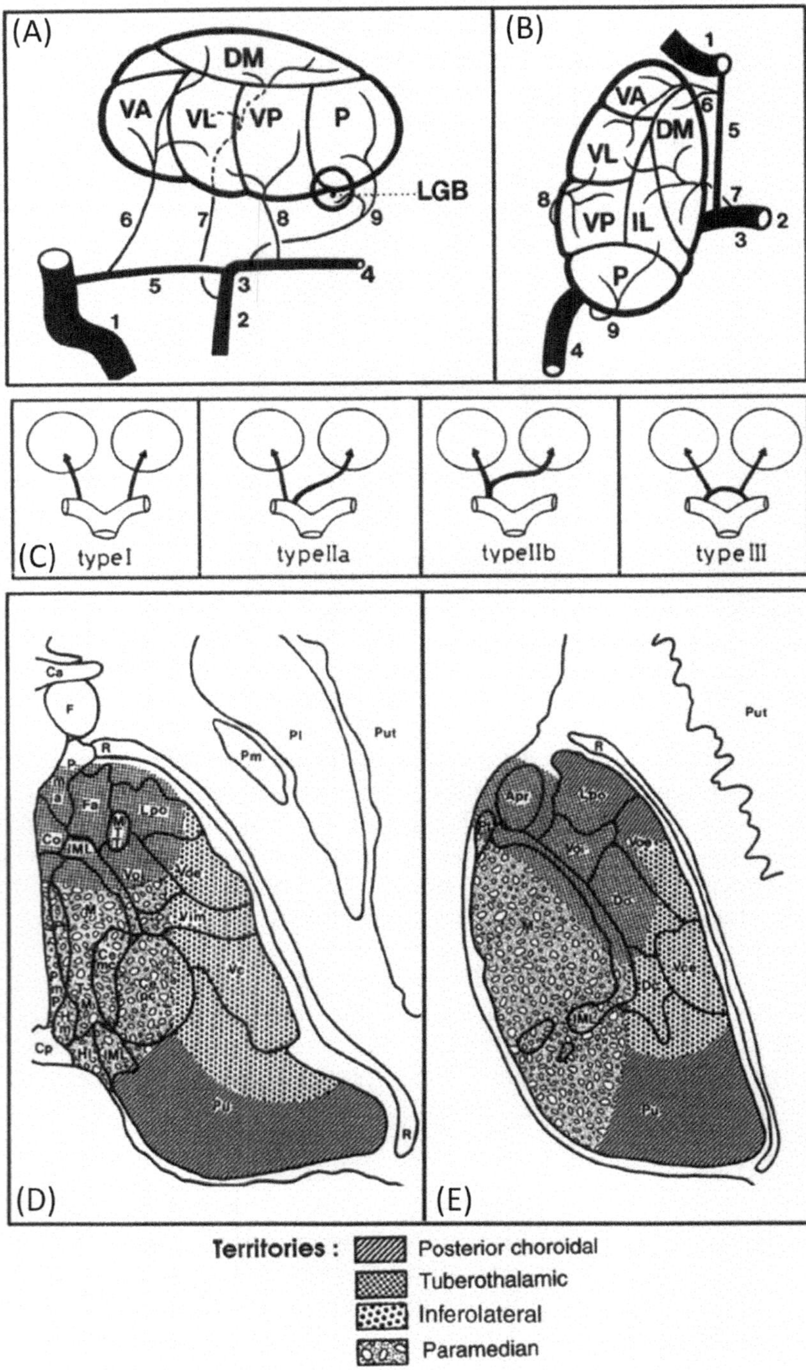

FIGURE 1.25 Thalamic vascular supply. Schematic diagram of lateral (A) and dorsal (B) views of the four major thalamic arteries and the nuclei they irrigate, according to

(continued)

1.6.3 Clinical implications of thalamic stroke syndromes

Table 1.5 gives an overview of the different thalamic arteries and the resulting stroke syndromes. A stroke of the tuberothalamic artery may result in unilateral memory deficits, such as verbal memory deficits after left hemisphere strokes. However, patients with strokes affecting the paramedian (posteromedial) artery may also show memory impairments, even though the anterior thalamic nucleus is not supplied by this artery. Von Cramon, Hebel [40] published a study of a small patient group with such strokes. They demonstrated that these patients were unimpaired in simple working memory tests. However, two-thirds of them showed impairments in paired-associate learning and on the Auditory Verbal Learning Test. Remote memory

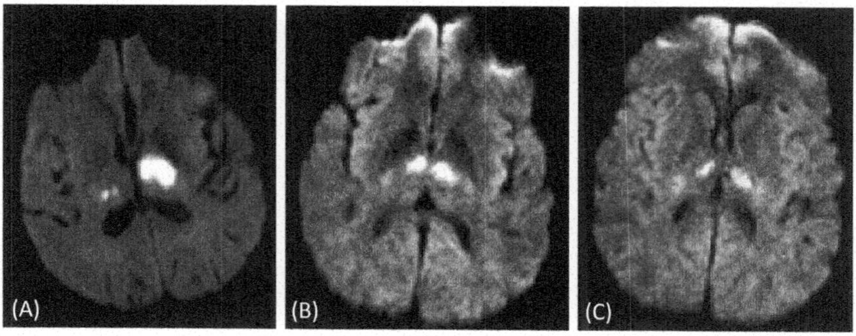

FIGURE 1.26 Clinical scans of thalamic stroke patterns. Diffusion-weighted MRI of acute thalamic infarction in two patients. (A) Extensive infarction in the territory of the left tuberothalamic artery (right of image), as well as small lesions in the territory of the inferolateral arteries on the right. (B) and (C) Bilateral infarction in a teenager with patent foramen ovale. The infarcted region is located within the tuberothalamic artery territory, although this pattern of bilateral stroke is more commonly observed following paramedian artery infarcts. This case is likely an example of the paramedian artery supplying both the paramedian and tuberothalamic "territories." The patient made a complete recovery, and follow-up MRI scans revealed only minor lesions. *From Schmahmann J.D. Vascular syndromes of the thalamus. Stroke 2003;34(9):2264–2278.*

Bogousslavsky et al. [21] Numbers indicate the following: 1, carotid artery; 2, basilar artery; 3, P1 region of the posterior cerebral artery (mesencephalic artery); 4, posterior cerebral artery; 5, posterior communicating artery; 6, tuberothalamic artery; 7, paramedian artery; 8, inferolateral artery; and 9, posterior choroidal artery; (C) depicts the varying patterns of origin of the paramedian artery arising from the mesencephalic/P1 artery; (D and E) illustrate the patterns of thalamic arterial irrigation supplying the thalamic nuclei. *From Schmahmann J.D. Vascular syndromes of the thalamus. Stroke 2003;34(9):2264–2278.*

TABLE 1.5 Thalamic strokes and associated syndromes.

Artery	Origin	Supplies	Clinical manifestations
Paramedian thalamic arteries	Posterior cerebral artery (PCA) or basilar artery	Central thalamic nuclei (including the dorsomedial nucleus)	– Bilateral thalamic infarction if arising from the basilar artery – Memory impairments (may include anterograde amnesia; disconnection syndrome) – Dysexecutive syndrome (e.g., impaired planning and set shifting issues) – Vertical gaze paresis (if the midbrain is involved)
Tuberothalamic artery	Posterior communicating artery	Anterior thalamus (including the anterior nucleus)	– Left hemisphere stroke: verbal memory impairments – Right hemisphere stroke: visuospatial memory deficit
Thalamogeniculate artery	Posterior cerebral artery (PCA)	Lateral thalamus including the ventral posterolateral (VPL) and ventral posteromedial (VPM) nuclei	– Sensory deficits (loss of pain/tactile perception) – Thalamic pain syndrome
Anterior choroidal artery	Internal carotid artery or middle cerebral artery (MCA)	Anterolateral thalamus and parts of the internal capsule	– Motor and sensory impairments (depending on internal capsule involvement)
Posterior choroidal artery	Posterior cerebral artery (PCA)	Posterior thalamus, parts of the internal capsule, and optic radiations	– Visual field deficits (due to damage to the optic radiations) – Sensory impairments (if the VPL/VPM nuclei are affected) – Thalamic hand syndrome (proprioceptive dysfunction)

(i.e., information from the distant past) was unimpaired. Lesion reconstruction revealed that, in impaired patients, the mammillothalamic tract was part of the lesion, whereas this tract was spared in unimpaired patients. These findings suggest that the memory impairment observed in patients with paramedian thalamic strokes may represent a disconnection syndrome, resulting in deafferentation of the anterior thalamic nucleus from afferent projections arising from the mammillary bodies.

The dorsomedial nucleus of the thalamus is also supplied by the paramedian artery. Therefore patients may show executive deficits because this nucleus has bidirectional connections with the ipsilateral prefrontal cortex. Accordingly, assessment of higher order working memory, planning, and set shifting should be part of the comprehensive neuropsychological evaluation of patients with corresponding MRI findings.

There is another important deficit, which is often associated with strokes affecting the paramedian thalamic artery. This artery also supplies nuclei of the midbrain [42]. Therefore a remarkable proportion of these patients suffer from a vertical gaze paresis, because the oculomotor nucleus or the rostral interstitial nucleus of the medial longitudinal fasciculus is lesioned.

The geniculate artery supplies the ventral posterolateral (VPL) and ventral posteromedial (VPM) nuclei. Both are projection zones for the medial lemniscus and the anterolateral funiculus, meaning that tactile and pain perception are relayed through these nuclei before reaching the postcentral gyrus and the insular cortex. Patients with strokes affecting this artery may develop dystonia due to the loss of proprioceptive afferent input. Some of these patients exhibit a thalamic hand syndrome, characterized, for example, by extended fingers held at an angle of approximately 90 degrees relative to the hand. Often, the hand is experienced as heavier than before. Another important issue is a reduced pain threshold. Lastly, cognitive impairments are generally not expected following geniculate artery strokes.

Posterolateral thalamic strokes resulting from occlusions of the posterior choroidal artery are rarely associated with visual field defects. When present, these deficits are usually caused by involvement of the optic radiations which originate from the lateral geniculate nucleus and project to the occipital cortex. In some patients, the stroke is restricted to specific parts of the optic radiations, producing arrow-like defects pointing toward the center of the visual field. Therefore, visual field examination should be performed in all patients with posterior thalamic strokes.

1.7 Vascularization of the basal forebrain

The basal forebrain is a region located in the anterior part of the brain, just anterior to the hypothalamus and posterior to the ventral parts of the orbitofrontal cortex (Fig. 1.27). It is characterized by various structures that are connected to the Papez circuit, but are not themselves part of it [17]. Fiber bundles originating in this part of the brain include the rostral portions of the precommissural fornix, the stria terminalis, and the stria medullaris thalami. The basal forebrain hosts essential cerebral cholinergic cell groups, which are integral to cognitive processes, especially memory formation, learning, and attention. Cholinergic cell groups can be found in the diagonal band of Broca and the substantia innominata, which contains the nucleus basalis of Meynert [17]. Even though additional cholinergic cell groups can be found in the brainstem, many cortical areas, as well as the amygdalae and hippocampus, receive their cholinergic projections exclusively from the basal forebrain.

1.7.1 Basal forebrain blood supply

The basal forebrain is supplied by the perforating subcallosal artery, which arises from the anterior communicating artery. This artery is often a single vessel initially and then divides to supply both hemispheres (Fig. 1.28). It should be noted that the columns of the fornix are also

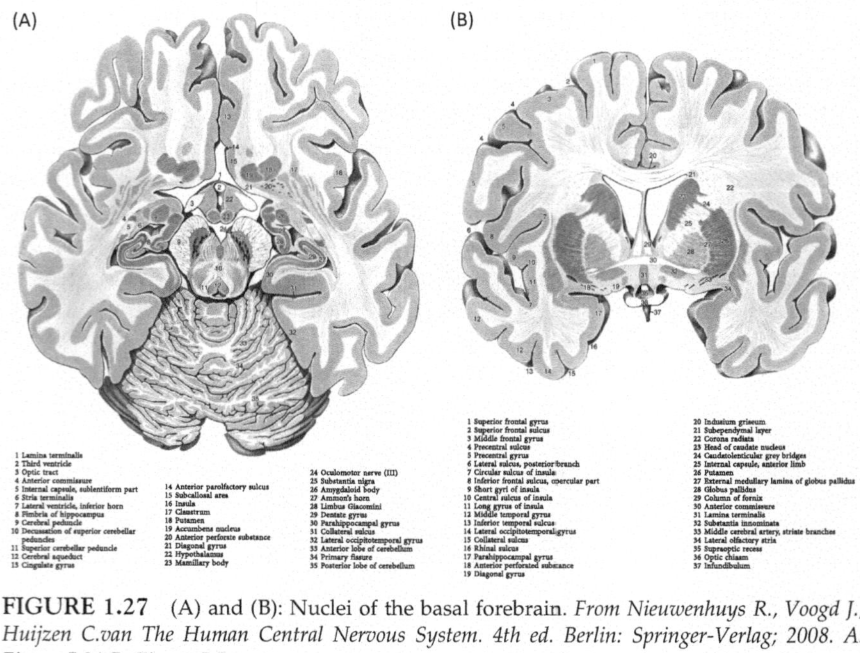

FIGURE 1.27 (A) and (B): Nuclei of the basal forebrain. *From Nieuwenhuys R., Voogd J., Huijzen C.van The Human Central Nervous System. 4th ed. Berlin: Springer-Verlag; 2008. A: Figure 5.34 B: Figure 5.5.*

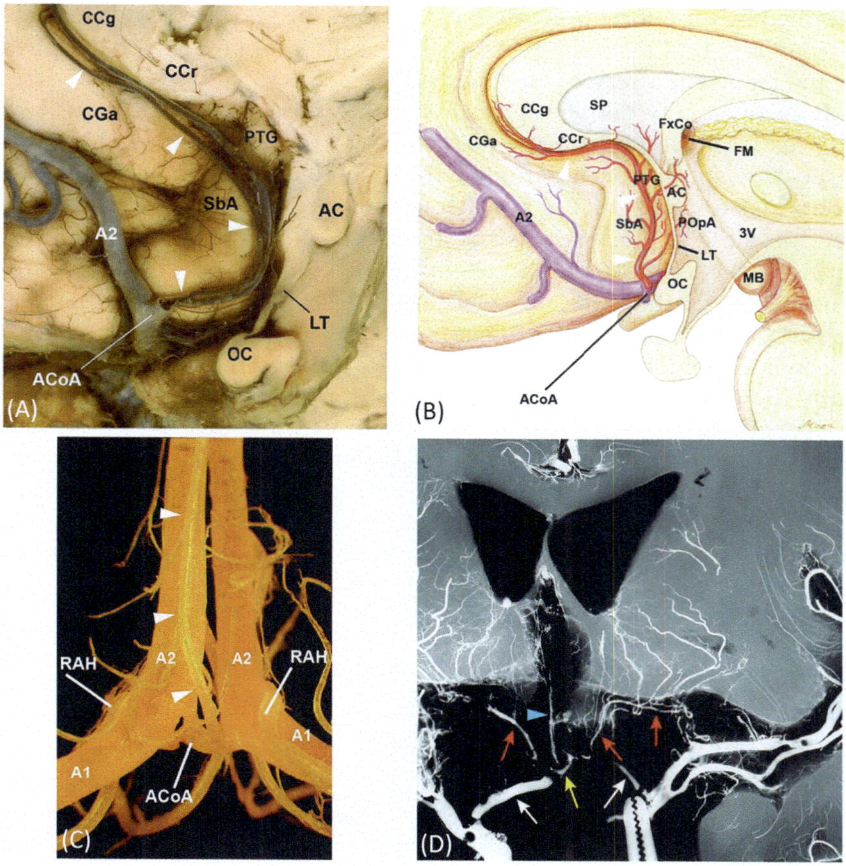

FIGURE 1.28 Vascularization of the basal forebrain. (A) Specimen shows the subcallosal artery. The unpaired subcallosal artery (*arrowheads*) originates from the posterosuperior aspect of the aneurysm of the anterior communicating artery (ACoA), divides into two stems, and ascends dorsally into the lamina terminalis (LT) cistern, then curves upward and forward along the LT, paraterminal gyrus (PTG), subcallosal area (SbA), the rostrum (CCr), and genu (CCg) of the corpus callosum, and the anterior cingulate gyrus (CGa), thus exhibiting a characteristic S-shaped curve. OC indicates optic chiasm. (B) Illustrative figure of the subcallosal artery (*arrowheads*) supplying the basal forebrain on the basis of our previous study regarding the microsurgical anatomy of the artery [14]. The subcallosal artery originates from the posterosuperior aspect of the ACoA, ascends dorsally into the LT cistern, and supplies the eight regions of the basal forebrain as follows: preoptic area (POpA), PTG including a part of the septum pellucidum (SP), SbA, anterior commissure (AC), and column of fornix (FxCo), then curves forward and upward to supply the CCr, CCg, and CGa. FM indicates foramen of Monro; MB, mammillary body; A2, A2 segment of the anterior cerebral artery; 3V, third ventricle. (C) Specimen of the anterior cerebral and ACoA complex injected with methacrylic resin viewed from the posterior side. The subcallosal artery (*arrowheads*) is seen arising from the ACoA, A1, right and left A1

(*continued*)

supplied by the subcallosal artery before they turn posteriorly toward the mammillary bodies. Some parts of the basal forebrain are also supplied by the recurrent artery of Heubner [43].

It is unclear whether there are anastomoses between these two arteries (subcallosal artery and recurrent artery of Heubner). In this respect, it should be mentioned that isolated strokes of the orbitofrontal cortex and/or the basal forebrain are extremely rare events. One possible explanation is the presence of the anterior communicating artery, which might be large enough to provide collateral blood flow to the adjacent orbitofrontal cortex of the contralateral hemisphere, but too small to compensate for the reduced blood flow following occlusion of the A2 segment or the pericallosal artery. The same may hold true for the basal forebrain: because the subcallosal artery arises from the anterior communicating artery, it receives blood from both the left and right A1 segments, potentially compensating for unilateral proximal ACA occlusions. Another reason may be that such small strokes can hardly be detected with conventional clinical MRI scanning, and such lesions often do not produce motor deficits.

1.7.2 The basal forebrain's vulnerability to subarachnoid hemorrhage

The basal forebrain is localized directly anterior to the optic chiasm, where the Circle of Willis is completed by the anterior communicating artery. The anterior communicating artery is the segment of the cerebral arterial system with the highest risk for brain aneurysms (approximately 40% of all brain aneurysms are located here (Fig. 1.4) [11]). Thus the risk of involvement of the basal forebrain in cases of nontraumatic subarachnoid hemorrhage (SAH) is high. Such hemorrhage leads to a sudden

segments, and A2, right and left A2 segments, of the anterior cerebral arteries. (D) Coronal microangiogram of the RAH on both sides and the unpaired subcallosal artery (reproduced, with permission, from Takahashi S, Goto K, Fukasawa H, et al. Computed tomography of cerebral infarction along the distribution of the basal perforating arteries. Part I. striate arterial group. *Radiology* 1985;155:107–18). Both internal carotid arteries have been retracted inferiorly to demonstrate the cisternal course of the RAH (*red arrows*), which follows a curved or tortuous course along the A1 segment of the anterior cerebral artery (*white arrows*). The branches of the RAH are distributed to a part of the basal forebrain. The subcallosal artery (*arrowhead*) is also seen arising from the ACoA (*yellow arrow*). *From Mugikura S., Kikuchi H., Fujii T. et al. MR imaging of subcallosal artery infarct causing amnesia after surgery for anterior communicating artery aneurysm. AJNR Am J Neuroradiol 2014;35(12):2293–2301.*

drop in blood flow distal to the affected artery. Moreover, blood pressure may be high enough to disrupt the pia mater and cause hemorrhagic extension into the adjacent brain tissue. Yet another mechanism contributing to focal lesions is vasoconstriction of vessels traversing this segment of the subarachnoid space.

Fig. 1.29 shows the cCT of a nontraumatic SAH. The star-like white structure indicates the clipping of the aneurysm (Fig. 1.29 upper line, fourth image from the left). Following the sequence of axial slices from ventral (upper outermost left image) to dorsal (lower outermost right image), one can observe a bilateral hypodensity left and right anterior to the dark symmetric lateral ventricles. This indicates involvement of the cingulate gyri of both hemispheres. In the most dorsal images, it becomes evident that the ACA stroke is more extensive on the right side (corresponding to the left hemisphere) than on the left side (corresponding to the right hemisphere). Such patients often suffer from apathy or akinetic mutism if being right-handed (see Chapter 9 for an explanation). The images also show a ventriculoperitoneal shunt, which can be followed from the interventricular foramen to the point where it exits the brain (visible as a light spot in the upper outermost right image gradually shifting leftward in the lower slices).

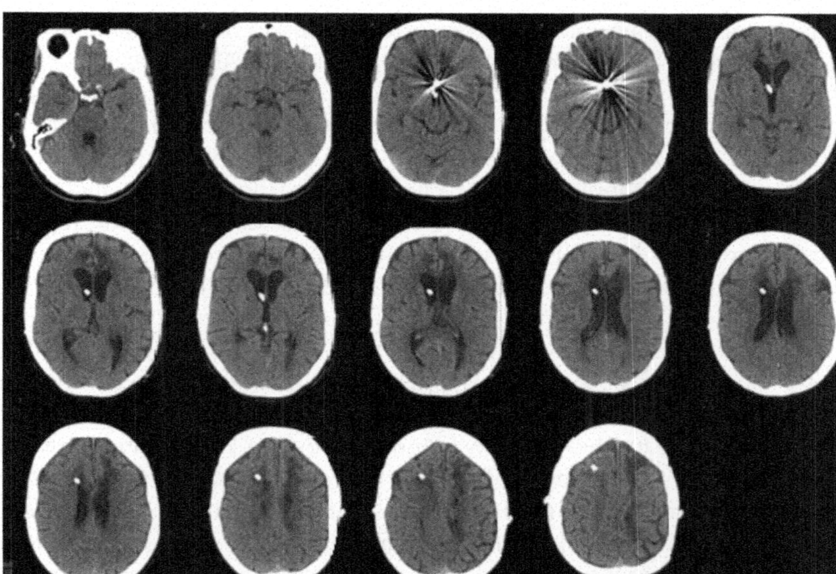

FIGURE 1.29 Clinical cranial computer tomography scan of a clipped anterior communicating artery aneurysm with bilateral cingulate stroke.

1.7.3 Basal forebrain lesions as a risk factor for confabulations

Confabulation is the production of fictitious, objectively false events or information that have no connection to reality but are believed to be true at that moment. Confabulations may result from the patient's acute clinical condition (e.g., as part of a delirium), or they may be related to the location of the brain lesion. Right ventrolateral prefrontal strokes and rupture of an anterior communicating artery aneurysm may lead to confabulations. Confabulating patients are not primarily restless; they do not typically show motor disinhibition (e.g., nesting movements) or suffer from severe attentional fluctuations as would be the case for those in a delirium. Another difference between delirium-related and lesion-related confabulation lies in the clinical course: delirium-related confabulations tend to remit within a few days, whereas confabulations associated with lesions of the basal forebrain, ventral right orbitofrontal cortex, and the ventromedial frontal cortex also tend to remit, but much more slowly.

In recent years, several different models have been developed to provide a cognitive explanation for the development of confabulations [44–47]. One neuropsychological model of confabulation can be found in (Hildebrandt, 2019) [48]. First, impaired inhibition may result in an inappropriate sense of correctness. This component has been conceptualized as disinhibition of a fast and automatic feeling of correctness, which has been linked to the orbitofrontal cortex [49]. Rupture of an aneurysm of the anterior communicating artery often leads to hemorrhage into the orbitofrontal cortex and may therefore contribute to the development of confabulations. A second, additional lack of inhibition is impaired postretrieval monitoring [50,51]. The right mid-ventrolateral prefrontal cortex may play a major role in retrieval monitoring [52]. Notably, blood within the subarachnoid space around the subcallosal artery and other branches of the pericallosal artery may lead to strokes in this region. Third, there may be a disorganized search strategy related to memory contents that are associated with this automatic feeling of correctness. As a result, patients may be unable to critically evaluate memory content and often fail to respond reasonably to evidence or arguments that contradict their confabulations. This deficit is also thought to be related to (right) frontal cortex dysfunction (especially the right ventrolateral prefrontal cortex, which is supplied by the MCA, not the ACA). In combination with impaired postretrieval monitoring, this may promote the formation of partially fantastic and highly associative combinations of ideas. These often stem from different episodes from the patient's past and lead to a more or less coherent confabulation. Many confabulating patients tell stories in which they occupy a central role in an important task or responsibility. Such confabulations may partly reflect the patient's attempt to cope with the threat posed by the current situation and the event that led to it, and the attempt to preserve their integrity and autonomy [45].

A seminal study of confabulation in patients following rupture of an anterior aneurysm was published by Schnider (2001, 2003, 2005) [53–55]. To characterize the confabulations observed in this patient group more precisely, Schnider et al. proposed a distinction between provoked confabulation, which occurs when individuals attempt to retrieve more information from memory than is available [49,53]. The retrieved information may also be real but misplaced in its chronological context. Spontaneous confabulation, in contrast, is characterized by loose associations and seemingly bizarre ideas, often accompanied by severe disorientation, references to earlier experiences, and a profound misinterpretation of the current situation. Spontaneous confabulations are characteristic of patients with lesions involving the medial prefrontal cortex, whereas provoked confabulations are more commonly observed in patients with (right) lateral prefrontal lesions. The patient described by Schnider and Bonvallat [55] exhibited dense amnesia 10 weeks after the SAH. After 3–5 months, neuropsychological assessment documented preserved intellectual functioning, but persistent amnesia and disorientation. The patient was discharged after 7 months. After 17 months, the confabulations had resolved. However, the patient's concept of reality continued to be determined by memories that were 15–20 years old, indicating a marked retrograde amnesia spanning this period.

Confabulations following rupture of an anterior communicating artery aneurysm may be caused directly by the underlying brain lesion; however, in some cases they may also result from hydrocephalus. In contrast to normal pressure hydrocephalus, which is characterized by the triad of slow gait, urinary incontinence, and cognitive slowing, patients with subacute onset of hydrocephalus due to SAH may develop signs of confusion, motor restlessness, and confabulation [56]. If confabulations and motor restlessness are increasing weeks after the aneurysm rupture, one should consider the possibility of hydrocephalus and perform a cCT scan.

Treatment approaches for confabulations from a functional perspective will be described in Chapter 7.

1.8 Veins of the brain

1.8.1 Location of the brain's sinuses

There are small and large veins located on the brain's surface and within the brain [17]. While the arteries supply the brain with oxygenated blood, the veins are responsible for draining deoxygenated blood. The smaller veins of the brain are divided into different branches that run mainly in the sulci on the cortical surface. These veins are often named after the adjacent cerebral gyri (Fig. 1.30). The system of larger veins, termed "sinuses," also runs along much of the cortical surface, although there are some exceptions. Their names are generally not associated with

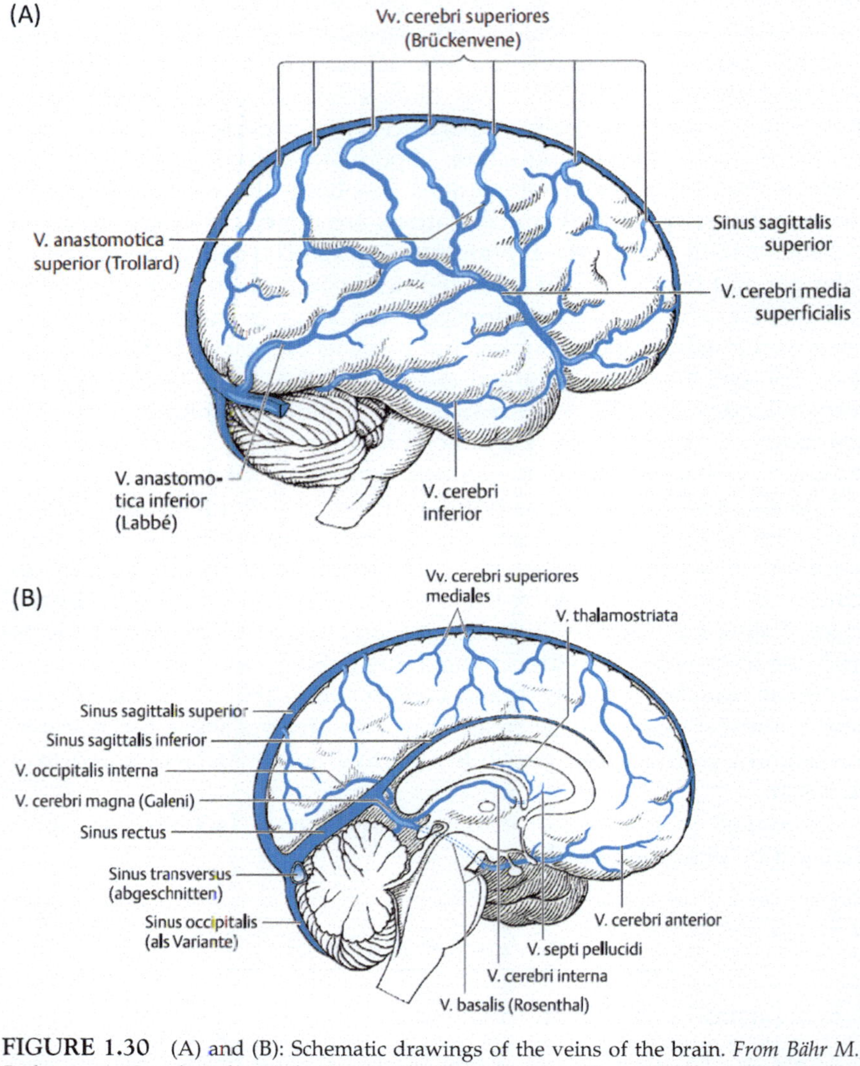

FIGURE 1.30 (A) and (B): Schematic drawings of the veins of the brain. *From Bähr M., Bechmann I. Neurologisch-topische Diagnostik: Anatomie - Funktion - Klinik.* 11 überarbeitete Auflage Thieme *2021. Figures. 11.13 and 11.14.*

the surrounding brain structures. The following segments of the sinuses can be distinguished:

(1) The superior sagittal sinus, the longest venous sinus of the brain, is located within the longitudinal fissure (also termed interhemispheric fissure), separating the left and right hemispheres. It extends from the frontal pole to the occipital pole. At the occipital pole, five sinuses converge: (2) the superior sagittal sinus, (3) the inferior sagittal sinus, which drains subcortical structures adjacent to the corpus callosum and the thalamus, (4) the occipital sinus, starting at the lowest level of the cerebellum, and (5) the transverse sinus, which collects venous blood from regions adjacent to the lateral (Sylvian) fissure. The transverse sinus drains into the (6) sigmoid sinus, and the blood is then drained from the brain by the internal jugular vein and the deep cervical vein.

Chapter 2 describes how to identify the sinuses on clinical MRI scans.

1.8.2 Venous drainage disorders ("Cerebral venous sinus thrombosis")

Venous drainage disorders most commonly result from cerebral venous sinus thrombosis (CVST), often associated with inflammation [2,7,57]. Initial symptoms include headache, visual disturbances, and epileptic seizures. It is not uncommon for hemorrhage to occur as a consequence of CVST. In general, however, CVST is relatively uncommon, and only about 1% of all patients admitted with stroke have CVST. However, this does not apply to individuals between 20 and 50 years of age, among whom stroke is rare and CVST is more common.

The neuropsychological consequences of CVST depend on the specific vein involved in the occlusion. Fig. 1.31 shows an MRI scan demonstrating thrombosis of the left vein of Labbé (a small vein near the Sylvian fissure). In contrast to ischemic stroke, the lesion is less well demarcated and more diffuse (reflecting venous congestion and secondary hemorrhagic transformation which does not follow typical arterial territories). Based on the location of the lesion (see Chapter 2 for lesion localization) in the left inferior and middle temporal cortex (regions important for language processing) and in the left lateral occipital cortex, one would expect visual and language deficits. However, neither Wernicke's aphasia nor complete hemianopia would be expected, because the optic radiation runs more medially through the white matter of the temporal and occipital lobes, sparing the regions typically associated with these syndromes.

Goldmann perimetry and visual field assessment using the test of attentional performance (TAP) did not reveal any visual field defect. However, there was a reading impairment: spontaneous reading behavior was characterized by slow letter-by-letter decoding of words and a

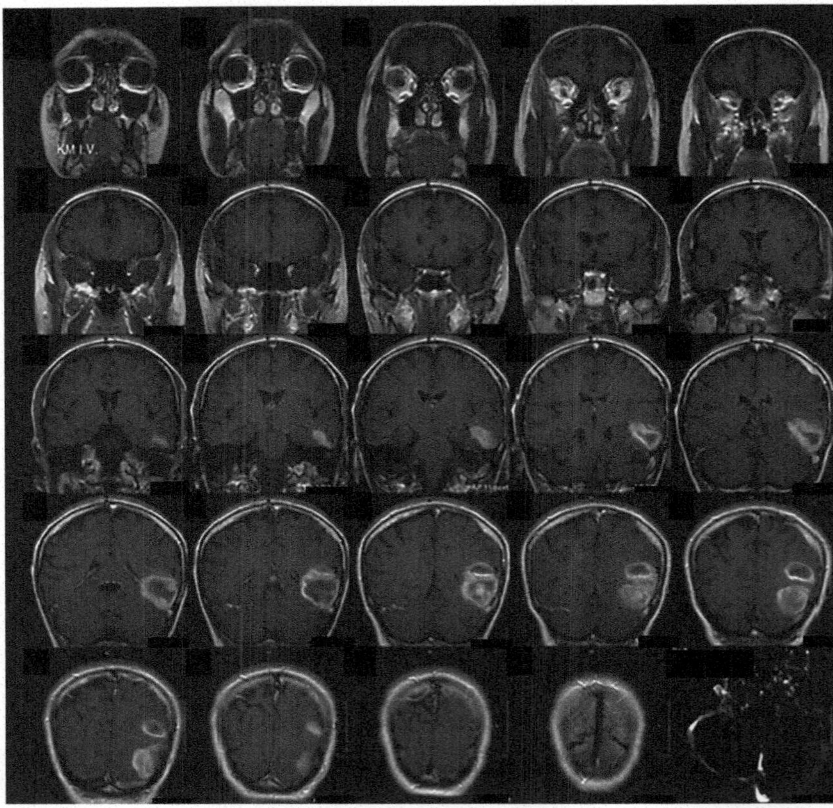

FIGURE 1.31 Clinical MRI scan of cerebral venous sinus thrombosis.

reliance on grapheme-phoneme conversion (e.g., reading vase as "v-a-s-e") before identifying the word). Furthermore the word recognition latency increased with word length, irrespective of word frequency: four-letter words =1.1 seconds, seven-letter words: 2.7 seconds. However, there was no clear dependence of the reading speed on word length for words containing fewer than four letters or on font type. In other words, reading speed decreased as word length increased, suggesting that words were processed serially rather than being recognized as whole units. The most probable diagnosis, therefore was central surface dyslexia with letter-by-letter reading. This interpretation is supported by the observation that font type did not influence reading performance (as would be expected in pure alexia) and because the lingual gyrus was not affected by the lesion (however, the left fusiform gyrus is still involved, and therefore pure alexia cannot be excluded solely on the basis of MRI findings).

1.9 Production and drainage of cerebrospinal fluid

The cerebrospinal fluid (CSF) is not strictly a component of the cerebrovascular system [17]. However, CSF is drained through the venous sinuses, surrounds the cerebral arteries within the subarachnoid space, and plays an important role in processes related to neuronal repair and regeneration. The volume of CSF is between 120 ml and 150 ml. It is renewed about two to three times a day. It is produced by the choroid plexus of the lateral ventricles, as well as by the third and fourth ventricles. The choroid plexus of the lateral ventricles is visible on clinical MRI scans and serves as a landmark for localizing structures such as the hypothalamus, hippocampus, and the body and columns of the fornix. Chapter 2 describes how to identify the choroid plexus on clinical MRI scans.

Table 1.6 gives an overview of the distribution of the CSF in the brain, its circulation, and its functions. The CSF is partly located in the interstitial space between neurons and glial cells. It supports the metabolic processes of these cells. Waste products of cellular activity are deposited in the interstitial space and are transported out of the brain with the flow of the CSF [58]. Another portion of the CSF is located inside the ventricles. Lastly CSF also fills the subarachnoid space. Apart from the transport of waste products from the interstitial space, a second important function of the CSF is the protection of the brain during concussions. This function is realized by the movement of CSF within the ventricles and subarachnoid space in response to sudden acceleration or impact.

1.9.1 Neuroanatomical structures for production, circulation, and drainage of cerebrospinal fluid

The ventricular system consists of the two lateral ventricles, each comprising the frontal horn, cella media, posterior horn, and temporal horn (the use of these structures for orientation on clinical MRIs will be described in Chapter 2).

At the interventricular foramen, the lateral ventricle is connected to the third ventricle (Fig. 1.32). The third ventricle is readily identifiable on most clinical brain scans and is an important landmark for neuroanatomical orientation because it is located medial to the two thalamic nuclei. The cerebral aqueduct, which connects the third ventricle with the fourth ventricle, can be identified on axial MRI scans as a small structure at the level of the midbrain. The choroid plexus of the fourth ventricle is located in the caudal pons. Just superior to the choroid plexus, the fourth ventricle communicates with the subarachnoid space through three openings (not visible on clinical MRI scans). These openings include

TABLE 1.6 Cerebrospinal fluid within the brain and its function.

Locations of cerebrospinal fluid (CSF) and its functions		
Location	**Description**	**Function**
Interstitial space (between neurons and glial cells)	CSF is partly present within the interstitial space between neurons and glial cells.	Metabolic support: Facilitates the transport of metabolic waste and byproducts out of the brain.
Ventricles (lateral, third, and fourth ventricles)	CSF is produced by the choroid plexus and circulates through the ventricular system: – Lateral ventricles: Contain the frontal horn, central part (cella media), posterior horn, and temporal horn. – Third ventricle: Located between the thalamic nuclei. – Cerebral aqueduct: Connects the third and fourth ventricles. – Fourth ventricle: Located between the brainstem and cerebellum and connected to the subarachnoid space.	CSF production and circulation: CSF flows through the ventricles, transporting nutrients and removing waste.
Subarachnoid space	Space between the pia mater and arachnoid mater, CSF flows around the brain and spinal cord after passing from the fourth ventricle via the lateral and median apertures.	Shock absorption and buoyancy: Protects the brain from mechanical damage by cushioning it.
Cisterns (e.g., cisterna magna, quadrigeminal cistern)	Expanded subarachnoid spaces are located near specific brain structures, following the sulci and gyri.	CSF reservoirs: Serve as landmarks in neuroimaging and help regulate CSF flow.
Arachnoid granulations	Structures involved in CSF absorption into the venous circulation, primarily via the superior sagittal sinus.	Drainage of CSF: CSF is reabsorbed into the bloodstream, primarily driven by pressure gradients and arterial pulsations.

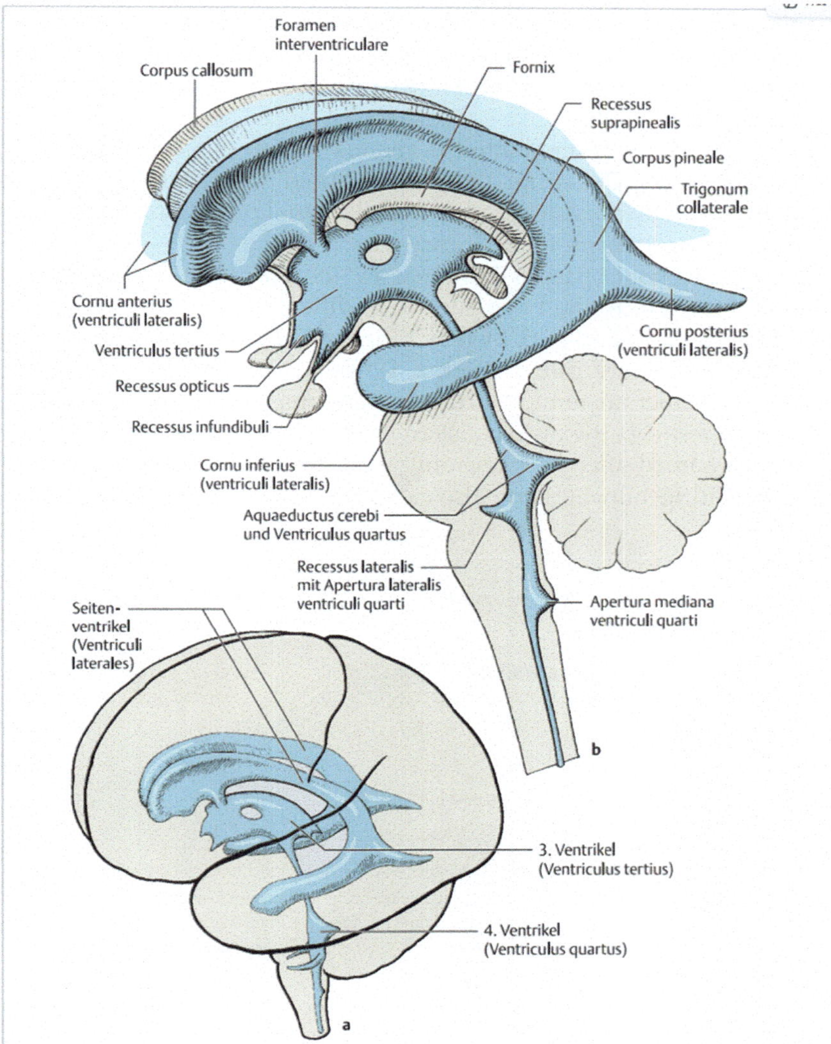

FIGURE 1.32 Ventricles of the brain. *From Bähr M., Bechmann I. Neurologisch-topische Diagnostik: Anatomie - Funktion - Klinik.* 11 überarbeitete Auflage Thieme *2021. (Fig. 10.3).*

the two lateral apertures and the median aperture. A substantial proportion of the CSF exits the fourth ventricle and enters the subarachnoid space through these openings. The median aperture is an important landmark for identifying the transition between the pons and medulla oblongata because, at this level, the pons gives way to the medulla oblongata on axial images. Entering the subarachnoid space through the lateral and median apertures, CSF flows around the brain and spinal cord where it is ultimately reabsorbed, for example, in the arachnoid granulations.

CSF is ultimately drained into the venous system (Figs. 1.33 and 1.34). The movement of CSF from the subarachnoid space into the venous system is driven by pressure gradients and arterial pulsations. There is no active pump mechanism for CSF clearance.

The subarachnoid space is bordered by the pia mater and arachnoid mater. Both adhere to the brain surface in different ways, and follow the contours of the sulci and gyri, thereby forming CSF-filled spaces of varying size. These spaces are called cisterns. When located adjacent to specific sulci, gyri, or other anatomical structures, cisterns are named according to these structures (e.g., the insular cistern or the frontal sulcus cistern). Some cisterns are named after their anatomical location or associated structures (e.g., the quadrigeminal cistern, also called the cistern of the great cerebral

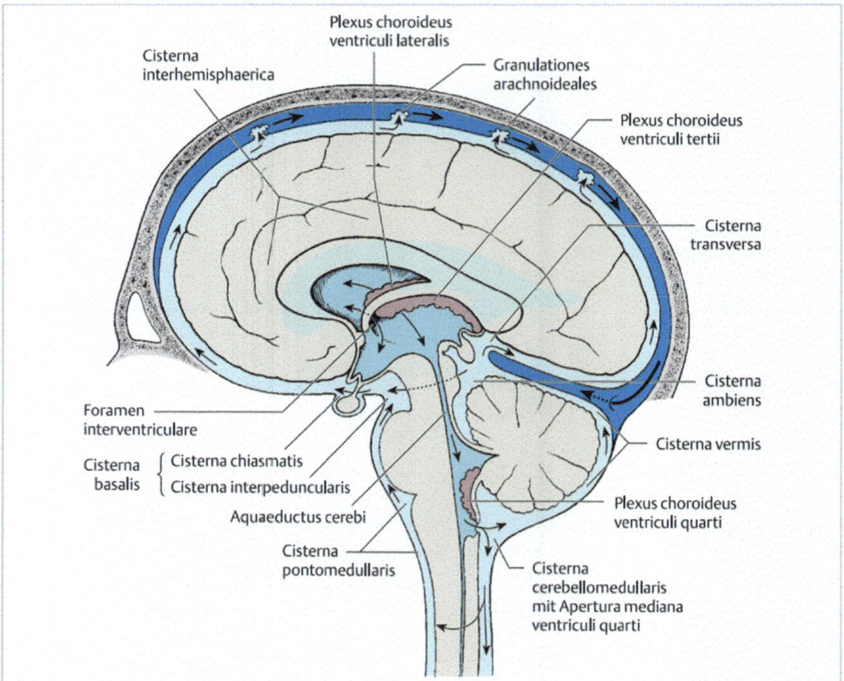

FIGURE 1.33 Circulation of cerebrospinal fluid in the brain. *From Bähr M., Bechmann I. Neurologisch-topische Diagnostik: Anatomie - Funktion - Klinik.* 11 überarbeitete Auflage Thieme *2021. (Figure 10.4).*

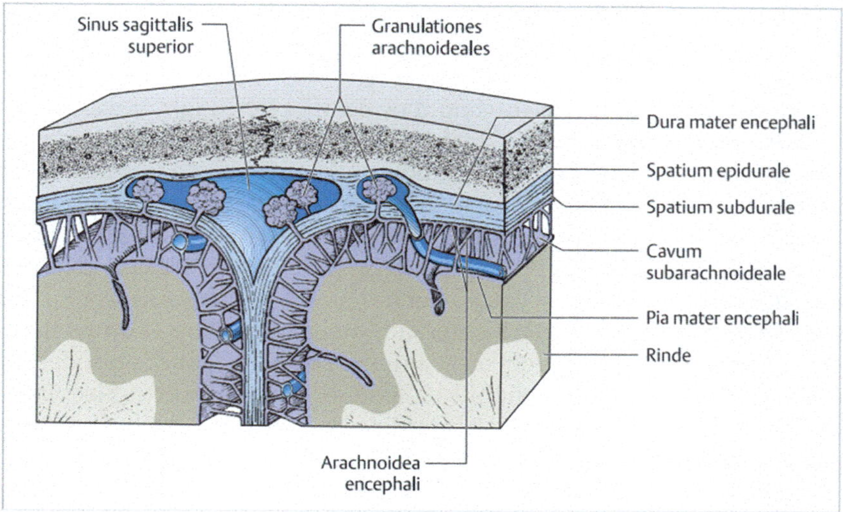

FIGURE 1.34 Schematic coronal picture of granulationes arachnoidalis. *From Bähr M., Bechmann I. Neurologisch-topische Diagnostik: Anatomie - Funktion - Klinik.* 11 überarbeitete Auflage Thieme *2021. Figure 10.1.*

vein). The cisterns serve as landmarks for neuroanatomical orientation on clinical scans, which will be described in Chapter 2.

Proper drainage of CSF from the interstitial space into the subarachnoid space, through the cisterns, and ultimately into the venous system is important not only for preventing normal pressure hydrocephalus (see Hildebrandt [59] for this syndrome and its neuropsychological assessment) but also for maintaining normal cortical and subcortical neuronal function. Adequate CSF drainage is necessary for the prevention of waste accumulation in the interstitial space. During sleep, the interstitial space expands as blood pressure decreases. This enables the clearance of metabolic waste products through CSF circulation.

1.9.2 Cerebrospinal fluid and sleep

Many (up to 70%) patients suffer from sleep apnea during the acute phase after stroke, and it has been estimated that up to 30% of patients still suffer from sleep apnea or other forms of sleep-disordered breathing in the chronic phase of a stroke [60,61]. Patients with sleep-disordered breathing often experience sleepiness, excessive daytime sleepiness, and increasing difficulties in attention and memory. Even if this disorder can be treated by lifestyle changes and continuous positive airway pressure

(CPAP) therapy, CPAP therapy alone may not fully reverse all cognitive deficits if recurrent breathing interruptions were present for extended periods.

Clinical neuropsychologists should be aware of the high prevalence of sleep-disordered breathing in stroke patients. Certain brainstem strokes may directly cause sleep apnea, although this is relatively uncommon. For most patients, other factors, such as obesity, are more common causes, which means that they have obstructive rather than central sleep apnea. Still, this disorder appears to increase the risk of stroke and stroke mortality, irrespective of its cause. Consequently, the neuropsychological assessment interview should include questions of snoring and breathing pauses during sleep. Moreover, daytime sleepiness and episodes of unintended daytime sleep should be assessed. The Epworth Sleepiness Scale (ESS) can be used for a standardized assessment. Such an assessment is particularly important in patients with mild memory disorders and deficits on higher-order working memory tasks. Signs of obesity should prompt the neuropsychologist to inquire about sleep disordered breathing and encourage patients to obtain information about their nighttime breathing from other patients sharing the same room or nursing staff. However, not all patients with sleep apnea snore, which means that marked daytime sleepiness alone may indicate sleep apnea. If sleep-disordered breathing is suspected, ambulatory screening should be recommended, and informing patients about the risk for developing cognitive deficits may help motivate adherence to treatment.

1.10 Vascularization and strokes of the brainstem

1.10.1 Blood supply and structure of the brainstem

The vascular supply of the brainstem (midbrain, pons, and medulla oblongata) is provided by the paired vertebral arteries and the unpaired basilar artery (Fig. 1.35A) [14,42,62,63]. The vertebral arteries are divided into four segments (V1, V2, V3, V4), but only V4 supplies the medulla oblongata, the lowest part of the brainstem, as well as the inferior cerebellum. A major branch arising from the V4 segment is the posterior inferior cerebellar artery (PICA), which supplies the lateral medulla and the inferior cerebellum. The two paired V4 segments of the vertebral arteries merge to form the basilar artery. The basilar artery supplies the pontine nuclei and major tracts traversing the pons. Its branches can be divided into the paramedian and lateral pontine arteries, and the anterior inferior and superior cerebellar arteries. The cranial nerve nuclei are supplied by branches of the vertebral arteries (cranial nerves X–XII) and

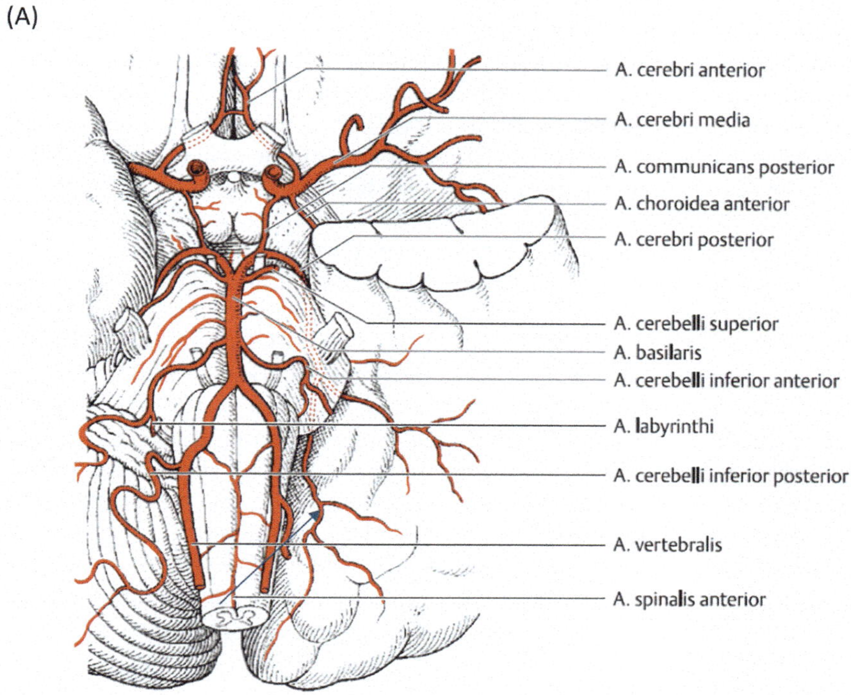

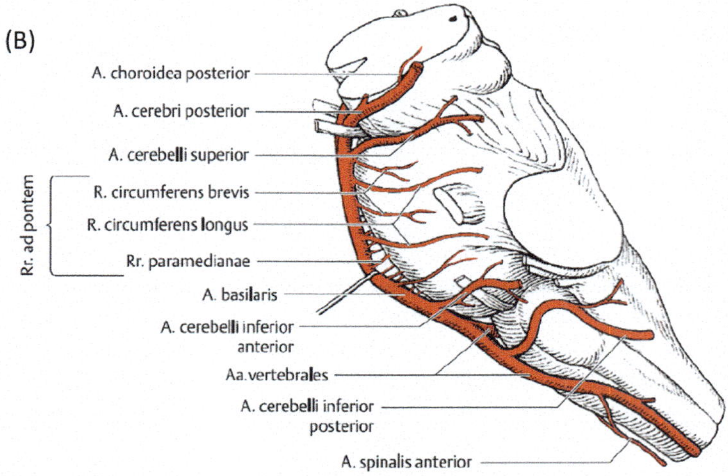

FIGURE 1.35 (A) and (B): Vascularization of the brainstem. *From Bähr M., Bechmann I. Neurologisch-topische Diagnostik: Anatomie - Funktion - Klinik.* 11 überarbeitete Auflage Thieme *2021. Figure 4.57.*

the basilar artery (cranial nerves IV–IX). Strokes at the pontine level (and in the upper medulla) may produce bilateral symptoms because most cranial nerve pathways remain ipsilateral, whereas the corticospinal tract decussates at the pyramidal decussation. Thus, patients may present with sensory deficits on one side of the body and motor deficits on the other, which will be discussed in more detail later. The pattern of impairments often allows relatively precise lesion localization. Fig. 1.35B illustrates the vascular supply of the brainstem in a lateral view.

The brainstem can be divided into two zones: a medial core zone and a lateral zone (Fig. 1.37) [17]. The medial core zone contains the ascending reticular activating system (ARAS), crucial for wakefulness, alertness, and pain perception. This system consists of loosely interconnected nuclei, through which sensory and motor fibers pass, forming a mesh-like structure. The ARAS includes several monoaminergic cell groups that release serotonin, adrenaline, norepinephrine, and acetylcholine. Fibers from these monoaminergic cell groups both ascend (towards the cerebrum) and descend (towards the spinal cord). Rostral cell groups in the pons and midbrain project to cerebral structures, whereas caudal cell groups in the pons and medulla project to nuclei in the lower brainstem and spinal cord. However, both groups innervate autonomic brainstem centers [17].

Fig. 1.38 shows three schematic axial sections of the brainstem at the level of the medulla and pons. The orientation of these sections differs from that typically seen on clinical MRI scans. In these schematic illustrations, the pons appears below the central portion of the brainstem, whereas on clinical MRIs, it appears above.

The first section shows the level of the pyramidal decussation, where the corticospinal tract crosses to the contralateral side. Adjacent to the pyramidal tract, the gracile and cuneate fasciculi are shown. The location of the ARAS is indicated by small gray dots. Fibers conveying pain information run within the anterolateral funiculus. The second section on the left is found on the level of the cranial nerves 10 and 12. It also shows the crossing of the sensory information from the gracile and cuneate nuclei to the lemniscus medialis, which is the major projection tract for tactile and proprioceptive information. The ARAS is again represented by the small gray spots. Mesial to all other structures, the raphe nucleus magnus can be found ("R"), bordered by the medial longitudinal fasciculus. The raphe nuclei remain in a central position throughout the brainstem; however, they may be subdivided into different subnuclei depending on their neuroarchitectural structure and their projections. The third section shows the nucleus of the facial nerve and of the abducens. Moreover, the position of the corticospinal tract inside the pons is indicated.

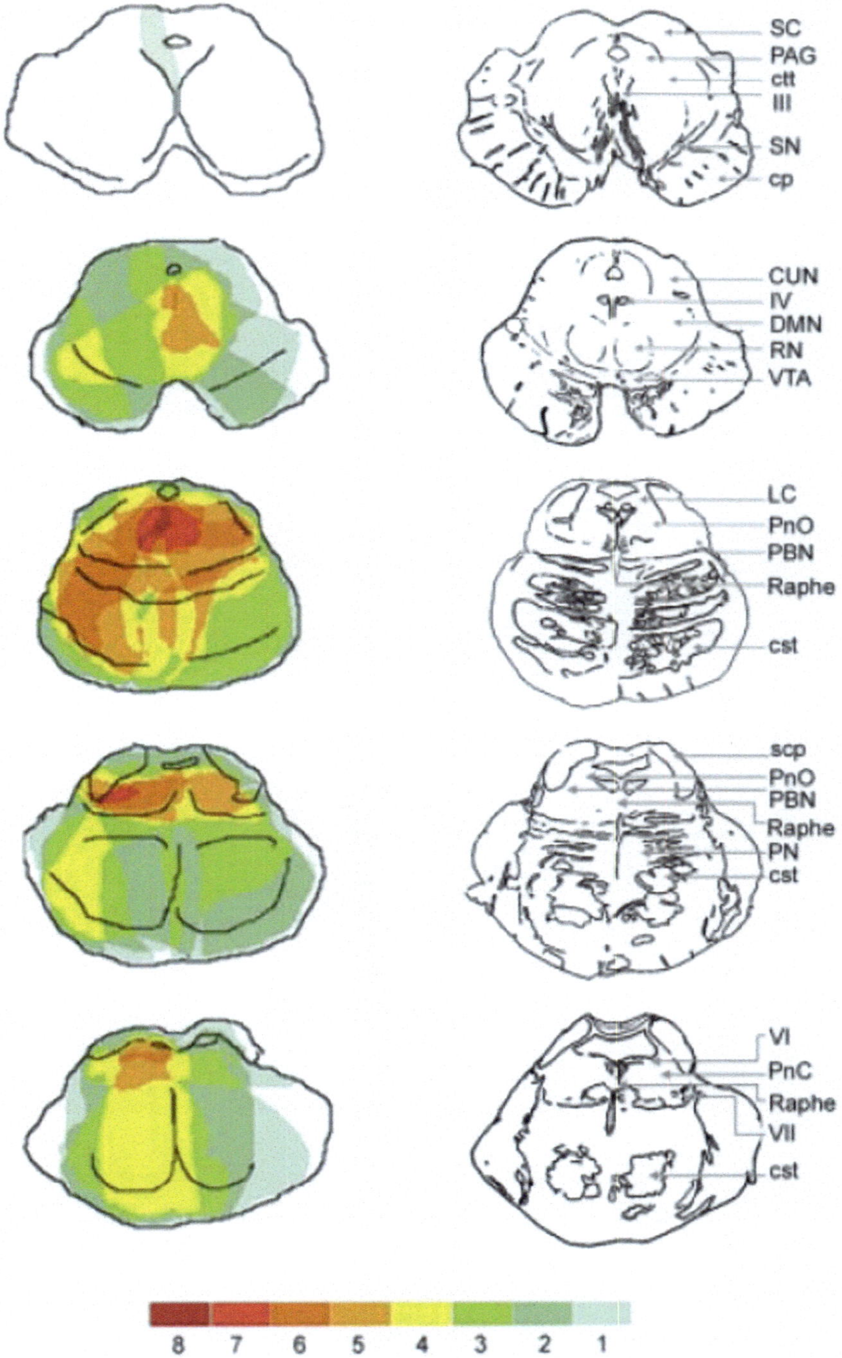

FIGURE 1.36 Medial brainstem strokes in patients with coma. Schematic transversal section through the brain stem Parvizi and Damasio [64]. SC = colliculus superior, PAG = periaqueductal gray matter, III = oculomotorius nucleus, SN = substantia nigra, cp = cerebral pedunculi, CUN = nucleus cuneiformis, IV = nucleus trochlearis, DMN = nucleus dorsomedialis, RN = Nucleus raphe, VTA = ventral tegmental area, LC = locus coeruleus, PnO = Nucleus pontis oralis, PBN = nucleus parabrachialis, cst = corticospinal tract, scp = pedunculus cerebelli superior.

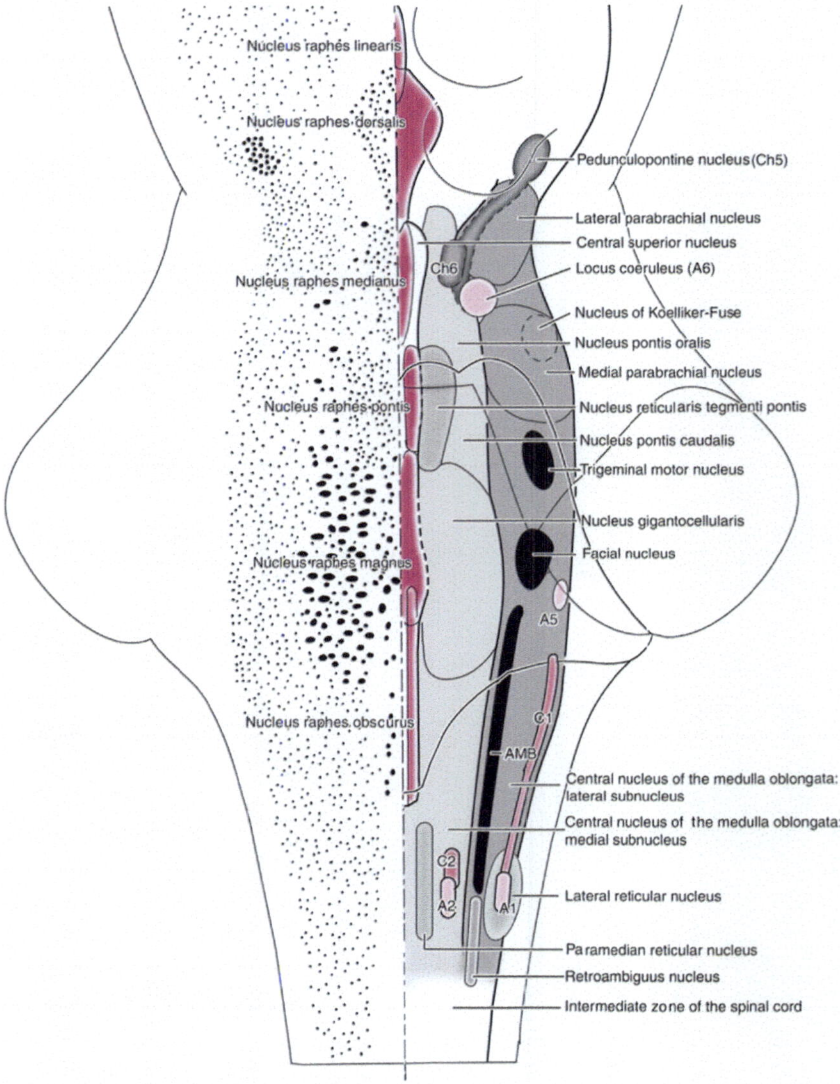

FIGURE 1.37 Medial zone of the brainstem and the relevant cell groups. *From Nieuwenhuys R., Voogd J., Huijzen C.van The Human Central Nervous System. 4th ed. Berlin: Springer-Verlag; 2008. Figure 22.1.*

1.10.2 Brainstem strokes

1.10.2.1 Strokes of the medial pontine core zone, apallic syndrome

Strokes involving the paramedian branches of the pontine arteries may affect the central nuclei of the brainstem [42,62,63]. If the stroke affects

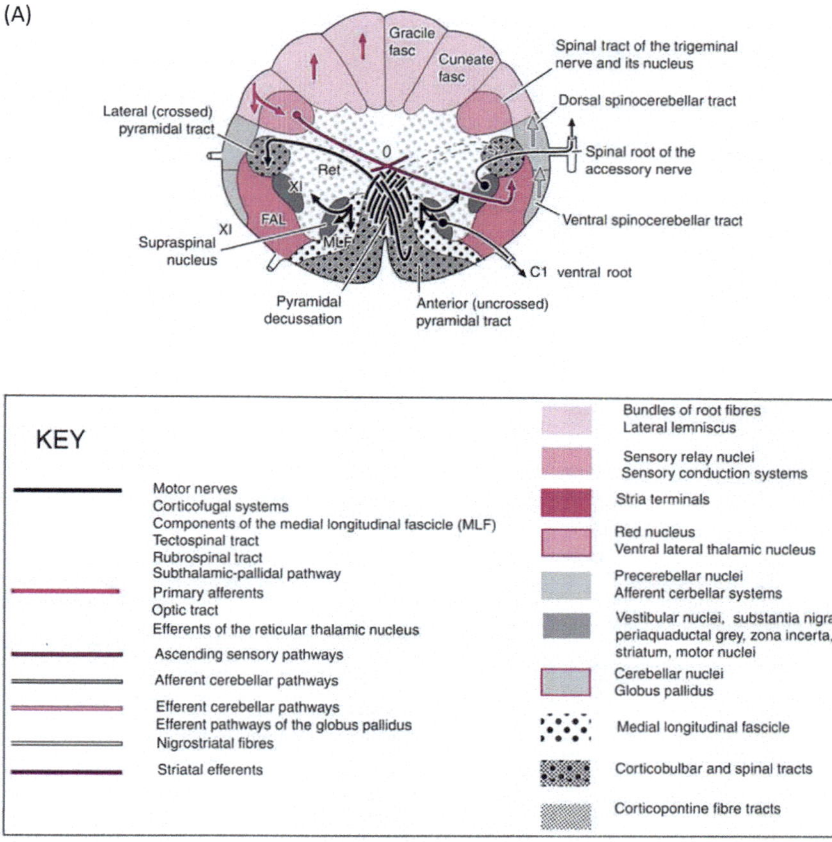

FIGURE 1.38 (A) and (B) and (C): Schematic drawings of axial sections through the brainstem. *From Nieuwenhuys R., Voogd J., Huijzen C. van The Human Central Nervous System. 4th ed. Berlin: Springer-Verlag; 2008. Figures 6.13 and 6.15.*

both sides of the brainstem, the cerebral cortex becomes deprived of ascending serotonergic and noradrenergic input, which corresponds to the classical concept of the apallic syndrome, nowadays referred to as unresponsive wakefulness syndrome (Chapter 9 discusses these states and their treatment). Patients typically show no signs of awareness, purposeful movements, or responses to stimuli. Such strokes are rare and, in contrast to global hypoxia (which causes cortical neuronal necrosis), a brainstem stroke primarily disrupts the ascending neuromodulatory input to the cerebral cortex.

Parvizi and Damasio [64] reported findings from patients who developed coma due to brainstem strokes. The neuroanatomical evaluation showed that in seven of the nine comatose patients, the raphe nuclei

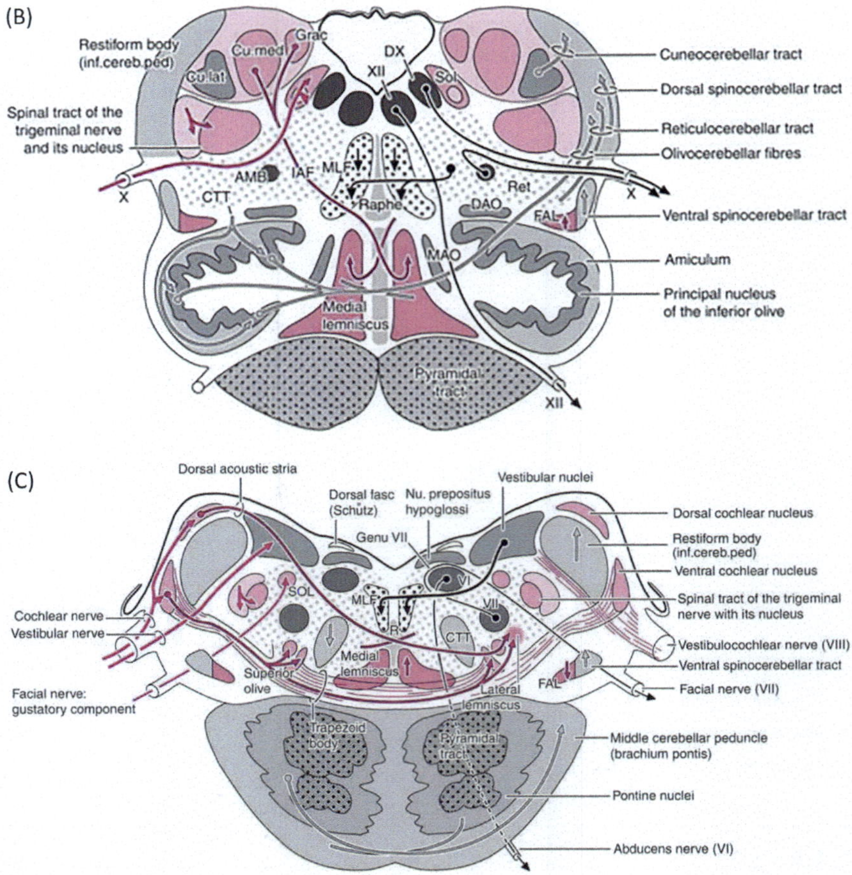

FIGURE 1.38 (*continued*).

were involved bilaterally; the remaining two had unilateral lesions of the raphe nuclei (Fig. 1.36). Six of the nine patients showed bilateral lesions of the locus coeruleus, which is the principal noradrenergic nucleus of the brainstem, and the same number showed bilateral lesions of the parabrachial nucleus, which is a higher-order brainstem center for autonomic nervous system functions. The cholinergic laterodorsal tegmental nucleus was involved bilaterally in five patients and unilaterally in two patients. This small series therefore supports the importance of the medial pontine core system for arousal. The frequent involvement of the raphe nuclei may suggest a particularly important role for serotonergic modulation in maintaining consciousness. However, because the serotonergic nuclei are considerably larger than the locus coeruleus, they are inherently more likely to be affected by brainstem lesions. Consequently, it remains unclear which role ascending fibers may have played in the development of the comatose state [64].

1.10.2.2 Cognitive deficits after brainstem stroke of various localizations

Brainstem strokes are usually not associated with specific cognitive syndromes, although isolated reports have described visuospatial neglect [65,66] and memory disorders [67,68]. Instead, their most important cognitive consequences are cognitive slowing, increased somnolence, and reduced vigilance, particularly with increasing task duration and task difficulty [69].

Allen, Houston [70] assessed 24 patients with Chiari Malformation type I, which is associated with compression of the medulla oblongata due to downward displacement of the inferior cerebellum. The most prominent finding was prolonged response times during incongruent colour naming in the Stroop task. However, slowing was already present in the congruent condition, and the study did not examine whether the incongruent condition produced an additional slowing or merely reflected a general reduction in processing speed.

Garrard, Bradshaw [71] published a case series of patients with brainstem injury and documented attentional deficits, which became more pronounced when executive demands were added to otherwise simple tasks. They did not find a relationship between lesion location and the resulting cognitive deficits. One limitation of this study is that some patients had lesions in the midbrain and not only in the pons or medulla. Van Zandvoort, De Haan [72] assessed 17 patients with lacunar strokes in the brainstem. Again, tests based on reaction time measures showed differences between age-matched healthy controls and patients, whereas performance on tasks without time restrictions or speed measures revealed no differences. In a study on attentional deficits after stroke, Rinne and Hassan [73] found alertness deficits in patients whose strokes involved the upper brainstem. One may therefore speculate that lesions involving the ARAS reduce the optimal modulation of cortical activity, resulting in cognitive slowing. Unfortunately, the impact of brainstem stroke on vigilance decrements has not yet been investigated explicitly. Consequently, neuropsychological assessment of patients with brainstem stroke should include tests that are sensitive to processing speed and vary in task difficulty. Moreover, some of these tests should include a prolonged monotonous condition to assess sleepiness (i.e., vigilance or alertness tests).

We assessed a 33-year-old male patient, with a university degree, who worked as an IT developer in the field of mechanical engineering. He experienced sentinel hemorrhages from a basilar aneurysm, presenting with headache. The aneurysm was detected before a major rupture occurred and was successfully treated by coil embolization without major complications. The patient reported residual symptoms including increased anxiety, mild depressive symptoms, and sleep disturbance. In addition, he reported uncertainty regarding possible cognitive deficits. Neuropsychological assessment showed unimpaired performance across a broad range of memory, attentional, and executive tasks (the California Verbal Learning Test (CVLT), paired-associate learning of object-location associations, divided attention, incompatibility, auditory vigilance, object alternation, and spatial working memory). However, performance on a two-back working memory task declined considerably following the vigilance test. At baseline, reaction time (RT) was 689 ms (PR = 21), with 5 omissions (PR = 10), 1 commission error (PR = 73). After approximately 1 hour: RT increased to 980 ms (PR = 3), omissions increased to 7 (PR = 2), and no commission errors occurred. These findings suggest impaired compensation for the effects of prolonged performance on a monotonous task. The clinical MRI scan showed a lesion or compression of the right caudal medulla (Fig. 1.39).

In conclusion, brainstem strokes typically do not cause specific cognitive syndromes but often lead to cognitive slowing, increased somnolence, and attentional deficits, especially in tasks requiring reaction speed, with impairments worsening under prolonged monotonous conditions.

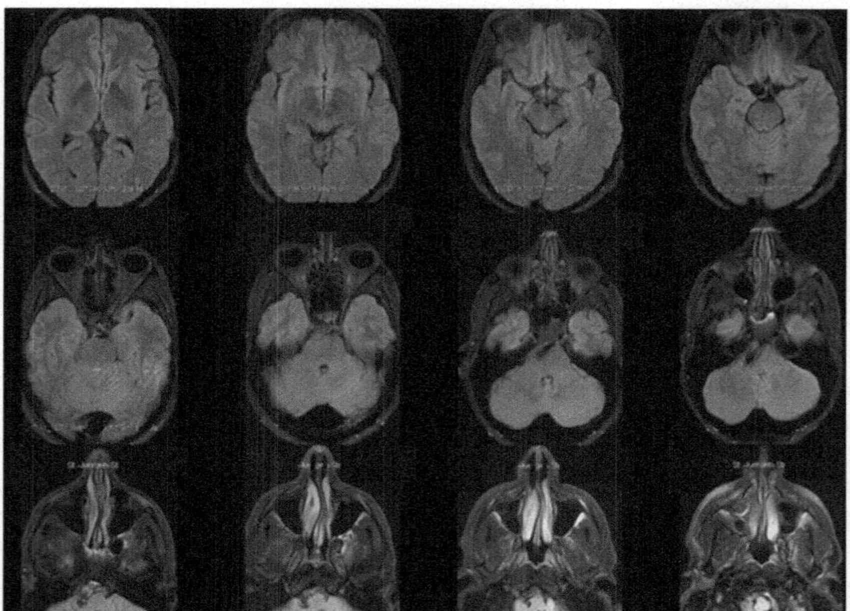

FIGURE 1.39 Right medullary brainstem lesion.

1.10.2.3 *Mood changes after stroke*

It is well established that serotonergic modulation of the cortex plays a role in depression and mood regulation. Cortical serotonergic modulation is mediated primarily by activity in the dorsal raphe nucleus, whereas the more caudal raphe nuclei are involved in the modulation and inhibition of functions such as pain perception. Numasawa and Hattori [74] enrolled 19 patients with a first-ever acute unilateral isolated brainstem infarction in an observational cross-sectional study. Depressive disorder was diagnosed according to the diagnostic and statistical manual of mental disorders (DSM-5) and a Montgomery–Åsberg Depression Rating Scale (MADRS) score of 12 or greater. Diffusion tensor imaging and proton density-weighted imaging were used to identify damage to the raphe nuclei, and patients were subsequently classified according to whether the raphe nuclei were damaged or intact. Depressive disorders were more frequent among patients with raphe lesions ($n = 6$) than among patients with brainstem lesions that spared the raphe nuclei ($n = 13$). MADRS scores were higher among patients with raphe lesions (17.5 ± 7.9) than without (7.0 ± 4.4). Fig. 1.40 presents the MRI images from the four separate subgroups (with vs. without depression and with vs. without raphe lesions). These findings suggest that neuropsychological assessment of patients with lesions involving the pontine core region should include a thorough evaluation of depressive symptoms.

1.10.2.4 *Autonomic nervous system deficits after stroke*

The nuclei involved in autonomic nervous system control are located within the medial core and in more lateral regions of the brainstem. Fig. 1.41 illustrates the location of a few of these nuclei. Two examples are highlighted here. First, the ventrolateral superficial reticular area interacts with the ventral and dorsal respiratory cell groups involved in respiratory control. Strokes affecting these brainstem structures may cause central hypoventilation syndrome, also known as Ondine syndrome, which is characterized by respiratory arrest during sleep. This condition represents one cause of central sleep apnea.

Lesions in the ventrolateral superficial reticular area of the brainstem may also cause paroxysmal neurogenic hypertension (Fig. 1.42). This phenomenon may result from increased sympathetic activity and baroreflex dysfunction. Blood pressure regulation is essential during standing and other abrupt changes in head and body position. To compensate for fluctuations in blood pressure, baroreceptors in the carotid sinus and aorta monitor arterial blood pressure. If blood pressure increases, the vessels dilate; if blood pressure drops, the vessels constrict. The autonomic control centers are located in the ventrolateral superficial reticular area, and the regulation depends on the reciprocal interaction of the parasympathetic and sympathetic nervous systems. It has been proposed

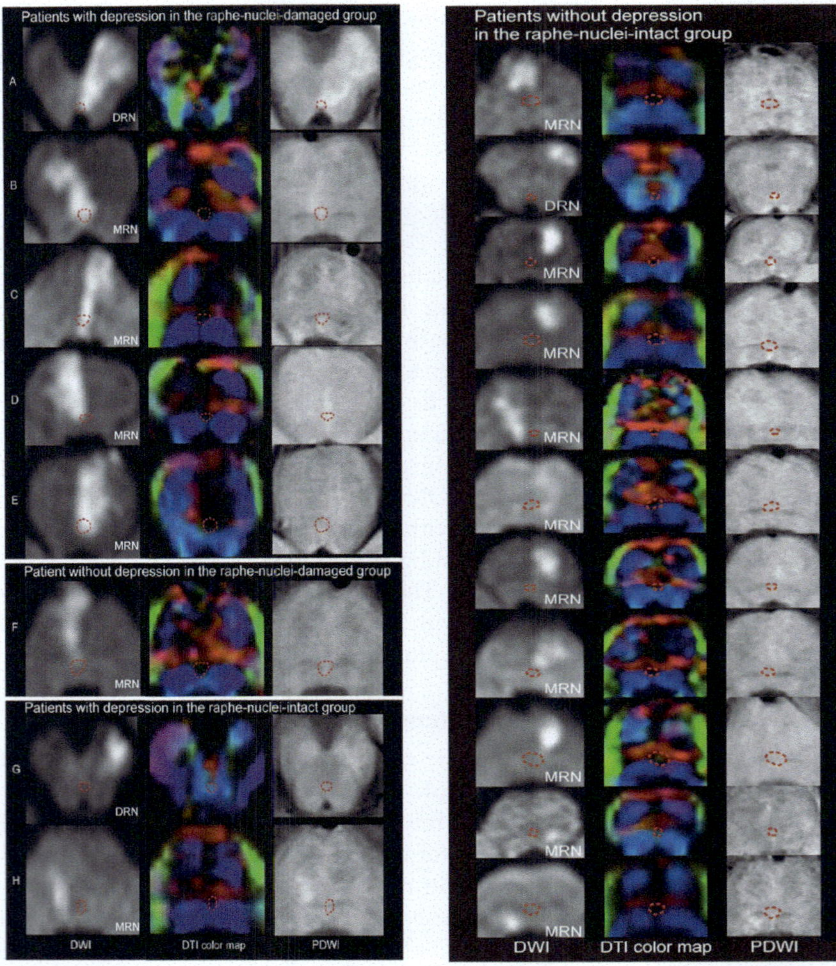

FIGURE 1.40 Location of the raphe nuclei in the brainstem and depression-related stroke areas. *From Numasawa Y., Hattori T., Ishiai S. et al. Depressive disorder may be associated with raphe nuclei lesions in patients with brainstem infarction. J Affect Disord 2017;213:191–198.*

that postural tachycardia syndrome, which may occur as part of the long-term effects of COVID-19, is related to dysfunction of this system.

1.10.3 Brainstem strokes of the corticospinal tract: the locked-in syndrome

The brainstem contains all major projection fiber tracts between the cerebrum and the spinal cord (Fig. 1.43). These tracts carry motor commands

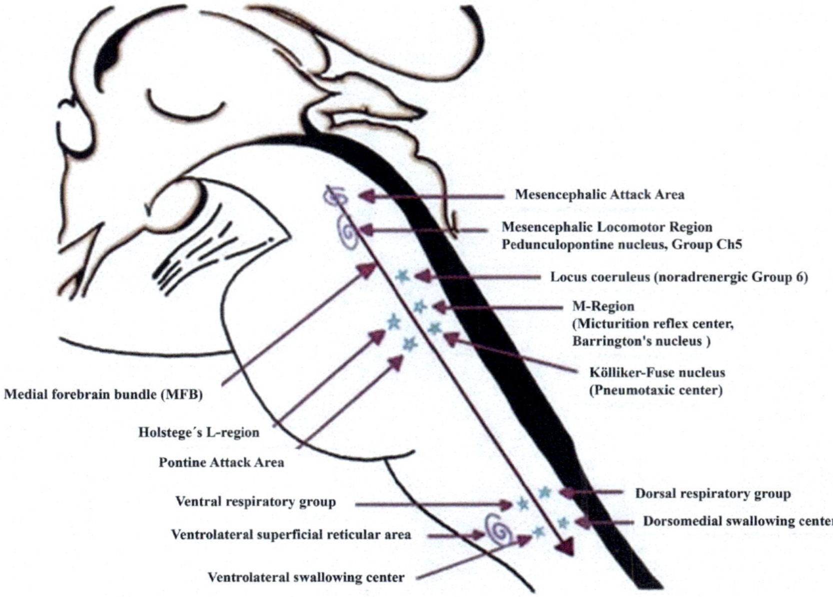

FIGURE 1.41 Major autonomic nuclei of the brainstem.

from the brain to the body and sensory information from the body to the brain. They can be distinguished by their origin (e.g., cortical or subcortical) and by whether they are relayed within the brainstem. Moreover, they can be classified according to whether they terminate in cranial nerve nuclei within the brainstem or continue toward the spinal cord. Those tracts that originate in the cortex and project to the cranial nerve nuclei of the brainstem are called corticonuclear tracts. The tract that descends through the brainstem to project to the ventral motor root of the spinal cord is called the corticospinal tract.

The nuclei of ten of the twelve cranial nerves are located in the midbrain, the pons, and the medulla oblongata. The oculomotor and trochlear nuclei are located in the midbrain; the trigeminal, abducens, and facial nuclei are located in the pons; the vestibulocochlear nuclei are located just below the pons; and the glossopharyngeal, vagal, accessory, and hypoglossal nuclei are located in the medulla (see Chapter 2 for guidance on identifying cranial nerves on MRI scans using MRIcron). The cranial nerves with nuclei in the medulla are involved in chewing and swallowing, taste perception, head turning, and autonomic and homeostatic functions (the vagus nerve in particular). Facial muscles are innervated by the facial and trigeminal nerves.

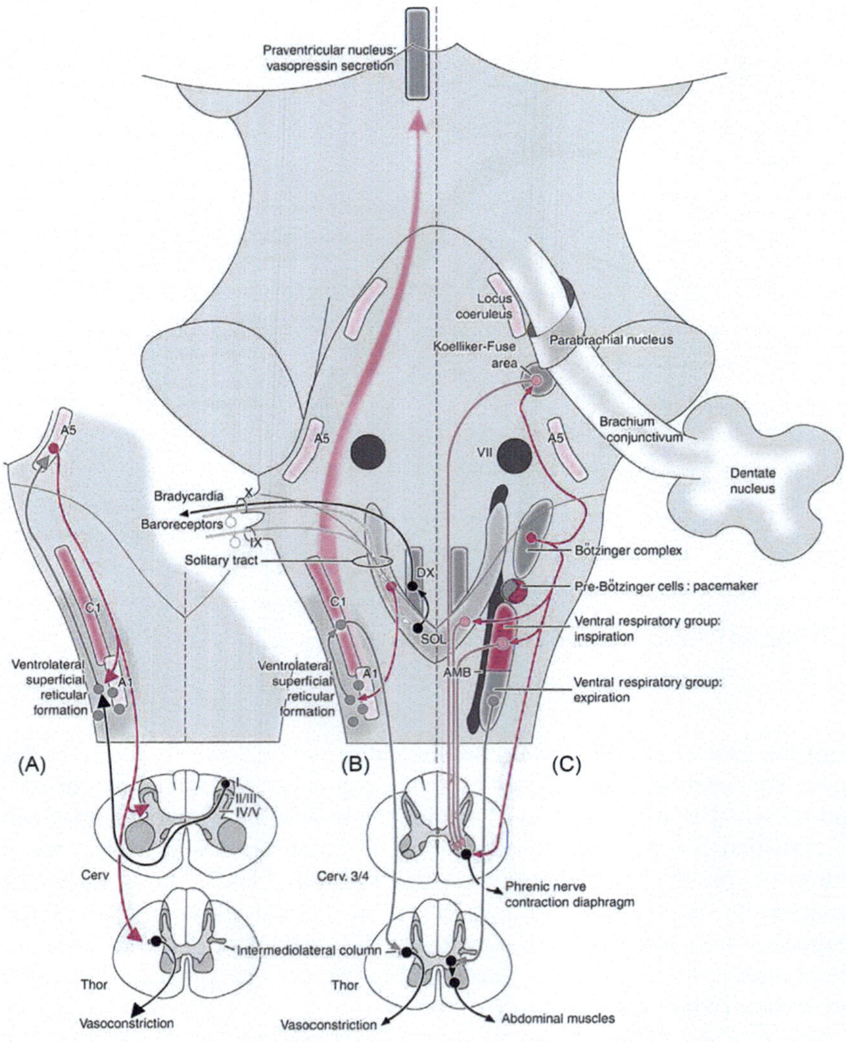

FIGURE 1.42 Brainstem nuclei for blood pressure control. (A) Descending pain-modulatory pathways; (B) Baroreceptor reflex circuitry; (C) Brainstem respiratory network and respiratory rhythm generation. *From Nieuwenhuys R., Voogd J., Huijzen C.van The Human Central Nervous System. 4th ed. Berlin: Springer-Verlag; 2008. Figure 22.4.*

The location of the cranial nerves and their nuclei helps explain the characteristic features of a syndrome resulting from a bilateral pontine stroke that damages the corticospinal and corticonuclear tracts at the pontine level. Specifically, such a stroke typically causes locked-in

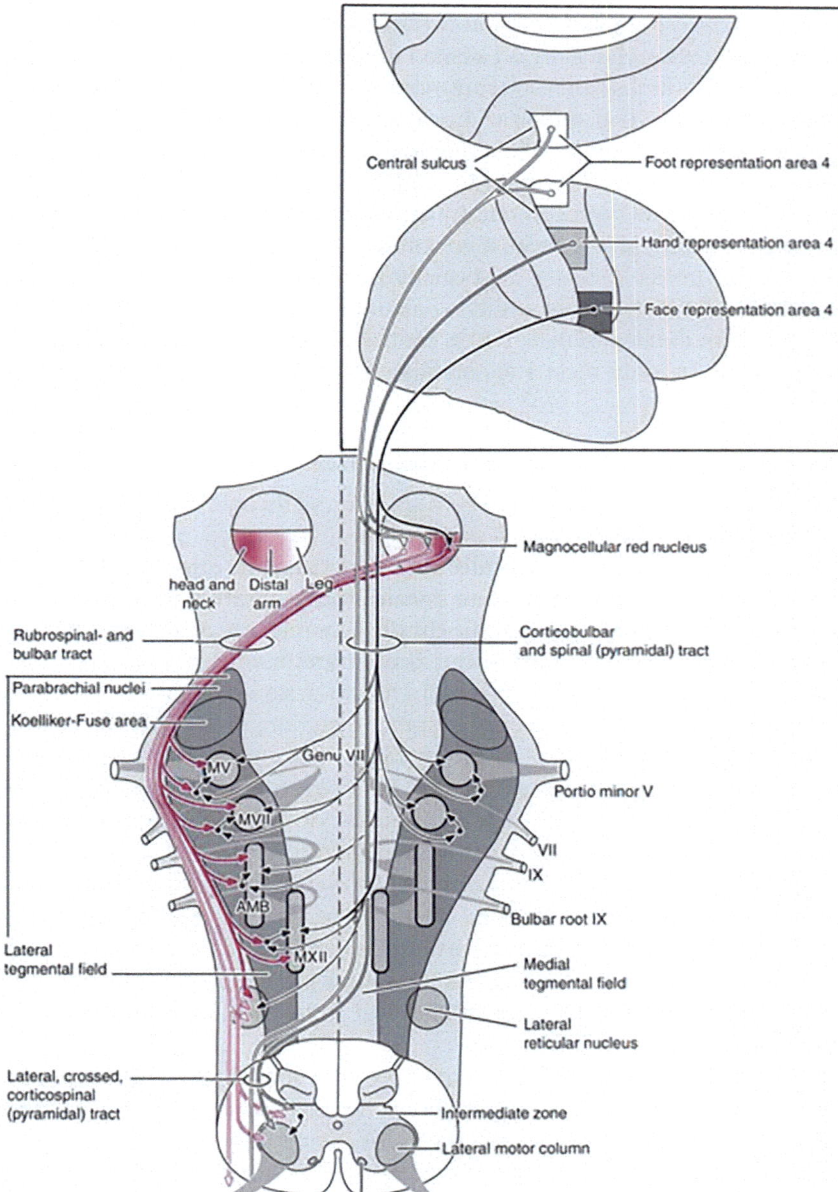

FIGURE 1.43 Cortical and subcortical tracts of the brainstem. *From Nieuwenhuys R., Voogd J., Huijzen C.van The Human Central Nervous System. 4th ed. Berlin: Springer-Verlag; 2008. Figure 21.3.*

syndrome [75–77]. Patients remain awake (although arousal may fluctuate rapidly) and comprehension is preserved. However, they exhibit complete paralysis of the limbs and facial muscles, because of the disruption to the corticospinal and corticonuclear tracts involved in those functions. The oculomotor (CN III) and trochlear (CN IV) nerves are spared, because their nuclei are located in the midbrain above the pons. Thus patients with locked-in syndrome typically retain vertical eye movements, a coordinated movement mediated by these two cranial nerves. Communication may therefore be possible using vertical eye movements (upwards for yes, downwards for no). If this ability is also lost, a brain-computer interface (BCI; a system that translates brain activity into communication commands) may provide the only means to establish communication.

1.10.3.1 Case study of locked-in syndrome

A 37-year-old patient with basilar artery thrombosis who had a tracheostomy cannula in place at admission, exhibited marked fluctuations in arousal and was typically unable to sustain attention for more than 5 minutes. During postacute rehabilitative treatment, spasticity of the trunk and legs increased significantly, whereas the arms were largely spared. Spelling-based communication attempts using an alphabet board printed on an A4 sheet of paper and clinical gaze observation indicated that the patient was able to understand questions and provide appropriate responses. However, communication through clinical interpretation of gaze direction was extremely time-consuming. Automated eye-tracking was not possible due to a ptosis of the left eye (caused by complete left oculomotor paresis), which therefore remained closed, and because the right eye could only be moved slightly in horizontal directions. Attempts to use a steady-state visual evoked potential (VEP)-supported brain-computer interface were ultimately unsuccessful, because of fluctuating attention. As a result, assisted communication, the primary goal of the neuropsychological intervention, could not be established.

Fig. 1.44 shows sagittal MRI scans several weeks after the thrombosis. The image in the upper left corner shows the left hemisphere, and the last image, in the bottom row shows the right hemisphere.

The scans show extensive pontine damage, with relative sparing of the most dorsal parts of the brainstem at this level.

Fig. 1.45 shows diffusion tensor imaging (DTI) tractography at the level of the midbrain (only a partial stroke), revealing two dense fiber tracts. Regions of interest (ROIs) placed in the lower brainstem revealed interruption of the fibers at the level of the stroke, with only a few residual fibers left that could be traced from the medulla to the midbrain.

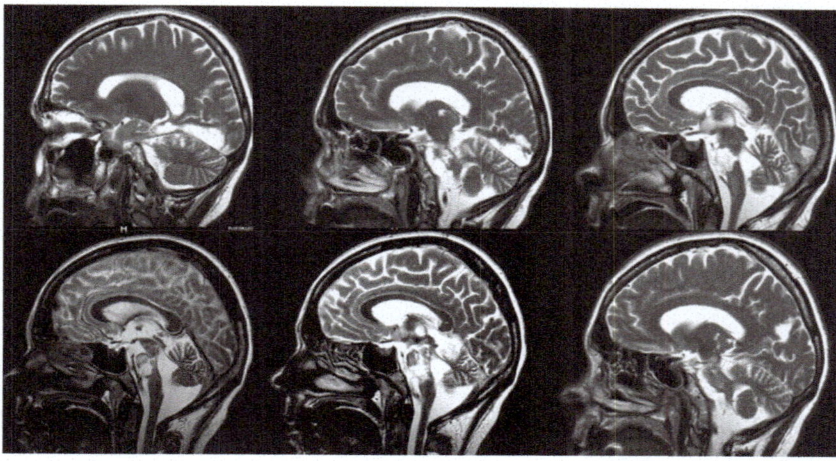

FIGURE 1.44 Clinical MRI scan of a patient with locked-in syndrome.

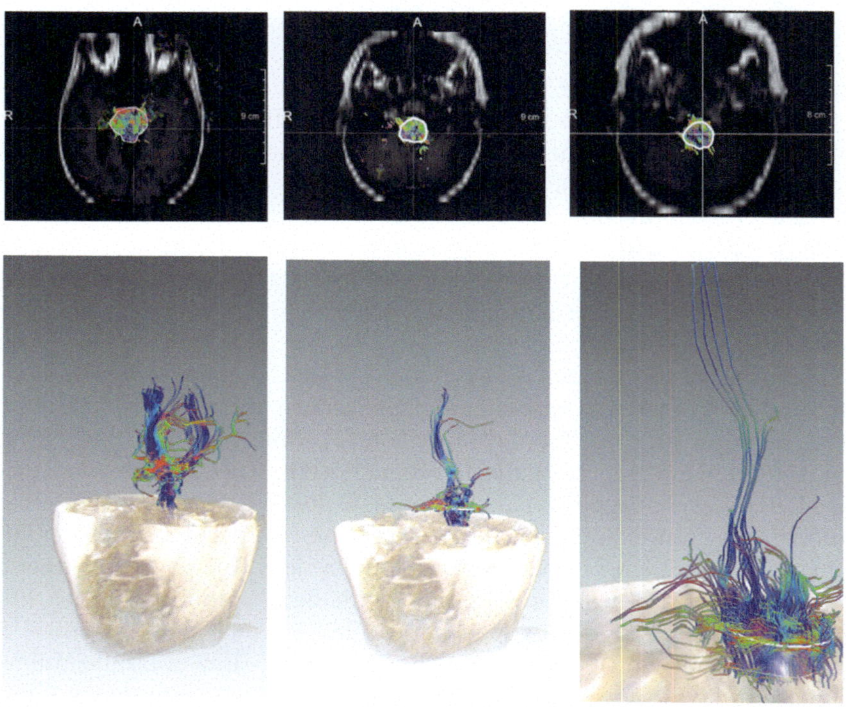

FIGURE 1.45 Seed ROIs (upper row) and reconstructed fiber tracts (lower row) of a patient with locked-in syndrome.

1.10.4 Brainstem stroke: crossed syndromes focusing on gaze disorders

The corticospinal and corticonuclear tracts cross at different levels of the nervous system. Most cranial nerves do not cross and instead innervate muscles on the same side or receive afferent input from ipsilateral structures. This can give rise to crossed (in the sense of different but bilateral) deficits following unilateral brainstem stroke [16]. These deficits reflect involvement of the affected cranial nerve (resulting in ipsilesional symptoms) together with damage to the corticospinal tract before decussation (resulting in contralesional impairment). Moreover, cerebellar motor control depends on ipsilateral afferent pathways. Damage to these cerebellar afferents caused by a unilateral stroke may thus result in motor disorders ("ataxia") contralateral to the corticospinal tract paresis.

Eye movement control is essential for clear vision, and visual function is a central topic of neuropsychological assessment and treatment. The following section introduces three crossed midbrain and brainstem syndromes that involve gaze disorder.

1.10.4.1 Oculomotor nerve involvement

The first syndrome results from a stroke affecting the inferior or middle paramedian thalamic artery, causing an infarction at the level of the midbrain (Fig. 1.46). Because the affected medial lemniscus has already crossed at this level, such a stroke results in contralateral impairment of tactile and proprioceptive sensation. Because the stroke also involves the red nucleus and the substantia nigra, additional manifestations include contralateral hyperkinetic movements and akinesia.

The oculomotor nucleus is also located at this level. Its lesion leads to an internal and external ipsilesional oculomotor paresis. The oculomotor nerve contains two functional components. The internal one is part of the parasympathetic branch of the nervous system. This branch mediates rapid pupillary constriction in response to light. The parasympathetic branch of the autonomic nervous system (ANS) works together with the sympathetic branch, which means that a loss of parasympathetic modulation leads to an unopposed sympathetic activity. Because the sympathetic branch causes pupillary dilation, the patient shows a widened pupil, which does not respond to light (however, the unimpaired pupil will show an indirect response). The outer component of the oculomotor nerve controls eye muscles and the eyelid. Because of the lesion, some of the muscles responsible for eyelid elevation are no longer activated; therefore the ipsilesional eye will be (almost) closed, a

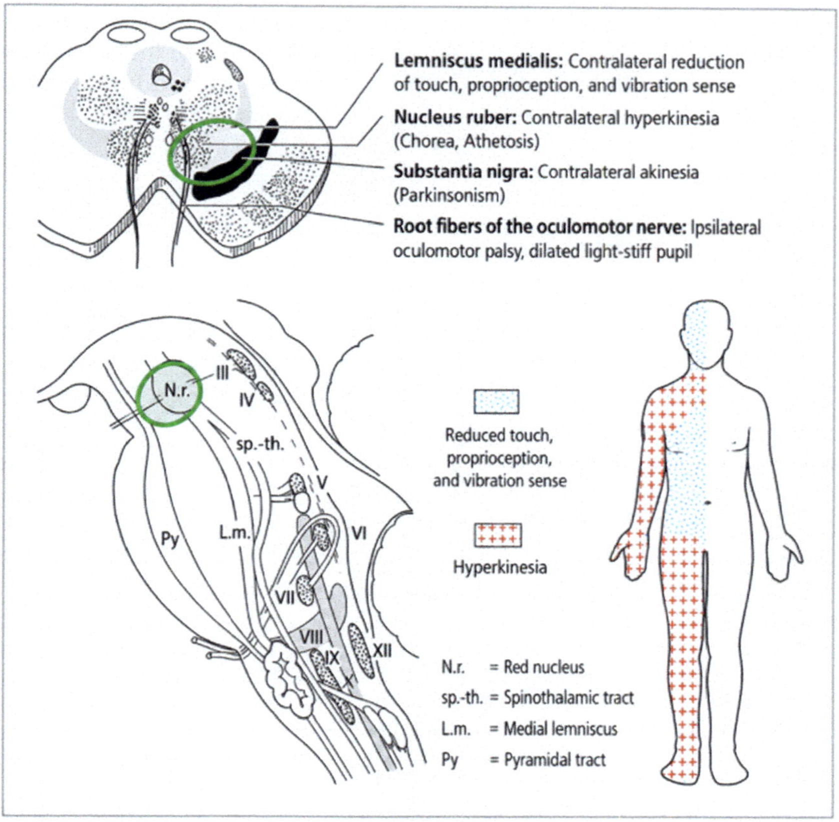

FIGURE 1.46 Brainstem stroke with crossed symptomatology and oculomotor involvement (Benedikt syndrome). *From Bähr M., Bechmann I. Neurologisch-topische Diagnostik: Anatomie - Funktion - Klinik.* 11 überarbeitete Auflage Thieme *2021. (Fig. 4.69).*

condition referred to as ptosis. The oculomotor nerve is also responsible for moving the eye upward, inward, and in certain rotational directions. When oculomotor innervation is lost, the actions of the remaining eye muscles become unopposed. Thus the eye may deviate downward (due to the uninhibited activity of the trochlear nerve) and laterally (due to the uninhibited activity of the abducens nerve).

Complete ptosis is not an inevitable consequence of oculomotor paresis. In the absence of ptosis, patients may experience diplopia (i.e., double vision, depending on the degree of ocular dominance). Some patients have difficulty integrating the spatial information from one of the two perceived images into motor control. In such a case, a characteristic spatial disturbance may be observed including past pointing, impaired reaching and grasping, and even the risk of collisions with walls and furniture because spatial information from the wrong eye is used for motor guidance. Patching of one eye may be helpful to reduce past-pointing in situations when other rehabilitation goals take priority. Patients should also be informed that, if diplopia persists, surgical correction may be used to restore ocular alignment. However, such surgery (e.g., shortening of the eye muscles) is usually deferred during the first year after stroke.

Conjugate eye movements can be trained, and this can be easily incorporated into daily life, even without continuous supervision by a therapist. The patient may fixate on a target on the opposite wall of the room and then rotate the head until a head position is reached at which diplopia disappears. Such a position usually exists, because the impaired nerve plays only a minor role in this direction of gaze. For example, in the case of an oculomotor paresis of the left eye, the head must be turned to the right until ocular alignment is achieved (or the fixated object disappears for the right eye due to the nose). The patient should then slowly move the eyes to the right while maintaining ocular alignment. If ocular alignment begins to deteriorate, the eyes should be moved slightly back to the left until single vision is restored, and the procedure should be repeated. If patients perform this exercise twice daily for 15 minutes, diplopia may gradually improve (Fig. 1.47) [16,18].

1.10.4.2 *Abducens nerve involvement*

Strokes affecting the lateral pontine arteries may lead to a crossed neurological syndrome involving the abducens nerve. As a result, the patient may develop weakness on the contralesional side of the body, because the corticospinal tract crosses below this level. The medial lemniscus crosses immediately rostral to the pyramidal decussation. Therefore tactile, proprioceptive, and pain sensation are impaired on the contralesional side. In contrast, the corticonuclear tracts of the facial nerve cross far rostral to the pyramidal decussation, above the level of the lesion. Consequently, weakness of the facial muscles affects the ipsilesional side of the face. Whereas the oculomotor nerve pulls the eye into a nasal direction, the abducens nerve (the sixth cranial nerve) pulls the eye in the opposite direction. Lesions of the abducens nerve in strokes affecting the lateral pontine arteries therefore fixate the eye in a nasal position, preventing the patient from looking toward the affected side. Thus one eye remains in a medial position and is unable to move outward, leading to double vision (diplopia) particularly when looking toward the affected side. The functional and surgical treatment of this gaze disorder is similar to that used for oculomotor palsy.

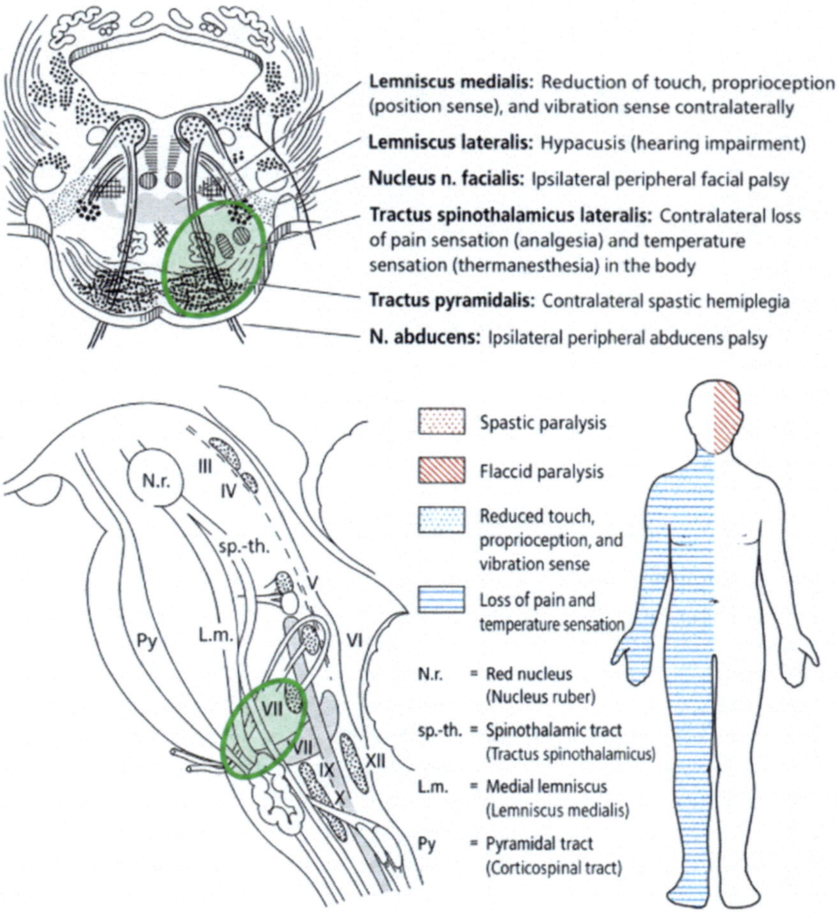

FIGURE 1.47 Brainstem stroke with crossed symptomatology and abducens nerve involvement (Millard–Gubler syndrome). *From Bähr M., Bechmann I. Neurologisch-topische Diagnostik: Anatomie - Funktion - Klinik.* 11 überarbeitete Auflage Thieme *2021. (Fig. 4.64).*

1.10.4.3 *Horner's syndrome*

A stroke affecting the lateral medulla oblongata may produce Horner's syndrome [16]. It is characterized by the following three symptoms: (1) miosis: paralysis of the pupil dilator muscle, (2) ptosis: paralysis of the superior tarsal muscle causing drooping of the eye, (3) enophthalmos or pseudo-enophthalmos, which may result from denervation of the orbital muscle. The sympathetic pathways supplying the eye originate in the lateral medulla oblongata. Consequently, a stroke affecting these pathways leaves parasympathetic influences relatively unopposed. As a result the pupil constricted. This becomes particularly apparent in a darkened room, when pupillary dilation is assessed: only the unaffected pupil dilates normally, whereas the affected pupil remains constricted. There are two additional symptoms often associated with Horner's syndrome, namely anhidrosis (decreased or absent sweating) on the affected side of the face and vasodilation (sympathetic nerve damage that interrupts signals that constrict facial blood vessels), causing the affected side of the face to appear redder compared to the unaffected side.

Because of the location of the lesions, autonomic centers are often affected as well. Possible symptoms include tachycardia and (sleep-)disordered breathing. Moreover, the patient may experience loss of taste, dysphagia, and dysarthria. Tactile and proprioceptive sensation is impaired on the contralesional side of the body, while sparing the face. Loss of cerebellar afferent input involved in movement control may result in limb ataxia.

1.11 Cerebellar strokes

The cerebellum is located posterior to the brainstem. It consists of a cortex, subcortical nuclei, and white matter. It is considerably more structured than the cerebral cortex, and its white matter fibers are organized more homogeneously. Different regions of the cerebellum are associated with distinct functions (Fig. 1.48) [17,78,79].

The rostro medial structures of the cerebellum—the culmen, declive, and vermis—are involved in integrating gravitational and vestibular information for postural control during movement and gait.

The caudal medial structures—collectively referred to as the vestibulocerebellum and encompassing the flocculonodular lobe—receive input from the vestibular system and project back to the vestibular nuclei. These structures are involved in the control of balance and gaze stabilization, particularly the maintenance of visual fixation on a target.

The lateral zones of the cerebellum receive input from the cerebral cortex and pontine nuclei and project to the thalamus and red nucleus. They do not appear to be involved in balance control, and play only a minor role in gait control. However, they play a major role in controlling voluntary limb movements. These areas therefore regulate the coordination of muscle activation and are important for visually guided movements. The lateral cerebellar cortex exhibits a topographic organization of motor functions, although this organization is less strictly linked to the specific effectors compared with the cortical homunculus. The role of the cerebellum in cognitive and affective functions remains a matter of debate (see below) [67,80–82].

(A)

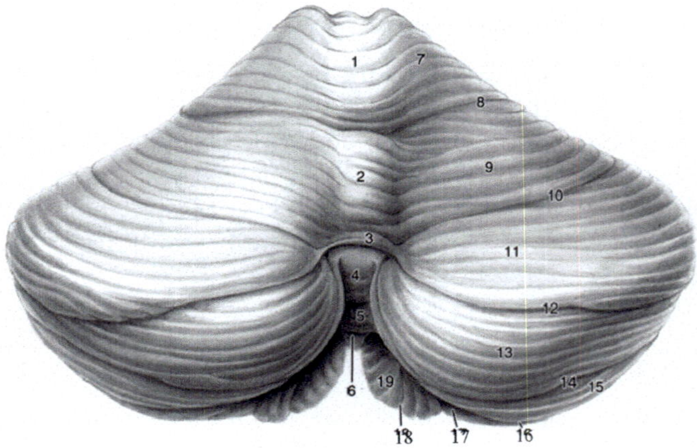

1 Culmen
2 Declive
3 Folium vermis
4 Tuber vermis
5 Pyramis
6 Uvula
7 Quadrangular lobule
8 Primary fissure
9 Lobulus simplex
10 Posterior superior fissure
11 Superior semilunar lobule
12 Horizontal fissure
13 Inferior semilunar lobule
14 Pregracile fissure (variable)
15 Gracile lobule
16 Prebiventral fissure
17 Biventral lobule
18 Secondary fissure
19 Tonsil

(B)

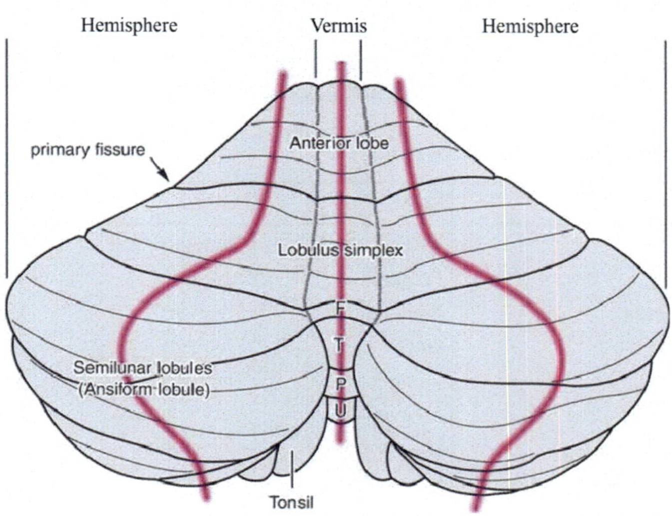

FIGURE 1.48 Schematic drawing of cerebellar areas in dorsal view. (A) Major lobules and fissure; (B) folial chain organization of the vermis and cerebellar hemispheres. *From Nieuwenhuys R., Voogd J., Huijzen C.van The Human Central Nervous System. 4th ed. Berlin: Springer-Verlag; 2008. Figure 3.11.*

1.11.1 Cerebellar blood supply

The cerebellum is supplied by the basilar artery [14,15,83]. Three major arteries contribute to its blood supply: (1) the PICA, (2) the anterior inferior cerebellar artery (AICA), and (3) the superior cerebellar artery (SCA) (Fig. 1.35). Cerebellar strokes are relatively uncommon, accounting for approximately 2% to 5% of all strokes. Most cerebellar infarctions occur in the PICA territories, followed by the AICA, whereas SCA infarctions are the least common.

1.11.2 Symptoms after cerebellar stroke

During the acute phase of stroke, the most common symptoms of cerebellar stroke include dysarthria, impaired coordination, limb weakness, dizziness/vertigo, gait and postural instability nausea or/and vomiting, nystagmus, dysphagia, and headache. Ataxia and tremor are also frequently observed [15,83]. However, brainstem structures are often affected as well, making it difficult to determine the precise anatomical basis of the observed deficits. Moreover, edema occurring during the acute phase may compromise brainstem functioning because of the limited space at this level of the brain.

Table 1.7 provides an overview of the frequency of symptoms associated with occlusion of the different cerebellar arteries. It should be noted that the clinical manifestations of isolated cerebellar infarctions

TABLE 1.7 Cerebellar stroke symptoms.

Symptoms	SCA	AICA	PICA
Deafness	Absent	Frequent	Absent
Dizziness	Frequent	Absent	Frequent
Drowsiness	Frequent	Frequent	Uncommon
Tinnitus	Uncommon	Frequent	Absent
Vertigo	Frequent	Frequent	Very common
Nausea/vomiting	Frequent	Very common	Frequent
Hallucinations	Uncommon	Uncommon	Absent
Headache/facial pain	Uncommon	Absent	Uncommon
Pain In limbs/trunk	Absent	frequent	Absent
Sleep disturbances	Uncommon	Absent	Absent

Abbreviations: AICA: anterior inferior cerebellar artery; PICA: posterior inferior cerebellar artery; SCA: superior cerebellar artery.

From Manto, Cerebellar stroke. In: Manto M., Manto M.U., editors. Cerebellar disorders: a practical approach to diagnosis and management. Cambridge: Cambridge University Press; 2010. pp. 88–101.

in the three major cerebellar vascular territories are largely similar. Nevertheless, dysarthria is most commonly associated with lesions in the SCA territory, whereas vertigo and lateropulsion are more frequently observed in lesions involving the PICA territory. Audio-vestibular symptoms are characteristic of lesions in the AICA territory.

Dysmetria is a cardinal sign of cerebellar motor dysfunction. Patients with cerebellar lesions attempting to perform goal-directed limb movements often either overshoot (hypermetria) or undershoot (hypometria) the target. This may also impact reaching and grasping movements. Dysmetria, decomposition of movements, and tremor (both intention and kinetic tremor) result in trajectory curvatures, an increased number of corrective movements, slowed and highly variable velocity profiles of the hand transport component, as well as increased grasp apertures and multiple peaks in grasp aperture when patients with cerebellar lesions reach for and grasp an object [80].

For a long time, the presence of cognitive symptoms following cerebellar lesions was disputed. It was not until the 1990s that researchers [84,85] began to argue for the existence of such impairments. Overall, the cognitive deficits associated with cerebellar stroke include impairments of executive functions (disorders of planning, set shifting, abstract reasoning, working memory, and perseveration), visuospatial disintegration with disorganized figure drawing, and language disturbances such as anomia, agrammatic speech, and impaired syntactic structure. Moreover, personality changes have been observed characterized by disinhibited behaviors such as overfamiliarity, flamboyant and impulsive actions, inappropriate humor, and a flattening or blunting of affect [82,84,85]. A consensus paper published in 2016 concluded that cognitive deficits are a recognized consequence of cerebellar stroke [80].

However, the empirical evidence for Schmahmann's syndrome (a constellation of executive, visuospatial, language, and affective disturbances following cerebellar damage) following stroke remains controversial. Hoche, Guell [82], for example, assessed 77 patients and reported no impairment on the mini mental state examination (MMSE) or the montreal cognitive assessment (MoCA), although mild cognitive and behavioral abnormalities consistent with Schmahmann's syndrome were observed. However, only 11 of these patients had experienced a stroke or hemorrhage; the remaining had genetic or neurodegenerative disorders affecting the cerebellum. Two further studies [67,81] suggested that posterolateral and medial structures of the cerebellum may play a greater role in the subtle cognitive impairments during the postacute phase than the anterior cerebellar zone.

1.11.3 Recovery of cerebellar stroke

Recovery from motor and most other somatic symptoms following cerebellar stroke is generally favorable and is often nearly complete after one year [86]. In contrast, cognitive symptoms may persist beyond this period.

Similar findings have been reported for nonmotor deficits. Taskiran-Sag, Uzuncakmak Uyanik [81] reassessed patients with cerebellar strokes four months after the event. They found that affective disturbances, except for depressive symptoms, recovered completely. Impairments in executive functions, attention, working memory, processing speed, and language persisted throughout the follow-up period, whereas memory performance improved. In addition, cognitive impairment was more common in patients with medial or posterolateral infarcts. Muller Ewald, Deifelt Streese [67] extended the follow-up period to more than one year. At follow-up, patients with cerebellar stroke no longer differed significantly from the control group. However, small differences remained in Stroop test performance (reading and naming), verbal learning, and motor function. These findings suggest that long-term recovery of cognitive functions may be comparable to recovery of motor functions.

1.12 Results and limitations of large-scale cerebral stroke studies

It should be emphasized that deficits such as pure dyslexia, visual agnosia, dynamic aphasia, or optic ataxia can only be detected if assessment tools sensitive to these specific syndromes are employed. The same applies to more specific forms of memory impairments, which may result either from lesions of the Papez circuits affecting consolidation or from frontal lesions disrupting retrieval processes rather than consolidation. Consequently, research investigating the cognitive consequences of stroke based on lesion location would require extensive assessment batteries to capture the full range of cognitive functions. As a result, the conclusions that can be drawn from large lesion-localization studies are limited, because they depend on the variety and specificity of neuropsychological tests employed. Another challenge is that stroke severity restricts the range of patients who can be assessed. For example, severe aphasia excludes a substantial proportion of patients with left-hemispheric lesions because they are unable to follow task instructions. Similarly, severe neglect limits the assessment of visuoconstructional abilities and reading and may reduce test performance.

Despite these limitations, the following two studies included such large patient cohorts that they warrant brief discussion. In the first study, including 1080 stroke patients, a small number of relatively simple and classical clinical neuropsychological tests were administered (Fig. 1.49) [87]. Factor analysis showed that test performance could be explained by four factors: a language factor, a global memory factor, a visuospatial processing factor, and a verbal learning factor. The language factor was associated with left-hemispheric lesions, including lesions involving the head of the caudate nucleus. The visuospatial factor was associated with right-hemispheric lesions; the global memory factor was the only factor related to parahippocampal and hippocampal lesions. However, the limitations of this approach become evident when examining lesions associated with factors 2 and 4: they clearly indicate visual field defects due to strokes affecting the P4 segment of the PCA. Because visual field deficits were not assessed, they could not contribute to the factor analysis

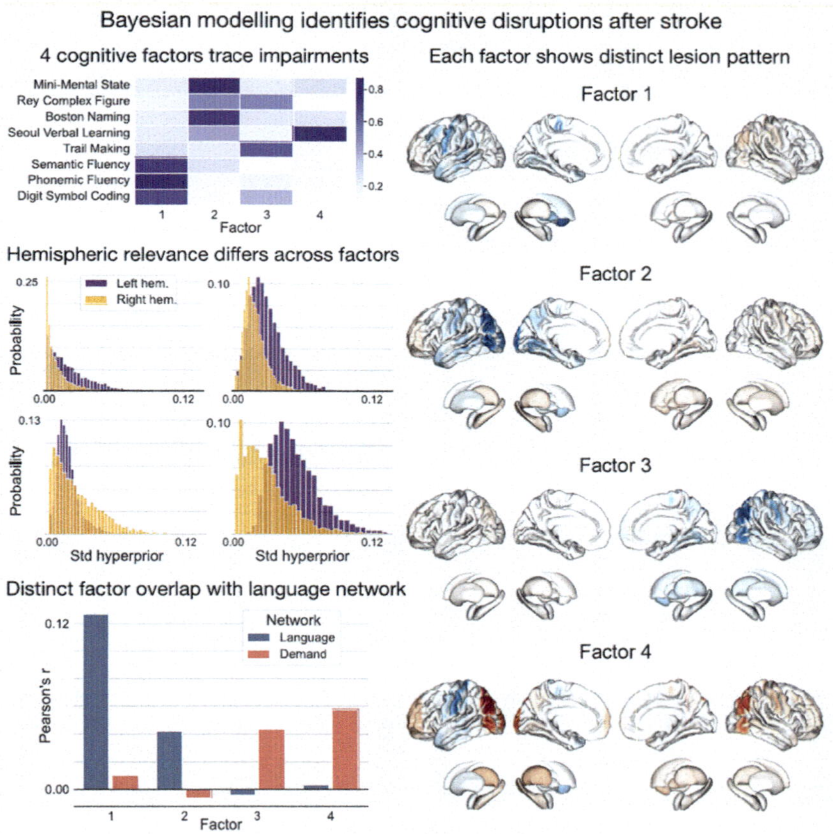

FIGURE 1.49 Cognitive factors and stroke localization. *From Hartwigsen G., Lim J.S., Bae H.J. et al. Bayesian modelling disentangles language versus executive control disruption in stroke. Brain Commun 2024;6(3):fcae129.*

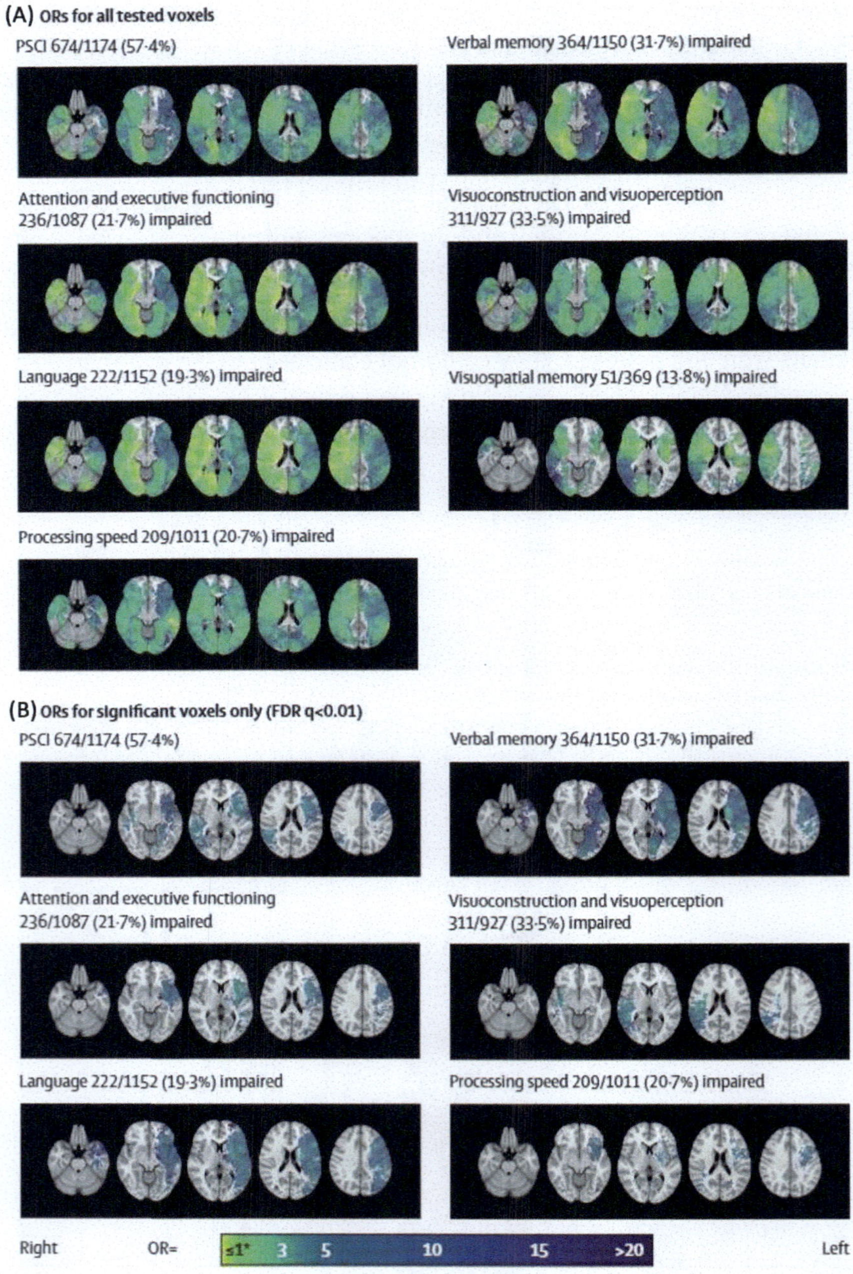

FIGURE 1.50 Overlapping stroke lesions and cognitive deficits. *From Weaver N.A., Kuijf H.J., Aben H.P. et al. Strategic infarct locations for post-stroke cognitive impairment: a pooled analysis of individual patient data from 12 acute ischaemic stroke cohorts. Lancet Neurol 2021;20(6):448–459.*

and therefore could not be localized as a consequence of stroke. The same limitation applies to deficits such as impaired spatial memory, divided attention, or disinhibition.

Fig. 1.50 shows the result of the second study, including 2950 (!) patients with stroke [88]. The findings largely reflect what would be expected based on the vascular anatomy of the brain. Most strokes affect the MCA and the lesion overlap maps predominantly reflect MCA strokes. Verbal learning and language functions are impaired following left-hemispheric strokes. Visuoconstructional and visuoperceptual abilities are more commonly affected following right- hemispheric lesions. Strokes affecting the left PCA are associated with verbal learning deficits. Finally, ACA strokes appear to be associated with relatively few cognitive deficits. However, this is likely to reflect an assessment bias: some patients may be too akinetic and apathetic to participate, and executive function impairments that cannot be adequately assessed using tasks such as word fluency or trail making test (TMT) B were not included in the study. Consequently, large-scale stroke studies face a trade-off between using more sensitive tests to identify specific deficits and including larger patient cohorts to ensure sufficient statistical power.

References

[1] Bogousslavsky J, Caplan LR. Stroke syndromes. *Cambridge University Press*; 2001.
[2] Poeck K. Neurologie. Berlin - Heidelberg - New York: Springer Verlag; 1992.
[3] Tariq N, Khatri R. Leptomeningeal collaterals in acute ischemic stroke. J Vasc Interv Neurol 2008;1(4):91–5.
[4] Guglielmi V, Quaranta D, Masone Iacobucci G, et al. Basal ganglia ischaemic infarction after thrombectomy: cognitive impairment at acute stage. Eur J Neurol 2023;30(12):3772–9.
[5] Liu CS, Bryan RN, Miki A, Woo JH, Liu GT, Elliott MA. Magnocellular and parvocellular visual pathways have different blood oxygen level-dependent signal time courses in human primary visual cortex. AJNR Am J Neuroradiol 2006;27(8):1628–34.
[6] Hildebrandt H, G C, Ebke M, Spang K. Differential impact of parvocellular and magnocellular pathways on visual impairment in apperceptive agnosia? Neurocase 2004;10(3):207–14.
[7] Netter FH. Netters neurologie. *Stuttgart: Thieme Verlag*; 2001.
[8] Dengler K, Fischer J, Kastrup A, Elsner1 M, Hildebrandt H. Was wird aus patienten mit Mediainfarkt bzw. -blutung und Behandlung in der Phase B der neurologischen Rehabilitation? Ergebnisse des Einjahres-Follow-ups. Neurol Rehabil 2015;21(1):13–22.
[9] Ringelstein EB, Stögbauer F. Border zone infarcts. In: Bogousslavsky J, Caplan LR, editors. Stroke syndromes. 2 ed.Cambridge: Cambridge University Press; 2001. p. 564–82.
[10] Momjian-Mayor I, Baron JC. The pathophysiology of watershed infarction in internal carotid artery disease: review of cerebral perfusion studies. Stroke 2005;36(3):567–77.
[11] Gijn Jv JE, Rinkel G. Subarachnoid hemorrhage syndromes 3 ed In: Caplan LR, van Gijn J, editors. Stroke syndromes3ed.Cambridge: Cambridge University Press; 2012. p. 534–41.
[12] Estol CJ, Caplan LR. Intracranial arterial dissections 3 ed In: Caplan LR, van Gijn J, editors. Stroke syndromes3ed.Cambridge: Cambridge University Press; 2012. p. 566–73.

[13] Keser Z, Meschia JF, Lanzino G. Craniocervical artery dissections: a concise review for clinicians. Mayo Clin Proc 2022;97(4):777–83.
[14] Tatu L, Moulin T, Bogousslavsky J, Duvernoy H. Arterial territories of human brain. In: Bogousslavsky J, Caplan LR, editors. Stroke syndromes. 2 ed.Cambridge: Cambridge University Press; 2001. p. 375–404.
[15] Amarenco P. Cerebellar stroke syndromes. In: Bogousslavsky J, Caplan LR, editors. Stroke syndromes. 2 ed.Cambridge: Cambridge University Press; 2001. p. 540–56.
[16] Duus P. Neurologisch-Topische diagnostik. Stuttgart New York Fifth Edition: Thieme Verlag; 1990.
[17] Nieuwenhuys R, Voogd J, Huijzen Cvan. The human central nervous system. 4th ed Berlin: Springer-Verlag; 2008.
[18] diagnostik: anatomie - funktion - Klinik. *11 überarbeitete Auflage Thieme* 2021.
[19] Pullicino P. Lenticulostriate arteries. In: Bogousslavsky J, Caplan LR, editors. Stroke syndromes. 2 ed.Cambridge: Cambridge University Press; 2001. p. 428–38.
[20] Vuadens P, Bogousslavsky J. Anterior choroidal artery territory infarcts. In: Bogousslavsky J, Caplan LR, editors. Stroke syndromes. 2 ed.Cambridge: Cambridge University Press; 2001. p. 451–60.
[21] Neau J-P, Bogousslavsky J. Superficial middle cerebral artery syndromes. In: Bogousslavsky J, Caplan LR, editors. Stroke syndromes. 2 ed.Cambridge: Cambridge University Press; 2001. p. 405–27.
[22] Brust JCM, Sawada T, Kazui S. Anterior cerebral artery. In: Bogousslavsky J, Caplan LR, editors. Stroke syndromes. 2 ed.Cambridge: Cambridge University Press; 2001. p. 439–50.
[23] Chung C-S, Lee H-S, Caplan LR. Caudate infarcts and hemorrhages. In: Bogousslavsky J, Caplan LR, editors. Stroke syndromes. 2 ed.Cambridge: Cambridge University Press; 2001. p. 469–78.
[24] Kumral E, Evyapan D, Balkir K. Acute caudate vascular lesions. Stroke 1999;30(1): 100–108.
[25] Dahms C, Brodoehl S, Witte OW, Klingner CM. The importance of different learning stages for motor sequence learning after stroke. Hum Brain Mapp 2020;41(1):270–86.
[26] Roth RH, Ding JB. Cortico-basal ganglia plasticity in motor learning. Neuron 2024; 112(15):2486–502.
[27] Russo C, Veronelli L, Casati C, et al. Explicit motor sequence learning after stroke: a neuropsychological study. Exp Brain Res 2021;239(7):2303–16.
[28] Minematsu K, Yamaguchi T. Putaminal hemorrhages. In: Bogousslavsky J, Caplan LR, editors. Stroke syndromes. 2 ed.Cambridge: Cambridge University Press; 2001. p. 590–8.
[29] Chaves CJ, Caplan LR. Posterior cerebral artery. In: Bogousslavsky J, Caplan LR, editors. Stroke syndromes. 2 ed.Cambridge: Cambridge University Press; 2001. p. 479–89.
[30] Hildebrandt H, Giesselmann H, Sachsenheimer W. Visual search and visual target detection in patients with infarctions of the left or right posterior or the right middle brain artery. J Clin Exp Neuropsyc 1999;21(1):94–107.
[31] Spang K, Hildebrandt H, Schwendemann G, Fahle M. Component perimetry and cortically caused visual defects. Perception 2001;30:109–10.
[32] Szabo K, Forster A, Jager T, et al. Hippocampal lesion patterns in acute posterior cerebral artery stroke: clinical and MRI findings. Stroke 2009;40(6):2042–5.
[33] von Cramon DY, Hebel N, Schuri U. Verbal memory and learning in unilateral posterior cerebral infarction. A report on 30 cases. Brain 1988;111(Pt 5):1061–77.
[34] Braak H, Braak E. Diagnostic criteria for neuropathologic assessment of Alzheimer's disease. Neurobiol Aging 1997;18(4 Suppl):S85–8.
[35] Braak H, Del Tredici K. The preclinical phase of the pathological process underlying sporadic Alzheimer's disease. Brain 2015;138(Pt 10):2814–33.
[36] Benke T, Bodner T, Wiesen D, Karnath HO. The amnestic syndrome of posterior cerebral artery infarction. Eur J Neurol 2022;29(10):2987–95.

[37] Kraft A, Grimsen C, Kehrer S, et al. Neurological and neuropsychological characteristics of occipital, occipito-temporal and occipito-parietal infarction. Cortex 2014;56:38–50.
[38] Burgess N, Becker S, King JA, O'Keefe J. Memory for events and their spatial context: models and experiments. Philos Trans R Soc Lond B Biol Sci 2001;356(1413):1493–503.
[39] Barth A, Bogousslavsky J, Caplan LR. Thalamic infarcts and hemorrhages. In: Bogousslavsky J, Caplan LR, editors. Stroke syndromes. 2 ed.Cambridge: Cambridge University Press; 2001. p. 461–8.
[40] von Cramon DY, Hebel N, Schuri U. A contribution to the anatomical basis of thalamic amnesia. Brain 1985;108(Pt 4):993–1008.
[41] Schmahmann JD. Vascular syndromes of the thalamus. Stroke 2003;34(9):2264–78.
[42] Hommel M, Besson G. Midbrain infarcts. In: Bogousslavsky J, Caplan LR, editors. Stroke syndromes. 2 ed.Cambridge: Cambridge University Press; 2001. p. 512–9.
[43] Mugikura S, Kikuchi H, Fujii T, et al. MR imaging of subcallosal artery infarct causing amnesia after surgery for anterior communicating artery aneurysm. AJNR Am J Neuroradiol 2014;35(12):2293–301.
[44] Destreri DG, Farina N, Calabrese E, Pinardi E, Imbornone G, Mariani E. C. Frontal impairment and confabulation after herpes simplex encephalitis: a case report. Arch Phys Med Rehabil 2002;83(3):423–6.
[45] Fotopoulou A. False selves in neuropsychological rehabilitation: the challenge of confabulation. Neuropsychol Rehabil 2008;18(5-6):541–65.
[46] Fotopoulou A, Conway MA, Solms M. Confabulation: motivated reality monitoring. Neuropsychologia 2007;45(10):2180–90.
[47] Glowinski R, Payman V, Frencham K. Confabulation: a spontaneous and fantastic review. Aust N Z J Psychiatry 2008;42(11):932–40.
[48] Hildebrandt H. Cognitive rehabilitation of memory. *Academic Press*. Elsevier; 2019.
[49] Schnider A. Orbitofrontal reality filtering. Front Behav Neurosci 2013;7:67.
[50] Hayama HR, Rugg MD. Right dorsolateral prefrontal cortex is engaged during post-retrieval processing of both episodic and semantic information. Neuropsychologia 2009;47(12):2409–16.
[51] Rugg MD, Henson RN, Robb WG. Neural correlates of retrieval processing in the prefrontal cortex during recognition and exclusion tasks. Neuropsychologia 2003;41(1):40–52.
[52] Barredo J, Oztekin I, Badre D. Ventral fronto-temporal pathway supporting cognitive control of episodic memory retrieval. Cereb Cortex 2015;25(4):1004–19.
[53] Schnider A. Spontaneous confabulation, reality monitoring, and the limbic system–a review. Brain Res Brain Res Rev 2001;36(2-3):150–60.
[54] Schnider A. Spontaneous confabulation and the adaptation of thought to ongoing reality. Nat Rev Neurosci 2003;4(8):662–71.
[55] Schnider A, Bonvallat J, Emond H, Leemann B. Reality confusion in spontaneous confabulation. Neurology 2005;65(7):1117–9.
[56] Hildebrandt, H. Cognitive rehabilitation of memory: a clinical-neuropsychological introduction. 2019.
[57] Mawet J, Crassard I, Bousser M-G. Cerebral venous thrombosis 3 ed In: Caplan LR, van Gijn J, editors. Stroke syndromes3ed.Cambridge: Cambridge University Press; 2012. p. 542–53.
[58] Ghanizada H, Nedergaard M. The glymphatic system. Handb Clin Neurol 2025;209:161–70.
[59] Hildebrandt H. Neuropsychological tools for dementia: differential diagnosis and treatment. 1. ed. *Elsevier*; 2020.
[60] Liu X, Lam DC, Chan KPF, Chan HY, Ip MS, Lau KK. Prevalence and determinants of sleep apnea in patients with stroke: a meta-analysis. J Stroke Cerebrovasc Dis 2021;30(12):106129.
[61] Baillieul S, Dekkers M, Brill AK, et al. Sleep apnoea and ischaemic stroke: current knowledge and future directions. Lancet Neurol 2022;21(1):78–88.

[62] Chung C-S, Caplan LR. Pontine infarcts and hemorrhages. In: Bogousslavsky J, Caplan LR, editors. Stroke syndromes. 2 ed.Cambridge: Cambridge University Press; 2001. p. 520–33.
[63] Norrving B. Medullary infarcts and hemorrhages. In: Bogousslavsky J, Caplan LR, editors. Stroke syndromes. 2 ed.Cambridge: Cambridge University Press; 2001. p. 534–9.
[64] Parvizi J. Damasio AR. Neuroanatomical correlates of brainstem coma. Brain 2003;126(Pt 7):1524–36.
[65] Cazzoli D, Kaufmann BC, Ruhe H, Geiser N, Vanbellingen T, Nyffeler T. A case study of left visual neglect after right pontine lesion: pathophysiological evidence for the infratentorial involvement in human visual attention. J Neurophysiol 2023;129(6):1534–9.
[66] Hildebrandt H, Spang K, Ebke M. Visuospatial hemi-inattention following cerebellar/brain stem bleeding. Neurocase 2002;8(4):323–9.
[67] Muller Ewald VA, Deifelt Streese C, Bruss JE, et al. Neuropsychiatric outcomes following strokes involving the cerebellum: a retrospective cohort study. Front Neurosci 2023;17:1203488.
[68] Fu X, Lu Z, Wang Y, et al. A clinical research study of cognitive dysfunction and affective impairment after isolated brainstem stroke. Front Aging Neurosci 2017;9:400.
[69] Wang Y, Wang C, Wei Y, et al. Abnormal functional connectivities patterns of multidomain cognitive impairments in pontine stroke patients. Hum Brain Mapp 2022;43(15):4676–88.
[70] Allen PA, Houston JR, Pollock JW, et al. Task-specific and general cognitive effects in Chiari malformation type I. PLoS One 2014;9(4):e94844.
[71] Garrard P, Bradshaw D, Jager HR, Thompson AJ, Losseff N, Playford D. Cognitive dysfunction after isolated brain stem insult. An underdiagnosed cause of long term morbidity. J Neurol Neurosurg Psychiatry 2002;73(2):191–4.
[72] van Zandvoort M, de Haan E, van Gijn J, Kappelle LJ. Cognitive functioning in patients with a small infarct in the brainstem. J Int Neuropsychol Soc 2003;9(3):490–4.
[73] Rinne P, Hassan M, Goniotakis D, et al. Triple dissociation of attention networks in stroke according to lesion location. Neurology 2013;81(9):812–20.
[74] Numasawa Y, Hattori T, Ishiai S, et al. Depressive disorder may be associated with raphe nuclei lesions in patients with brainstem infarction. J Affect Disord 2017;213:191–8.
[75] Bender A. S3-LL Neurologische rehabilitation bei Koma und schwerer Bewusstseinsstörung im Erwachsenenalter. 2022.
[76] Golaszewski S, Florea C, Wutzl B, et al. The locked-in-plus-syndrome. Eur J Neurol 2016;23:725.
[77] Kondziella D, Bender A, Diserens K, et al. European academy of neurology guideline on the diagnosis of coma and other disorders of consciousness. Eur J Neurol 2020;27(5):741–56.
[78] Park IS, Lee NJ, Rhyu IJ. Roles of the declive, folium, and tuber cerebellar vermian lobules in sportspeople. J Clin Neurol 2018;14(1):1–7.
[79] Cerebellar stroke. In: Manto M, Manto MU, editors. Cerebellar disorders: a practical approach to diagnosis and management. Cambridge: Cambridge University Press; 2010. p. 88–101.
[80] Bodranghien F, Bastian A, Casali C, et al. Consensus paper: revisiting the symptoms and signs of cerebellar syndrome. Cerebellum 2016;15(3):369–91.
[81] Taskiran-Sag A, Uzuncakmak Uyanik H, Uyanik SA, Oztekin N. Prospective investigation of cerebellar cognitive affective syndrome in a previously non-demented population of acute cerebellar stroke. J Stroke Cerebrovasc Dis 2020;29(8):104923.
[82] Hoche F, Guell X, Vangel MG, Sherman JC, Schmahmann JD. The cerebellar cognitive affective/Schmahmann syndrome scale. Brain 2018;141(1):248–70.
[83] Mazighi M, Amarenco P. Cerebellar infarcts 3 ed In: Caplan LR, van Gijn J, editors. Stroke syndromes3ed.Cambridge: Cambridge University Press; 2012. p. 469–79.

[84] Schmahmann JD. An emerging concept. The cerebellar contribution to higher function. Arch Neurol 1991;48(11):1178–87.
[85] Schmahmann JD, Sherman JC. Cerebellar cognitive affective syndrome. Int Rev Neurobiol 1997;41:433–40.
[86] Kelly PJ, Stein J, Shafqat S, et al. Functional recovery after rehabilitation for cerebellar stroke. Stroke 2001;32(2):530–4.
[87] Hartwigsen G, Lim JS, Bae HJ, et al. Bayesian modelling disentangles language versus executive control disruption in stroke. Brain Commun 2024;6(3):fcae129.
[88] Weaver NA, Kuijf HJ, Aben HP, et al. Strategic infarct locations for post-stroke cognitive impairment: a pooled analysis of individual patient data from 12 acute ischaemic stroke cohorts. Lancet Neurol 2021;20(6):448–59.

CHAPTER

2

Localizing brain lesions on clinical brain scans

2.1 Landmarks for neuroanatomical orientation in clinical scans

2.1.1 Introduction

Basic functional neuroanatomy is a central part of neuropsychological education, and there are some excellent textbooks on this topic [1,2]. In the following, such basic knowledge about brain functions will be assumed and not discussed in detail.

Localizing specific areas and structures in clinical images is crucial in the work of a neuropsychologist. Despite its clinical relevance, this advanced skill is typically not taught in neuropsychological university courses. For instance, clinical brain scans may display a visible lesion, but reports typically lack information on its precise neuroanatomical location needed to determine functional outcome and prognosis prediction. Only in specialized centers, there sometimes is a brief description in the neuroradiologist's report. However, at least in Germany, this is an exception and not the rule.

Importantly, brain imaging in clinical practice is primarily performed to guide acute medical treatment. Consequently, scans and the corresponding reports are not optimized to address the questions most relevant for neurorehabilitation. This leads to a gap between the education at the university (and for neuroradiology in acute stroke treatment) and clinical neuropsychology (and neurorehabilitation). Nevertheless, they can provide crucial information for neuropsychologists, for example, by helping to frame and guide neuropsychological assessment and treatment planning (for a similar attempt to integrate information from clinical scans and neuropsychology, compare Prosiegel et al. [3]).

One way to bridge this gap is to use the available clinical scans, even though they were acquired for different purposes, and to practice

Applied Neuropsychology of Cerebrovascular Diseases
DOI: https://doi.org/10.1016/B978-0-443-45450-9.00012-6

localizing visible brain lesions in terms of functional neuroanatomy. This is the focus of this chapter: providing practical tasks that help readers practice localizing brain lesions in clinical scans and apply functional neuroanatomical knowledge.

2.1.2 Using MRIcron to train neuroanatomical orientation and lesion localization

2.1.2.1 Installing and using MRIcron

For practicing the localization of brain lesions, we will use the free software MRIcron, which can be downloaded from the following link: https://www.nitrc.org/projects/mricron.

After having installed the software, MRIcron should be started twice independently to run two instances in parallel. One version should use the ch2.nii.gz template, which can be loaded using the file menu (Fig. 2.1). The other version should use the aal.nii.gz template. Having loaded these two templates, use the view menu to yoke both versions by clicking on "yoke." Now, reduce the windows of the two running versions so that both are visible at the same time on your screen. Any scrolling through the different slices of the ch2.nii.gz template, will now be followed by an identical movement through the aal.nii.gz template. You can also move through the template more precisely if you use the x, y, z slots directly below the menu line. If you click into any cortical area in the first template, the corresponding brain area can be identified in the aal.nii.gz template directly below the upper border of the software window. This is an easy way to learn to localize brain areas in a cranial magnetic resonance imaging (cMRI) scan, and we will provide some examples later.

2.1.3 Some background information for localizing brain lesions on clinical scans

2.1.3.1 Some neuroanatomical terms

Before showing clinical examples of strokes, it is necessary to introduce some terms that will be used when referring to the neuroanatomical locations in clinical brain scans. The two most commonly used brain scan methods are cMRI, which uses strong magnetic fields and radio waves to generate highly detailed images of brain structures and soft tissues, and cranial computed tomography (cCT) scans, which use X-rays to create cross-sectional images of the brain.

Several anatomical terms are essential for describing the localization of brain lesions, and a summary can be found in Figs. 2.2 and 2.3, upper right text window. The two easiest terms are lateral (toward the side) and

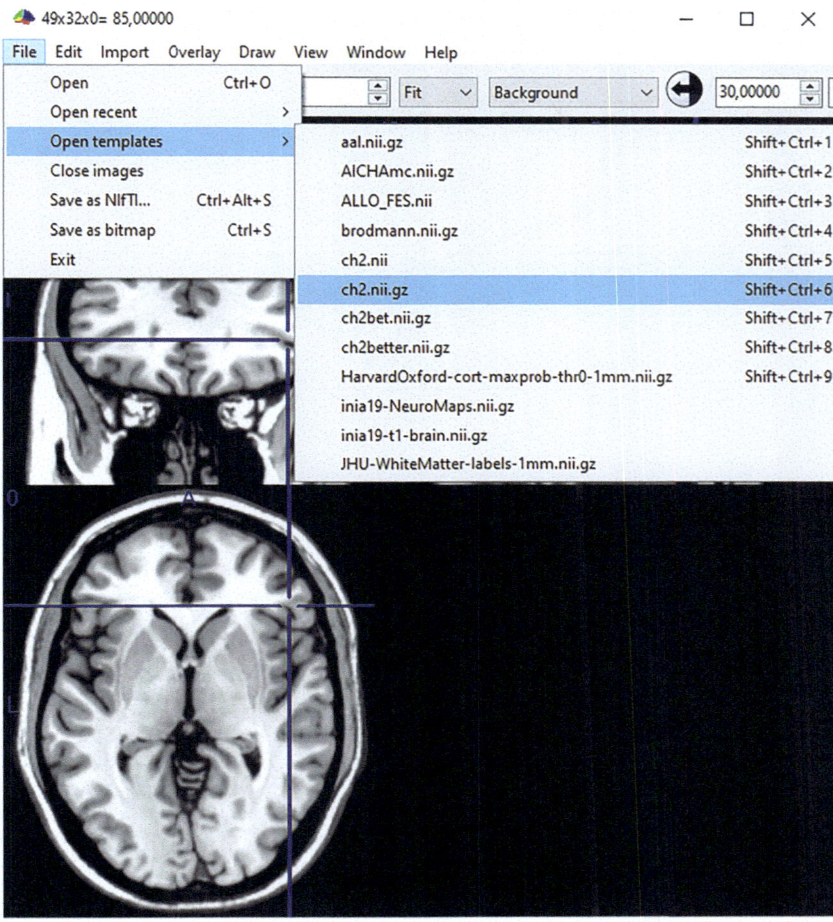

FIGURE 2.1 MRIcron menu.

medial (toward the center). Mesial refers to a fixed anatomical location rather than a position. For example, the term mesial temporal lobe refers to a fixed location on the inner side of the temporal lobe (including structures such as the hippocampus), whereas terms such as lateral or anterior describe directions relative to other points. Two other corresponding simple terms are inferior (downward) and superior (upward). However, these two terms are context-dependent. At the level of the cortex, they mean toward the vertex of the brain and toward the brainstem. However, in the case of the brainstem, they also may mean toward the cerebellum or toward the pons. This is because in animals the cerebrum is not tilted as in humans, where the frontal cortex is rotated

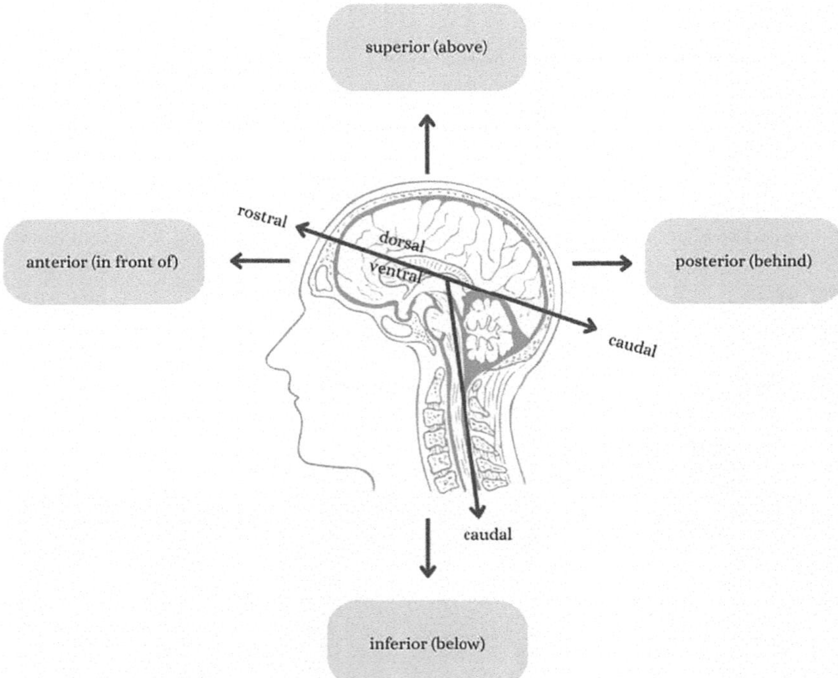

FIGURE 2.2 Terms for specifying neuroanatomical orientation and location.

about 90 degrees and therefore not identical with the vertex. This is the reason that two other terms are also not unequivocal: dorsal and ventral mean the same as superior and inferior at the level of the cerebrum, but not on the level of the brainstem, where dorsal means the direction toward the back and ventral toward the belly.

The same shift of meaning concerns the terms rostral (toward the snout) and caudal (toward the tail). The first one is identical to anterior (or frontal) on the level of the cerebrum, and the second one to the posterior. However, at the level of the brainstem, rostral means in the direction of the vertex and caudal in the direction of the spinal cord.

Clinical reports about the patient's lesion also use the terms supratentorial and infratentorial. Supratentorial means superior or above the cerebellum, because the tentorium is a dent-like structure between the cerebrum and the cerebellum, infratentorial below this structure, meaning that the lesion will be localized in the brainstem or in the cerebellum.

However, the most important terms for understanding the following chapter concern the directions in which clinical images cut through the brain. Therefore they will be repeated here:

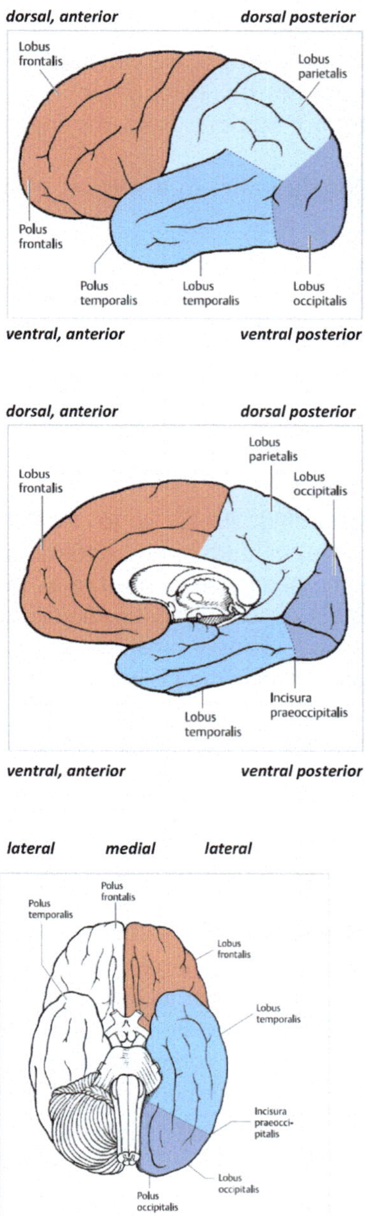

Some terminology for the orientation in neuroanatomical structures (at the level of cerebrum, which means supratentorial, above the brainstem)

Dorsal, superior =
upwards, on the top

ventral, inferior =
downwards, below

anterior, rostral, frontal =
in front of, at the front

posterior, caudal =
behind of, at the back

lateral =
sideways, toward the left or right of the centre

medial, mesial =
toward the center/middle, in the middle

FIGURE 2.3 Gross anatomy of lobuli and terminology for orientation. *Bähr and Bechmann [4], Figures 9.4, 9.5 and 9.6.*

- Axial or transverse (or in a horizontal orientation): from the forehead to the occiput, parallel to a level that roughly aligns with both ears. We will almost exclusively use slices performed in this orientation.
- Coronal or frontal (in a vertical orientation): sections from the top of the head down to the neck.
- Sagittal (longitudinal orientation): sections parallel to a section from the nose to the occiput.

Most clinical brain scans include these different cut directions (especially in cCT scanning), but not all viewing programs allow you to scroll through and compare these planes simultaneously (as explained in the following section).

2.1.3.2 *Cranial computed tomography vs cranial magnetic resonance imaging—what can be seen and when to use it*

The primary goal of cCT scans in suspected stroke is to exclude hemorrhage since this contraindicates thrombolysis and thrombectomy, as this could, for instance, provoke or worsen the hemorrhage. Strokes in the acute stage without hemorrhage are not visible on cCT scans immediately because, among other reasons, early structural changes are subtle, and cytotoxic edema takes hours to develop. Thus they become visible only after a few days. However, there are indirect signs that indicate a stroke. These signs include sulcal effacement in the affected region and compression of the adjacent ventricles. Stroke may lead to cerebral swelling and the consequences (e.g., compression of surrounding structures) can be used to conclude its existence.

cCT and cMRI scans not only differ in respect of sensitivity to acute events (stroke or hemorrhage) (see Table 2.1). They also differ in terms of spatial resolution. In cCT scanning, the distance between the slices will be, in most instances, at least one centimeter, and the thickness of one section encompasses several millimeters. This is far above the values of MRI scanning, where the distance between the images is smaller, allowing for a better resolution of small structures. However, this comes at a cost of longer scan times for cMRI. Another important difference between cCT and cMRI scans concerns the direction of the transverse slices. MRI scans are, in most cases, aligned to the anterior and posterior commissures. It is easily possible to locate these structures and then to initiate the scanning procedure. This is not possible with cCT scans. Because of the adverse side effects of the X-rays, scanning time should be as short as possible. Therefore skull structures reducing the number of necessary slices while still standardizing the images somewhat are often used. Fig. 2.4 shows the MRI orientation of a transverse cut as black line B and two different cCT conventional orientations as blue or gray lines. The K-line is chosen because

TABLE 2.1 Clinical meaning of different brain imaging sequences and techniques.

Aspect	Cranial computed tomography	Cranial magnetic resonance imaging
Primary clinical use	First-line in acute stroke to **exclude hemorrhage**, especially before thrombolysis/thrombectomy.	Broad diagnostic use: stroke (ischemic/hemorrhagic), neurodegeneration, tumors, inflammatory lesions, trauma.
Sensitivity in acute stroke	Low in the first hours: only **indirect signs** (sulcal effacement, compressed ventricles, swelling). Ischemia becomes visible after 24–72 h.	High: **DWI** detects ischemia within minutes; **FLAIR** shows subacute changes; multiple sequences can differentiate lesion types.
Resolution	(Not always) lower: slice distance ≥1 cm, thickness several mm → small structures less visible.	Higher: thinner slices, smaller distances → small structures (hippocampus, white matter lesions) better detected.
Orientation	Standardized via skull landmarks (K-line, etc.); transverse slices differ from MRI orientation. Midbrain comparable, but anterior/posterior slices differ.	Standardized to the anterior-posterior commissure line (AC–PC), more consistent across scans and patients.
Available orientations/ sequences	Typically, one acquisition is reconstructed in transverse, coronal, and sagittal planes.	Multiple sequences in different orientations: • **FLAIR/T2** → sensitive to most lesions • **DWI** → acute stroke • **T1/T2 coronal** → hippocampal atrophy (e.g., AD) • Additional specialized sequences (contrast, perfusion, susceptibility-weighted images (SWI), etc.).
When to use	• Acute stroke (rule out **hemorrhage**) • Emergency settings (fast, accessible) • Patients with MRI contraindications (pacemaker, claustrophobia, metal implants).	• Acute ischemia (DWI) • Neurodegeneration (hippocampal atrophy) • Tumors, demyelination, trauma, subtle lesions • When high resolution is required.
Limitations	• Ionizing radiation exposure • Lower sensitivity for ischemia in the hyperacute phase • Poor hippocampal visualization • Limited resolution for small lesions.	• Longer scan times • Contraindications (implants, severe agitation) • Less available in acute emergencies compared to CT.

at this position the distance between the frontal and occipital tips is largest. The different orientation of cCT and cMRI scans is important to know because images will show the same structures at a mesial position (in the case of the figure, the two lines meet in the mid-brain), but quite different structures for more rostral and more caudal positions. For example, with the K-line orientation used in cCT, the cerebellum is visible on the image, whereas it is not included in the corresponding MRI slice acquired in the B orientation. Still, for the midbrain, the same neuroanatomical structures are shown. Regions lateral to the z-axis are also not affected by the differences in the transverse slices comparing cCT and cMRI scans. Because the midbrain is very helpful as a clinical landmark, it should be kept in mind that at the midbrain, the difference between MRI and cCT images is minimal, whereas it is maximal when inspecting the anterior or posterior segments of the images.

Fig. 2.4 shows the orientation of MRI (black) and cCT transverse slices in the brain.

Cranial CT scanning typically provides images in a single sequence, displayed in three orientations (transverse, coronal, sagittal). In contrast, clinical cMRI scans often include multiple sequences acquired in different orientations. This raises the question of which sequence and orientation should be used for lesion localization. As a general rule, it is advised to begin with transverse images. Usually, there will be one file depicting the patient's brain in transverse or axial orientation using a fluid attenuated inversion recovery sequence (FLAIR) or a dark trim T2 sequence. These

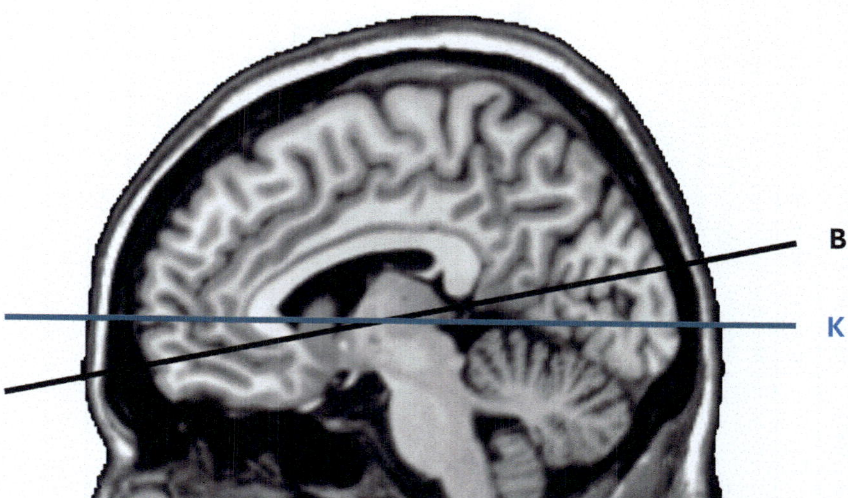

FIGURE 2.4 Difference between the orientation of transverse cMRI and cCT slices.

sequences are sensitive to any kind of lesion and thus represent the best starting point for neuropsychologists.

However, there are clinical questions where the transverse FLAIR is not the first choice or at least not the only sequence one should look for. When analyzing the acute stroke's extension, one should also look for diffusion weighted images (DWI), which is the most sensitive sequence immediately after the stroke (in terms of minutes, whereas cCT scans in the acute state only show indirect indications of the stroke and even the FLAIR sequences are not sensitive enough to represent the whole area involved in the stroke).

In terms of neurodegenerative disorders, other sequences and slices should be considered. In Alzheimer's disease, for instance, coronal slices through the hippocampus are important, and one may use T1 or T2 sequences for the inspection of possible hippocampal atrophy. It should be noted that the difference in orientation also affects the coronal orientation of the cCT scans (z-axis in Fig. 2.4) and therefore the hippocampus is less well visualized on cCT scan, which—among other limitations—restricts the use of this technology for imaging neurodegenerative diseases.

2.1.4 Clinical landmarks of cranial computed tomography and cranial magnetic resonance imaging for neuroanatomical orientation

Lesion localization as a part of clinical routine practice is a skill that is of immense importance for neuropsychological assessment and treatment planning. However, it is also a skill that must be trained because brain scans of different individuals look different, scanning of the brain follows different conventions, and large lesions often only allow indirect conclusions, about which brain areas are involved (due to massive distortions of the shape by swelling or by craniectomy).

To localize lesions on clinical scans, it is necessary to recognize landmarks, indicating the localization of important neuroanatomical structures, and to know the position of other structures relative to these landmarks. This is especially the case because clinical MRIs and cCTs are not always coregistered, which means that only the information of two dimensions is at hand; the third dimension must be extrapolated from the series of images. This increases the difficulty of finding the different sulci of the brain, which, on the other hand, are highly important to localize cortical lesions. Fig. 2.3 presents the main sulci of the cortex from different perspectives on the brain (lateral view, medial view, caudal view). To illustrate the problems of localizing cortical sulci, have a look at the Sylvian fissure, which is the lateral sulcus or the one separating the temporal from the frontal lobe. Now, imagine a series of sections through the brain from frontal to posterior, running from ventral to dorsal. For the lowest of these transverse images, the Sylvian fissure will be located in the anterior part of the image. However, this position will change in more dorsal images, and on the most dorsal level, the Sylvian fissure will be in the posterior part of the image. Something similar can be expected for the central sulcus, separating the frontal and the parietal lobes, although the position change will be smaller than for the Sylvian fissure, because the main direction of the sulcus goes from dorsal to ventral. The intraparietal sulcus offers another example of a structure that changes its position and orientation considerably across transverse slices. In most of the images, this sulcus will be present at almost the same position (posterior and somewhat laterally to the interhemispheric fissure). However, in the most ventral and most dorsal figures, the intraparietal sulcus will gain a lateral position, and depending on the specific direction of the section, it will be visible at different positions on the same image.

2.1.4.1 Ventricles and localization of basal ganglia and amygdala

Let's start with a short introduction on how to localize subcortical structures on clinical transverse scans to proceed to cortical sulci and gyri later. Fig. 2.5 shows a clinical cMRI produced with a FLAIR sequence, which is sensitive to lesions and should be used to get a first impression.

Now, the easiest structure to be recognized on clinical scans is the ventricles (Chapter 1, Figure 1.33). Starting from a dorsal position, the lateral ventricles become visible at the level of the centrum semiovale (Fig. 2.5, line 2 column 2), which consists of white matter tracts connecting the different cortical areas but also motor and sensory fibers to and from the brainstem and the thalamus. The ventricles visible at this dorsal position are the body of the lateral ventricles. On FLAIR and on cCT images, they are presented as two parallel black structures in the medial part of the image. They develop into two mirrored sickle-like structures and then split into two parts: one in an anterior position and one in a posterior position (Fig. 2.5, line 2 column 4). These parts are called the horns of the lateral ventricle, and the anterior split is the frontal horn. In the image showing this split, a thin black line directly in the middle of the brain becomes visible, which is oriented in an anterior-posterior direction. This is the third ventricle. In even more ventral slices, the frontal part of the lateral ventricles is vanishing, and the two posterior parts reach their most caudal position (Fig. 2.5, line 3 column 1 and 2). This is called the posterior horn of the lateral ventricles. At the same time, a small line becomes visible connecting the posterior horn of the lateral ventricles with a small sickle in the center of the temporal lobe (Fig. 2.5, line 3 column 4). This line and the sickle are called the temporal horn of the lateral ventricle. On the level where the temporal horn becomes visible, there is a small black dot directly in the middle of the image in a structure that looks like a butterfly (Fig. 2.5, line 3, column 3). This dot is part of the aqueduct connecting the third and fourth ventricles of the

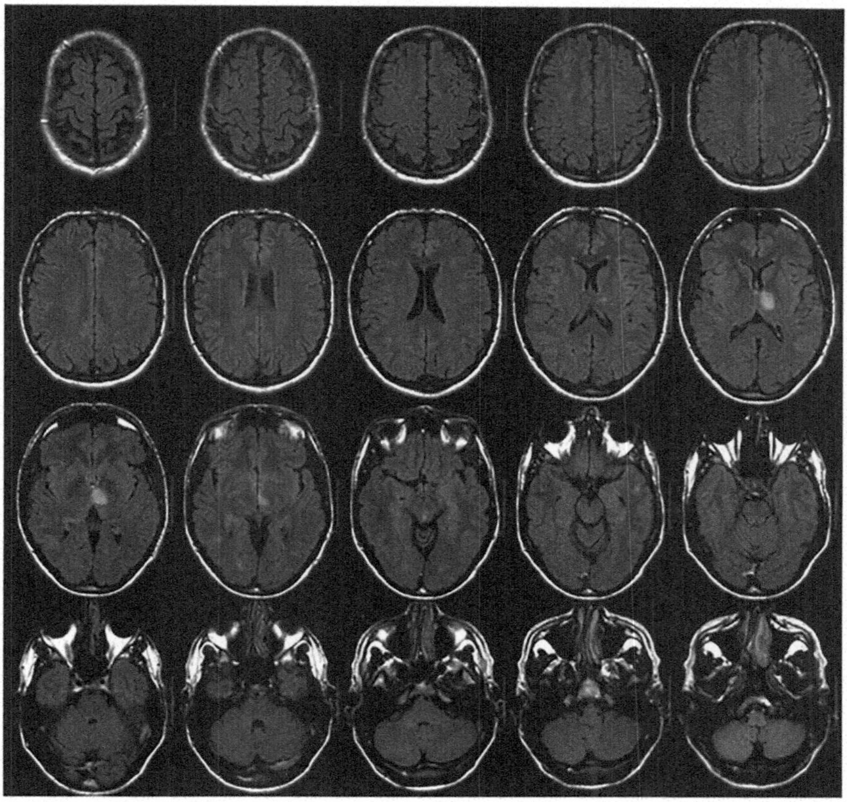

FIGURE 2.5 A clinical fluid attenuated inversion recovery sequence cranial magnetic resonance imaging scan showing the transverse images of a relatively young patient, who suffered a left anterior thalamic stroke (white egg-like area, please, note that on clinical MRI scans, left is right and vice versa).

brainstem. The fourth ventricle is visible in the lowest row, first as a black half-circle and more inferiorly as a curved line in the middle, separating the cerebellum and the brainstem.

Now, the ventricular system of the brain allows to identify some subcortical and cortical structures. Starting again with the most dorsal position of the lateral ventricles at the level of the centrum semiovale, immediately adjacent to the ventricles, one can find parts of the body of the caudate nucleus (Fig. 2.5, line 2 column 2 and line 2 column 3), which is an essential structure of the basal ganglia. The body and head of the caudate nucleus are a little bit lighter structures, directly adjacent to the lateral ventricle. On the images where the lateral ventricles split (they do not really split—this is only an effect of the transverse direction of the section), there are small egg-like lighter structures adjacent to the frontal parts of the lateral ventricles. These are the bilateral heads of the caudate nucleus (Fig. 2.5, line 2 column 4 and 5). It is possible to follow these lighter structures for another two or more images in a ventral direction (meaning that one moves to the two next images in this line). At this point, the ventral part of the caudate head is located, which also encompasses the nucleus accumbens. The ventral parts of the caudate head are involved in emotional regulation, whereas the dorsal parts of the caudate head take part in the cognitive basal ganglia loops (and the body in the motor loops).

Fig. 2.6 shows the position of the basal ganglia in the brain. The caudate nucleus, the putamen, and the globus pallidus are separated by the internal capsule, which is a structure that comprises corticosubcortical and corticospinal fibers (and vice versa) and also fibers connecting the thalamus with the frontal cortex. The internal capsule is composed of three major substructures: (1) the anterior limb, (2) the genu, and (3) the posterior limb. Most of the corticospinal fibers run through the genu and the posterior part of the internal capsule. In FLAIR MRIs and cCT, the internal capsule is darker than the basal ganglia separated by it (Fig. 2.5, line 2 column 4 and 5, line 3 column 1). On the most dorsal image, adjacent to the internal capsule, the putamen (Fig. 2.5, line 2 column 4) is visible. The globus pallidus takes over this adjacent position on Fig. 2.5, line 2 column 5, line 3 column 1, and the putamen moves in a more lateral position. The globus pallidus may be, but is not always, differentiated by a separate darker line from the putamen. As discussed in the first chapter, the basal ganglia receive their blood supply from perforating branches of the MCA and anterior cerebral artery (ACA) (the medial and lateral anterocentral arteries) and are often involved in strokes, because the perforating arteries are small and located inside the brain where no leptomeningeal anastomoses are present.

The tail of the caudate is invisible on MRI scans and in any case on cCT, because of clinical limitations for imaging. However, it is located laterally and directly adjacent to the temporal horn of the lateral ventricle and can be expected exactly there, even without being visible (Fig. 2.5, line 3 column 4). The black line inside the temporal lobe ending together with the small sickles—which was already introduced as the temporal horn of the lateral ventricle (Fig. 2.5, line 3 column 3 and column 4)—are important landmarks to localize the hippocampi and the amygdala. The hippocampus is located for most of its parts directly adjacent to the temporal horn, forming the medial and the posterior border of it. Only a small portion of the hippocampus can be found directly laterally and anterior to the sickle. Moreover, anterior and inferior to the sickle, the different nuclei of the amygdala are located.

The third ventricle, displayed as a thin or bold line directly in the middle of the brain below the image, where the lateral ventricle splits, offers another important landmark for orientation on clinical scans. It is bordered by the

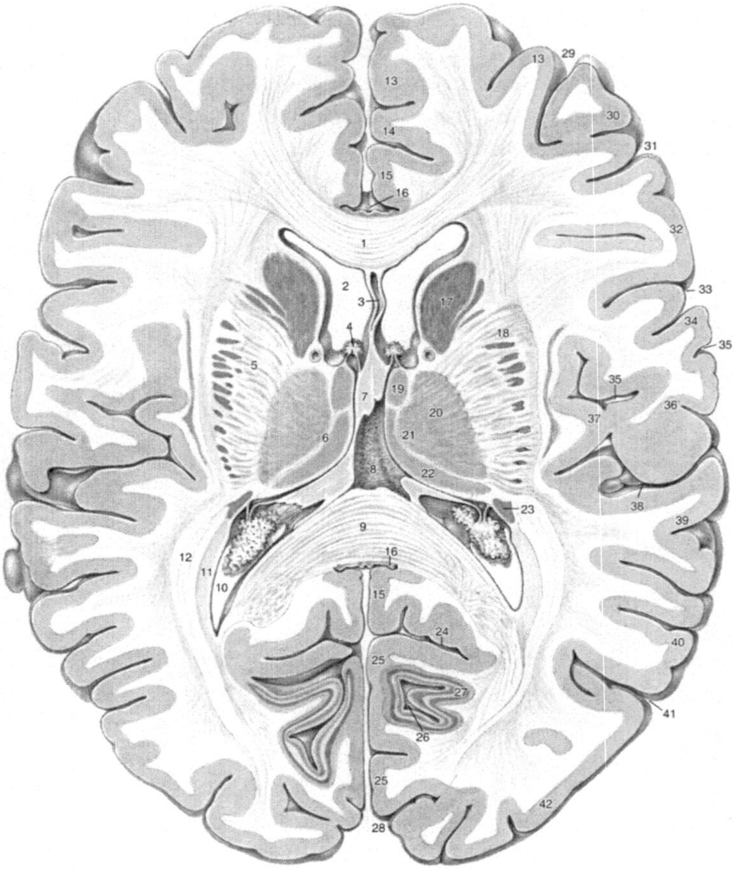

Nieuwenhuys [5]

1 Genu of corpus callosum
2 Lateral ventricle, anterior horn
3 Cave of septum pellucidum
4 Choroid plexus of lateral ventricle
5 Internal capsule
6 Internal medullary lamina
7 Fornix
8 Roof of third ventricle
9 Splenium of corpus callosum
10 Lateral ventricle, posterior horn
11 Tapetum
12 Optic radiation
13 Superior frontal gyrus
14 Cingulate sulcus
15 Cingulate gyrus
16 Indusium griseum
11 Tapetum
12 Optic radiation
13 Superior frontal gyrus
14 Cingulate sulcus
15 Cingulate gyrus
16 Indusium griseum
17 Head of caudate nucleus
18 Caudatolenticular grey bridges
19 Anterior thalamic nucleus
20 Ventral nuclei of thalamus
21 Mediodorsal thalamic nucleus
22 Lateral dorsal thalamic nucleus
23 Tail of caudate nucleus
24 Parieto-occipital sulcus
25 Cuneus
26 Calcarine sulcus
27 Striate area
28 Lunate sulcus
29 Superior frontal sulcus
30 Middle frontal gyrus
31 Inferior frontal sulcus
32 Inferior frontal gyrus
33 Precentral sulcus
34 Precentral gyrus
35 Central sulcus
36 Postcentral gyrus
37 Long gyrus of insula
38 Lateral sulcus, posterior branch
39 Superior temporal gyrus
40 Middle temporal gyrus
41 Anterior occipital sulcus
42 Occipital gyri

FIGURE 2.6 Clinical brain image of cerebral structures on a transverse slide at the level of the striatum. *Nieuwenhuys [5], Fig. 5.30.*

two thalamic nuclei, which, again, on FLAIR scans are somewhat lighter than the rest of the structures. Importantly, the anterior nucleus of the thalamus can be found on the most dorsal images showing the thalamus (Fig. 2.5, line 2 column 5, in this case identical with the light stroke lesion sign), whereas the pulvinar (involved in visual attention) and the lateral geniculate nucleus (part of the thalamus involved in the visual pathway) can be found on more ventral images located in the posterior thalamus.

2.1.4.1.1 Using MRIcron to localize the basal ganglia, hippocampus, and the amygdala

Open MRIcron two times, one with the ch2.nii.gz template and one with the aal.nii.gz template. Yoke the two versions of MRIcron as described above and look for the most dorsal slice showing the lateral ventricles. Scroll down until you can see two gray lines immediately adjacent to the lateral ventricles. Click into these gray lines (e.g., x = 109, y = 123, z = 96). Now, the MRIcron version with the aal.nii.gz version will show a green area here, and you can find the name of the area written in the upper left corner (using MS Windows), which is caudate_R. It should be noted that MRIcron does not reverse the left and the right as clinical MRI scans. Now, it is possible to follow anteriorly the caudate down to x = 102, y = 136, z = 62, which is called the ventral head of the caudate. The putamen can be found, for example, at x = 119, y = 131, z = 74, and the globus pallidum at x = 112, y = 126, z = 74. But even MRIcron does not show the tail of the caudate, which is localized lateral to the temporal horn of the lateral ventricle.

As already mentioned, if hippocampal thickness is of primary interest, one should use a coronal slice. Fig. 2.7 on the left shows the hippocampus combining both slices' orientation into one view. Immediately anterior to the temporal horn of the lateral ventricle, the amygdala can be found (x = 118, y = 128, z = 52).

On the coronal image, the dorsal parts of the lateral ventricles are visible as two black structures in a central position. Diagonally downwards from the lateral ventricles, a tiny gray structure is visible on both sides. These are the bodies of the caudate nucleus. Mesially, there is a light structure with two light points surrounded by tiny black lines. The tiny black lines form the interventricular foramen or foramen of Monro, which connects the lateral and the third ventricle, and the bilateral light structure is the fornix.

2.1.4.2 Ventricles and localization of Papez circuit

At the level of the split of the lateral ventricle into an anterior and posterior part, there are two other important landmarks. The first one can be found *inside* the central and posterior part of the lateral ventricle, and it looks a little bit scattered (Fig. 2.5, line 2 column 4). This is the choroid plexus of the lateral

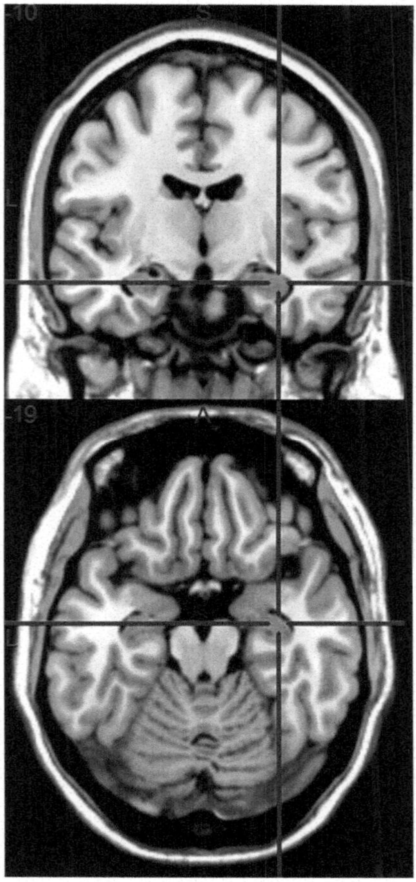

FIGURE 2.7 Localization of the hippocampus using coronal and transverse slices in MRIcron. The temporal horn of the lateral ventricle can be traced through the temporal lobe, starting, for example, at x = 127, y = 119, z = 52. The hippocampus is located medial and posterior to the temporal horn (x = 124, y = 117, z = 52). It can be traced up to x = 109, y = 92, z = 82. However, due to the directions of sectioning, it moves to a medial and anterior position of the posterior horn of the lateral ventricle, starting about x = 125, y = 97, z = 54. Still, the hippocampus can easily be found in clinical cranial magnetic resonance imaging scans, knowing that it is located medial and posterior to the temporal horn of the lateral ventricle in most of the slices.

ventricle. The fornix, as a part of the Papez circuit (Chapter 1, Figure 1.23, shows the Papez circuit and some remarks on its meaning for memory), runs directly below the choroid plexus. The fornix is the continuation of the fimbria hippocampi, a bundle of the hippocampus, which fans out in the coronal plane, and then condenses again into a round fiber tract, which runs medially above the corpus callosum. How to localize the position of the corpus callosum on clinical scans will be introduced in some paragraphs later. Now, at the level where the thalamus becomes visible, it is often possible (at least in MRI scans) to see a tiny paired central structure, which is located inside the two frontal parts of the lateral ventricle and anterior and medial to the upper part of the thalamus. These are the columns of the fornix (Fig. 2.5, line 3 column 5). The position of the columns is also marked by two paired tiny black lines that connect the frontal horn of the lateral ventricle with the third ventricle, which is called the foramen of Monro or interventricular foramen, which has already been localized on a coronal image above. It allows the cerebrospinal fluid (CSF) to flow from the lateral ventricle to the third ventricle. Irrespective of stroke, colloid cysts of the third ventricle growing here will impair CSF circulation, leading to a hydrocephalic increase of the lateral ventricle and eventually compressing the columns of the fornix, leading to specific memory deficits [6]. The resection of the colloid cysts may involve a transection of the fornix if the cysts adhere to the columns of the fornix.

Following the thin or bold line in the center of the transverse image, indicating the third ventricle, in a ventral direction, a butterfly-like structure directly in the middle of the brain becomes visible (Fig. 2.5, line 3 column 3, Fig. 2.8 in the center). Just before the "butterfly" starts to separate by black lines from the temporal lobes, anterior to it, there is a small point indicating the ventral tip of the third ventricle. This ventral tip is bordered by the hypothalamus on both sides. On MRI scans, it is often possible also to see two small circle-like structures somewhat lighter (or darker on T2 sequences) than the rest of the brain at this level. The two circle-like structures are the mammillary bodies and border the posterior part of the ventral tip of the third ventricle (Fig. 2.8). Described from an opposite perspective, whereas the thalamus borders the dorsal parts of the third ventricle, the ventral parts are bordered by the hypothalamus. And the two mammillary bodies border the posterior tip of the third ventricle.

There are two additional structures related to the lateral ventricles, which are helpful landmarks for the orientation in clinical MRI and cCT scans. The first one is visible at the level of the choroid plexus, that is, where the lateral ventricles begin to divert. Directly anterior to the lateral ventricles, there is a somewhat darker structure, not interrupted by the interhemispheric fissure (Fig. 2.5, line 2 column 2–5). The same holds on this level directly caudal to the posterior part of the lateral ventricle (Fig. 2.5, line 2 column 3–5). These two structures connect both hemispheres and are the genu of the corpus callosum (at the anterior position) and the splenium of the corpus callosum (at the posterior position). The corpus callosum is a clamp-like structure in the medial part of the brain. It is possible to follow it up in the dorsal direction to the level where the lateral ventricle disappears (Fig. 2.5, line 2 column 1). At this dorsal

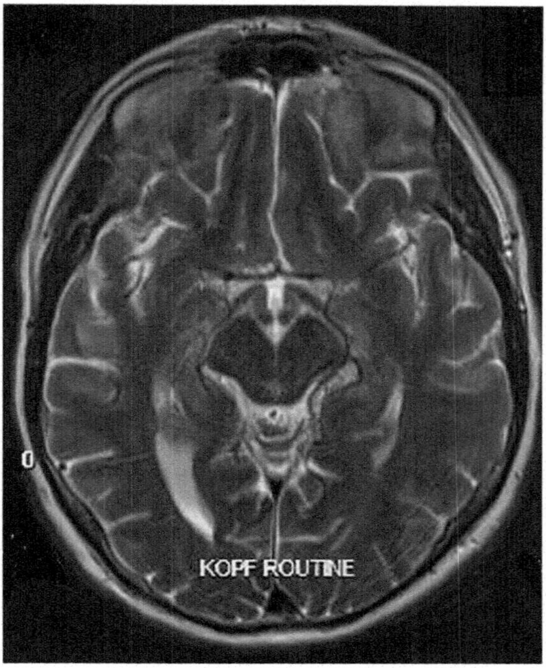

FIGURE 2.8 Clinical transverse MRI scan showing the midbrain.

position, the two hemispheres are separated again by the interhemispheric fissure. Now, the cingulate gyrus is a clamp-like structure directly surrounding the corpus callosum. This means that having identified the corpus callosum immediately informs about the position of the cingulate gyrus, which is localized directly rostral of the genu of the corpus callosum and directly caudal to the splenium of the corpus callosum and at the level where the interhemispheric fissure becomes visible again above the lateral ventricle and the corpus callosum.

The cingulate gyrus contains the cingulum and the indusium griseum (stria longitudinalis medialis and lateralis), which are two fiber tracts that close the Papez circuit and contribute to memory consolidation. These fiber tracts originate in the anterior thalamic nucleus or the basal forebrain and project toward the hippocampal structure in the basomedial areas of the temporal lobes or to the amygdala. Even if they are not visible as separate fiber tracts on clinical scans, their position can be estimated using this information.

Table 2.2 gives an overview of the ventricles and related neuroanatomical structures.

TABLE 2.2 .

Structure	Location in transverse scans	Key characteristics on Fig. 2.5 (FLAIR MRI scan)	Reference in Fig. 2.5
Lateral ventricles (body)	On dorsal images, located medially	Black parallel structures on dorsal images	Line-col. 2.2, 2.3
Lateral ventricles (cornua or horns)	Frontal horn: in front of the choroid plexus and thalamus posterior horn: medial border of the temporal and parietal lobes Temporal horn: mediobasal position inside the temporal lobe	Black paired sickle-like on medial images Black triangles on medial images Black lateral paired sickle-like on inferior images	Line-col. 2.4, 2.5 Line-col. 3.1, 3.2 Line-col. 3.3, 3.4
choroid plexus	Inside the body part of the lateral ventricle and inside the third and fourth ventricles	Scattered appearance on images. Starting point for the division between the frontal horn and the body of the lateral ventricles on the most dorsal images	Line-col. 2.4
Third ventricle	Midline, below the body of the lateral ventricles	Thin/bold black line in anterior-posterior direction	Line-col. 3.2, 3.3
Foramen of Monro	Between the frontal horn of the lateral ventricle and the third ventricle	Tiny paired black lines	Line-col. 3.5
Fourth ventricle	Inferior images, between brainstem and cerebellum	Initially a black half-circle, later a curved line on ventral images	Line-col. 4.1–4.5
Aqueduct	Midline, ventral to the third ventricle	Small black dot in the posterior part of the "butterfly" structure of the midbrain	Line-col. 3.3
Basal ganglia, motor fibers			
Caudate nucleus (Body)	Adjacent to the lateral ventricles at centrum semiovale level	Lighter structure next to body of the lateral ventricles on FLAIR	Line-col. 2.2, 2.3
Caudate nucleus (Head)	More ventral, adjacent to the anterior lateral ventricles	Egg-like lighter structure next to the frontal horn of the lateral ventricle	Line-col. 2.4, 2.5

Tail of the caudate	Laterally adjacent to the temporal horn of the lateral ventricle	Not visible on MRI/CT	~ Line-col. 3.4
Nucleus accumbens	Ventral to the caudate head	Not visible on MRI/CT, inside the lighter V-like medial structure below the head of the caudate nucleus	Line-col. 3.1, 3.2
Putamen	Lateral to the internal capsule	Lighter structure lateral and posterior to the head of the caudate	Line-col. 2.5, 3.1
Globus pallidus	On ventral images medial to the putamen	Sometimes not well differentiated from the putamen	Line-col. 2.5, 3.1
Internal capsule	Medial to the caudate nucleus, putamen, and lateral to thalamus	Darker than the basal ganglia and thalamus, it contains corticospinal fibers	Line-col. 2.4, 2.5, 3.1
Limbic system			
Hippocampus	Medially adjacent to the temporal horn of the lateral ventricle	Forms medial/posterior border of temporal horn	Line-col. 3.3, 3.4
Amygdala	Anterior/inferior to the temporal horn	Lighter structure, but not touching the midbrain	Line-col. 3.3- 3.4
Fornix	Below choroid plexus, runs medially	Part of the Papez circuit, involved in memory	Line-col. 2.4
Columns of the fornix	Anterior of the thalamus, inside frontal horn of lateral ventricle.	On the two inferior images lateral to the third ventricle	Line-col. 2.5, 3.1, 3.2
Thalamus	borders the third ventricle	On FLAIR scans, lighter than the internal capsule	Line-col. 2.5, 3.1, 3.2
Anterior nucleus (thalamus)	Dorsal imaging showing the thalamus	Inside the stroke visible in Fig. 2.5	Line-col. 2.5
Hypothalamus	Borders ventral tip of the third ventricle	Small liplike structure anterior to the "butterfly" structure of the midbrain	Line-col. 3.3
Mammillary bodies	Posterior to the ventral tip of the third ventricle		Line-col. 3.3

(*Continued*)

TABLE 2.2 (Continued)

Structure	Location in transverse scans	Key characteristics on Fig. 2.5 (FLAIR MRI scan)	Reference in Fig. 2.5
		Posterior border of the lip-like structure anterior to the "butterfly" structure of the midbrain	
Visual system			
Lateral geniculate nucleus (thalamus)	Borders anterior part of the posterior horn of the lateral ventricle	Part of the visual pathway	Line-col. 3.1, 3.2
Optic radiation	Posterior of the lateral geniculate nucleus. Splits into two parts.	Dorsal part: remains medial and curves somewhat dorsal and posterior to reach the medial occipital lobe. Ventral part (Meyer's loop): turns anteriorly and somewhat laterally to get into a lateral position of the posterior horn of the lateral ventricle to reach the medial occipital lobe	Line-col. 3.4
Pulvinar (thalamus)	Posterior thalamus, adjacent to quadrigeminal cistern	Visible posterior to the stroke in Figure 3.1	Line-col. 3.1, 3.2
Dorsal core structures			
Corpus callosum (genu and splenium)	Anterior (genu) and posterior (splenium) to the lateral ventricles	Because connecting the hemispheres, the corpus callosum is visible as a homogenous structure without interruption by the interhemispheric fissure	Line-col. 2.2–2.5
Cingulate gyrus	Surrounding the corpus callosum	Either anterior, posterior, or directly superior to the corpus callosum	Line-col. 1.4–2.5

Structures of the brain and how to find in clinical MRI scans. Part I.

2.1.4.2.1 Using MRIcron to localize the Papez circuit

The Papez circuit is a fiber tract (white matter structure), and the aal.nii.gz atlas was developed to distinguish between cortical but not white matter structures. Therefore close the aal.nii.gz template and load the JHU-WhiteMatter-labels-1mm.nii.gz template. The fornix is displayed in the center of the brain and can be traced in both directions, starting, for example, with x = 90, y = 121, z = 86. The reconstruction of the fornix ends on the level of z = 73. However, using the ch32.nii.gz template, it is possible to follow the fornix as two light points down to x = 89, y = 125, z = 64 until the fornix reaches both mammillary bodies on x = 95, y = 121, z = 58. Directly anterior to the mammillary bodies, the hypothalamus is visible. Posterior to the mammillary body, the butterfly-like structure of the midbrain can be seen.

2.1.4.3 *Using cisterns of the brain as landmarks for the visual system*

CSF cannot only be found in the ventricles but also inside the subarachnoid space of the brain (Chapter 1). If the subarachnoid space expands in relation to the different sulci or gyri of the brain, the space filled with CSF is termed a cistern. Cisterns serve as reservoirs for CSF and help with its circulation. The names of cisterns are specified according to the adjacent structure (e.g., insular cistern, cistern of the frontal sulcus, cistern of the tectal lamina, etc.). Some of the cisterns are named according to their surface structure (e.g., "quadrigeminal cistern," also called the cistern of the great cerebral vein). The five most prominent cisterns, their names, and localization are shown in Fig. 2.9.

Fig. 2.9 offers the opportunity to find the different ventricles and the cisterns on a transverse clinical MRI scan.

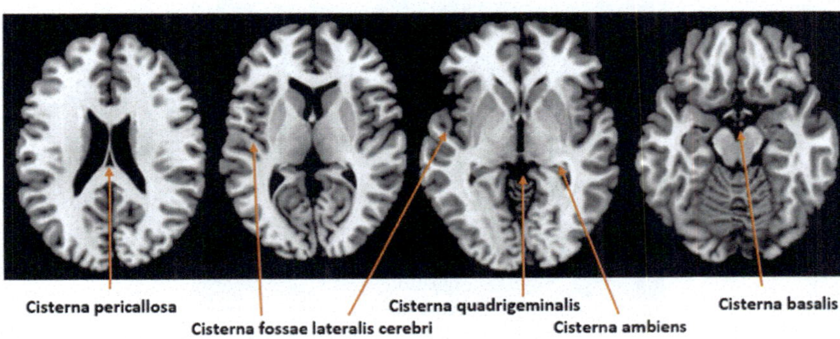

FIGURE 2.9 Cisterns of the cerebrum.

The *pericallosal cistern* is not always visible on clinical images. Importantly, this cistern separates the corpus callosum from the cingulate gyrus dorsal to the splenium of the corpus callosum.

The *insular cistern* is located lateral to the insular cortex and is bordered by the frontal and the temporal cortex. Fig. 2.5 shows the insular cistern on line 2, column 4 and 5, and on line 3, column 1 and 2. Anteriorly, the insular cistern shows a transition into the Sylvian fissure (see below). At its most dorsal and posterior position, the posterior ascending ramus starts. It can be detected and followed dorsally and ventrally in MRIcron on z = 69, x = 141, and y = 136.

The *pericallosal cisterns* border the corpus callosum and the cingulate, dorsal cortex, the genu and the splenium of the corpus callosum. These cisterns are not visible in the brains of young people, being too small to be visible.

The dorsal parts of the *interpeduncular cistern* host the two mammillary bodies (the MRIcron coordinates of the mammillary body are mentioned in the section above). The mammillary bodies are not always visible on clinical MRI scans, because of being too small. However, the somewhat darker gray structure directly anterior to the mammillary bodies and extending in an anterior-posterior direction is always visible and shows the hypothalamus. For localizing the hypothalamus, therefore the interpeduncular cistern in front of the midbrain (butterfly-like structures) plays a major role (Fig. 2.10). In Fig. 2.5 the hypothalamus

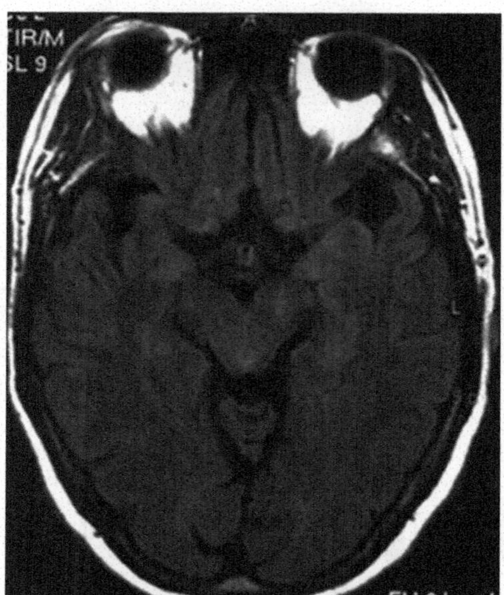

FIGURE 2.10 Cistern interpeduncularis in front of the midbrain.

can be found in line 3, image 3. At the most caudal position of the hypothalamus, it seems possible to detect two small points, which might represent cross-sections of the mammillary bodies. Diagonally above the mammillary bodies, two gray lines point medially and look like the tip of an arrow. These are parts of the optic nerve beyond the optic chiasm. Following their posterior extension, not visible as specific structures on the clinical MRI scan, they border the butterfly-like midbrain structure before turning inside. At this level, they form the optic tract projecting toward the lateral geniculate nucleus. The *interpeduncular cistern* is bordered anteriorly by the optic chiasm, which is often visible on clinical scans (but not on Fig. 2.5). One would expect the optic chiasm between line 3, image 3, and image 4, but it was not captured on these slices, probably being located directly between the two slices. Mammillary bodies, hypothalamus, and the optic tract are visible on the single image of a clinical MRI scan on the left.

This figure also shows the *quadrigeminal cistern,* which is located directly posterior and inferior to the superior colliculi. The superior colliculi are displayed posterior to the aqueduct on this figure as two small hills pointing posteriorly. They play a major role in spatial orientation and attention.

The quadrigeminal cistern borders the lateral geniculate nucleus (Fig. 2.5, line 3, column 1) and, more dorsally, the pulvinar (Fig. 2.5, line 2, column 5). Lesions of the lateral geniculate nucleus and fibers running posteriorly to it will cause visual field deficits, whereas lesions localized inside the pulvinar will produce visual attentional deficits.

The posterior horn of the lateral ventricle (Fig. 2.5, line 3, column 1), visible on this image only in the left hemisphere (i.e., on the right), is an important landmark to localize the optic radiation. Meyer's loop, which is responsible for transmitting visual information to the visual cortex, runs laterally to the posterior horn projecting to the calcarine sulcus. Strokes of the middle cerebral artery (MCA) and of the PCA often involve the optic radiation and produce visual field deficits. Therefore lesions adjacent to the posterior horn call for visual field assessment.

Table 2.3 gives an overview of the cranial cisterns and related neuroanatomical structures.

2.1.4.3.1 Using MRIcron to localize the visual system

To follow the visual system, it is possible to start directly with the optic nerve, which can be found in MRIcron on x = 65, y = 173, z = 38. It is possible to track the optic nerve projecting to the optic chiasm image-wise, for example, on x = 80, y = 147, z = 44. The optic chiasm can be found in MRIcron on x = 94, y = 134, z = 52 as a light, laterally oriented structure. This

TABLE 2.3 Where to find cranial cisterns and related neuroanatomical structures.

Structure	Location in transverse scans	Key characteristics on *FLAIR* MRI	Reference in Fig. 2.5
Ambient cistern	Dorsal to the splenium of the corpus callosum, separating it from the cingulate gyrus	Not always visible in clinical scans	Line-col. 9
Insular cistern	Lateral to the insular cortex; bordered by frontal and temporal cortex	Black structure with posterior-anterior direction. Loses its solid shape on more dorsal images.	Line-col. 9 Line-col. 5: line 2: images 4 and 5; line 3, images 1,2
Pericallosal cistern	Dorsal to the genu and splenium of the corpus callosum, bordering the cingulate cortex	Too small to be visible in young individuals	Line-col. 9
Interpeduncular cistern	Anterior to the midbrain (in front of the "butterfly-shaped" structure)	directly anterior to the hypothalamus (always visible as a lighter medial gray matter extending in anterior-posterior direction)	Line-col. 9, Line-col. 10 Line-col. 5: Line 3, Image 3, and 4
Optic chiasm	Anterior border of the interpeduncular cistern	Often visible in clinical scans, but not in Fig. 2.5 (likely between image 3.3 and 3.4)	Line-col. 7, two medial structures in light color
Optic tract	Extending posteriorly from the optic chiasm, surrounding the midbrain ("butterfly-shaped" structure)	Not distinctly visible; projects toward lateral geniculate nucleus	Line-col. 10 [Line-col. 5: line 3, image 3]
Quadrigeminal cistern	Posterior to the superior and inferior colliculi, anterior to the cerebellar vermis	Dark medial structure behind the "butterfly-shaped" midbrain and ventral thalamus	Line-col. 9 Line-col. 5: line 3, image 1–5
Lateral geniculate nucleus	Directly anterior to the quadrigeminal cistern	Small light structure anterior to the most lateral extension of the quadrigeminal cistern.	Line-col. 5: line 3, image 1 and 2
Pulvinar	Large posterior part of the thalamus is anterior and dorsal to the lateral geniculate nucleus	Borders the dorsal and anterior parts of the quadrigeminal cistern	Line-col. 5: line 1, image 1
Posterior horn of the lateral ventricle	Black structure lateral to the quadrigeminal cistern is shaped like a triangle.	Inside the dark triangles, often some crumpled structure is visible, which is part of the choroid plexus	Line-col. 5: line 3, image 1 and 2
Optic radiation (Meyer's loop)	Lateral to the posterior horn of the lateral ventricle, projecting to the calcarine sulcus	Not directly visible	[Line-col. 5: line 3, image 1 and 2]

structure borders the hypothalamus anteriorly, but on more dorsal images, it curves posteriorly, and touches the midbrain as optic tract (x = 79, y = 122, z = 60). Some of its projections reach the superior colliculi anterior to the quadrigeminal cistern. The right superior colliculus can be found at coodinates x = 87, y = 96, z = 68. At the same slice, more laterally, a gray structure can be found bilaterally, which is called lateral geniculate nucleus and which receives most of the projections of the optic tract. At this point, a second version of MRIcron should be started, and the JHU-WhiteMatter-labels-1mm.nii.gz should be loaded. Starting with x = 55, y = 86, z = 81 in this template, it is possible to learn the projections of the optic radiation, which is located laterally to the posterior horn of the lateral ventricle. It should be clear that the template does not show all parts of the optic radiation, because the reconstruction neither reaches the lateral geniculate nucleus nor the calcarine sulcus. To localize this structure, the aal.nii.gz can be loaded, and one may start at x = 88,y = 33,z = 72 to get an impression about the extension of this area (compare Fig. 2.12 below for a left PCA stroke involving the optic radiation and the medial occipital cortex).

2.1.4.4 *Cortical landmarks to identify cortical areas*

Knowing the position of the different parts of the cerebral ventricles helps to localize different cortical and subcortical structures important for neuropsychologists. However, it does not inform where the major sulci and cortical gyri are localized. For a definition of landmarks of the major sulci, we start with the Sylvian fissure or lateral sulcus, which is the border between the frontal and the temporal lobes.

2.1.4.4.1 The Sylvian fissure

The temporal lobe can be easily detected starting from a ventral position and looking for two lateral structures that are similar to each other and on the next few dorsal images (Fig. 2.5, line 4 column 1 and 2). They are separated at this vertical position by the brainstem in the center of the section and partly by the cerebellum, extending in a posterior direction, showing a more parallel structuring and homogeneous pattern.

The temporal lobe develops during the following dorsal images, extending posteriorly into the occipital lobe, which surrounds the dorsal parts of the cerebellum on these dorsal images (Fig. 2.5, line 3 column 3–5). The most dorsal tip of the cerebellum, the cerebellar vermis, vanished at the level of the butterfly-like structure (the midbrain, Fig. 2.5, line 3 column 3). The superior colliculi are localized at this level directly anterior to the cerebellar vermis. At the same level as the most lateral position, a small fissure becomes visible, which runs from anterior to posterior, separating a lateral wedge-like part of the brain from the more central major part. Medial to this wedge-like structure, the insular cortex is located (Fig. 2.5, line 2 column 5, line 3 column 1 and 2). The front of the wedge-like structure is the Sylvian fissure. From this image on, one can follow the Sylvian fissure for some images in the dorsal direction. On the following dorsal images, all brain structures directly connected to the part of the brain and posterior to the wedge belong to the temporal lobe (as most of those structures below the most ventral image showing the wedge). The position of the Sylvian fissure moves from anterior to a more posterior position on these transverse images because of its extension from the inferior frontal lobe to the highest posterior tip of the temporal lobe. This is important because all the structures anterior to the Sylvian fissure belong to the frontal cortex, even if they extend into the posterior half of the images. The first sulcus anterior to the Sylvian fissure is either the postcentral sulcus or, more ventrally, the central sulcus. The one anterior to the central sulcus is the precentral sulcus (Fig. 2.3A, first sulcus anterior to the central sulcus dividing the parietal lobe (light blue) from the frontal lobe (orange). Just anterior to the precentral sulcus on the left, Broca's area is located and can be followed for several sections from its most ventral to its most dorsal position. Broca's area plays a major role in language production, grammar, and verbal working memory (Chapter 1). To localize Broca's area, it is helpful to imagine what happens if one cuts axially through the brain at the level of the exit of the anterior ascending ramus from the Sylvian fissure. You will find this ramus on Fig. 2.3A as the sulcus inside the frontal lobe (orange). It starts directly superior of the temporal lobe (blue) and is oriented dorsally. Broca's area is part of the gyrus surrounding the anterior ascending ramus. Images dorsal to the exit of the anterior ascending ramus should show three parallel medially oriented sulci, and the Broca's area should be caudal and rostral to the most anterior one of these sulci. Such a pattern can be easily detected in Fig. 2.5, line 2, column 5. Broca's area extends to the dorsal images at line 2, column 3, and it is possible to follow the ascending ramus up to those images.

The Sylvian fissure itself loses its connection to the insular cistern, which was responsible for the posterior parts of the wedge-like structure, as one moves to more dorsal slices. It becomes a sulcus running directly medial (Fig. 2.5, line 2 column 4). At this level, Heschl's gyrus is located containing the primary auditory cortex (Stroke area of Fig. 2.11, line 2, column 3–5; Fig. 2.5 line 2 column 3, (right side of the brain, left side of the image) at a position of 9:45, looking like a finger). At the level where the Sylvian fissure loses contact with the insular cistern and starts to show a medial course, directly posterior to the fissure, one can find the dorsal parts of Wernicke's area. The Wernicke's area plays a major role in holding and interpreting phonological representations according to their meaning. The clinical consequences and functional treatment of lesions in this area will be discussed in Chapter 6. Many MRI scans show a dorsal extension of the

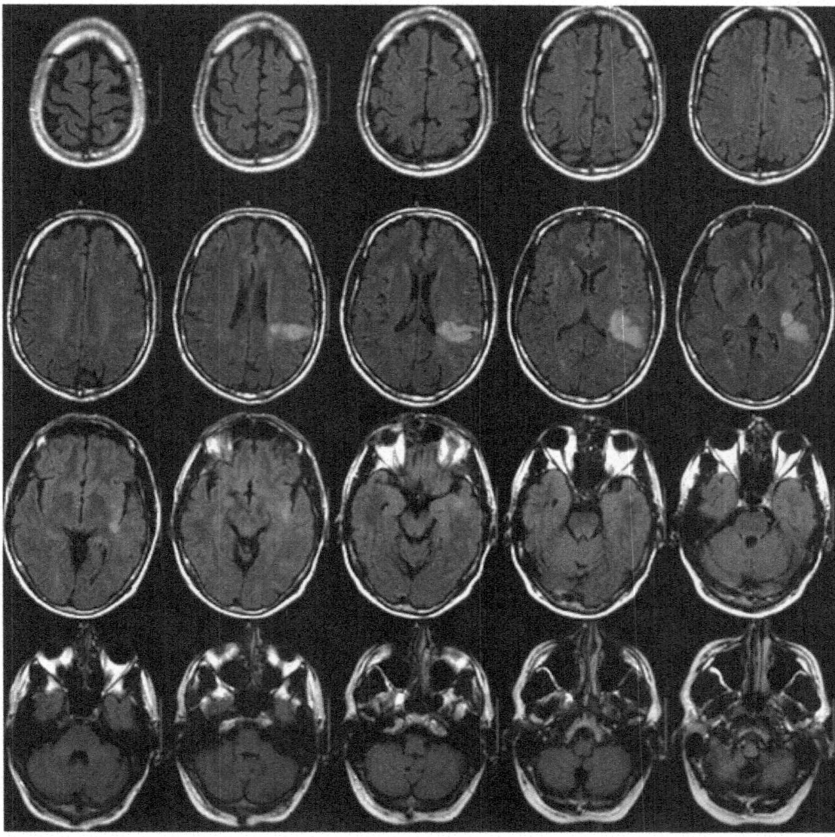

FIGURE 2.11 Stroke involving the primary auditory cortex on the left and the posterior ascending ramus of the Sylvian (capital "S") fissure.

Sylvian fissure, which does not lose its anterior-posterior position from here on anymore (Fig. 2.5, line 2 column 4 and 5, line 3 column 1–3, especially on the right side at the position of 3:15). This part of the fissure is called the posterior ascending ramus and around the posterior ascending ramus the supramarginal gyrus or the parietotemporal junction is located, a supramodal integration center important for phonological decoding and reading on the left and visuospatial attention on the right (as part of the ventral spatial attention system). Figure 2.11 shows a stroke located at the position of the posterior ascending ramus and the supramarginal gyrus.

The part of the supramarginal gyrus posterior to the ascending ramus of the Sylvian fissure is the most ventral starting point of the parietal lobe. There are no lateral sulci separating the parietal lobe from the occipital lobe; therefore these two lobes cannot be clearly defined with the help of clinical MRI scans. However, there is no major problem in distinguishing between the medial parts of the parietal lobe and the occipital lobe (see below).

2.1.4.4.2 Using MRIcron to localize auditory processing and the Wernicke's area

The two neuroanatomical structures for processing auditory information, which can be detected on clinical MRI scans are the two inferior colliculi. Using MRIcron, one of the two inferior colliculi is located around x = 86, y = 94, z = 62. The auditory radiation crosses the internal capsule at its posterior extension. To localize Heschl's gyrus, one may use x = 146, y = 119, z = 79 as a starting point. As already mentioned, it looks like a finger pointing diagonally and laterally.

We argued that there are two landmarks that can be used to find the Wernicke's area: the Heschl's gyrus and the direction change of the Sylvian fissure at the position of the posterior ascending ramus. The structures directly anterior to Heschl's gyrus belong to the frontal cortex, whereas the structures posterior to the Heschl's gyrus are the superior temporal gyrus and the most dorsal parts of the middle temporal gyrus. The Wernicke's area is located inside the posterior segments of the superior temporal gyrus and the posterior segments of the middle temporal gyrus. If we now move dorsally to a z-level of 90, we can follow a medially oriented large sulcus, which corresponds to the posterior ascending ramus of the Sylvian fissure. The cortex directly posterior to this sulcus belongs to the superior temporal gyrus and is part of Wernicke's area (up to the level of z = 92 and down to about level 77). You can follow the Wernicke's area by starting, for example, at x = 141, y = 85, z = 81.

2.1.4.5 *The parieto-occipital sulcus*

The medial border between the parietal and the occipital lobe is defined by the parieto-occipital sulcus, which runs from the posterior surface of the cortex in an anterior and ventral direction (Fig. 2.3B). The starting point of this sulcus can be found approximately at the level of the most dorsal position of the lateral ventricles or even one or two sections more dorsally. In these sections, there is a laterally oriented sulcus (on both sides) starting at the interhemispheric fissure and in parallel to the posterior boundary of the brain (Fig. 2.5, line 2 column 2–5). This sulcus then moves in an anterior direction on the next ventral images and can be traced downwards up to the section where the splenium of the corporus callosi disappears (Fig. 2.5, line 3 column 1). All structures directly in front of the sulcus are parietal, and structures posterior to the sulcus belong to the occipital lobe. The occipital structures are called cuneus and play an important role in the integration of visual and motor coordinates for hand movements (as part of the dorsal visual processing system). At the level where the sulcus disappears (Fig. 2.3B, the sulcus bordering the light blue and grey area which disappears when it touches the blue temporal area), the calcarine sulcus

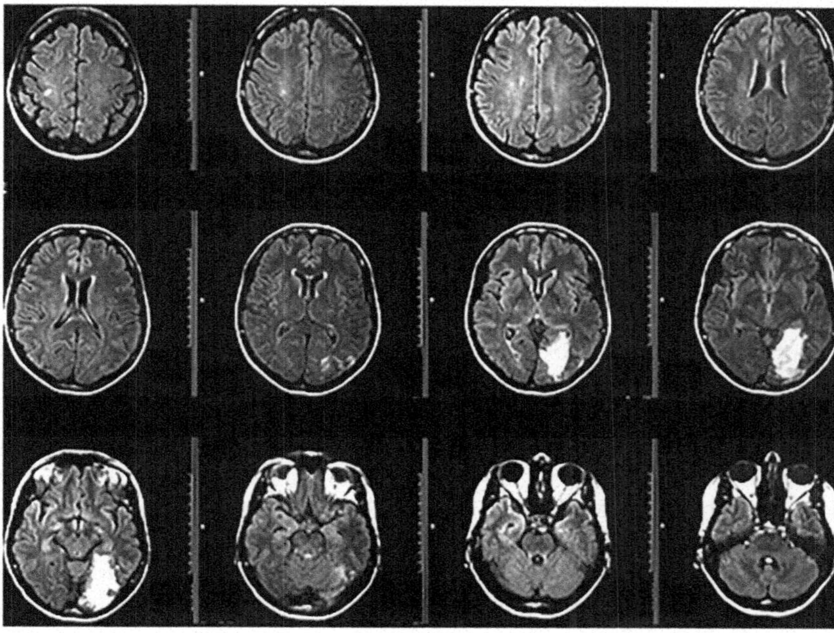

FIGURE 2.12 Stroke of the left posterior cerebral artery involving the optic radiation and parts of the primary visual cortex.

starts cutting through the primary visual cortex. At the level of the cerebellar vermis (see below), the lateral parts bordering the cerebellar vermis (Fig. 2.5, line 3 column 4 and 5) are the fusiform gyrus and the entorhinal or parahippocampal cortex, which play a major role in visual recognition and episodic memory integration. Figure 2.12, already shown in Chapter 1, shows the consequence of a PCA stroke in this area. The collateral sulcus is visible on Fig. 2.5, 3.1 on the nonimpaired left image side (right hemisphere), and it is involved in the lesion on the left hemisphere, which means the input from the entorhinal cortex would not reach the hippocampus anymore (as discussed in the chapter on the cognitive consequences of a PCA stroke). Parts of the hippocampus, medially and caudally to the temporal sickle of the lateral ventricle, are also involved. Importantly, the localization of the lesion as on Fig. 2.12, line 2 column 4 and line 3 column 1 and 2 (where the lesion vanishes) argues not only for the presence of a visual field defect but also for a possible visual associative agnosia and/or a pure alexia due to the involvement of the lingual gyrus and fusiform gyrus (Fig. 2.12).

2.1.4.5.1 Using MRIcron to localize the parieto-occipital sulcus

The sulcus parieto-occipitalis can be found and traced starting at $x = 109$, $y = 46$, $z = 118$. Areas anterior to this sulcus are part of the parietal lobe, areas posterior are part of the occipital lobe. The sulcus sticks to its medial position and lateral direction and can be followed downwards until z = 78. At this level, the precuneus, part of the parietal lobe, is still present but starts to be divided from the occipital lobe by a white matter structure. Posterior to the parieto-occipital sulcus, the calcarine sulcus is located.

2.1.4.6 *The intraparietal sulcus*

The parietal lobe is subdivided by the intraparietal sulcus into different areas (Fig. 2.3A, sulcus in the centre of light blue area). This sulcus divides the anterior and posterior parietal cortex and the superior and inferior parietal cortex. It is a sulcus without a dominant orientation and changes its direction from dorsal to ventral images. The sulcus can easily be found on the dorsal sections (Fig. 2.5, line 1 column 4 and 5), where the sulcus parieto-occipitalis becomes visible, as bilateral lines running from the posterior end of the image in a frontal direction not far away from the interhemispheric fissure. As can be seen on line 1, column 4, to line 2, column 1, the sulcus starts to split parts of the parietal lobe from the rest of the cortex. This split is not a real split but the effect of the transverse cutting series. Lateral to the intraparietal sulcus, for example, the angular gyrus is located, a tertiary integration center involved in the dorsal attention system and in reading, visuoconstruction, and mental imagery. Medial to the sulcus, the superior parietal cortex can be found, and lesions here may lead to optic ataxia. Along the intraparietal sulcus, the motor coordinates of different body parts are integrated with visual information. Thus lesions inside these regions may lead to ideomotor apraxia, but also mental rotation deficits, the inability to copy complex figures, and specific forms of body neglect.

Fig. 2.13 showing a stroke of the right angular branch of the MCA (the stroke area starts directly anterior to the intraparietal sulcus, Fig. 2.13: Line column 1.4 and 1.5 and 2.1).

2.1.4.6.1 Using MRIcron to localize the intraparietal sulcus

Going back to the starting position of the sulcus parieto-occipitalis at x = 109, y = 46, z = 118, another sulcus can be found, directly lateral to the most lateral extension of the sulcus parieto-occipitalis (x = 62, y = 48, z = 118). This sulcus changes the direction first running in an anterior direction and then turning to the left and splitting into two different rami. At the position of x = 44, y = 87, z = 128, the sulcus joins with another sulcus, which is the postcentral sulcus.

2.1.4.7 *The central sulcus*

The next major sulcus of the cerebrum is the central sulcus. This is difficult to locate on clinical scans. The central sulcus starts at its most

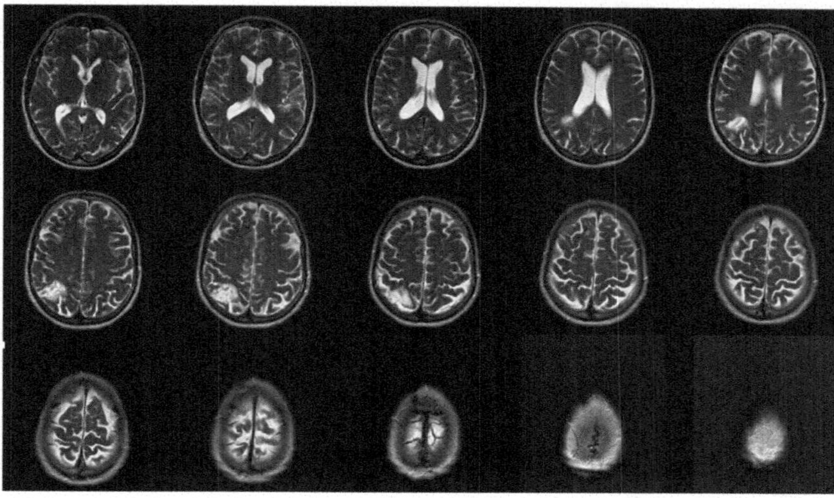

FIGURE 2.13 Stroke of the right angularis branch of the middle cerebral artery.

dorsal position lateral to the interhemispheric fissure without reaching the interhemispheric fissure completely, because of technical problems in visualizing the most dorsal millimeters of the brain. The position then moves on a series of transverse sections slightly in an anterior position.

There are three different features that can be used to identify the central sulcus. The first one is related to the two adjacent sulci, the precentral sulcus and the postcentral sulcus. Together, they form a structure of three parallel lateral sulci, which are visible on the dorsal transverse section. The central sulcus is the one in the middle of these three sulci. The second characteristic is the existence of the hand knob. Due to the fine motor performance humans can execute, the motor representation of the hand needs a place. We know from the homunculus that the representation of the hand follows that of the leg and body after about one-third of its extension from dorsal to ventral. This means that on the level of the corona radiata, that is, dorsal to the tip of the lateral ventricle, a half-circle (the hand knob) should be present (Fig. 2.14).

There is a third feature, which is very helpful for localizing the central sulcus. This feature is based on the representation of the superior frontal sulcus in transverse MRI or cCT sections. The superior frontal sulcus is a deep sulcus starting lateral to the interhemispheric fissure, becoming visible approximately on the same image, which shows the hand knob. It runs from anterior to posterior and can be recognized as a deep sulcus parallel to the interhemispheric fissure (visible in Fig. 2.5, line 1 column 2 or line 1 column 4 or Fig. 2.15, line 1 column 2, line 1 column 3; a closer view also shows the hand knob in 1.3). It divides the superior frontal gyrus from the middle frontal gyrus. The superior frontal sulcus divides

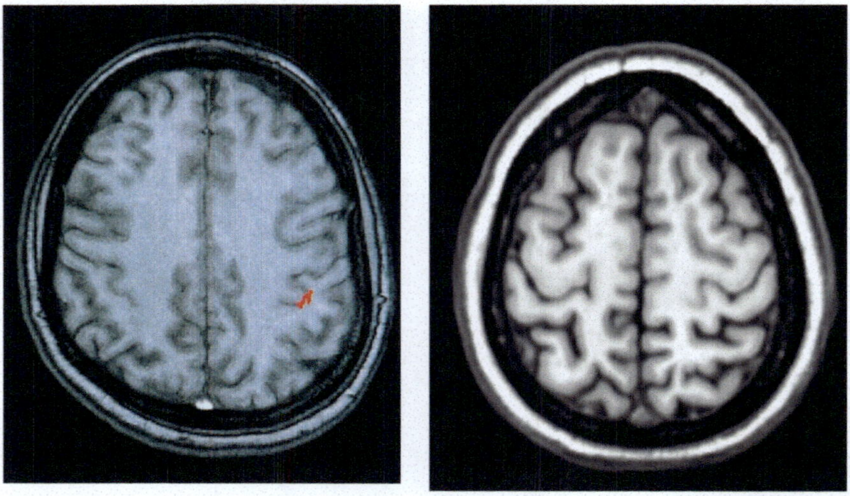

FIGURE 2.14 Hand knob of the central sulcus. Yousry, Schmid, Alkadhi, Schmidt, Peraud, Buettner and Winkler [7].

coarsely between those parts of the frontal cortex supplied by the MCA and the ACA. Medial to the superior frontal sulcus, supplied by the ACA, the representation of the leg, the supplementary motor cortex, and the presupplementary motor cortex can be found. Lesions of the supplementary motor cortex are often accompanied by akinetic symptoms, motor neglect (right hemisphere) or mutism (left hemisphere), and apathy (we will discuss these syndromes in Chapter 9). Caudal to this sulcus, the premotor and motor cortex are located. Anterior and more ventrally, the superior frontal sulcus borders the frontal pole and the Brodmann areas 9 and 10, which are important for action planning abilities.

Now, the posterior extension of the superior frontal sulcus reaches the precentral sulcus but not the central sulcus. Tracing this sulcus on the different transverse sections from dorsal to ventral, therefore allows us to identify the precentral sulcus, and the central sulcus is the next one in the posterior direction. Related to Fig. 2.15 line 1 column 2 shows the superior frontal sulcus with the largest posterior extension. Therefore we expect that the sulcus ends at the precentral sulcus. On the same image, three parallel sulci can be recognized, and the central sulcus is the one in the middle, which fits the expectation based on the extension of the superior frontal sulcus. Image 1.3 shows the hand knob; therefore we can be as sure as possible on the basis of a clinical MRI scan that this sulcus is the central sulcus. All parts anterior to the central sulcus then belong to the frontal cortex, and the parts posterior to the parietal cortex as long as not the temporal or the occipital lobe is reached.

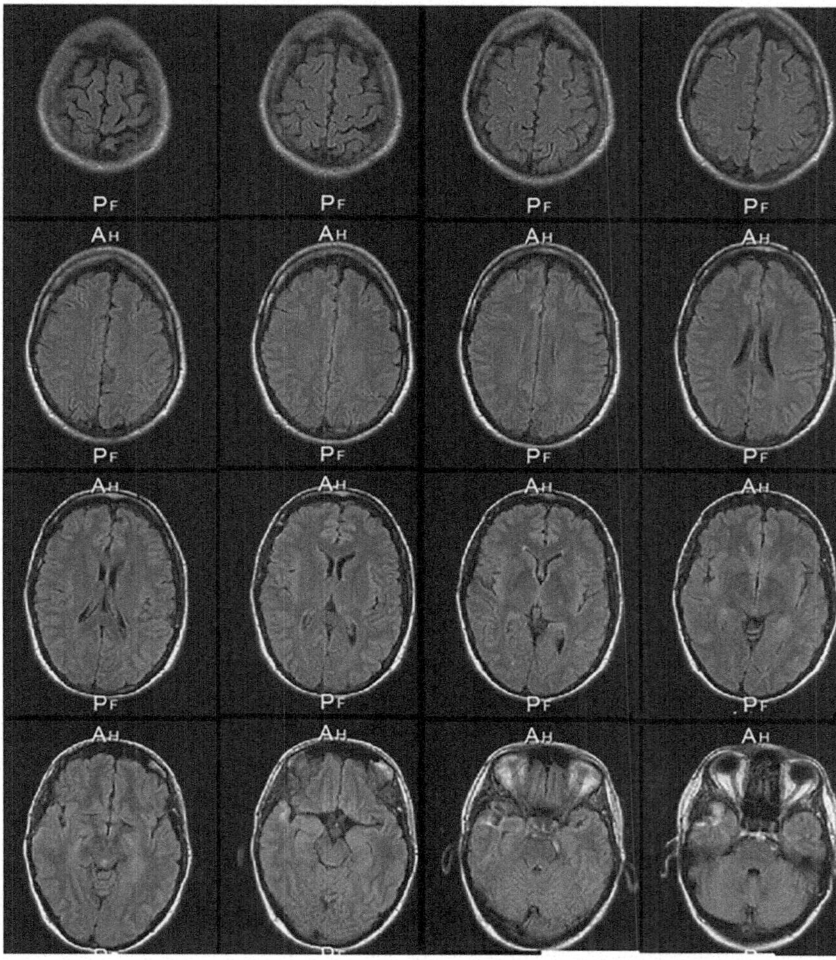

FIGURE 2.15 Clinical example for localizing the central sulcus.

2.1.4.7.1 Using MRIcron to learn the position of the central sulcus and the supplementary motor cortex

In the following, we will use the three landmarks for the identification of the central sulcus in MRIcron. If we start at a z-level of 130, we can easily detect two of them: first, there are three parallel sulci running in a medial direction (first at the position of x = 132, y = 119, and z = 130; second: x = 130, y = 98, and z=130, third: x = 127, y = 85, z = 130). Moreover, there is a sulcus running in the anterior part of the image parallel to the interhemispheric fissure on the left of the image. This is the superior frontal sulcus. Now this sulcus does not reach the second of the three sulci, which one should be the central sulcus. To check if this first identification is in accordance with the third landmark, we move to z-level 132, where at x = 119, y = 84, and z = 132, the hand knob, a distinctive feature of the precentral gyrus, can be found. This fits the results of the two other characteristics. Now, use the MRIcron yoked version to look if the identification based on clinical characteristics was correct.

As already mentioned at x = 70, y = 130, z = 130, the superior frontal sulcus is located. This sulcus can be traced down to z = 117 and upwards to x = 60, y = 123, z = 139. Most of the areas between the left and the right superior frontal sulcus belong to the supplementary motor cortex, which extends even more dorsally until z = 151.

2.1.4.8 *Dividing the prefrontal and orbitofrontal cortex*

Another important subdivision inside the frontal cortex is that between the prefrontal cortex and the orbitofrontal cortex. Whereas the prefrontal cortex is related to conditional learning, working memory, and planning, the orbitofrontal cortex biases decision-making and is involved in the processing of basic needs and emotions. There is only a rule of thumb at which level the orbitofrontal cortex ends, and the prefrontal cortex starts. This is especially the case because the distal parts of each transverse image are strongly influenced by the angle at which images are acquired. Now, this angle is more rotated downwards in cCTs than in MRI scans (and the realignment of MRI scans with both commissures is in clinical images far from being perfect). This means that the orbitofrontal cortex related to a central position (e.g., the thalamus) will start earlier in MRI scans compared to cCT scans. Nevertheless, the anterior commissure is located at a level where caudally the orbitofrontal cortex starts, whereas dorsally the prefrontal cortex is located. The anterior commissure is a fiber tract that connects the two hemispheres at the level of the most ventral thalamic structures. Because it is small, the connection between the hemispheres is invisible. Still, the MRI shows a long, somewhat curved line, representing the anterior commissure and being visible on Fig. 2.16 on the left just dorsal to the hypothalamus. The frontal parts ventrally to this section are images of the orbitofrontal cortex, whereas the images dorsally show the prefrontal cortex.

2.1.4.8.1 Using MRIcron to learn the position of the anterior commissure

The anterior commissure is visible in MRIcron at x = 91, y = 131, z = 67 as a light line connecting both hemispheres. It is possible to localize different segments of the orbitofrontal cortex (inferior, medial, superior, Gyrus rectus) by scrolling through the z levels and looking for the names of the structures in the aal.nii.gz atlas.

Table 2.4 gives an overview of cortical sulci and related areas.

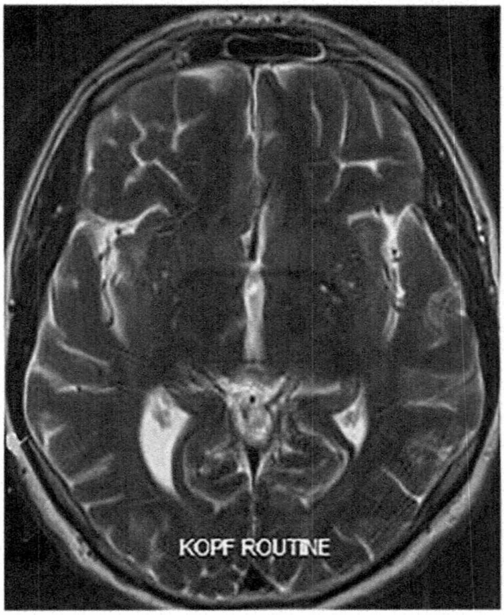

FIGURE 2.16 Anterior commissure as landmark for differentiating the prefrontal and orbitofrontal cortex.

2.1.4.9 Veins and ventricles

2.1.4.9.1 Using MRIcron to visualize the sinuses (veins) of the brain

The sinuses are visible on clinical cMRI scans with high resolution, but also in MRIcron. Using the ch2.nii.gz template and navigating to the x = 92, y = 53, z = 136 coordinates shows the superior sagittal sinus of the brain in the sagittal view (the gray unstructured hem above the sulci). On the coronal images, the superior sagittal sinus is visible at the tip as a gray structure between the brain halves. On the transverse images, it can be found at the most central frontal and posterior positions (x = 93, y = 163, z = 133; x = 98, y = 30, z = 92). The inferior sagittal sinus is visible as a small line starting directly above the cerebellum and running toward the right and upward, almost touching the splenium of the corpus callosum and ending at the dorsal level of the cingulate cortex if one chooses a sagittal view at the position of x = 91, y = 95, z = 118. It is easy to follow the superior sagittal sinus scrolling upwards in the transverse cut until a z-coordinate of 150 and above, observing how the frontal and postcentral parts of the sinus are joining there. Scrolling downward in the transverse cut shows how the different sinuses join posterior to the cerebellum and occipital lobe, starting at the z-level of 54 and flowing into the transverse sinus at the z-level of 46, which then moves down into the direction of the external jugular vein, which can be followed from a z-level of 16 to 8.

TABLE 2.4 Localization of the major cortical sulci and gyri as functional landmarks on clinical brain scans.

Structure	Location in transverse scans	Key characteristics of FLAIR MRI	Reference in figure
Sylvian fissure (fissura sylvii)	Between frontal and temporal lobes	Visible from ventral to dorsal; wedge-shaped lateral border; transforms into the medial sulcus dorsally	Figs. 2.3 and 2.5: Line 2, image 3 to line 3: image 3
Anterior ascending ramus	Branching from the Sylvian fissure, anteriorly	Surrounded by Broca's area; appears as a dorsally running sulcus	Figs. 2.3 and 2.5: Line 2, image 3–5
Broca's area	Left inferior frontal gyrus	Located around anterior ascending ramus; visible as a three parallel sulci pattern lateral to the anterior insula	Fig. 2.5: Line 2, image 3–5
Heschl's gyrus	Within lateral sulcus	Finger-like gyrus starting directly posterior to the dorsal insular cortex	Fig. 2.5: Line 2, image 4–5
Wernicke's area	Posterior to Heschl's gyrus	Located in the superior and middle temporal gyri, posterior and ventral to the posterior ascending ramus	Fig. 2.5: Line 2, image 4 to line 3, image 1
posterior ascending ramus	Dorsal extension of the Sylvian fissure	A dorsally oriented sulcus visible on different images at the same position coarsely above Heschl's gyrus	Figs. 2.3 and 2.5: line 2, image 3–5
Supramarginal gyrus	Anterior and posterior to the posterior ascending ramus	Extends dorsally beyond the ascending ramus	Fig. 2.5: Line 2, images 3–5 Line 3, image
Parieto-occipital sulcus	Medial sulcus runs from the parietal cortex toward the ventral splenium	visible first as two parallel, then horizontal sulci moving more and more anterior on more ventral images	Figs. 2.3 and 2.5 Line 2, images 3–5 Line 3, image 1
Cuneus	Posterior to the parieto-occipital sulcus	On images superior to the calcarine sulcus	Fig. 2.5: line 2, images 4–5
Calcarine sulcus	Starts ventral to the splenium	Irregular structure of sulci located medially in the occipital lobe	Figs. 2.3 and 2.5: line 3, images 1–4
Fusiform gyrus	Lateral to cerebellar vermis	Below the calcarine sulcus, first inside the posterior temporal lobe, and more ventrally as its medial-oriented surface	Fig. 2.5: line 3, images 4–5

Collateral sulcus	Sulcus inside the posterior temporal lobe	The orientation is first anterior-posterior, then more ventral, medial to lateral	Fig. 2.5: line 3, images 3–4
Intraparietal sulcus	Two parallel sulci starting in the posterior parietal cortex	Runs anteriorly, then splits and shows anterior and lateral direction	Figs. 2.3 and 2.5: line 1, image 3 to line 2, image 3
Angular gyrus	Lateral to intraparietal sulcus	Starting on images directly above the cingulate cortex, but posteriorly in the parietal lobe	Figs. 2.3 and 2.5: line 1, image 3–5
Central sulcus	Between precentral and postcentral sulci	Identified by three parallel sulci, the hand knob, and the most posterior extension of the sulcus frontalis superior	Fig. 2.5: line 1, image 1 to line 2, image 5
Hand knob	Central sulcus, dorsal levels	Half-circle shape; corresponds to hand motor representation	Figs. 2.5 and 2.14: line 1, image 3
Superior frontal sulcus	Anterior to the precentral sulcus	Starting from the dorsal frontal images and running on several images in a posterior direction	Figs. 2.3 and 2.5: line 1, image 2–4
Supplementary motor area	Most dorsal medial ACA territory	Medial and dorsal to the sulcus frontalis superior	
Orbitofrontal cortex	Ventral of anterior commissure	Anterior to the hypothalamus, posterior and medial to the two eyes	Figs. 2.5 and 2.16: line 3, image 2–4
Prefrontal cortex	Dorsal of anterior commissure	Anterior to the precentral gyrus	Fig. 2.5: line 1, image 2 to line 3, image 1

2.1.4.9.2 Using MRIcron to visualize the foramen of Monroi, the third and fourth ventricles

The lateral ventricle is readily recognizable, and, therefore it is not necessary to localize it with the help of MRIcron.

The foramen of Monro can be easily detected in MRIcron on a transverse cut of z = 74. The two symmetrical frontal horns merge at this position with one small structure directly at the center of the brain. This central dark line visible here is the upper boundary of the third ventricle. The line (=third ventricle) is opening a little bit, going down to z = 68, and the posterior border is moving somewhat in the frontal direction.

The third ventricle is easily detected on any brain scan and is an important landmark for a neuroanatomical orientation because it is located medial to the two thalamic nuclei. Between z = 68 and z = 65, a progressively smaller part of the line gets detached, moves posteriorly (as aqueduct), and becomes a larger separated dark structure on z = 51. The smaller structure is called the aqueduct, and it connects the third ventricle with the fourth ventricle. Where it increases in size, the upper part of the fourth ventricle has been reached. Around z = 39, a gray flat-like structure is visible in the lower part of the fourth ventricle. This is the choroid plexus of the fourth ventricle. Just above the plexus, the fourth ventricle communicates with the subarachnoid space (not visible on clinical MRI scans). These openings are called lateral apertures. Around z = 25, the median aperture is visible where the fourth ventricle is opening for a large cistern (black structure posterior to the fourth ventricle).

2.1.5 Localizing brainstem and cerebellar structures in clinical MRIs

2.1.5.1 A coarse orientation for brainstem and cerebellar structures

The parts of the brain ventral to the cerebrum can be divided into the midbrain, pons, medulla oblongata, and cerebellum. Unlike the cerebral cortex, these structures either lack a distinct layered structure or, if layers are present, their arrangement differs significantly from the layered structure of the cortex and its organization into gyri. These neuroanatomical differences will not be discussed in this book. It is enough to mention that these differences are visible when comparing the layers and differentiation of the cerebellum and the cerebral cortex, even in cCT and MRI scans. Figures 2.17 and 2.18 show the structure of the brainstem, cerebellum, and medulla oblongata in a schematic drawing and from a sagittal perspective.

For clinical landmarks, it is important to note that with and ventral to (or better caudal at this level of the brain) the midbrain, the brainstem starts and is enclosed anteriorly by the pons (see Fig. 2.18 (A)). Remember that the pons contains the afferent and efferent fibers of the cerebellum (apart from corticospinal and spinocortical tracts).

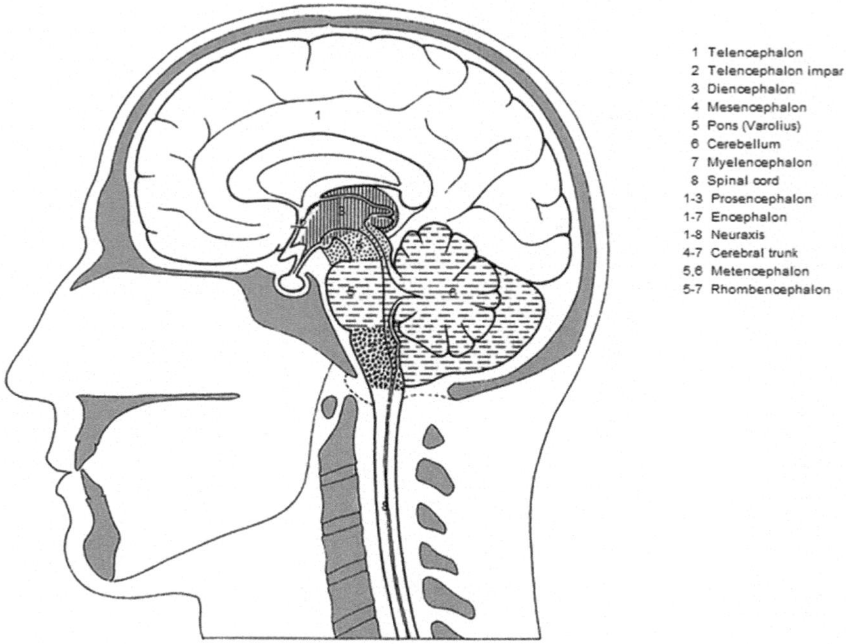

FIGURE 2.17 Sagittal drawing of the brainstem and the cerebellum. *Nieuwenhuys [5], Fig. 1.2.*

As you move caudally from the midbrain (butterfly-like structure) on transverse slides, there will be an increase in the diameter of the brainstem and a half-circle-like shape at the anterior side of the transverse image—this represents the pons. However, as soon as the medulla oblongata is reached, the brainstem's diameter decreases again, and the half-circle shape structure disappears.

Another important feature visible on this schematic drawing is that the sulci of the cerebellum, which are located posterior to the brainstem, are deep and much more symmetric compared to the somewhat erratic appearance of the cortical sulci (see Fig. 2.18 (B)). This leads to the expectation that images of the cerebellum should display a more homogeneous appearance compared to the cerebral cortex.

There are two other important expectations for transverse images that are based on Fig. 2.18B. This figure shows that there is something like an interhemispheric notch at the most anterior position of the pons, which should be visible on clinical scans. The second expectation is that there should be images where the cerebellum is connected to the pons by a continuous structure, which are termed cerebellar peduncles. There are three cerebellar peduncles: a superior, a middle, and an inferior peduncle.

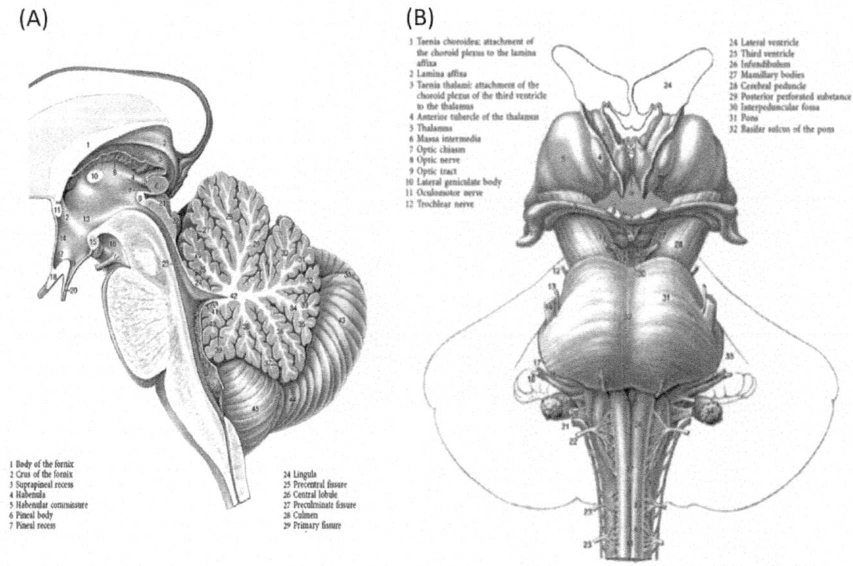

FIGURE 2.18 Two schematic drawings of the pons in (A) sagittal and (B) ventral view. *Nieuwenhuys [5], A: Fig. 3.8 B: Fig. 3.12.*

The superior cerebellar peduncle connects the cerebellum to the midbrain and is mainly efferent. The middle cerebellar peduncles connect the cerebellum to the pons and are composed entirely of afferent fibers. They form the largest of the three cerebellar peduncles and is always visible on clinical cCT and cMRI scans. The inferior cerebellar peduncle occupies the upper part of the medulla oblongata and has mainly afferent but also some efferent fibers. Together, they form the lateral border of the fourth ventricle. The expectation is that the cerebellar peduncles should be visible as continuous structures between the cerebellum and the pons (see Fig. 2.20 (B)).

The next Fig. 2.19 shows transverse clinical images of the midbrain, brainstem, the cerebellum, and the medulla oblongata (Fig. 2.19). The cerebellum becomes visible in line 1 on column 3, just in the center, and is marked by symmetrical sulci. Following this structure on more caudal images allows us to identify the middle cerebellar peduncle, connecting the cerebellum with the pons. It is visible first on line 2, column 1, and most clearly on line 2, column 2. The inferior cerebellar peduncle connecting to the medulla oblongata is visible on line 2, column 3. The cerebellum is the large structure directly posterior to the fourth ventricle in these images.

Having identified the cerebellum and the cerebellar peduncles (it is impossible to distinguish the superior cerebellar peduncle on these clinical images), the next question is where the pons starts and where the medulla

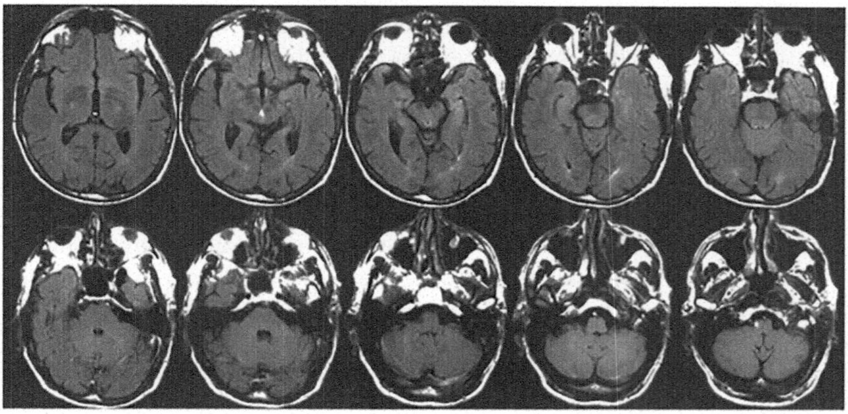

FIGURE 2.19 A transverse clinical scan showing the brainstem and the cerebellum.

oblongata can be found. Now, the pons should appear like a half-circle structure with a notch in the middle surrounding the brainstem. Such a structure is visible on the clinical scan, starting in line 1, column 5, to line 2, column 2. At line 2, column 3, this structure disappears, and an elongated, somewhat more rectangular-like structure becomes visible. This is the level where the transverse images show the medulla oblongata, which can be followed down to the lowest caudal image.

2.1.5.1.1 Using MRIcron to localize coarse structures of the midbrain and brainstem

The midbrain starts from a dorsal position at the level of z = 66, where the superior colliculi can be distinguished at x = 88, y = 97. Moreover, the most dorsal part of the vermis (the coarse structure of the cerebellum is discussed in Chapter 1) is shown around x = 90, y = 76, z = 66. At level z = 53 the midbrain transitions into the pons/brainstem, and two millimeters below at x = 98, y = 89, z = 51, the superior cerebellar peduncle can be found. Moreover, posterior to the peduncle, the different structure of the sulci and gyri of the cerebellum compared to the cerebrum becomes evident. At level z = 42, the large middle cerebellar peduncles and the inferior border of the fourth ventricle laterally are visible. The pons starts to vanish at level z = 29 and to disappear at z = 23. At this level, the transverse images only display the medulla oblongata.

2.1.5.2 Localization of cranial nerves in the brainstem

Ten of the 12 cranial nerves are located in the brainstem. Increasing the resolution of the clinical scan of Fig. 2.19 and focusing on line 1, image 3, and line 2, image 1, each shows a very tiny gray line running in a posterior-anterior direction in front of or adjacent to the midbrain or brainstem. These tiny structures represent the third (oculomotor) and the fifth (trigeminal) cranial nerve.

Lesions of the cranial nerves produce enduring and clinically well-defined impairments. Figure 2.20 shows schematically the localization of cranial nerves related to the surface of the brainstem. Two of the three cranial nerves responsible for eye movements exit the midbrain; all other cranial nerves exit more caudally. One of these two eye movement nerves is the trochlear nerve, and this is the only nerve that exits in a posterior direction before curving around the midbrain to reach the two eyes. The other cranial nerve is the oculomotor nerve. These two nerves join to travel to the two eyes, before they split again to innervate different eye muscles.

There is only one cranial nerve that exits the pons, which, moreover, is the largest in diameter: this is the trigeminal nerve, mainly responsible for tactile and pain perception of the face. The next three nerves can be found directly at the transition of the pons to the medulla oblongata, whereby the nuclei of these nerves are located inside the pons (but not their exit). These nerves are the abducens nerve (horizontal eye movements, moving the eyes laterally), the facial nerve, and the vestibulocochlear nerve. The ninth to 12th cranial nerves exit the medulla oblongata. A short description of the functional consequence of lesions involving these cranial nerves can be found in Chapter 1. Clinical MRI scans only occassionally show some of these nerves, but their localization can be traced in MRIcron at least for the most important one.

2.1.5.2.1 Using MRIcron to localize cranial nerves

Starting from the level of the medulla oblongata and moving in a rostral (upward) direction, the first cranial nerve becomes visible as two medially curved lines leaving the medulla for taking a lateral direction ($x = 80$, $y = 92$, $z = 16$). Because the starting point of the nerve is on the front of the medulla, this is the 12th cranial nerve, called hypoglossal nerve. Lesions related to this cranial nerve will induce immobility of the tongue and a swallowing disorder. At $x = 105$, $y = 93$, $z = 94$, the next cranial nerve can be detected. It starts more dorsally from the posterior part of the medulla, which argues that this is the 10th cranial nerve, the vagus nerve. The vagus nerve is part of the parasympathetic nervous system and controls several autonomic functions, but also regulates the swallowing process. It coordinates the movements of the tongue, throat muscles, and esophagus to ensure smooth and efficient passage of food and liquids. At the transition zone between the medulla and the pons, which is located between $z = 28$ and $z = 30$, different cranial nerves exit the brainstem. From a posterior position, the vestibulocochlear nerve is visible at $x = 106$, $y = 91$, $z = 28$ on the left, and on $z = 29$ on both sides.

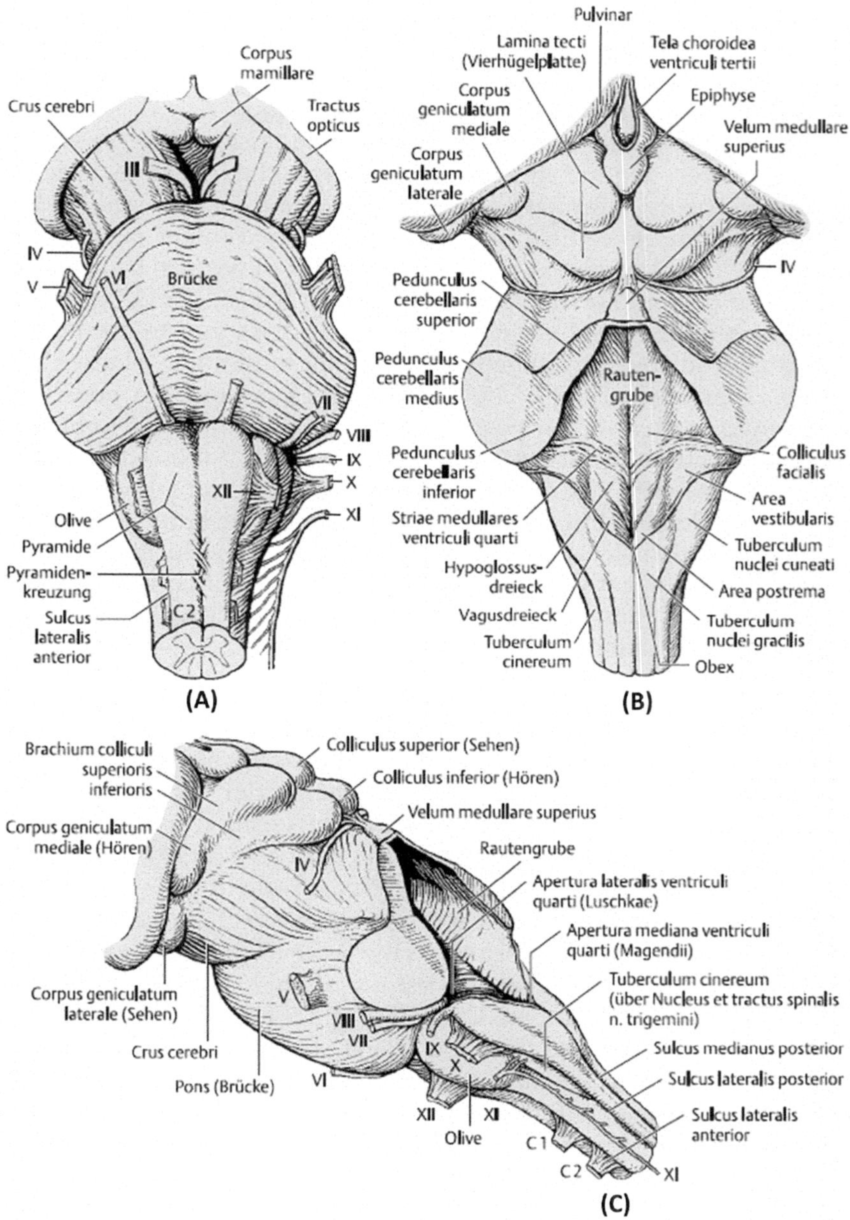

FIGURE 2.20 Different views of the brainstem and cranial nerves Bähr and Bechmann [4] Abb. 4.1.

A lesion of this cranial nerve will cause unilateral hearing loss and balance problems. It is also possible to detect the sixth cranial nerve exiting from a ventral position on x = 82, y = 110, z = 28. This nerve is responsible for moving the eye into a lateral position.

At z = 38, the trigeminal nerve can be found, a cranial nerve with a large diameter, exiting the pons laterally. The trigeminal nerve processes sensory information of the face, head, and tongue, and is involved in muscle control for chewing. The two upper oculomotor nerves, the trochlear nerve and the oculomotor nerve, can be found at z = 50. The oculomotor nerve is displayed at x = 85, y = 118. Moving one or two images in the caudal direction, allows you to see how it originates from the ventromedial part of the midbrain, whereas the trochlear nerve (x = 79, y = 117, z = 50) curves around the pons and midbrain to reach a similar position as the oculomotor nerve to project into the direction of the eye, which can be nicely followed scrolling down to z = 44 (x90, y = 127). Lesions of these two cranial nerves will lead to well-defined but different eye movement disorders. It should be mentioned that strokes involving the cranial nerves, or their nuclei, directly show a negative prognosis for the function involved, because in most respects, there are no compensatory mechanisms that could be used for rehabilitation.

2.1.5.3 Core and lateral brainstem structures

From a clinical point of view, the following structures of the brainstem are of interest. First of all, the nuclei surrounding the aqueduct which remain in a similar medial position as long as the pons are visible. These inner parts of the brainstem host serotonergic and noradrenergic nuclei, which play a major role in pain perception, mood, and wakefulness (compare Chapter 1). Second, the corticospinal tract ("pyramidal tract") is located in the anterior part of the pons and the medulla oblongata. Bilateral lesions of this tract will induce a locked-in syndrome (compare Chapter 1 and 9 for a description).

Chapter 1 discusses the core and lateral structures of the brainstem. Although of immense significance for the clinical picture of the patients, these structures cannot be differentiated directly by cMRI scanning, and cCT scanning gives even less information about the localization of these centers. For localizing the lesions, it is necessary to transfer relative positions from schematic drawings on atlases to the clinical cMRI scans. Chapter 1 shows several such drawings or pictures from nonusual MRI scans, which can be used for such a comparison (see Fig. 2.21).

For the localization in clinical cMRI images, the following features are important. The aqueduct can be used to find the periaqueductal gray matter, which should also look gray on FLAIR scans. The second feature is that the

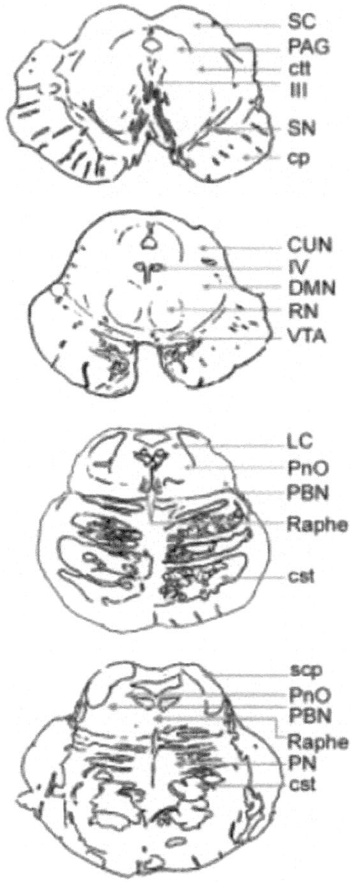

FIGURE 2.21 Schematic transverse section through the brainstem Parvizi and Damasio [8]. The upper picture starts at the level of the midbrain and is rotated 180 degrees compared to the usual view on a clinical MRI scan. Abbreviations: SC, colliculus superior; PAG, periaqueductal gray matter; III, oculomotorius nucleus; SN, substantia nigra; cp, cerebral peduncles; CUN, nucleus cuneiformis; IV, nucleus trochlearis; DMN, nucleus dorsomedialis; RN, Raphe nucleus; VTA, ventral tegmental area; LC, locus coeruleus; PnO, Oral pontine nucleus; PBN, nucleus parabrachialis; cst, corticospinal tract; scp, pedunculus cerebelli superior.

part of the brainstem is separated from the pons, which is lighter, and only encompasses a small area anterior to the fourth ventricle. Thirdly, the nuclei relevant for the release of noradrenaline and serotonin are located medially in the brainstem, and the corticospinal and spinocortical tracts are located inside the pons. Moreover, not displayed on the figure on the left, the pyramidal tract moves into a rostral position at the level of the medulla oblongata.

2.1.5.3.1 Using MRIcron to localize some focal midbrain and brainstem structures

The first image of Fig. 2.21 (above) corresponds with level z = 64 in MRIcron using the ch2.nii.gz template. The aqueduct is located at x = 92, y = 98, z = 64, and it is surrounded by an area somewhat distinguished by dark gray, which is the periaqueductal gray matter, important for pain perception and regulation of combined autonomic responses. At x = 83, y = 113, z = 64, a shallow diagonal line is visible, which indicates the position of the substantia nigra. The second image of Fig. 2.21 roughly corresponds to z = 60 of the ch2.nii.gz template. At this level, the ventral tegmental area, a structure rich in dopamine-expressing neurons, is visible as a curved diagonal line at x = 83, y = 114, z = 60. The z levels of the next two pictures cannot be indicated in MRIcron, because the transverse slice orientation deviates and there are no clear-cut features which could be used for a comparison. As already mentioned, the pons starts at z = 50, and the separation between the pons and the rest of the brainstem is visible in MRIcron, because the pons looks somewhat brighter than the brainstem. Moreover, the brainstem is located directly anterior to the fourth ventricle. The pyramidal tract can be localized again caudal to the pons as two light oval structures in front of the medulla oblongata, for example, at x = 88, y = 97, z = 22.

2.2 Clinical examples and how to use MRIcron to localize strokes on cranial magnetic resonance imaging and cranial computed tomography

2.2.1 Clinical examples

In the following section, multiple examples of stroke lesions as visualized through clinical cCT and cMRI scans will be discussed. These examples aim to illustrate the typical patterns and characteristics of brain lesions caused by stroke, highlighting how different types of strokes can be identified using imaging techniques.

For training localization on clinical images, the reader is invited to reconstruct the lesion on the appropriate MRIcron slices. Please, remember when doing this that the distance between the images of clinical scans is about 6–10 mm, whereas the distance between images in MRIcron is 1 mm. Therefore, you must leave out 6–10 images in MRIcron to reach the next images of a clinical scan. How to use MRIcron to localize the brain lesions is described above.

2.2.1.1 Case study 1: right MCA stroke

Figs. 2.22 and 2.23 show the lesion of the same patient in two different cCT scans in a postacute situation and 10 days later. The right middle cerebral

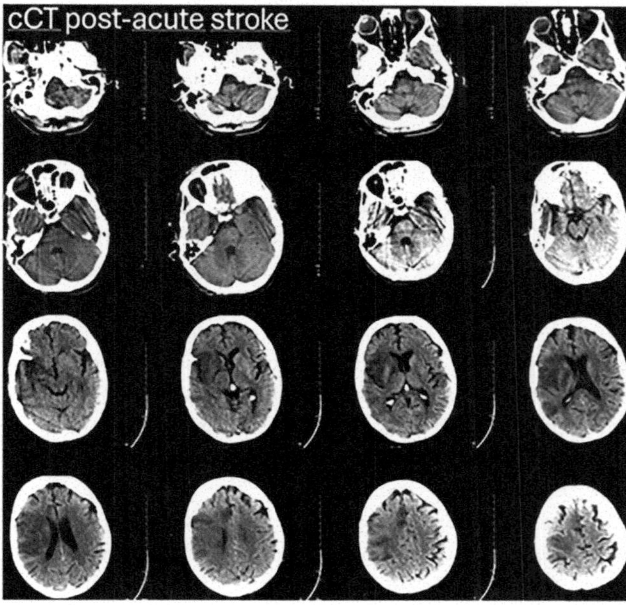

FIGURE 2.22 Large right middle cerebral artery stroke early in the post-acute phase.

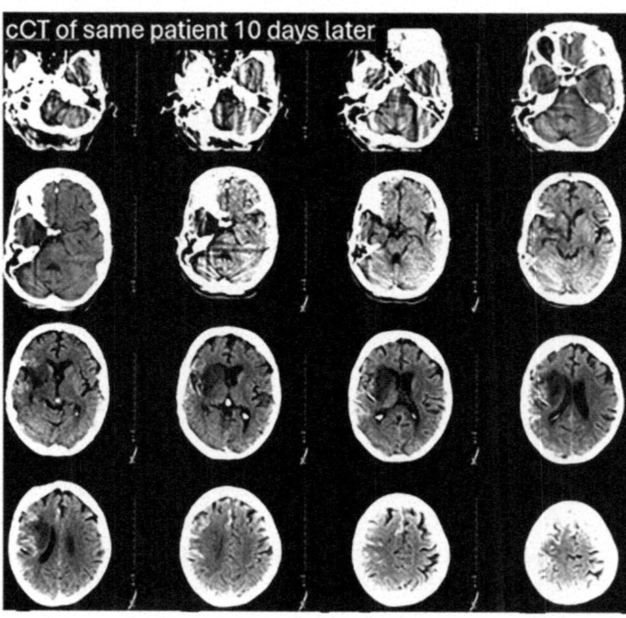

FIGURE 2.23 Large right middle cerebral artery stroke ten days later.

artery stroke is visible on the left side of the different slices (in clinical scanning, the brain halves are mirrored). One already sees the stroke by the relatively darker brain areas, starting dorsally on the picture in the lower right corner (Fig. 2.22, line 4, image 4) and then up to the third row on the outermost left images, showing a section through the midbrain. For the interpretation of a cCT scan, it is also important to mention the indirect signs visible: the effaced sulci on the left (right half of the cerebrum), especially for the dorsal slices, and compared to the right, which indicate stroke-related brain swelling in these regions. If such swelling reaches a specific intensity, it might compress vessels and induce additional damage to the brain. Secondly, the somewhat compressed lateral ventricle (long black symmetrical medial structure running from rostral to caudal). Ten days later, the sulci start to open again on the left. The lateral ventricles are still somewhat crushed, but the head of the patient is also a little bit turned, which contributes to a different width.

There is another important difference between the two cCT scans, and this difference is that the orientation of the transverse images varies between scans due to a lack of precise landmarks for the alignment of sections. The whole second row of the second scan shows the frontal cortex, which is even visible on the outermost right slide of the first row. Now, on the first scan 10 days earlier, the frontal cortex is visible only on the outermost right image of the second row. This shows the impact the tilting of the transverse orientation has in presenting rostral and caudal brain structures of the same cut with a reference to the midbrain (see Fig. 2.4).

Fig. 2.23 shows that the post-acute, right-hemisphere stroke involved the head of the caudate, putamen, and globus pallidus, the centrum semiovale, corona radiata, and the anterior insula. There is also a small chronic stroke of the right posterior cerebral artery. Note that on the level of mid-brain structure the frontal cortex is not visible anymore in direct contrast to Fig. 2.23.

2.2.1.2 Case study 2; Chronic stroke of the left middle cerebral artery and sub-acute stroke of the right posterior cerebral artery

The next figure shows a FLAIR sequence of another patient. The butterfly-like structure of the midbrain is visible in the third line, third column from the left. Here, again, the ventral level of the frontal cortex is reached as in Fig. 2.22 but not in Fig. 2.23: further inferior images do not show the frontal cortex anymore.

The cMRI of Fig. 2.24 documents two strokes for different time points. On the right side (left brain half), there is an old MCA stroke of one of the frontal branches. The sign for a *chronic* stroke is the presence of a scar: a very light and sharp structure adjacent to black holes. Microglia are building a wall around the stroke to protect against inflammation and CSF leakage. In the postcentral part of the slides, one also sees light areas, without black

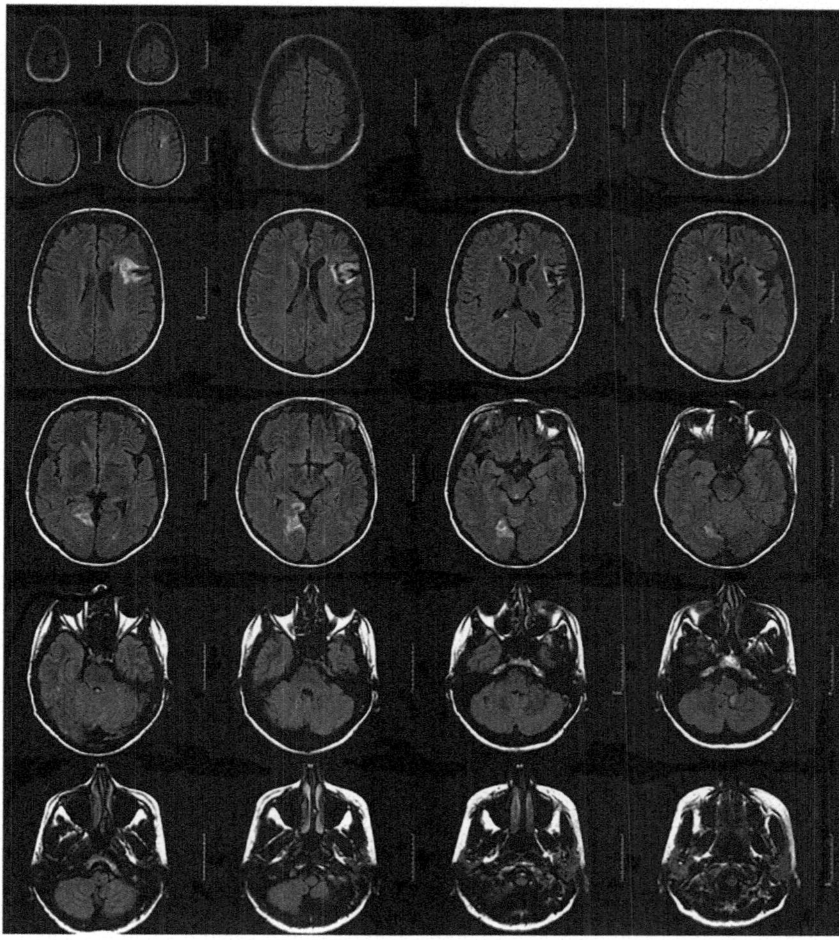

FIGURE 2.24 Post acute stroke of the right posterior cerebral artery and chronic stroke of the left middle cerebral artery.

holes, and not as white as in the frontal cortex. This is how postacute stroke is represented on FLAIR images.

The acute stroke is localized in the ventral part of the lingual cortex and the fusiform gyrus; the chronic lesion involves the anterior and superior parts of the insular and also Broca's area.

2.2.1.3 Case study 3: right hemisphere MCA stroke

Figure 2.25 shows a cMRI scan of a right hemisphere MCA stroke of the parietal and temporal branches (Fig. 2.25). Obviously, some anastomoses were able to rescue parts of the rostral middle and superior

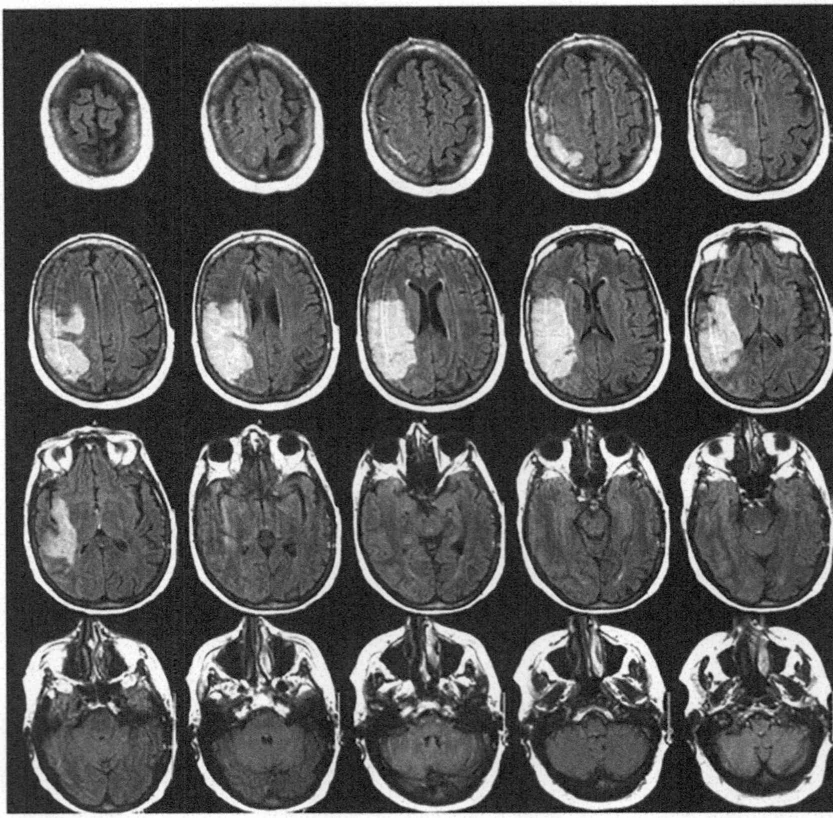

FIGURE 2.25 Large right hemisphere middle cerebral artery stroke.

temporal lobe, which are usually also supplied by the MCA. Now, involving these branches of the MCA means that one should expect sensory (and motor) deficits of the left body half, maybe sparing the leg and foot, because their areas are supplied by the ACA and consequently not involved in the stroke. Moreover, because the right parietal cortex is involved, one would also expect contralateral visuospatial neglect and problems with mental rotation and visuospatial construction. The patient might suffer from hemianopia or at least a field loss of the left lower quadrant, because the upper part of the optic radiation is involved (image line 3, column 1). Moreover, decreased prosody and decreased understanding of complex messages may be a consequence.

2.2.1.4 Case study 4: MCA stroke in the anterior right insular cortex

The next example of an MCA stroke on Fig. 2.26 demonstrates a lesion in the anterior right insular cortex (Fig. 2.26). It is a relatively small lesion, and the right anterior insula does not have (primarily) cognitive functions. Therefore one would expect unimpaired test results. Please note that there are also only a few unremarkable signs of microangiopathy in the white matter, which also argues against any cognitive impairment. On the other hand, the anterior right insula plays a major role in the regulation of autonomic responses, for example, for the rhythmicity of the heart rate, pain evaluation, and other somatic markers. Thus in these patients, the risk for heart attacks is increased.

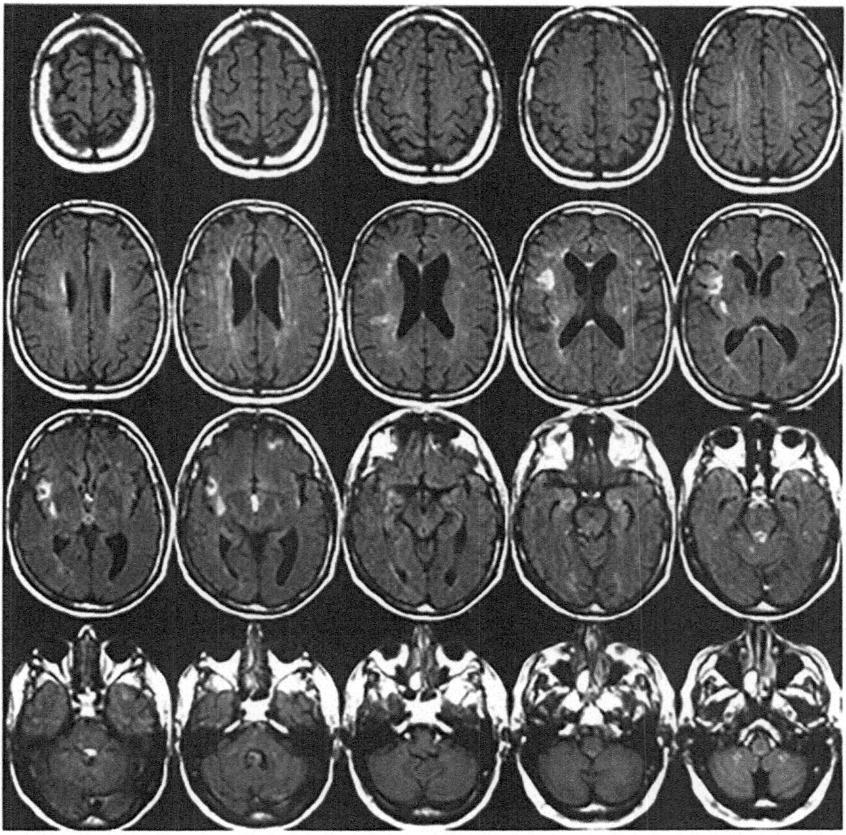

FIGURE 2.26 Small stroke of the right insular cortex.

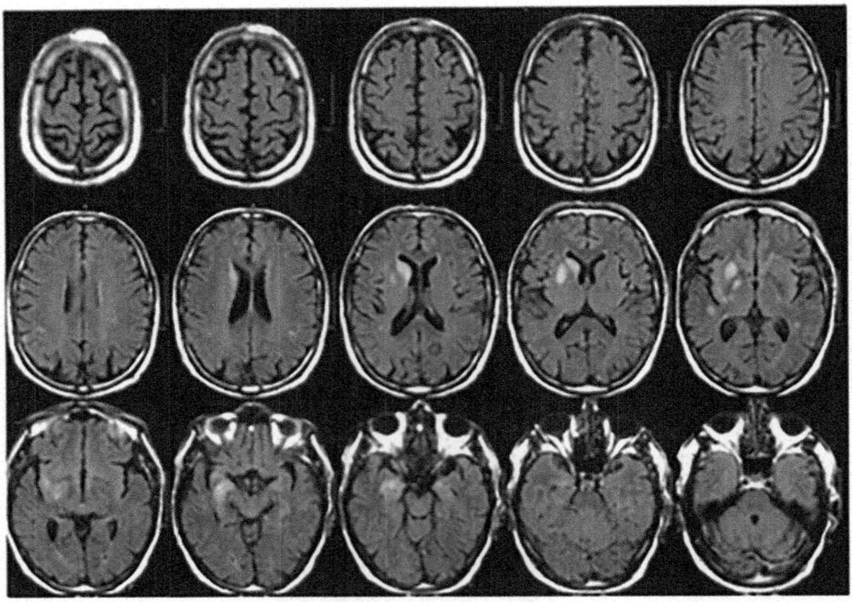

FIGURE 2.27 Right basal ganglia stroke.

2.2.1.5 *Case study 5: right hemisphere basal ganglia stroke*

The last clinical example (see Fig. 2.27) shows a T2 dark trim cMRI scan of a right hemisphere basal ganglia stroke (Fig. 2.27). The lesion involves the head of the caudate nucleus, the anterior part of the body of the caudate, the anterior compartments of the putamen, and also the posterior part of the internal capsule. The ventral structures of the head of the caudate are spared from the stroke. This arrangement argues that an anterolateral branch of the right MCA was involved. The scan also shows a typical consequence of successful thrombolysis and thrombectomy. There are some cortical spots located in the right insular cortex, and the medial temporal pole, but not in any other branches of the MCA, arguing for effective collateral anastomoses to prevent extended cortical damage.

2.2.2 How to use MRIcron to localize clinical brain lesions: two examples

Let's use the clinical MCA FLAIR image of case study 4, introduced above, for a first training of neuroanatomical knowledge on the localization of lesions in clinical MRI scans (Fig. 2.26).

The scan shows a right hemisphere MCA stroke located in the insula and a small left frontal lesion (on the right side of the image, visible on row 3, column 3 and 4). To find out where the small left hemisphere hyperintensity is located, we first have to find the z-coordinates of the corresponding MRI slices in MRIcron. The z-level, shown above the MRI scans and below the menu of MRIcron, indicates the position of a transverse image according to the dorsoventral dimension. The z-coordinate can be changed either in the z-coordinate window below the MRI images or by clicking on the transverse images and using the up and down arrow keys. Please note that clinical MRIs have an interslice spacing/slice interval between 6–10 mm, whereas in MRIcron, the distance between the images is exactly 1 mm. Therefore, adjusting the level in MRIcron means looking for a probable z-level. To increase neuroanatomical transfer learning, one should focus only on the transverse slices, which can be achieved in the MRIcron view menu, under "display" and activating "axial only."

Now, which exact z-coordinate corresponds to one of the images showing the left frontal lesion? The choice of that coordinate must be based on the clinical landmarks we introduced before. One landmark, which is helpful for orienting in this case, is the choroid plexus of the lateral ventricle, which produces the CSF of the brain (compare Chapter 1, on ventricles, veins, and cisterns). The choroid plexus can be seen at a z-level of 92. It is the gray structure inside the black lateral ventricles in the center of the image. You will find the corresponding structure in line two, image four of the clinical example. This image also shows the genu and the splenium of the corpus callosum, which can be seen in the clinical MRI scan. Using this as a reference, the next dorsal clinical image corresponds to a z-coordinate of 100, and the two ventral images to $z = 84$ and $z = 76$ (with an in-between image distance of 8 mm). The visible hyper-intense area in the left frontal cortex, visible on row 3, column 2, should therefore be found on a z-level of 68 (Fig. 2.28). If you go to the z-coordinate in MRIcron, you will see that the two brains differ, and probably also the angle of the transverse slices. But still, it is possible to localize the hyperintensity on the scale of gyri. Clicking on the analogous position in MRIcron (left side of Fig. 2.29) gives you information about the corresponding z-value shown on the right side of Fig. 2.29: it is the left superior frontal cortex (remember that in clinical scans the sides are exchanged) as displayed at the upper left of the right figure.

Now, use the z-coordinates and the mouse to click in MRIcron on those positions that are the hyperintense stroke structures of the right hemisphere. This will give you the information about where it is located. For example, on z-level 84 (Fig 2.29), corresponding to row 2, column 5 of the clinical MRI scan (Fig. 2.26), you will find that the stroke involved the right insular cortex, and it is restricted to this area for all the other slides (again on the top left of the right figure). Now, think about which consequences you expect the patient to suffer from.

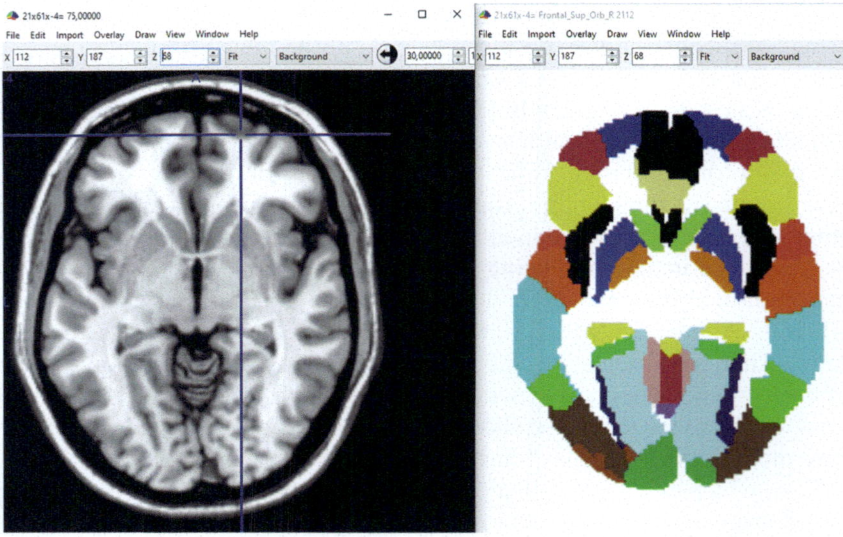

FIGURE 2.28 Reconstruction of the small left hemisphere lesion of Figure 2.26 in MRIcron.

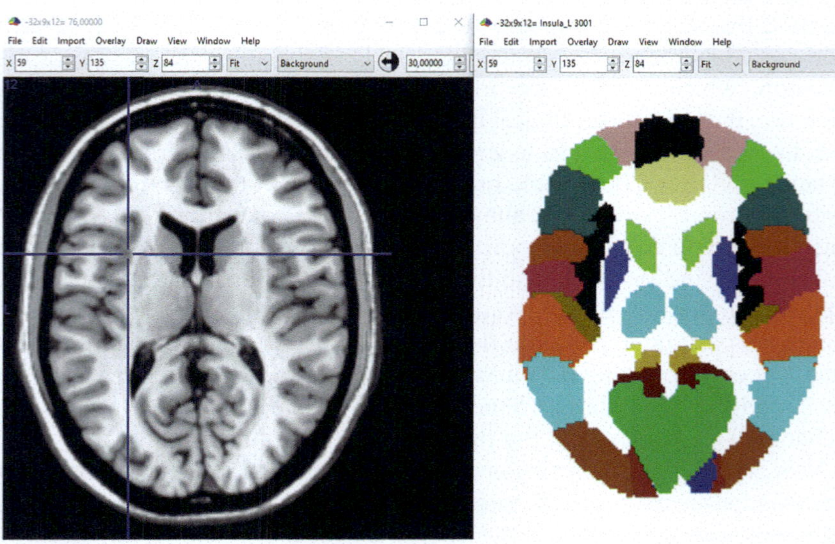

FIGURE 2.29 Reconstruction of the insular cortex lesion of Figure 2.26 in MRIcron.

For the second case, we will use Fig. 2.30.

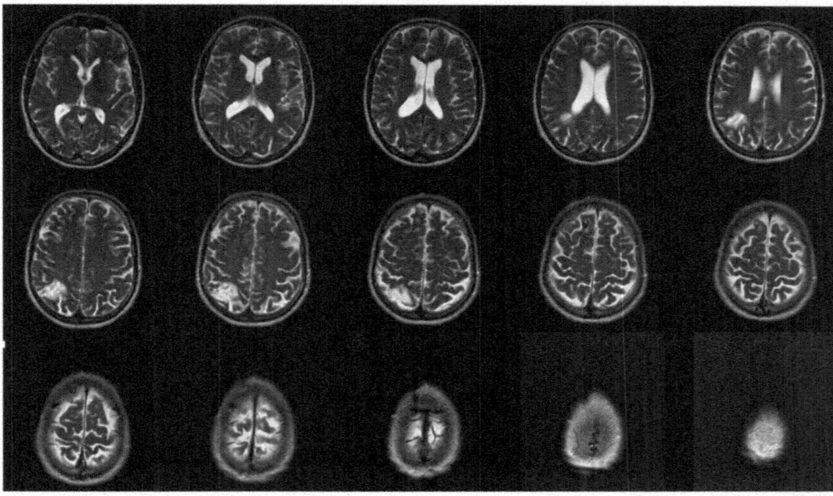

FIGURE 2.30 Right parietal stroke lesion used as example for localizing the lesion.

In this case, the MRI scan was done in the chronic phase, months after the stroke, and the main question was about its precise extent. The patient who suffered this stroke was a surgeon and the question was whether he would be able to work again in his profession. Therefore the distance between two slices is relatively small. If we use the choroid plexus as a landmark, image 3 of the first line gives us the information about the corresponding z-coordinate of 92 for MRIcron. Now, the first clear sign of the stroke can be found in row 2, the first image, which then corresponds to a z-coordinate of 104, 110, 116, and 122. Transferring the position of the stroke from the clinical scan to the MRIcron templates shows that the stroke is localized inside the angular gyrus and the superior parietal gyrus of the right hemisphere. This suggests possible cognitive deficits, for example, in visuo-construction and alertness. One might also think of optic ataxia for grasping with the left hand toward the left when holding a central fixation.

Repeat that with the other clinical images, and this will give you a first feeling of finding neuroanatomical structures in the brain.

2.2.3 Summary and knowledge test

Test your knowledge, use MRIcron to localize, and try to localize the stroke areas of the following figure (Fig. 2.31). Which arteries are involved? What will be the main clinical syndromes of the patient? Is there a lesion of the orbitofrontal cortex?

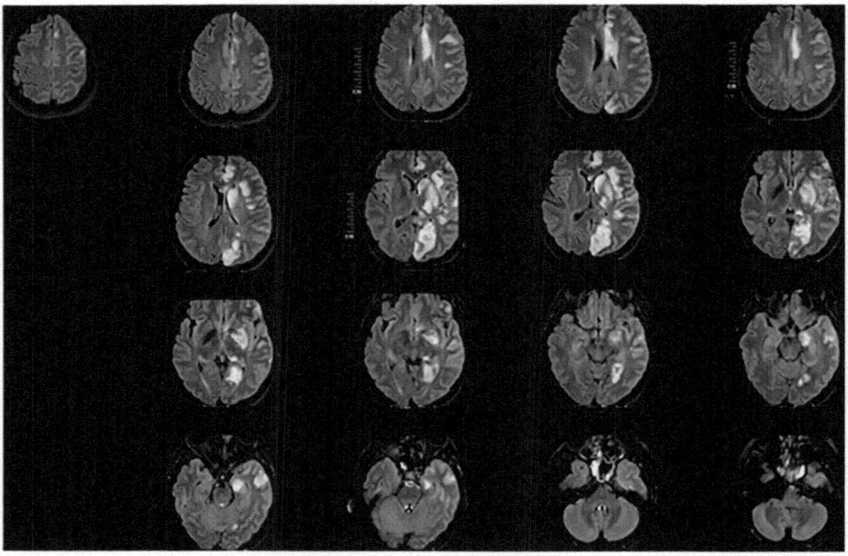

FIGURE 2.31 Training example for practicing lesion localization.

References

[1] McCarthy RA, Warrington EK. Cognitive Neuropsychology: A Clinical Introduction. San Diego: Academic Press; 1990.

[2] Kolb B, Whishaw IQ. Fundamentals of Human Neuropsychology. New York: Worth Publishers/Macmillan Learning; 2021.

[3] Prosiegel M, Paulig M, Böttger S, Radau J, Winkler P. Klinische Hirnanatomie. Funktion und Störung Zentralnervöser Strukturen. Bad Kissingen: Pflaum; 2002.

[4] Bähr M., Bechmann I. Neurologisch-topische diagnostik: Anatomie - funktion - klinik. *11. überarbeitete Auflage*. Thieme. 2021.

[5] Nieuwenhuys R, Voogd J, Huijzen C, van. The Human Central Nervous System. 4th ed. Berlin: Springer-Verlag; 2008.

[6] Tsivilis D, Vann SD, Denby C, Roberts N, Mayes AR, Montaldi D, et al. A disproportionate role for the fornix and mammillary bodies in recall versus recognition memory. Nat Neurosci 2008;11:834–42.

[7] Yousry TA, Schmid UD, Alkadhi H, Schmidt D, Peraud A, Buettner A, et al. Localization of the motor hand area to a knob on the precentral gyrus. A new landmark. Brain 1997;120(Pt 1):141–57.

[8] Parvizi J, Damasio AR. Neuroanatomical correlates of brainstem coma. Brain 2003;126:1524–36.

CHAPTER

3

How to perform neurorehabilitation: answers based on artificial middle cerebral artery strokes in animals

3.1 Introduction

In 2019, patients with neurological disorders were the third largest group in need of rehabilitation worldwide, and stroke patients had the highest need for neurorehabilitation [1]. As the population ages, the incidence of strokes is expected to rise, making effective neurorehabilitation increasingly important. Despite considerable progress in the treatment of acute stroke, progress in neurorehabilitation has been slow. Basic questions about how to design neurorehabilitation most effectively remain unanswered. This concerns, for example, when to start (very early after the event, early, or late), how intense to intervene (many sessions blocked or dispersed over a longer period), training embedded in everyday activities or focused on specific functional deficits. Additionally, relevant neurobiological outcome parameters are difficult to assess in humans: for example, myelination and remyelination of (perilesional) stroke areas, the basic process of recovery, cannot be measured accurately in living organisms, although new MRI techniques offer some possibilities to estimate myelin concentration in brain structures. Another topic concerns poststroke inflammatory processes around the lesion and inside the brain, which can only be analyzed in animals. Thus as research is limited in depth due to ethical reasons, animal studies are powerful tools to generate plausible hypotheses about basic principles of neurorehabilitation.

Strokes affecting the middle cerebral artery (MCA) are the most common cause of focal brain lesions in humans. Therefore the following studies focus

Applied Neuropsychology of Cerebrovascular Diseases
DOI: https://doi.org/10.1016/B978-0-443-45450-9.00011-4

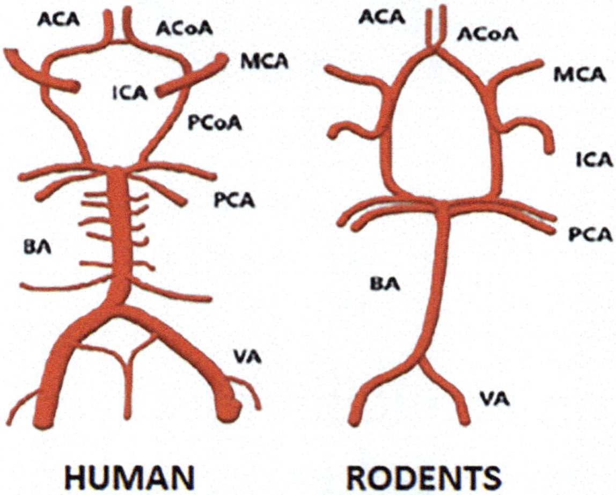

FIGURE 3.1 Cerebral arteries in human and rodent.

on artificial MCA strokes in rodents (rats or mice). The organization of cerebral supply is broadly similar in humans and rodents (Fig. 3.1). The same applies to the functional organization of many brain areas. For instance, mice and humans are similar in the way they process sensory information and control motor functions, as both species exhibit a comparable organization of cortical areas and lateralization of these functions.

However, there are also important differences between rodents and humans, which limit the generalization of findings from animal studies to human neurorehabilitation. For ethical reasons, humans cannot be forced to participate in rehabilitation interventions, whereas animal studies permit experimental interventions that would not be ethically acceptable in human participants. At the same time, it is possible to inform humans about the intention of interventions, and this understanding may enhance their motivation to train specific skills and functions. However, it is impossible to establish a shared understanding with rodents on a rational level. Consequently approaches to neurorehabilitation will necessarily differ between species.

In rodents, an enriched environment (EE) is one of the most widely used interventions. EE refers to a housing condition in which animals can move freely, explore, and are provided with opportunities for movement (e.g., running wheels), as well as hiding. Typically, animals are housed in an EE together with other animals of their species for at least approximately 6 hours per day. EE provides cognitive, motor, and social stimulation without requiring the animals to perform specific behaviour. As a control condition, a group housed in standard cage housing (SCH) is included, where no specific stimuli are provided (Fig. 3.2).

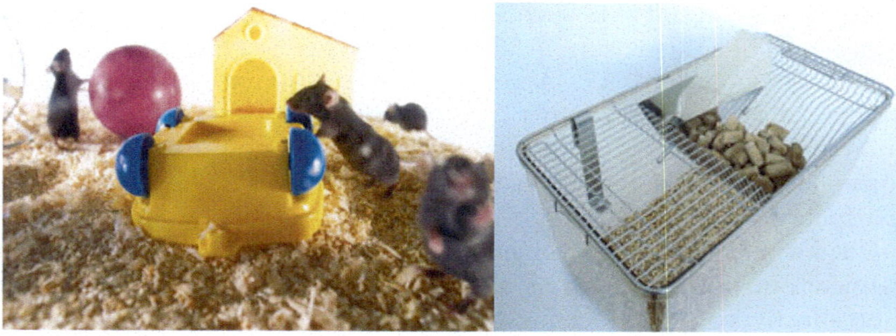

FIGURE 3.2 Standard cage housing versus enriched environment.

In terms of human neurorehabilitation, EE can be viewed as a nonspecific, voluntary treatment, which can hardly be offered as a single intervention. EE offers the possibility of training and relearning. However, because it is completely voluntary, the execution of behavior is not under scientific control and will differ between animals, leading to high inter-individual variation. From the perspective of human neurorehabilitation, EE-related behavior depends on motivation elicited by everyday tasks. Motivation and training in meaningful behavior are two variables that are highly interesting in human neurorehabilitation. At the same time, their impact on the outcome of neurorehabilitation remains unanswered. Furthermore, in humans, neurorehabilitation efforts without any therapeutic guidance and structure, as in EE, would not be reimbursed.

Thus a direct translation of EE to human neurorehabilitation is impossible. Treating humans in a manner comparable to rodents in SCH (the control condition in EE studies) is, at least during the subacute stage, not feasible. One might argue that waiting list control groups in the chronic phase resemble standard cage conditions. However, waiting list control groups without any intervention are feasible only in the chronic stage and carry a high risk of a negative placebo effect, as patients may expect little or no improvement when no treatment is provided.

Similar challenges arise when attempting to translate findings from exercise studies, which are often used in animal research as an alternative to EE, particularly when rehabilitation focuses on motor or sensorimotor deficits. Both are common consequences of MCA stroke, and these functions show a relatively similar neuroanatomical organization in rodents and humans and can be assessed using comparable measures. Exercise-based rehabilitation studies often involve placing animals on running wheels and requiring them to run at a predetermined speed ("running exercise"). Another approach is to reduce the amount of food available so that the animals must reach for food pellets ("grasping training"). The results of such training are then compared with the performance of animals kept in SCH and, in a few studies, also with that of animals housed in EE. Apart from the difference in the control condition discussed above, this type of training appears highly authoritarian and narrowly focused on a single function from a human neurorehabilitation perspective. Human patients would be unlikely to participate in such rigid exercise studies without expecting substantial benefits for recovery. Moreover such expectations could already influence treatment outcomes through recruiting bias (patients who do not believe in the effectiveness may decline participation).

Finally, it should be noted that the prospects for rehabilitation may depend on the extent to which a specific brain area or fiber tract associated with a particular function has been damaged. In this regard, leptomeningeal anastomoses and interindividual variations in the Circle of Willis may lead to differences in lesion size and localization, even among strokes affecting the same cerebral artery. Furthermore although the brains of humans and rodents share a similar lateralization of sensory and motor functions, important differences exist due to the development of language and hand function. For example, human MCA strokes involving the corticospinal tract may completely impair reaching performance while allowing some recovery of gait, because hand movements are more strongly lateralized than leg movements. Such a pronounced distinction between the upper and lower extremity does not exist in rodents. In addition, verbal functions, which are predominantly localized in the left hemisphere in humans, have no equivalent in rodents. Consequently the impact of extensive damage to specialized brain areas on the prospects for neurorehabilitation cannot be adequately answered based on (unilateral) MCA strokes in animals. Addressing such questions would require selective surgical disruption of specific nuclei or strategic fiber tracts and the assumptions of functionally homologous brain specilizations.

These considerations illustrate the challenges associated with translating findings from animal neurorehabilitation studies to human neurorehabilitation. At the same time, it should be emphasized that there are also compelling reasons why such studies are highly relevant. Perhaps the most important advantage is that these studies allow for a neurobiological analysis of the effects of such interventions, which cannot be performed humans [2]. Historically, Bryan Kolb's book [2] on brain plasticity, which was largely based on animal studies, was an important source of inspiration for numerous neurorehabilitation research studies and contributed to the hope that outcomes for patients with brain lesions could be improved.

In the following sections, we will start with a focus on memory impairment and examine the effects of partial and extended lesions of memory-relevant brain structures on recovery and training outcomes [3]. We will then turn to the rehabilitation of MCA strokes, including motor paresis, based on artificial stroke studies and surgical interventions in rodents. Subsequently, we will discuss the optimal timing of rehabilitative interventions, the effects of global EE and specific forced motor training, and the role of training intensity in recovery after artificial MCA strokes in rodents. Finally, we will review findings on the effects of rehabilitation on poststroke (re-)myelination and inflammation.

3.2 Effects of enriched environment, lesion localization, and intensity of training on memory rehabilitation

3.2.1 MCA stroke studies

Among the studies reviewed here, five studies reported behavioral data on learning and memory performance following an artificial unilateral MCA stroke in rodents [4–8]. The duration of EE exposure varied between 2 and 4 weeks. In all studies, memory performance was assessed using the Morris water maze test (MWM) (Fig. 3.3). The MWM is a test of spatial learning that relies on distal cues to navigate from various starting locations in an open swimming arena to locate a submerged escape platform. Spatial learning is assessed by measuring the swim time and swim distance required to reach the invisible platform from different

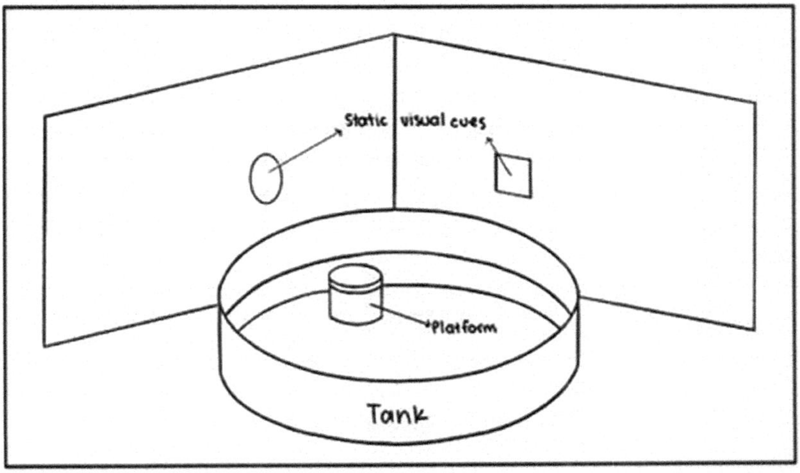

FIGURE 3.3 Morris water maze test. The platform is hidden beneath the water surface during swimming. The rodents are placed at different positions within the tank. Swim path and escape latency serve as measures of episodic-like memory performance.

starting locations. There is broad consensus that the MWM is a form of episodic memory test in animals. All but one study demonstrated that after 14 days, the learning and retention performance of the animals housed in EE had returned to prestroke levels compared to the sham group (i.e., no significant differences between stroke rodents and those without MCA occlusion), whereas those in SCH showed significantly poorer memory performance.

Three additional studies used bilateral occlusion of either the MCA or the internal carotid artery [9–11], either partially or completely. The duration of EE exposure was 14 days in one study and 28 days in the other two. In the study with the longest duration of hypoxia, EE did not result in complete recovery of memory performance even after 28 days of treatment. Nevertheless, the EE group performed significantly better than the stroke group in SCH. The other two studies, which used a shorter duration of bilateral occlusion, yielded similar findings to those observed after unilateral MCA occlusion, namely a substantial recovery of memory performance.

In summary: EE significantly improves memory recovery after MCA stroke, with most studies showing near-normal performance after 14 days in unilateral stroke models, whereas bilateral occlusion models required longer treatment durations and showed substantial but incomplete recovery.

3.2.2 Surgical lesion studies

16 studies have investigated the effects of surgical lesions of the extended hippocampal system or the Papez circuit (the Papez circuit is described in Chapter 1). Across these studies, both lesion location and lesion size determined the severity of impairment and the extent to which recovery could be achieved with EE. Complete bilateral hippocampal lesions showed no evidence of recovery, whereas partial lesions allowed for limited improvement, and a longer period of EE exposure suggested a dose–response relationship, particularly in animals with incomplete lesions.

After complete bilateral lesions of the hippocampal fimbria and fornix or both hippocampi, no recovery was observed. In contrast, bilateral incomplete lesions of the hippocampus, subiculum, and basal forebrain cholinergic nuclei generally allowed for partial recovery with EE. However, because these lesions produced severe memory impairments, researchers often used simpler behavioral tasks than the MWM (e.g., The T-maze, in which animals learn to choose or alternate between different paths, is such a simpler memory test). Indeed, at least one study demonstrated that improvements in these simpler tests were not associated with improvements in more demanding MWM [12].

Two studies [13,14] explicitly examined the long-term effects of EE (210 days or 1 1/4 years). In both studies, there was a partial improvement following EE, but only after a considerable period of time, suggesting a dose–response relationship. In the study by Kelche et al. (1988) [13], which involved complete bilateral lesions of the fimbria hippocampal fimbria and fornix, extending EE after an initial 2-month period for a further 3 months did not lead to additional improvement. However, the total duration of 150 days was substantially shorter than in studies of Kelche et al. (1995) [15] and Paban et al. (2005) [14], in which beneficial effects became apparent only after 210 days or longer[16]. In contrast, the same study showed that in animals with incomplete lesions limited to the dorsal hippocampus, the effects of EE emerged early and reached a plateau during the following weeks. This study also compared multimodal EE exposure with social cage housing and SCH. Only multimodal EE exposure resulted in improved, and possibly even a normalization of, performance, highlighting the importance of EE intensity for treatment effectiveness. Finally, the study by Kapgal et al. (2016) [17] similarly demonstrated additional benefits when EE exposure was combined with specific stimulation and a specialized diet.

Dalrymple-Alford et al. [18] reviewed studies investigating selective lesions of the anterior thalamic nuclei. Notably, most of these experiments assessed working memory performance using the T-maze, rather than memory performance in the MWM. Lesions of the anterior thalamic nuclei resulted in persistent working memory deficits when task performance required the use of allocentric (external landmarks) rather than repetitive egocentric (i.e., body-centered spatial strategies) cues. Although the duration of EE exposure was not systematically varied, the effects of immediate versus delayed EE onset (40 days after lesion induction) were examined. The timing of EE onset did not influence the outcome. In both conditions, SCH did not improve performance, whereas EE exposure resulted in significant improvement, although performance remained below that of sham-operated animals.

In summary: bilateral surgical lesions of the Papez circuit show only limited recovery even after prolonged periods of EE treatment.

3.2.3 Practical implications

Taken together, the findings from the two lesion models and the available evidence on dose–response relationships suggest the following conclusions. For lesions that do not affect key memory structures, there appears to be no clear linear relationship between the amount of EE exposure and the degree of functional improvement. Rather functional improvement seems to occur once a certain threshold of EE exposure has been reached and reaches a level close to the pre-lesion. Possible explanations include an early ceiling effect or a period of heightened neuroplasticity that is largely restricted to the immediate post-lesion phase [19]. However, a certain amount of EE exposure appears to be essential for improvement, as SCH seems to prevent recovery, whereas motor exercise alone has produced inconsistent results.

In contrast, partial lesions affecting key memory structures (i.e., lesions that do not completely disrupt the memory network), provide some evidence for a dose–response relationship: greater therapy intensity and longer treatment durations appear to contribute to improved outcomes. However, it remains unclear whether delaying therapy onset has a significant impact on recovery.

For complete lesions affecting the Papez circle or the hippocampal system, EE exposure failed to produce measurable improvement [20–22], or any benefits were limited to performance on tasks that were substantially less demanding than MWM. Moreover, considerably longer periods of EE exposure may be needed to reveal beneficial effects after bilateral strategic lesions.

These findings provide a strong rationale for shifting the therapeutic focus at an early stage in memory-impaired patients with extensive bilateral lesions (e.g., following hypoxia) from attempts to restore memory function toward teaching the effective use of external memory aids, as discussed in Chapter 7 on memory rehabilitation.

3.3 Enriched environment and the optimal time to start rehabilitation

The optimal timing of rehabilitation remains a matter of debate. Based on the literature available up to 2013, the reviews of Schmidt et al. (2014) [23] argue that there is a time window shortly after, but not too early, following a brain lesion during which neuroplastic processes are enhanced and rehabilitation may therefore be particularly effective. Exactly when this optimal time window begins and ends remains uncertain. Following stroke, neurogenesis and dendritic sprouting is initially increased, followed by a decline between 14 days and 28 days. In general, the period for spontaneous recovery in rodents lasts approximately 30 days and is presumed to be around 3 months in humans. Moreover, EE exposure may become less effective when initiated more than 30 days after stroke.

3.3.1 Very early versus early start of rehabilitation

Several recent studies have examined the question of the optimal timing of rehabilitation in greater detail. For example, Wahl et al. (2019) [24] compared the effects of early versus delayed onset of EE exposure following a large MCA stroke. EE exposure either began on the day of the artificial stroke and continued for 14 days, or it began on day 14, lasting for the following 14 days. Both groups were compared in terms of their performance on the 28th day. The result showed that the very early beginning of compulsory EE exposure was associated with poorer outcomes. The group with the delayed onset of EE exposure achieved a higher gripping accuracy. The authors concluded that immediately following a stroke, there may be a phase of recovery during which the organism clears damaged tissue while simultaneously generating new neurons. Delaying the onset of training may facilitate the stabilization of these newly generated neurons and their integration into functional networks. One somewhat unusual aspect of this study was that the rats remained in the EE throughout the day, and obtained food only through their performance within the environment. Thus, participation in the EE was not entirely voluntary. In addition, improvement was assessed with regard to motor performance, not memory function.

Zhang et al. [25] compared the effects of forced running training initiated 24, 48, 72, or 96 hours after stroke (Fig. 3.4). They concluded that training initiated within the first 24 hours was ineffective, whereas later initiation promoted functional recovery, with no differences in efficacy between the later time points. In the context of nonforced, voluntary EE exposure, Lee et al. (2022) [26] showed that, following a large stroke, an early onset of rehabilitation (i.e., only 1 rather than 5 days after the artificial stroke) significantly reduced its effectiveness. Moreover, larger infarctions were associated with a delayed onset of recovery compared to smaller infarctions. Tan et al. [27] similarly compared the effects of EE exposure and SCH when introduced on day 5 after stroke and investigated the influence of EE exposure on hippocampal neurogenesis. EE exposure was shown to promote hippocampal neurogenesis and facilitated recovery from neurological deficits and impairment in spatial memory. Taken together, these studies support the conclusions of earlier reviews that rehabilitation initiated within the first 24 hours after a stroke may be associated with more adverse effects than interventions introduced at a later stage [23,28].

3.3.2 Extension for starting intervention to later periods

Several recent studies have investigated the effectiveness of interventions initiated at later points. In the study by Li et al. (2022) [30], training began 14 days after an MCA stroke induction. Treatment did not consist of

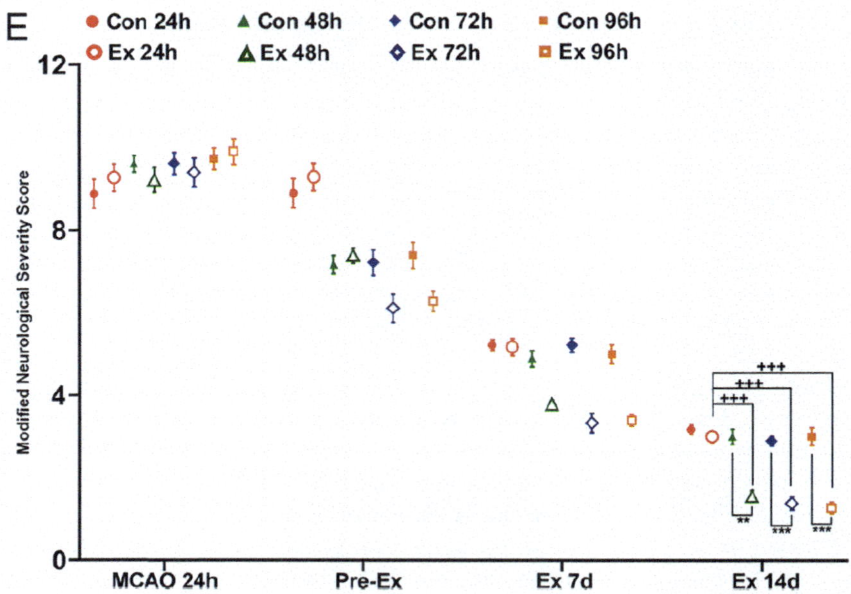

FIGURE 3.4 Four different time points for the initiation of neurorehabilitation in rodents. Rehabilitation initiated within the first 24 hours after a middle cerebral artery stroke) revealed no improvement after 14 days. In contrast, rehabilitation initiated on the 2nd, 3rd, or 4th day after stroke was associated with improved performance on a rodent-adapted neurological assessment scale [29].

EE exposure, but rather of either grasping training of the affected front paw or of running exercise. The training was more intensive than in most other studies and continued for 6 weeks. Both interventions were effective, although they benefited different functional domains. Running exercise increased grip strength to a greater extent than grasping training, and both interventions were superior to SCH. In contrast, spatial memory performance improved significantly more following grasping training than running exercise, and both interventions outperformed SCH. If grasping is considered the more complex motor performance, these findings may suggest a trade-off between gains in grip strength and the transfer of training effects to cognitive functions such as memory.

de Boer et al. [31] investigated the effects of a negative regulator of axonal guidance that was administered shortly after stroke. However, this intervention proved ineffective. Of greater interest was the placement of rats in an EE, which began on day 16 after stroke and continued until day 63. Outcome measures included the ability to remain on a rotating platform and the accuracy of front paw placement while crossing a horizontal ladder. Rats housed in an EE significantly improved in their ability to remain on the rotating plate, but not in the precision of front paw placement. These findings suggest that delayed intervention may also be effective and that EE exposure may improve overall motor performance without enhancing fine motor function. Thus both studies indicate that EE exposure remains effective when initiated at a later stage, although it should be noted that both interventions involved comparatively long treatment periods.

In summary, these studies indicate the existence of an extended time window during the subacute phase in which intervention remains effective. Whether there is an upper limit beyond which training no longer produces beneficial effects remains unclear. However, initiating rehabilitation too early appears to have an adverse effects on outcome. One possible explanation for the negative impact of too-early intervention is the presence of inflammatory processes (see below).

3.4 Specific motor training versus enriched environment

3.4.1 Constraint-induced motor treatment for the affected limb: timing and effectiveness

Constraint-induced motor treatment (CIMT) is one of the most effective and well-studied methods of neurorehabilitation. It is based on the observation that many patients develop compensatory strategies after stroke to cope with their impairments. These strategies rely on the use of preserved functions, for example, preferential use of the unaffected hand for everyday activities. As a consequence, residual abilities of the stroke-affected limb are used less frequently, resulting in a phenomenon known as learned nonuse. This secondary nonuse may negatively affect the recovery of function in the affected limb.

For independence in daily living and quality of life, compensatory use of the unaffected side of the body plays a central role. Therefore, for each individual patient, it must be carefully considered whether and when a CIMT of the affected limb is appropriate [32]. To address this issue, Nemchek et al. (2021) investigated whether compensatory training during the early phase after stroke compromises the effectiveness of later, specific training of the affected limb. Specifically, they compared the effect of grasping training on the unaffected side of the body with voluntary running training and SCH in rodents. Training began 4 days after the artificial stroke and training continued for 14 days. Subsequently, all three groups received 5 days of training with the affected front paw. Remarkably, after the first day of training with the affected front paw, no differences in performance were observed between the groups. Hence neither running exercise nor training of the unaffected forepaw during the initial 14-day period transferred immediately to performance of the affected forepaw. After four additional days of training, the group that had previously received running exercise improved, while the training group with previous training on the unaffected front paw remained at the level of the SCH group. These findings suggest that grasping training of the unaffected front paw does not transfer to skilled use of the affected front paw. Moreover voluntary activation after stroke may extend the time window during which specific training remains effective into a more chronic phase (3–4 weeks after stroke). These results indicate that an initial reliance on compensatory strategies may not be associated with adverse effects on subsequent recovery of the affected limb, provided that general rehabilitative activation occurs in parallel. This raises the question of whether CIMT may be most effective when introduced during the chronic phase, because two previous metaanalysis of animal experiments on the CIMT (mainly during the subacute stage) did not show any positive effect [23,33].

3.4.2 Effects of specific motor training versus enriched environment

While studies on environmental enrichment or enriched environment (EE) have consistently shown improvements in overall motor function and compensatory abilities, EE exposure does not seem to enhance fine motor skills such as grasping. Improvements in fine motor function appear to require specific training [34]. For example, Schneider et al. (2014) compared the effects of running exercise and CIMT of the front paw on grasping performance of rats and found significant improvements only after specific training. Another study has compared specific training with EE (Fig. 3.5) [35]. In this study, both interventions were equally effective in improving motor performance, whereas memory performance improved only following EE.

A second study found that EE and grasping training had comparable effects on accurate front paw placement while crossing a horizontal ladder [36]. However, fine motor grasping performance was not assessed directly in this study. A third study investigated the effects of EE on running performance after stroke [31]. EE significantly increased the animals' running speed. However, a detailed analysis of movements of the affected front paw revealed no significant improvement. Notably, studies investigating task-specific training of the paretic forepaw have also yielded inconsistent findings.

3.4.3 Effects of specific motor interventions on memory performance

The vast majority of studies show that EE improves compensation ("International Classification of Functioning, Disability and Health"-based performance) and episodic-like memory, but not fine motor skills.

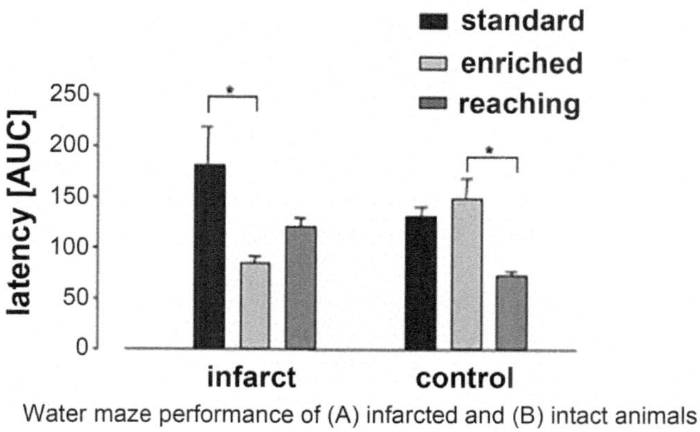

FIGURE 3.5 Enriched environment reduces memory impairment in stroke animals. *From Wurm F., Keiner S., Kunze A., Witte O.W., Redecker C. Effects of skilled forelimb training on hippocampal neurogenesis and spatial learning after focal cortical infarcts in the adult rat brain. Stroke 2007;38(10):2833–2840. https://doi.org/10.1161/STROKEAHA.107.485524.*

If *specific* motor intervention increases memory performance, it is less clear Li et al. [30] compared the effect of running and grasping training. Both led to improvements compared to the SCH. However, the effect of grasping training on memory performance was significantly higher than that of running exercise. In contrast, Wurm et al. [35] did not show a generalization of grasping training on memory performance. Marin et al. [37], unlimited, voluntary running exercise affected biological recovery in young mice, but not in old ones. Pure grasping training was not effective in this study Pan et al. [38] compared light, moderate, and intensive forced running training on running and memory performance. The start of this training was already on the 2nd day after the stroke, and the animals were forced to do the training. The study demonstrated that only light and moderate training had an effect. These two interventions also generalized to memory performance Geng et al. [39] achieved a completely analogous result in terms of memory performance comparing moderate and intensive running training Li et al. [40] also intervened by employing running training. A distinctive feature of this study is that the rats were trained for 12 weeks, which is a very long period. The training consisted of forced running for 30 minutes a day. There were significant improvements in grasping, running, and memory performance. Taken together, the effects of specific motor training on memory are inconsistent—some studies suggest grasping training enhances memory, while others find only light to moderate running exercise improves both motor and memory performance, especially when applied early and over a long duration.

Unfortunately, only one study explicitly compared EE with forced exercise. Jeffers and Corbett [41] incorporated three groups: EE, grasping training, and EE plus grasping training. Training began 1 week after the stroke and was carried out for 4 weeks. Animals without a stroke, but with EE and grasping training, served as a comparison group. After the 4th week of training, the two stroke groups with either EE or grasping training showed similar recovery rates. The combined treatment group outperformed both single treatment groups at some measurement points and reached the grasping performance of the sham group at the end of the training.

Thus the comparative effectiveness of EE and specific training is still somewhat unclear [42]. EE, compared to SCH, always influences "everyday motor" and memory performance. Whether EE has an effect at the impairment level is questionable. Studies on running exercise also show an effect on everyday motor performance and memory (depending on the intensity, duration, and time of start of the training). It should be noted, however, that most EEs include a running wheel, which means that the difference between running exercise and EE is one of spontaneous or forced use of the wheel. The results for grasping training are contradictory, but this training seems to be effective for improving performance at the impairment level. EE combined with specific training is the most promising method compared to either alone.

For human neurorehabilitation, these findings argue that physiotherapeutic or occupational treatment of the upper extremities alone will not necessarily improve memory performance. Only the memory-related cognitive challenges provided by EE promote memory recovery after stroke.

3.5 Environmental complexity and training intensity

The daily schedule and duration of rehabilitation remain uncertain in neurorehabilitation. Some studies have focused on the importance of therapy intensity, while others have looked at how the rehabilitation process should be structured.

Several studies have begun to systematically increase the difficulty of EE. Instead of just one EE, two or three levels with different objects are used, which are unlocked on a weekly basis. The rationale is that the complexity of the environment should be systematically increased progressively as functions improve. The results are impressive in absolute terms, but a head-to-head comparison without complexity increase is still pending.

Above, it was argued that intensity plays a role, especially when the lesion affects areas that are essential for the performance in question. Lee et al. [26] analyzed the effect of treatment intensity in respect to stroke size. They compared four groups: sham control non stroke, stroke

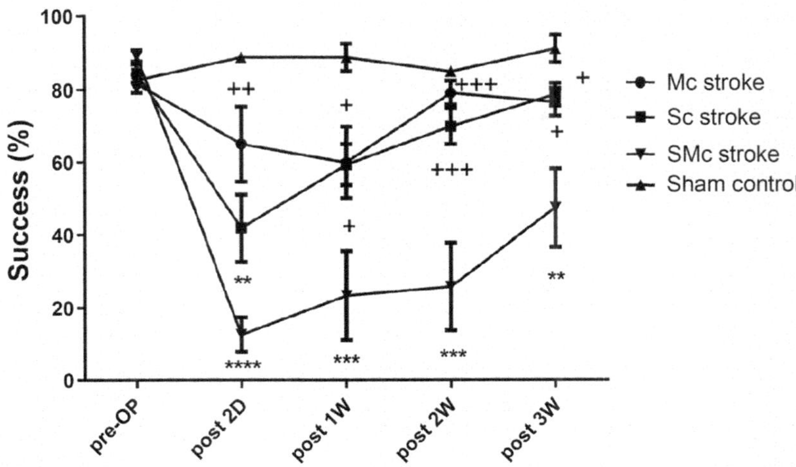

FIGURE 3.6 Dynamics of functional recovery from stroke and size of the lesion. *From Lee K.H., Jeong E.H., Joa K.L. Effects of stroke lesions and timing of rehabilitation on the compensatory movement patterns during stroke recovery. Am J Phys Med Rehabil 2022;101(11):1031–1037. https://doi.org/10.1097/PHM.0000000000001968.*

restricted to the motor cortex, stroke restricted to the sensory cortex, and stroke encompassing sensory and motor cortex (Fig. 3.6). Training started early or late (2 days after the stroke, 5 days after stroke or 2 weeks after the stroke). Larger stroke size led to higher impairment and delayed, but not reduced overall extent of improvement. However, due to the larger impairment, the group with large stroke needed 3 weeks to achieve a similar performance as the two other groups after 1 week (Fig. 3.4). The other important information was that the earliest starting point was detrimental for recovery in the group with large stroke, but not in the groups with small strokes.

This would mean that large strokes need extended treatment schedules for recovery, because recovery is delayed but will take place later on. Paradoxically, in humans, neurorehabilitation is organized in the opposite way. Patients with large lesions are admitted to early rehabilitation units. However, patients with small lesions and limited impairment may go home first, to start with neurorehabilitation later. Even, if the reason for this difference is related to the amount of nursing care for patients with large strokes from a neurorehabilitation perspective, the timing of rehabilitation for these two groups should perhaps be reversed.

Concerning the intensity of training in artificial stroke, Pan et al. [38] showed that light or moderate running training is superior to intensive training in terms of effectiveness on motor performance. The study by Hase [43], which used a model of bilateral internal carotid artery stenosis, compared, 3 hours of EE per day with full-time EE against SCH. The different durations of the EE showed no effect on the magnitude of the effect on memory performance. Radabaugh et al. [44] investigated the extent to which the distribution of EE times over the day could affect rehabilitation success. Although this study used a rodent model of traumatic brain injury (TBI) rather than stroke, it is discussed here because of its potential clinical relevance. The two conditions (bundled over 6 hours or spread over 2 × 3-hour throughout the day) were equally effective. These studies suggest that moderate exercise intensity could be sufficient. However, it must be noted that EE implies that the activity level is determined by the animals themselves, which is not the case with forced training. Pan et al. [38] compared cortisol levels in the animals 30 and 60 minutes after forced exercise with different intensities. The cortisol level was increased for all groups with stroke compared to the sham group. However, for the group with intensive training, the cortisol level was also increased compared to the other groups with lower intensity schedules. At the same time, the high-intensity group showed reduced treatment success. The results argue that forced training is unfavorable above a certain intensity. In conclusion, moderate exercise intensity is generally more effective than high-intensity training, with forced high-intensity training potentially increasing stress and reducing treatment success.

The study by Wang et al. [45], which used animals with artificial TBI, not with stroke, started with forced running training for 2 weeks. To avoid excessive demands, the extent of forced training was adaptively increased. This was done because a significant number of animals showed depression-like symptoms at the beginning, so some degree of external prompting seemed necessary in order not to succumb to functional nonuse. In the 3rd week, one group received EE, that is, a voluntary amount of global stimulation. The other group continued with adaptive forced running training. The findings clearly demonstrated the following: the largest reduction in neurological impairment was shown by the group with initially forced and then later self-directed training through EE exposure. This group also had significantly lower cortisol levels. However, the two groups did not differ in their memory performance. In their review of research published until 2018, Xing et al. [28] also concluded that voluntary training may be superior to compulsory training. However, conclusive studies are still lacking.

3.6 Effects on (re-)myelination

Most studies on stroke do not show an effect of training on lesion size. However, the studies on remyelination of axons after stroke offer more optimistic results [46], and myelination or remyelination are the neurobiological basis for compensatory processes.

3.6.1 Stroke-induced demyelination

Stroke-induced neuronal death and reduced myelination are closely linked. Oligodendrocytes, a type of glial cells responsible for producing and maintaining myelin, are just as dependent on oxygen as nerve cells and are therefore affected by MCA stroke independently of neuronral injury. It is unclear whether there is an interaction: neuronal death certainly leads to demyelination and destruction of axons. However, their demyelination could also affect the number of nerve cells that are dying (Fig. 3.7). Now, remyelination takes place continuously in healthy brains, for which oligodendrocyte precursor cells (OPCs) are formed [47]. However, the ability to form such progenitor cells or differentiate into oligodendrocytes decreases with age, and age is a risk factor for stroke.

Stroke does not lead to loss of the ability to form OPCs. However, their differentiation into oligodendrocytes and their ability to set up myelin sheath seem to be blocked Cheng et al. [48] study found, in a mouse MCA stroke model, that OPCs failed to mature into oligodendrocytes in the lesion area. Instead, there was an increased number of stripped axons. Stroke, thus leads to the death of oligodendrocytes and demyelination, and, under appropriate conditions, they can also reduce the possibility of differentiation and maturation of OPCs.

The highly interesting results of Pan et al. [38] were all collected on mice after MCA stroke *without* stimulation, that is, living in SCH. In this respect, the question arises whether rehabilitation could affect remyelination. This is because (re-)myelination depends on neuronal activity, and glutamate

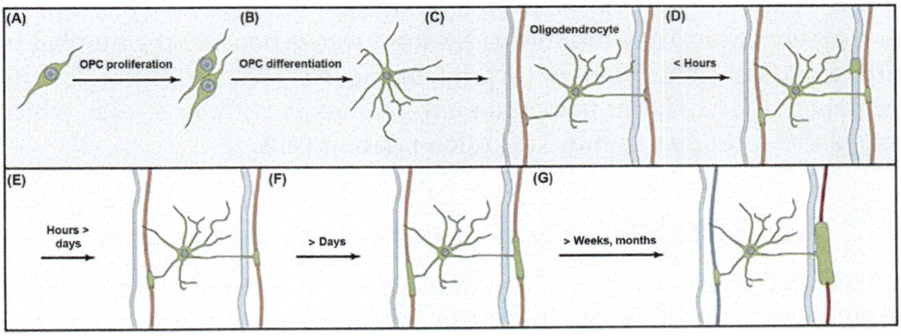

FIGURE 3.7 Processes of (re-)myelination. *From Sampaio-Baptista C., Johansen-Berg H. White matter plasticity in the adult brain. Neuron 2017;96(6):1239–1251. https://doi.org/10.1016/j.neuron.2017.11.026.*

expression, as a sign of neuronal activity, is a decisive trigger for the maturation of OPCs into oligodendrocytes [47,49,50].

3.6.2 Rehabilitation and its impact on remyelination

It should be evident that myelination and remyelination are of central importance for neurorehabilitation, because myelination is an important biological basis for learning and neurorehabilitation depends on rewiring of cortical and subcortical connections. A summary of the studies on myelin repair after stroke before 2019 can be found in Jia et al. [50]. Since then, several studies have dealt with this question again. Li et al. [40] investigated the effect of EE on white matter integrity using different types of imaging. They found that EE prevents white matter volume loss without affecting the lesion size. It also promoted the differentiation of OPCs into oligodendrocytes and subsequent remyelination of axons.

Zhang et al. [25] investigated the effect of a global reduction in oxygen availability in the brain analogous to bilateral internal carotid stenosis. As a result, there was a significant loss of myelin in the corpus callosum, which was significantly lower in the EE group. The concentration of the myelin basic protein, a main component of the myelin sheath, was increased in this group compared to the comparison group with SCH, but at the same time also lower than in animals operated on sham. EE also improved memory performance and depressive-like mood.

Guo et al. [51] investigated the effects of EE beginning one week after stroke. They found significantly improved memory performance 4 weeks after the infarction compared to SCH. In the EE group, hippocampal myelination and myelin basic protein levels were higher than in the SCH group, but lower than in the sham group. The result was quite analogous to that of [25].

Han et al. [52] used biochemical methods to investigate the effect of EE on remyelination. They found that EE for 4 weeks boosted the number of differentiating OPCs and of myelinated axons when compared with animals in the SCH, but not compared to animals without stroke, which have an even higher number of differentiating cells.

3.6.3 Age-related differences in remyelination after stroke

Two studies dealt with the dependence of the differentiation of OPCs on the age of the animals. The study by Dingman et al. [53] compared young and old mice after an artificial stroke concerning the formation of OPCs and their differentiation into oligodendrocytes. In young mice, there was a significant increase in OPCs in the 1st weeks after stroke, but this was not the case in older animals. In addition, the study showed that even in the young mice, the OPCs differentiated less frequently into mature oligodendrocytes. Therefore this study anticipated the results of Marin et al. and Chen et al. [37,54] that living in standard cages reduces or blocks neuroplastic processes. Moreover, it argued that there may be a specific window of opportunity for rapid rehab gain, which could be based on the increased production of OPCs, at least in young animals.

The study by Marin et al. [37] compared young and old mice that received either specific reaching training, access to a blocked running wheel, or unlimited access to a complex running wheel. Only the latter leads to significant OPC maturation—and only in younger mice. Electrophysiological recordings further confirmed enhanced conduction speed in remyelinated axons. However, no direct correlation was found between OPC maturation and functional recovery, highlighting the complexity of this relationship. In the study by [55], it was shown that stroke led to higher performance losses in older animals, but the absolute effect of EE on recovery was similar for the 2 age groups.

The result of these studies can be summarized as follows: after stroke OPCs are generated, which could be used for subsequent remyelination. This is especially the case in younger animals. There is a certain period for the formation of OPCs, which expires after a few weeks, although even after that (as in healthy brains), OPCs are still permanently formed for repair processes on axons, but outside the (peri-) lesional area. EE and free, unlimited access to running wheels lead to a differentiation of OPCs. If there is no motor and cognitive stimulation during this period (i.e., in a condition such as SCH), the OPCs do not differentiate towards mature oligodendrocytes. However, the exact relationship between OPC differentiation and functional improvement is still unclear, because the behavioral effect of EE in older animals does not differ from that in younger animals.

3.7 Poststroke inflammation

As a consequence of stroke, three phases of inflammatory processes can be distinguished. The initial phase is marked by a strong inflammatory reaction right after the stroke. This is followed by a period of immunosuppression, which gradually transitions into a late phase characterized by a resurgence of inflammatory activity. The second phase, often persisting for weeks, is particularly relevant to stroke recovery, as it may exert sustained effects on neuroplasticity and tissue repair [56] (Fig. 3.8).

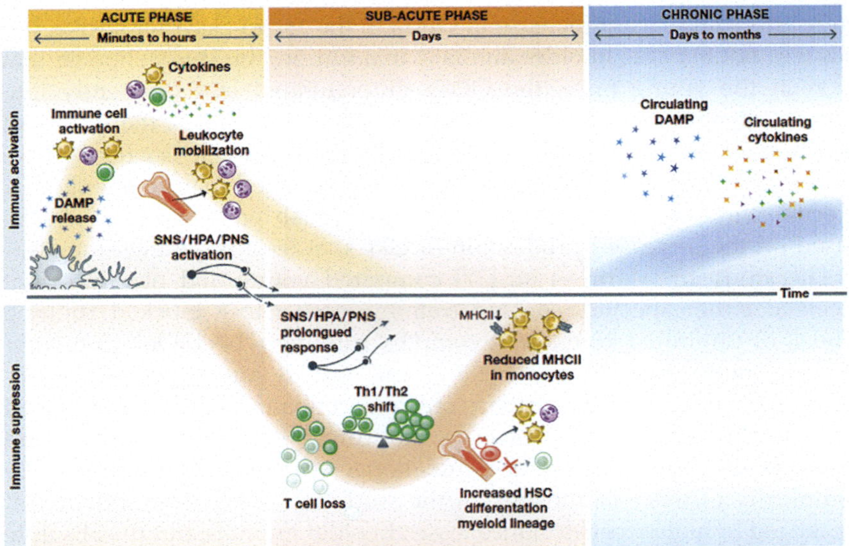

FIGURE 3.8 Phases of poststroke inflammation. *From Simats A., Liesz A. Systemic inflammation after stroke: implications for post-stroke comorbidities. EMBO Mol Med 2022;14(9):e16269. https://doi.org/10.15252/emmm.202216269.*

Three new studies have examined how EE modulates these late inflammatory processes, focusing specifically on changes in interleukin concentration, which we will limit ourselves to here. Guo et al. [51] investigated the effect of EE on remyelination, memory performance, and IL-1ß and IL-6 as markers of inflammatory pathways 4 weeks after infarction. Notably, animals housed in EE conditions showed significantly reduced concentrations of pro-inflammatory cytokines IL-1β and IL-6 compared to animals maintained in standard cages, though levels remained elevated relative to sham-operated controls. This suggests that while EE attenuates inflammation, it does not fully normalize it.

Han et al. [52] followed a similar experimental design. Their results also demonstrated cognitive improvements in the EE group, alongside a decrease in IL-1ß concentration and TNF-α levels compared to the standard group. Furthermore, EE animals exhibited elevated levels of antiinflammatory cytokines IL-4 and IL-10. For the antiinflammatory IL-4 and IL-10, there was an increase in the EE group compared to SCH. In this respect, EE was again effective in reducing the late immune response.

Zhang et al. [25] compared the effects of very early and early onset on forced running (see above). The result showed that training reduces the concentration of pro-inflammatory cytokines (IL-1α, IL-1ß, and TNF-α), except for the earliest start of training. Interestingly, all training groups, regardless of start time, showed a decrease in IL-10 concentrations, suggesting a complex relationship between timing, inflammation, and neuroimmune modulation.

Taken together, these findings indicate that EE and structured physical activity can reduce late poststroke inflammation, but the timing of intervention is critical. While both strategies modulate inflammatory cytokines in a beneficial direction, premature initiation may attenuate these effects. Thus tailoring the onset of rehabilitative interventions appears crucial for optimizing neuroimmune outcomes.

3.8 Conclusions for the following chapters and translational perspectives

This scoping review of recent animal studies on stroke rehabilitation supports several important conclusions relevant to neurorehabilitation:

1. Rehabilitation efforts change behavior, they also change the brain in many ways. These include cell differentiation, remyelination, vascular remodeling, and a reduction of focal inflammation. Such changes reflect the multifaceted biological basis underlying functional recovery.
2. Brain plasticity and the effects of neurorehabilitation differ related to phases of recovery. Most findings support an inverted U-curve, where plastic potential peaks in the postacute phase and declines thereafter. This underscores the need for timely intervention.
3. Interventions too early may have a detrimental effect by increasing inflammatory processes and triggering stress-related pathways that impair recovery. Therefore careful timing of rehabilitation is crucial.
4. Strokes (and other brain lesions) often lead to secondary passivity, which may reduce motivation and engagement in rehabilitation. Encouraging patients to actively participate in structured treatments can help rebuild self-confidence and self-agency. However, distinguishing between primary and secondary passivity remains a clinical decision, that must be addressed through careful patient interaction and observation.
5. Motivated animals in a complex environment such as EE adapt their behaviour to compensate for the consequences of brain lesions. Yet, these solutions do not mean that the fine structure of the behavior is changed. Such a tuning of the fine structure depends on specific training interventions (which does not guarantee per se a broader adaptation).
6. The effect of rehabilitation efforts depends on the severity of the lesion. Lesions that occur outside of highly specialized brain areas are more

amenable to plasticity-driven compensation, whereas damage to core functional hubs or their connections significantly limits the potential for recovery.

7. Functionally relevant brain plasticity is relatively large after nontotal destruction of specialized brain areas, but low if specialized areas or their connections are completely destroyed.
8. Interventions for restitution should be stopped if the lesions destroyed the strategic areas completely, and as soon as the patient is able to accept that (often external) compensation is the only realistic goal.

The following chapters on neuropsychological rehabilitation of stroke syndromes will therefore distinguish the phase of the recovery (postacute and chronic) and severity of the impairment as important decision criteria for treatment.

Most animal research is focused on biochemical and physiological processes. Below, some questions are outlined, which are important from the perspective of a *clinical-rehabilitative* practitioner, and which would profit from animal findings.

1. The most widely used model for influencing the course of stroke continues to be EE. However, EE is a complex intervention, because—as a spontaneous behavior—it depends on motivation, the basic rate of spontaneous behavior ("personality traits"), the design of the EE ("degree of complexity"), and the degree of impairment, restricting possible interaction with the environment. For a targeted transfer into everyday clinical practice, it would be necessary to vary these different aspects separately.
2. As far as motivation is concerned, it would be interesting to know whether 1 or 2 days of observation would help to identify animals for which pure EE is not beneficial because they show too little spontaneous behavior.
3. New studies have begun to adapt the complexity of EE more systematically to the performance of the animals concerned. This procedure corresponds to the targeted design of systematic rehabilitation. However, there is still a lack of studies investigating whether increasing environmental complexity is itself a relevant factor and how this increase should best be implemented.
4. Another unresolved issue is whether EE leads to improved compensation of the deficit, while structured training reduces specific impairments. Clarifying this distinction is crucial for understanding the limits of generalization across domains and for designing optimal treatment pathways.
5. While early intervention is generally beneficial, emerging findings caution against initiating stimulation prematurely. Inflammatory

processes may be a key factor in determining this threshold. It would therefore be extremely interesting to identify laboratory markers that could guide clinical decisions about when and at what intensity to initiate rehabilitation.

References

[1] Cieza A, Causey K, Kamenov K, Hanson SW, Chatterji S, Vos T. Global estimates of the need for rehabilitation based on the global burden of disease study 2019: a systematic analysis for the global burden of disease study 2019. Lancet 2021;396(10267):2006–17. Available from https://doi.org/10.1016/S0140-6736(20)32340-0.

[2] Kolb B. Brain plasticity and behavior. Lawrence Erlbaum Associates; 1995. Publisher description. http://www.loc.gov/catdir/enhancements/fy0745/94045561-d.html.

[3] Hildebrandt H. Was sagt der Tierversuch über die Dosis-Wirkungs-Beziehung bei der Rehabilitation von Lern- und Gedächtnisstörungen? Neurol Rehalbil 2017;23(1):33–8.

[4] Matsumori Y, Hong SM, Fan Y, Kayama T, Hsu CY, Weinstein PR, et al. Enriched environment and spatial learning enhance hippocampal neurogenesis and salvages ischemic penumbra after focal cerebral ischemia. Neurobiol Dis 2006;22(1):187–98. Available from https://doi.org/10.1016/j.nbd.2005.10.015.

[5] Ronnback A, Dahlqvist P, Svensson PA, Jernas M, Carlsson B, Carlsson LM, et al. Gene expression profiling of the rat hippocampus one month after focal cerebral ischemia followed by enriched environment. Neurosci Lett 2005;385(2):173–8. Available from https://doi.org/10.1016/j.neulet.2005.05.016.

[6] Xu X, Ye L, Ruan Q. Environmental enrichment induces synaptic structural modification after transient focal cerebral ischemia in rats. Exp Biol Med (Maywood) 2009;234(3):296–305. Available from https://doi.org/10.3181/0804-RM-128.

[7] Yu K, Wu Y, Zhang Q, Xie H, Liu G, Guo Z, et al. Enriched environment induces angiogenesis and improves neural function outcomes in rat stroke model. J Neurol Sci 2014;347(1-2):275–80. Available from https://doi.org/10.1016/j.jns.2014.10.022.

[8] Dahlqvist P, Ronnback A, Bergstrom SA, Soderstrom I, Olsson T. Environmental enrichment reverses learning impairment in the Morris water maze after focal cerebral ischemia in rats. Eur J Neurosci 2004;19(8):2288–98. Available from https://doi.org/10.1111/j.0953-816X.2004.03248.x.

[9] Gobbo OL, O'Mara SM. Impact of enriched-environment housing on brain-derived neurotrophic factor and on cognitive performance after a transient global ischemia. Behav Brain Res 2004;152(2):231–41. Available from https://doi.org/10.1016/j.bbr.2003.10.017.

[10] Briones TL, Rogozinska M, Woods J. Environmental experience modulates ischemia-induced amyloidogenesis and enhances functional recovery. J Neurotrauma 2009;26(4):613–25. Available from https://doi.org/10.1089/neu.2008.0707.

[11] Yang Y, Zhang J, Xiong L, Deng M, Wang J, Xin J, et al. Cognitive improvement induced by environment enrichment in chronic cerebral hypoperfusion rats: a result of upregulated endogenous neuroprotection? J Mol Neurosci 2015;56(2):278–89. Available from https://doi.org/10.1007/s12031-015-0529-2.

[12] Bindu B, Rekha J, Kutty BM. Post insult enriched housing improves the 8-arm radial maze performance but not the Morris water maze task in ventral subicular lesioned rats. Brain Res 2005;1063(2):121–31. Available from https://doi.org/10.1016/j.brainres.2005.09.044.

[13] Kelche C, Dalrymple-Alford JC, Will B. Housing conditions modulate the effects of intracerebral grafts in rats with brain lesions. Behav Brain Res 1988;28(3):287–95. Available from https://doi.org/10.1016/0166-4328(88)90131-3.
[14] Paban V, Jaffard M, Chambon C, Malafosse M, Alescio-Lautier B. Time course of behavioral changes following basal forebrain cholinergic damage in rats: environmental enrichment as a therapeutic intervention. Neuroscience 2005;132(1):13–32. Available from https://doi.org/10.1016/j.neuroscience.2004.11.024.
[15] Kelche C, Roeser C, Jeltsch H, Cassel JC, Will B. The effects of intrahippocampal grafts, training, and postoperative housing on behavioral recovery after septohippocampal damage in the rat. Neurobiol Learn Mem 1995;63(2):155–66. Available from https://doi.org/10.1006/nlme.1995.1016.
[16] Will B, Deluzarche F, Kelche C. Does post-operative environment attenuate or exacerbate symptoms which follow hippocampal lesions in rats? Behav Brain Res 1983;7(1):125–32. Available from https://doi.org/10.1016/0166-4328(83)90009-8.
[17] Kapgal V, Prem N, Hegde P, Laxmi TR, Kutty BM. Long term exposure to combination paradigm of environmental enrichment, physical exercise and diet reverses the spatial memory deficits and restores hippocampal neurogenesis in ventral subicular lesioned rats. Neurobiol Learn Mem 2016;130:61–70. Available from https://doi.org/10.1016/j.nlm.2016.01.013.
[18] Dalrymple-Alford JC, Harland B, Loukavenko EA, Perry B, Mercer S, Collings DA, et al. Anterior thalamic nuclei lesions and recovery of function: relevance to cognitive thalamus. Neurosci Biobehav Rev 2015;54:145–60. Available from https://doi.org/10.1016/j.neubiorev.2014.12.007.
[19] Zeiler SR, Krakauer JW. The interaction between training and plasticity in the poststroke brain. Curr Opin Neurol 2013;26(6):609–16. Available from https://doi.org/10.1097/WCO.0000000000000025.
[20] Galani R, Jarrard LE, Will BE, Kelche C. Effects of postoperative housing conditions on functional recovery in rats with lesions of the hippocampus, subiculum, or entorhinal cortex. Neurobiol Learn Mem 1997;67(1):43–56. Available from https://doi.org/10.1006/nlme.1996.3745.
[21] Kelche C, Dalrymple-Alford J, Will B. Effects of postoperative environment on recovery of function after fimbria-fornix transection in the rat. Physiol Behav 1987;40(6):731–6. Available from https://doi.org/10.1016/0031-9384(87)90275-7.
[22] Pacteau C, Einon D, Sinden J. Early rearing environment and dorsal hippocampal ibotenic acid lesions: long-term influences on spatial learning and alternation in the rat. Behav Brain Res 1989;34(1-2):79–96. Available from https://doi.org/10.1016/s0166-4328(89)80092-0.
[23] Schmidt A, Wellmann J, Schilling M, Strecker JK, Sommer C, Schabitz WR, et al. Meta-analysis of the efficacy of different training strategies in animal models of ischemic stroke. Stroke 2014;45(1):239–47. Available from https://doi.org/10.1161/STROKEAHA.113.002048.
[24] Wahl AS, Erlebach E, Brattoli B, Buchler U, Kaiser J, Ineichen BV, et al. Early reduced behavioral activity induced by large strokes affects the efficiency of enriched environment in rats. J Cereb Blood Flow Metab 2019;39(10):2022–34. Available from https://doi.org/10.1177/0271678X18777661.
[25] Zhang S, Zhang Y, Liu H, Wu F, Wang Z, Li L, et al. Enriched environment remodels the central immune environment and improves the prognosis of acute ischemic stroke in elderly mice with chronic ischemia. Front Immunol 2023;14:1114596. Available from https://doi.org/10.3389/fimmu.2023.1114596.
[26] Lee KH, Jeong EH, Joa KL. Effects of stroke lesions and timing of rehabilitation on the compensatory movement patterns during stroke recovery. Am J Phys Med Rehabil 2022;101(11):1031–7. Available from https://doi.org/10.1097/PHM.0000000000001968.

[27] Tan XD, Liu B, Jiang Y, Yu HJ, Li CQ. Gadd45b mediates environmental enrichment-induced neurogenesis in the SVZ of rats following ischemia stroke via BDNF. Neurosci Lett 2021;745:135616. Available from https://doi.org/10.1016/j.neulet.2020.135616.

[28] Xing Y, Yang SD, Dong F, Wang MM, Feng YS, Zhang F. The beneficial role of early exercise training following stroke and possible mechanisms. Life Sci 2018;198:32–7. Available from https://doi.org/10.1016/j.lfs.2018.02.018.

[29] Zhan Y, Li MZ, Yang L, Feng XF, Lei JF, Zhang N, et al. The three-phase enriched environment paradigm promotes neurovascular restorative and prevents learning impairment after ischemic stroke in rats. Neurobiol Dis 2020;146:105091. Available from https://doi.org/10.1016/j.nbd.2020.105091.

[30] Li C, Sun R, Chen J, Hong J, Sun J, Zeng Y, et al. Different training patterns at recovery stage improve cognitive function in ischemic stroke rats through regulation of the axonal growth inhibitor pathway. Behav Brain Res 2022;421:113730. Available from https://doi.org/10.1016/j.bbr.2021.113730.

[31] de Boer A, Storm A, Gomez-Soler M, Smolders S, Rue L, Poppe L, et al. Environmental enrichment during the chronic phase after experimental stroke promotes functional recovery without synergistic effects of EphA4 targeted therapy. Hum Mol Genet 2020;29(4):605–17. Available from https://doi.org/10.1093/hmg/ddz288.

[32] Nemchek V, Haan EM, Mavros R, Macuiba A, Kerr AL. Voluntary exercise ameliorates the good limb training effect in a mouse model of stroke. Exp Brain Res 2021;239(2):687–97. Available from https://doi.org/10.1007/s00221-020-05994-6.

[33] Janssen H, Speare S, Spratt NJ, Sena ES, Ada L, Hannan AJ, et al. Exploring the efficacy of constraint in animal models of stroke: meta-analysis and systematic review of the current evidence. Neurorehabil Neural Repair 2013;27(1):3–12. Available from https://doi.org/10.1177/1545968312449696.

[34] Schneider A, Rogalewski A, Wafzig O, Kirsch F, Gretz N, Kruger C, et al. Forced arm use is superior to voluntary training for motor recovery and brain plasticity after cortical ischemia in rats. Exp Transl Stroke Med 2014;6(1):3. Available from https://doi.org/10.1186/2040-7378-6-3.

[35] Wurm F, Keiner S, Kunze A, Witte OW, Redecker C. Effects of skilled forelimb training on hippocampal neurogenesis and spatial learning after focal cortical infarcts in the adult rat brain. Stroke 2007;38(10):2833–40. Available from https://doi.org/10.1161/STROKEAHA.107.485524.

[36] Keiner S, Wurm F, Kunze A, Witte OW, Redecker C. Rehabilitative therapies differentially alter proliferation and survival of glial cell populations in the perilesional zone of cortical infarcts. Glia 2008;56(5):516–27. Available from https://doi.org/10.1002/glia.20632.

[37] Marin MA, Gleichman AJ, Wei X, Whittaker DS, Mody I, Colwell CS, et al. Motor activity-induced white matter repair in white matter stroke. J Neurosci 2023;43(48):8126–39. Available from https://doi.org/10.1523/JNEUROSCI.0631-23.2023.

[38] Pan G, Cheng J, Shen W, Lin Y, Zhu A, Jin L, et al. Intensive treadmill training promotes cognitive recovery after cerebral ischemia-reperfusion in juvenile rats. Behav Brain Res 2021;401:113085. Available from https://doi.org/10.1016/j.bbr.2020.113085.

[39] Geng X, Wang Q, Lee H, Huber C, Wills M, Elkin K, et al. Remote ischemic postconditioning vs. physical exercise after stroke: an alternative rehabilitation strategy? Mol Neurobiol 2021;58(7):3141–57. Available from https://doi.org/10.1007/s12035-021-02329-6.

[40] Li M, Zhao Y, Zhan Y, Yang L, Feng X, Lu Y, et al. Enhanced white matter reorganization and activated brain glucose metabolism by enriched environment

following ischemic stroke: Micro PET/CT and MRI study. Neuropharmacology 2020;176:108202. Available from https://doi.org/10.1016/j.neuropharm.2020.108202.

[41] Jeffers MS, Corbett D. Synergistic effects of enriched environment and task-specific reach training on poststroke recovery of motor function. Stroke 2018;49(6):1496–503. Available from https://doi.org/10.1161/STROKEAHA.118.020814.

[42] Yuan M, Guo YS, Han Y, Gao ZK, Shen XY, Bi X. Effectiveness and mechanisms of enriched environment in post-stroke cognitive impairment. Behav Brain Res 2021;410:113357. Available from https://doi.org/10.1016/j.bbr.2021.113357.

[43] Hase Y, Polvikoski TM, Ihara M, Hase M, Zafar R, Stevenson W, et al. Carotid artery disease in post-stroke survivors and effects of enriched environment on stroke pathology in a mouse model of carotid artery stenosis. Neuropathol Appl Neurobiol 2019;45(7):681–97. Available from https://doi.org/10.1111/nan.12550.

[44] Radabaugh HL, Carlson LJ, O'Neil DA, LaPorte MJ, Monaco CM, Cheng JP, et al. Abbreviated environmental enrichment confers neurobehavioral, cognitive, and histological benefits in brain-injured female rats. Exp Neurol 2016;286:61–8. Available from https://doi.org/10.1016/j.expneurol.2016.09.015.

[45] Wang YL, Chen CC, Chang CP. Effect of stress on the rehabilitation performance of rats with repetitive mild fluid percussion-induced traumatic brain injuries. Cogn Neurodyn 2024;18(1):283–97. Available from https://doi.org/10.1007/s11571-023-09961-z.

[46] Yuan M, Zhang XX, Fu XC, Bi X. Enriched environment alleviates post-stroke cognitive impairment through enhancing alpha7-nAChR expression in rats. Arq Neuropsiquiatr 2020;78(10):603–10. Available from https://doi.org/10.1590/0004-282X20200081.

[47] Sampaio-Baptista C, Johansen-Berg H. White matter plasticity in the adult brain. Neuron 2017;96(6):1239–51. Available from https://doi.org/10.1016/j.neuron.2017.11.026.

[48] Cheng YJ, Wang F, Feng J, Yu B, Wang B, Gao Q, et al. Prolonged myelin deficits contribute to neuron loss and functional impairments after ischaemic stroke. Brain 2024;147(4):1294–311. Available from https://doi.org/10.1093/brain/awae029.

[49] Jia P, Wang J, Ren X, He J, Wang S, Xing Y, et al. An enriched environment improves long-term functional outcomes in mice after intracerebral hemorrhage by mechanisms that involve the Nrf2/BDNF/glutaminase pathway. J Cereb Blood Flow Metab 2023;43(5):694–711. Available from https://doi.org/10.1177/0271678X221135419.

[50] Jia W, Kamen Y, Pivonkova H, Karadottir RT. Neuronal activity-dependent myelin repair after stroke. Neurosci Lett 2019;703:139–44. Available from https://doi.org/10.1016/j.neulet.2019.03.005.

[51] Guo YS, Yuan M, Han Y, Shen XY, Gao ZK, Bi X. Effects of enriched environment on microglia and functional white matter recovery in rats with post stroke cognitive impairment. Neurochem Int 2022;154:105295. Available from https://doi.org/10.1016/j.neuint.2022.105295.

[52] Han Y, Shen X, Gao Z, Han P, Bi X. Enriched environment treatment promotes neural functional recovery together with microglia polarization and remyelination after cerebral ischemia in rats. Brain Res Bull 2024;209:110912. Available from https://doi.org/10.1016/j.brainresbull.2024.110912.

[53] Dingman AL, Rodgers KM, Dietz RM, Hickey SP, Frazier AP, Clevenger AC, et al. Oligodendrocyte progenitor cell proliferation and fate after white matter stroke in juvenile and adult mice. Dev Neurosci 2019:1–16. Available from https://doi.org/10.1159/000496200.

[54] Chen X, Wang W, Li H, Zhang X. Enriched environment alleviates neurological deficits via downregulation of Cx43 after experimental stroke. Brain Res 2023;1821:148619. Available from https://doi.org/10.1016/j.brainres.2023.148619.
[55] Gresita A, Mihai R, Hermann DM, Amandei FS, Capitanescu B, Popa-Wagner A. Effect of environmental enrichment and isolation on behavioral and histological indices following focal ischemia in old rats. Geroscience 2022;44(1):211–28. Available from https://doi.org/10.1007/s11357-021-00432-z.
[56] Simats A, Liesz A. Systemic inflammation after stroke: implications for post-stroke comorbidities. EMBO Mol Med 2022;14(9):e16269. Available from https://doi.org/10.15252/emmm.202216269.

CHAPTER

4

Rehabilitation of visual field defects

4.1 Introduction

Visual field deficits (VFDs) affect approximately 8%–25% of all stroke survivors [1–4]. These deficits may have debilitating effects on mobility, visuospatial orientation, higher perceptual or attentional functions, and reading. Although visual rehabilitative interventions suggest that homonymous hemianopia can be treated to some extent, complete restitution is rarely observed [2,5,6]. As spontaneous visual field recovery is very limited [3,4] during or absent after the first 3–6 months poststroke [5], the vast majority of VFD patients will suffer from a permanent and stable VFD.

4.1.1 Some remarks on terminology of visual field deficits and associated disorders

VFD can be distinguished into those affecting visual information from only one eye or both eyes, according to their size and according to their homogeneity for both eyes. Fig. 4.1 shows an overview of different patterns of blindness. Except for rare cases, enduring VFD after strokes concerns lesions at the level of C–F of the figure. However, an occlusion of the ophthalmic artery may affect only one eye, leading to its blindness, which is called amaurosis fugax. This indicates a higher risk of an impending stroke, though the condition is often reversible after a few hours.

Many textbooks provide detailed information about stroke-related visual field defects, their clinical implications, and methods of diagnosis [6–8]. In this context, we will briefly outline essential information about the syndrome and its prognosis, with a primary focus on rehabilitation.

Applied Neuropsychology of Cerebrovascular Diseases
DOI: https://doi.org/10.1016/B978-0-443-45450-9.00001-1

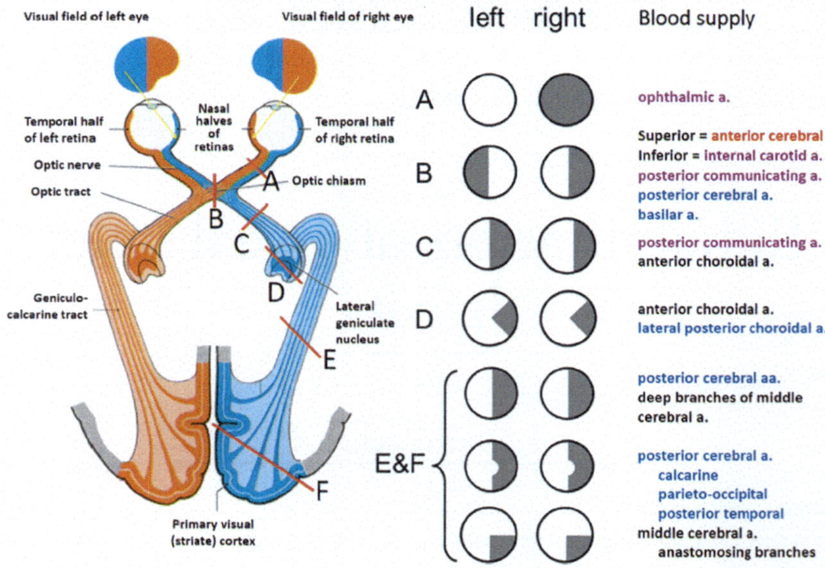

FIGURE 4.1 Different arteries' stroke and resulting visual field defect [7].

VFDs after a stroke are typically homogeneous, meaning that the size and structure of the visual field loss are similar when measured in either eye. In contrast, heteronymous visual field loss—where the location of the deficit varies depending on which eye is being examined—is always indicative of a prechiasmatic lesion [7]. This could be caused by conditions such as a tumor in the hypophysis or optic neuritis, provided the eye itself remains unaffected.

Strokes may lead to a complete loss of one-half of the visual field, which is called homonymous hemianopia. In most cases, the most central part of the visual field (the fovea) is spared (for the neuroanatomic reason see below). Sparing depends on the arteries involved and on their anastomosis. Diagnosing hemianopia should include information about the amount of the spared visual field. Sentences such as, sparing concerns "xx" visual degrees along the horizontal and "xx" visual degrees along the vertical meridian should be part of informing about the result of the assessment. Not infrequently, the field loss concerns only a quarter of the visual field. Such VFDs are called quadrantanopia. In the clinical routine, the extent of the VFD is often somewhat larger than a quadrant. In this case, the description should add a sentence like extending for "xx" degrees along the vertical meridian into the upper or lower quadrant.

There are several peculiarities associated with VFD after stroke that warrant attention. Fluent reading requires at least 2 to 4 degrees of visual angle to the left in order to identify the initial letters of a word [9,10].

Consequently, patients with complete hemianopia without foveal sparing often suffer from a specific reading disorder known as hemianopic dyslexia, characterized by difficulty locating the beginning or end of a word or line of text.

In addition, left sided posterior cerebral artery (PCA) strokes with or without hemianopia may involve the visual word form area [9,11]. Damage to this region can result in pure alexia, a disorder where patients read slowly and rely on letter-by-letter decoding. They often use copying of the letters to recognize them and struggle with identifying atypical letter forms. Pure alexia differs from surface dyslexia in that it stems from impaired visual recognition and is therefore classified as a peripheral dyslexia, while surface dyslexia arises from impaired lexical-semantic processing and is categorized as central.

In the case of a bilateral PCA stroke, hemianopia may spare the central foveal region, resulting in tunnel vision. In very rare cases, it may lead to complete cerebral blindness, although this is more commonly caused by global hypoxia rather than focal ischemia. Notably, some patients with cerebral blindness remain unaware of their deficit—a phenomenon known as Anton's syndrome—and may fabricate visual experiences when prompted, albeit with vague or inconsistent descriptions. Additionally, during the postacute phase, patients with hemianopia may experience visual illusions or visual hallucinations within their blind field.

4.1.2 Neurological basis of visual field deficits

The nervus opticus starts at the retina and projects in most of its fibers toward the corpus geniculatum laterale [12]. At the level of the chiasma opticum, where the fibers reorganize, the nervus opticus becomes the tractus opticus. Upon reaching the corpus geniculatum laterale, fibers extend toward the occipital cortex, which contains the primary visual areas. The radiatio optica connects the corpus geniculatum laterale and the visual areas.

The radiatio optica encompasses two major bundles (Chapter 1). The first bundle, known as Meyer's loop, travels ventrally and initially courses anteriorly before looping posteriorly [12]. It runs lateral to the temporal horn of the lateral ventricle and adjacent to the tail of the caudate nucleus, ultimately reaching the white matter of the occipital lobe. This bundle carries visual information from the upper contralateral visual field quadrant.

The second bundle takes a more direct path, projecting posteriorly with a smaller first dorsal and then a broadening ventral extension. It conveys information from the lower contralateral visual field quadrant.

VFDs are a common consequence of strokes affecting the temporal branch of the arteria cerebri media (ACM) and partly also of a parietal branch (Fig. 4.1) [13]. In such cases, the occipital visual cortex typically remains unaffected. However, the stroke interrupts one or both bundles of the radiatio optica, the fiber pathways that connect the corpus geniculatus laterale with the occipital cortex (Fig. 4.1, lesion at the level of E).

This disconnection is analogous to an internal capsule stroke, where the cortical sensorimotor area is spared, but the thalamocortical and corticospinal pathways are disrupted. Due to the complexity of neuronal connections, the likelihood of dendrites or axons successfully regrowing and reconnecting with the small, specific target neurons of the occipital lobe is essentially zero. As a result, biological restitution in the sense of rebuilt connections is not possible.

Another stroke pattern leading to VFD is an occipital stroke affecting the P4 segment of the PCA. In this case, the radiatio optica may be involved, likely at a more posterior level, along with the cortical visual areas (Fig. 4.1, lesion at level F). Rarely, the stroke affects exclusively the corpus geniculatum laterale, which leads to arrow-like visual deficits (Fig. 4.1, lesion at level D). Such strokes involve one of the choroidal arteries.

As mentioned above, many of these strokes spare the *foveal* visual field (Fig. 4.1), because the most polar part of the occipital lobe (and the gyrus calcarina) is also supplied by anastomoses of the ACM. Additionally, overlapping receptive fields of other neurons, which were not affected by the stroke, but have "sleeping" connections, leave room for recovery at the edges of the field loss. Thus from a therapeutic perspective, these two conditions argue for the possibility of different approaches to VFD: a purely top-down approach may be appropriate if the radiatio optica is affected, whereas restitution may be possible if the stroke is localized more cortically. It is worth noting that causes for VFD, such as traumatic brain injury (TBI) or encephalitis, rarely lead to complete functional losses as complete as those typically seen after stroke, which accounts for the vast majority of cases. Therefore from a theoretical point of view, these conditions may offer greater potential for functional restitution.

4.2 Methods of rehabilitation of visual field deficits

Two main methods of rehabilitation have been proposed [14].

4.2.1 Compensatory therapy—a top-down approach

Compensatory therapy (CT) argues for the necessity to train strategies to make more efficient and systematic saccades into the hemianopic field to indirectly expand the usable field of view. Therefore this approach is a cognitive, top-down approach, accepting the stance that postgeniculate strokes do not show any chance of direct improvement of vision anymore.

4.2.2 Restorative computerized training—a bottom-up approach

Restorative computerized training (RT) is based on visual detection tasks without execution of saccades, aiming for direct restoration of a portion of the visual field by stimulating preserved neuronal representations of the visual system. RT is typically a bottom-up based treatment approach, arguing that the mere number of trials will induce perceptual learning or reactivate functionally not working neurons.

Table 4.1 shows an overview of the two approaches and when they should be used. The evidence for CT is high, whereas evidence for RT is controversial (see below). Up to now, starting with compensatory training to increase the behavioral independence of the patients is indispensable.

However, some neurons, representing the outskirts of the visual blackout zone, might still function physiologically, changing their state only related to highly salient visual information and/or focused attention. Moreover, there might be neurons that have overlapping receptive fields that reach into the defect zone, which are "sleeping," because of a specialization of these neurons for information from outside the VFD. For these areas ("transition zones") restitutive training may be considered, if

TABLE 4.1 Two different approaches for the treatment of visual field defects.

State, stage of recovery	**Approach**	
	Top-down (compensatory therapy)	**Bottom-up (restorative computerized training)**
(Early) postacute visual field defect		Passive visual stimulation of the blind field with acoustic cuing (spatial synchronized tone position)
Postacute severe to moderate visual field defect	Training of large saccades inside the impaired visual field; learning a systematic search strategy. Increased checking behavior in fast changing and unknown environments, which should be avoided if possible.	Training of letter and word recognition, which moves in the direction of the visual field loss. Intensive training of target detection at the border of the field defect, if an amblyopic transition zone is present.
Chronic visual field defect	Transfer of compensatory strategies to different situations which are important for the patient. Advice concerning environmental re-arrangement if necessary.	Intensive training of target detection at the border of the field defect, if an amblyopic transition zone is present. Audio-visual stimulation of the blind field (spatial synchronized position).

visual awareness can be documented under optimal conditions (e.g., a dark room, bright light stimuli, and no interference), but not during daylight condition with static interference. However, without such a transition zone, the chance of a real recovery of the visual field is very low, which can also be concluded by analogy from motor rehabilitation, where a complete plegia (no visual awareness possible in any case) does not recover, whereas a paresis (visual awareness at least in optimal conditions) allows for some recovery.

4.2.3 Blindsight—another possible starting point of rehabilitation?

In contrast to neglect and memory rehabilitation, where interventions often combine top-down (cognitive-driven) and bottom-up (stimulus-driven) approaches, visual field rehabilitation still lacks integrated approaches. A notable exception may be *blindsight*, which could represent a promising, though underexplored, third approach in the treatment of VFD.

Blindsight refers to the implicit ability to respond to visual stimuli presented within a blind visual field, without conscious awareness of the stimuli [15]. This phenomenon is typically demonstrated by asking the patients with VFD to "guess" about the existence and nature of stimuli presented in their blind field. Many patients perform significantly above chance, suggesting residual processing capacity in affected areas. If conscious access to the processes underlying blindsight could be achieved, it might open the door to a combined bottom-up and top-down approach for addressing VFD.

From a neuroanatomical perspective, *blindsight* should be present in a considerable proportion of stroke patients, though estimates vary widely—from 5% to over 70% depending on assessment methods [16,17]. There is consensus that blindsight involves the extrastriate visual pathway, particularly the tractus opticus radix medialis, which branches off at the level of the tractus opticus and projects to midbrain structures such as the superior colliculus, pretectal region, and nucleus accessorius (Fig. 4.2) [12].

The independence of the radix medialis from the radix lateralis can be tested clinically. Even after complete hemianopia, the patients do respond to light presented inside their visual field loss with a direct and indirect pupil response and without becoming aware of the light. Moreover, even completely cortically blind patients suffering from a bilateral PCA stroke do show circadian modulation of melatonin production, because this is based on daily light experience processed by the autonomous visual system. Moreover, at the level of the colliculi superior, the extra striatal visual system also processes information about motion, position, and

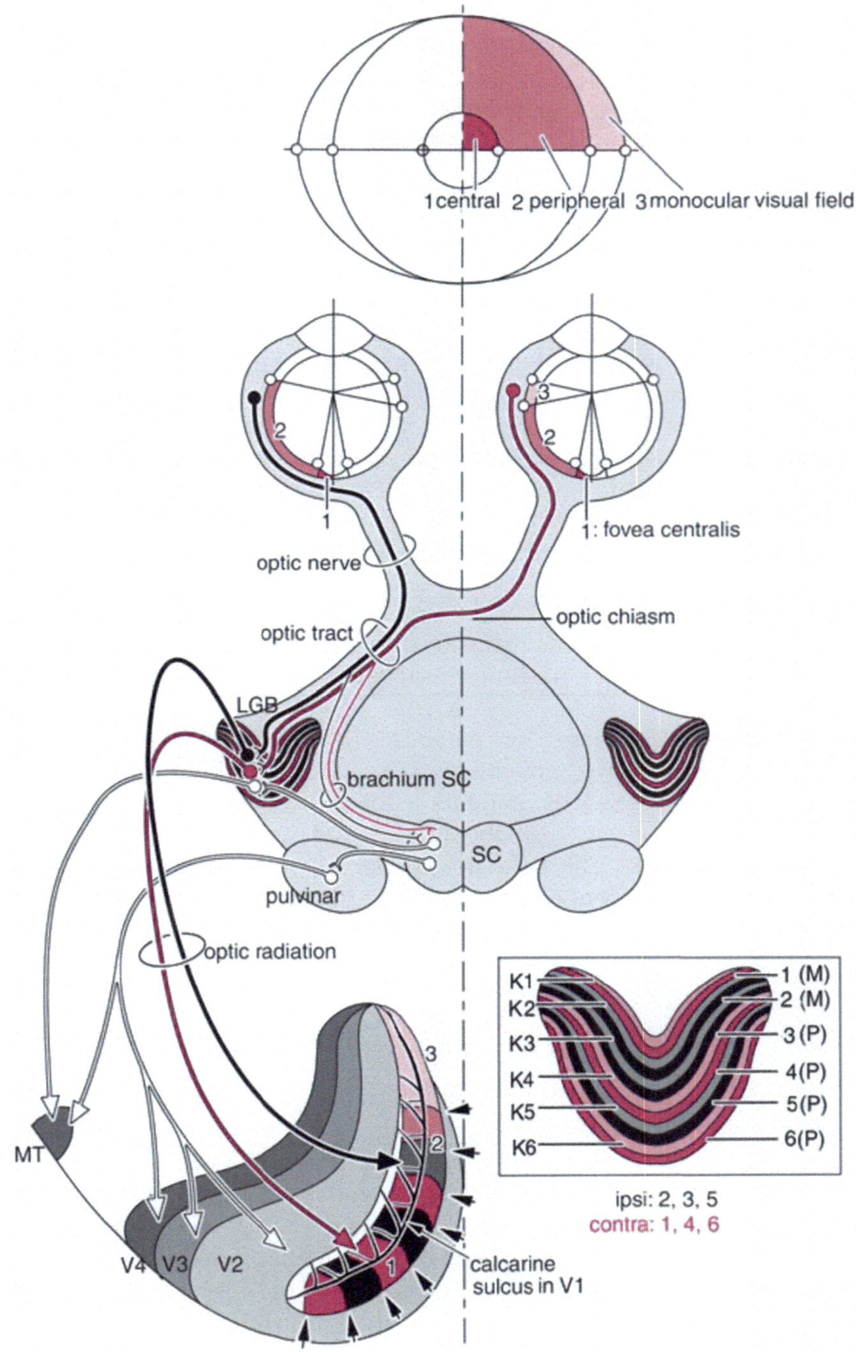

FIGURE 4.2 Neuroanatomical processing of visual information from the retina to the visual cortex. *From Nieuwenhuys R.V., van Huijzen J. Chris the Human Central Nervous System.* Berlin: Springer; *2008.*

luminance. Colliculi-fugal fibers feed this information forward to the pulvinar [18], and there seems also to exist an independent colliculi-fugal tract toward the amygdala for fearful objects [12]. The pulvinar, a large thalamic nucleus, which is involved in selective visuospatial attention and motion perception, also receives afferents directly from the retina, bypassing the superior colliculus but also the corpus geniculatum laterale.

There are also fiber tracts that exit the corpus geniculatum laterale and project directly to the secondary visual cortex, bypassing the primary visual cortex. Most of these tracts may not be affected by typical PCA and ACM strokes, potentially enabling implicit or partially conscious awareness of visual information in the impaired visual field. Since the seminal work of Weiskrantz and Weiskrantz [19], two forms of blindsight have been distinguished: type I, involving purely implicit visual processing without conscious awareness, and type II, where some level of conscious awareness is present. From a rehabilitative perspective, the central question remains whether this implicitly present visual processing can be used for improving abilities in everyday life.

4.3 Top-down compensation as treatment of hemianopia field deficits—saccades

Cognitive interventions for patients with VFD are based on the possibility of using eye movements (i.e., saccades) to compensate for visual loss. In other words, patients learn to execute saccades into the impaired visual field to use the unimpaired hemifield to detect the relevant information. The field defect, per se, is not impacted by this treatment. The main goal of compensatory training is to enlarge saccade amplitude and reduce saccadic reaction time when looking to the blind portion of the visual field [14,20].

4.3.1 Training saccades to compensate for visual loss

The Fig. 4.3 shows an example of the training of saccades taken from the Reha software "Rehacom, Magdeburg." The task of the patients is to start at the center of the screen (where the moon is located) and detect objects that are appearing predominantly on the side of the VFD. The size of the object and the distance from the center of the screen vary according to the level of compensation reached by the patients. Another component of compensation training is the introduction of a systematic search strategy, which should always start far enough inside the VFD to allow an efficient orientation and overview.

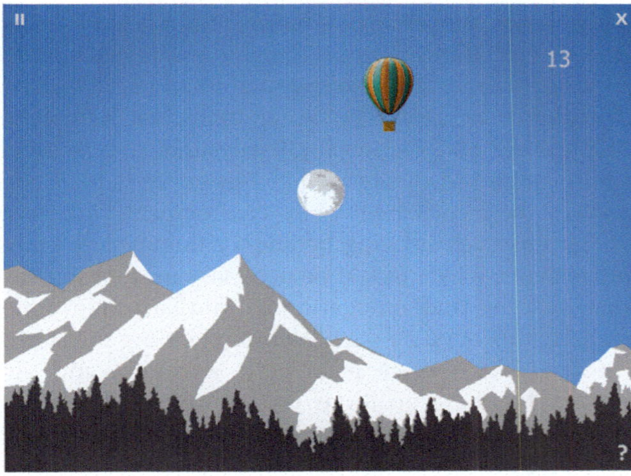

FIGURE 4.3 Screen for compensatory training in patients with visual field defects.

4.3.2 Visual search strategy and systematic scanning

Early visual search training typically used simplified displays, such as randomly positioned white targets embedded among distractor elements on a black background. These targets differed from distractors along a single dimension—such as form, size, or orientation size—allowing for controlled manipulation of target salience. To prevent participants from developing automatic response patterns, nontarget trials can be randomly interspersed.

Pambakian, Mannan, Hodgson, and Kennard [21] showed that compensatory visual scanning training led to improvements in visual search times and patient-reported quality of life, but no measurable change was observed in the extent of the VFD. In a similar study, Hayes, Chen, Clarke, and Thompson [22] replicated these findings and documented better orientation in a real-life course, requiring avoidance of obstacles. Again, the VFD remained unchanged. Both studies implemented approximately 20 one-hour sessions and found that the benefits persisted at follow-up, indicating the durability of the training effect. However, as both studies were simple pre and post trials without control groups, their findings should be interpreted with caution.

Nelles, Pscherer, de Greiff, Gerhard, Forsting, Esser, and Diener [23] used functional Magnetic Resonance Imaging (fMRI) to analyze the effects of compensatory training on the brain activity of stroke patients with hemianopia. They found an increased ipsilateral extrastriate activation of the intact hemisphere, without corresponding activation in contralateral striate areas—suggesting an ipsilesional reorganization of visual processing following stroke.

Thus several observational and smaller randomized controlled trials (RCTs) indicated that compensatory training improves visual scanning, gaining a quick and safe visual overview of a visual scene. Accordingly, the Cochrane review by Pollock, Hazelton, Rowe, Jonuscheit, Kernohan, Angilley, Henderson, Langhorne, and Campbell [3] states that compensation training can contribute to improved quality of life. Nevertheless, their effectiveness largely depends on the predictability of the environment. Unknown and fast-changing settings remain challenging, because no training will lead to fast and erratic eye movements, which would be necessary in such situations.

By contrast, reading and navigation in familiar environments is an ability that can be improved by such training. Finding the starting or end point of text lines takes place in a static situation, and visuospatial working memory for these positions can be used to guide and control saccades. The same holds for navigation in an office or at home, where furniture and objects do not move from their place.

The effectiveness of scanning training on search performance and saccadic behavior was reviewed recently by Postuma, Heutink, Tol, Jansen, Koopman, Cornelissen, and de Haan [24]. Spontaneous adaptations were characterized by more scanning repetitions, shorter saccades, and more frequent scanning of the blind hemispace. Training reduced the number of fixations and tended to decrease repetition and scanpath length. This was consistent across search and reading training. Moreover, the review showed that effective search behavior differs according to the environment: large saccades are important during driving, but unimportant for reading, where restricted saccade amplitudes towards the beginning of the line must be kept in working memory. This suggests that, during the chronic phase, interventions should be adapted to address the specific issues patients face at the outset of treatment.

4.3.3 Moving window training for hemianopic reading disorders

While saccadic and compensatory visual search training can improve reading performance in patients with hemianopic reading disorders, the observed effects are typically limited. Focusing directly on reading seems to be more effective [25].

A particularly promising compensatory treatment is *moving window training* for a comprehensive overview, see Kerkhoff and Kraft [26]. In this training, several lines of continuous text were presented, but only one word was highlighted in bright white, which is the target word that should be read out aloud. Once the patient presses a response button, the next word is illuminated while the previous ones fade to dark gray. The remaining words remain faintly visible, providing spatial orientation within the line and on the screen while minimizing visual crowding.

An alternative approach is *rapid serial visual presentation*, which displays single words or objects at high speed, encouraging fast saccades into the blind hemifield in order to promote improved spatial coverage. A third method, known as *floating line therapy*, involves the presentation of a single line of text that moves horizontally (right to left) through the center of the screen this helps to structure scanning movements in a predictable manner and supports consistent reading flow (indicated by the white arrow in Fig. 4.4, which is not visible during therapy).

Kerkhoff and Kraft [26] applied these training methods for treating patients with chronic hemianopic dyslexia (n = 27) and evaluated the effect using a single-case experimental design. Their results demonstrated significant and lasting improvements across all outcome measures. Notably, approximately 63% of the patients were able to return to work after the intervention. However, the study lacks detail regarding the exact number and duration of sessions and did not include an active control group.

Nevertheless, the reviews by Schuett [27] and Maeyama, Okada, and Sakai [25] support the superiority of compensatory over restorative training approaches for hemianopic reading disorders. Compensatory methods lead to selective, stable, and clinically meaningful improvements both subjectively and objectively. Moreover, they are more cost-effective and require significantly less time investment than restorative therapies.

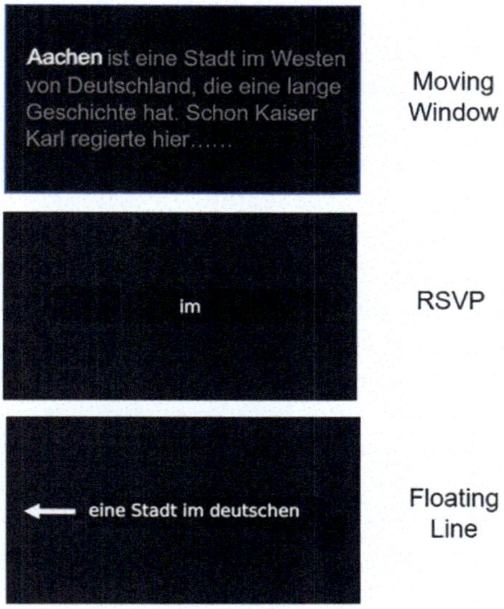

FIGURE 4.4 Schematic illustration of three reading trainings (Kerkhoff & Kraft) [26]. First rectangle: Reading with the help of highlighting the word. Second rectangle: short-term presentation of the sentence's words in the center of the screen. Third rectangle: Running of the sentence's words toward the left.

4.4 Bottom-up stimulation for treating hemianopic field deficits

Bottom-up approaches to VFD rehabilitation are based on the principles of perceptual learning and/or on activating functioning neurons, which get the visual information but were not involved in processing before, because other neuronal repertoires were more specialized. The core assumption is that high-repetition stimulation can recruit functionally silent or underutilized neurons near the lesion site by strengthening their involvement in visual processing, so that over time, the patient may experience some recovery of their vision. In the study by Casco, Barollo, Contemori, and Battaglini [28], for example, targets were systematically shifted toward the blind field, adapting dynamically to the patient's progress (Fig. 4.5).

4.4.1 Effectiveness of restitutive training

Subsequent investigations found that RT may mildly reduce VFD, on average, by less than 2 degrees [6–11]. One study found no improvement at all [12]. A Cochrane review concluded that there is currently no evidence supporting RT for improving outcomes in hemianopic patients and recommended prioritizing compensatory treatment. According to this review, future studies should compare compensatory and restitutive interventions against placebo, control, no treatment, or usual care [22].

One more recent non-RCT study analyzed the impact of intensive RT in patients with stroke over more than 10 months [29]. While field improvements were small (1–2 degrees), these gains were more pronounced in individuals who retained perilesional neurons capable of processing visual stimuli. The improvements were primarily limited to luminance and motion detection, with no evidence of recovery in shape recognition, which is essential for tasks such as reading or driving. These findings raise important concerns about the functional relevance of minor field expansions if they do not restore more complex perceptual capabilities.

Additional support for the significance of neural reserve comes from Elshout, Bergsma, van den Berg, and Haak [30], who provided 80 hours of RT to patients with poststroke hemianopia. Improvements were not restricted to regions in the primary visual cortex but also related to activity in higher-order visual areas. This finding aligns with the assumption of sleeping neurons and is related to earlier work demonstrating that restitutive training depends on an amblyopic transition field (area of residual vision) with partial correct response during testing, where the treatment should be focused. Poggel, Treutwein, Sabel, and Strasburger [31] noted as a result of their study that in such transition zones between the blind and intact areas where patients showed a between 20% and 80% of stimulus detection probability during pretraining testing, the improvement was marked. Still, the interindividual

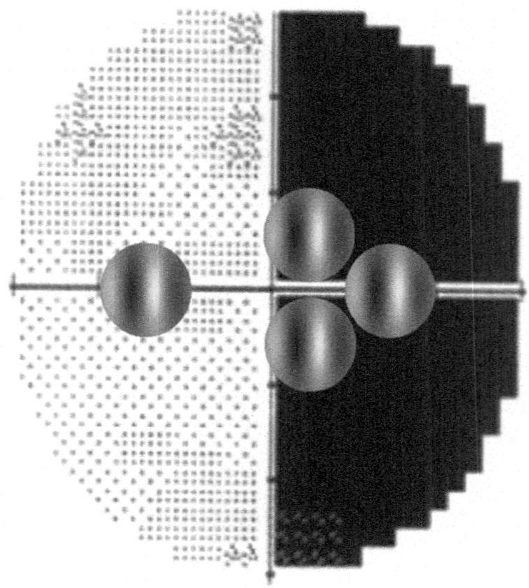

FIGURE 4.5 The figure shows one example of stimulus position: two stimuli along the hemianopic borders, one stimulus in the blind field, and one stimulus in the seeing field. Bear in mind that in a Gabor stimulus, the carrier is presented within a Gaussian envelope, which smooths the contrast at the border. *From Casco C., Barollo M., Contemori G., Battaglini L. Neural restoration training improves visual functions and expands visual field of patients with homonymous visual field defects. Restor Neurol Neurosci 2018;36:275–291.*

training outcome variability is very high, with some patients showing little change and others showing performance approaching that of healthy controls.

it also relates to prior studies trying to use prior cuing of target positions to enhance their detection inside the blind field [31]. documented that focusing attention on position inside the amblyopic transition field between normal vision and complete field loss changed topographic and temporal patterns of recovery as compared with uncued regions of the visual field, and the patients showed a higher shift of the visual field border toward the blind area.

Based on the results of [31] and [29,32] on the meaning of the amblyopic transition zone for efficacy, restitutive training should be started only if such a transition zone can be shown during the assessment. Such transition zones can be easily detected either by using larger and lighter spots for visual field testing and by comparing these results to those with small and low salient spots. Or by using, for example, the "Gesichtsfeldtest kurz" of the Testbatterie zur Aufmerksamkeitsprüfung [33] in a darkened room and comparing these results with those of the "Neglekt Test" of the TAP in a room with daylight. Fig. 4.6 shows the results of a patient with a large amblyopic transition zone in the left upper quadrant, which became

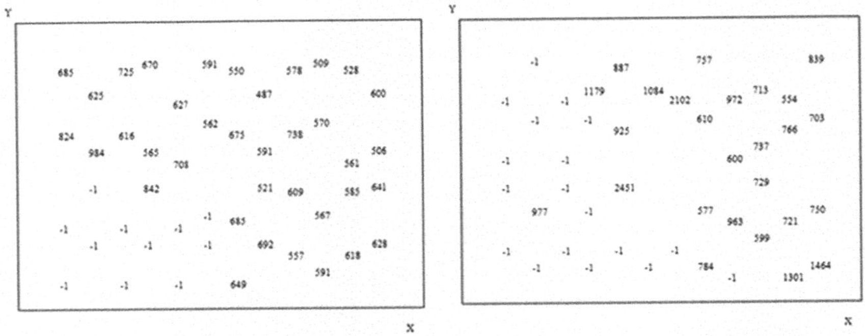

FIGURE 4.6 Different size of visual field defects dependent on the salience of targets.

evident when tested with the same task in two different conditions of visual salience and additionally controlling for any eye movements.

A third recent study compared the effect of performing the intervention in the postacute or chronic stage [32]. Patients in a postacute stage showed markedly faster progress than those in the chronic phase, achieving comparable outcomes with significantly fewer training sessions. This observation supports the idea that the window for effective RT may lie earlier in the recovery process than traditionally assumed.

Only a few studies have directly compared RT with compensatory treatment. In two groups of chronic brain damage patients with unilateral field defects, Roth et al. showed that compensatory treatment was superior to RT by decreasing search time at the follow-up investigation and by improving eye movement strategies.

Most studies have focused on chronic patients involving various causes of hemianopia. However, systematic early treatment offered early in the recovery process may be more effective than late-stage intervention, and outcomes may differ between stroke and TBI patients. In our own RCT, we evaluated 45 stroke patients with VFDs during inpatient rehabilitation [34]. Participants were assigned to either RT-using computer-based stimulation at the visual field border; to CT-involving computer-based visual search strategy training; or to occupational therapy (OT) as an active control focusing on compensatory strategies in daily life. The primary outcome measures were visual field expansion for RT, visual search performance for CT, and reading performance for both treatments. Visual conjunction search, alertness, and the Barthel Index served as secondary outcome measures.

All groups received 15 sessions over 3 weeks. CT employed the RehaCom "Exploration" task, adapted for the hemianopic side, where patients tracked a moving ring across a symbol matrix and responded upon detecting target items—especially placed on the blind side to promote exploration [34] (Table 4.2)

TABLE 4.2 Significant. Improvement per training group (only intragroup pre/post comparisons).

	Restitutional training	Compensatory treatment	Occupational treatment
Visual field enlargement (TAP, visual field assessment)	Yes (3.9 ± 4.9)[a,b]	Yes (2.9 ± 4.0)[a]	No (1.3 ± 4.7)[a]
Cancellation tasks of the BIT (omissions)	Yes (5.3 ± 10.5)	Yes (5.4 ± 5.2)	No (2.3 ± 5.0)
Reading performance (errors)	No (0.9 ± 2.4)	Yes (0.9 ± 1.1)	No (0.7 ± 1.0)
Attention (TAP, Alertness)	Yes (28.5 ± 56.9)	Yes (77.8 ± 112.9)	No (-13.3 ± 112.7)
Visual conjunction search (TAP, visual scanning)	No (2.7 ± 5.1)	Yes (7.0 ± 5.0)	No (3.5 ± 6.8)
Extended Barthel Index	Yes (1.5 ± 2.8)	Yes (3.3 ± 3.6)	Yes (1.8 ± 2.0)

Abbreviations: BIT, behavioral inattention test; TAP, testing battery for attention performance.
[a] *Number of additional detected stimuli during testing.*
[b] *The figures in parentheses show the difference score between t2 (after treatment) and 11 (before treatment) and the standard deviation for this difference score. Positive values indicate improvements, negative values indicate deteriorations.*

The patients receiving CT were informed of the meaning of large saccades toward the hemianopic visual field. Patients were informed why such a strategy is safe and effective for compensating for the VFD. Moreover, the meaning of systematic scanning behavior was introduced. The compensatory strategies were trained by computer-based training. On a dark background, different bright stimuli arranged in rows and columns were presented. A ring (diameter of 2 cm) moved line by line (interlaced) on a matrix unit over the field. The participant was instructed to follow the ring (starting point to an outmost fixation in the blind side) by eye movements and to identify a critical targeted icon. The targets were not always distributed homogeneously, but were clustered on the blind side. Thus the exploration in the hemianopic field was further promoted. The patients had to respond (by pressing a key) when the targeted icon was perceived in the circle. The program contained several difficulty levels. In levels 1–20, all lines were completely filled with symbols, whereas there were omissions in the rows of symbols in levels 21–30 to increase the difficulty.

The group receiving the RT used a perimeter-based training system (Teltra) tailored to each patient's visual field map. A series of colored targets presented on a blue screen appeared anywhere at one of 10 positions on the borderline. A randomly presented first fixation target (a rotating arrow) announced the second stimulus-target in the hemianopic border zone (basic principle of covert attention shift). It was required to respond to key presses upon detection (colored and flickering frames, beams, and spots). The program contained no adaptive difficulty levels. Eye movements were not allowed and were monitored.

The results were conclusive: patients performing the compensatory training improved in all primary and secondary outcome parameter, patients performing the restitutive training only for some. CT improved all primary and secondary outcomes. RT yielded limited gains and showed no field expansion advantage over OT. CT patients had better visual search performance, and overall, compensatory training enhanced functional outcomes more effectively. These results support current guidelines recommending CT as a first-line intervention [34]. Moreover, it is safe, easy, and can be based partly on supervised computerized training software. Our results fit those from many other studies, and teaching the patients compensatory strategies to cope with their problems related to the hemianopic field defect is recommended by different guidelines.

4.5 Improving visual awareness and visual guided behavior by blindsight?

4.5.1 Conceptual differences to RT and compensatory therapy

As already mentioned, blindsight refers to a form of implicit visual processing where individuals can respond to visual stimuli without conscious visual awareness—or in a qualitatively different way than typical perception. This phenomenon opens a potential third pathway for VFD rehabilitation that goes beyond traditional compensatory or restitutive strategies.

Unlike the compensatory approach, using blindsight as a starting point would try to gain access to unconscious processing and use this processing to reestablish a *kind* of seeing inside the field defect. In contrast to simple restitution training, blindsight training uses large, flickering gratings or moving stimuli, which are features that optimize the chance for detection by involving secondary visual processes known to be dependent also on extra-geniculate processing systems. In contrast to restitution training, the goal is not to stimulate receptive fields of functionally "sleeping" neurons, but to use extra-geniculate processes to improve visual perception.

These conceptual differences are crucial when designing the rehabilitative training. First, eye tracking integration is essential, both during training and outcome assessment, to control for microsaccades. This ensures that stimulus detection cannot be attributed to a gaze shift into intact visual field regions and that genuine processing within the blind field is being measured. Second, forced-choice paradigms between two or more response options are preferred over passive detection tasks (instead of just not responding, which may avoid decisions, which is the case in restitutive trainings).

Third, training protocols often include gamified and adaptive elements that keep patients engaged and gradually increase task complexity. Some studies also use performance feedback, enhancing motivation and reinforcing learning—even if responses are based on intuition rather than conscious awareness.

Fig. 4.7 illustrates a typical method for assessing blindsight: participants are shown a series of stimuli and either asked to indicate stimulus presence/absence (method 1) or to rate their perceptual awareness using a graded scale (method 2).

This allows comparisons between binary and graded awareness responses and enables correlations between subjective reports and actual stimulus presentation.

Fig. 4.7 also illustrates how different visual features can be tested to determine whether blindsight is present across all or only specific stimulus characteristics. Research suggests that blindsight is most reliable when it emerges in response to luminance and movement cues, while unconscious processing of form and color is considerably less common [36]. Another feature of stimuli that appears capable of triggering preconscious processing involves facial expressions, which may activate subcortical pathways linked to emotional and social perception, even in the absence of visual awareness.

4.5.2 Effectiveness of blindsight in rehabilitation

Willis, Caron, Cavanaugh, Starling, Ajina, Pestilli, Tamietto, Huxlin, Watkins, and Bridge [37] published a recent study on using blindsight-based rehabilitation for VFD. The study included 18 stroke patients with chronic,

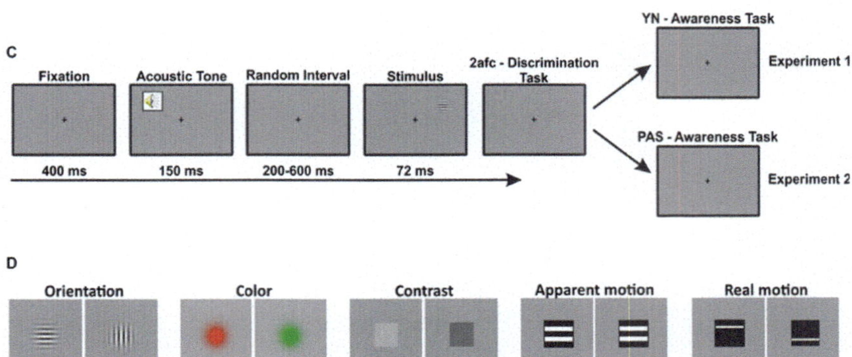

FIGURE 4.7 Typical design to test patients for blind sight [35].

unilateral VFDs from retrogeniculate brain lesions. Over 6 months, at least five times per week, participants completed daily motion discrimination tasks at home, targeting two nonoverlapping blind field locations. Posttraining assessments revealed improved motion discrimination and modest reductions in field defect on perimetry, though with substantial interindividual variability. Notably, improvements in motion discrimination performance predicted the extent of VFD recovery, while the pretraining deficit size did not. These findings support the idea that blindsight can generalize beyond the specific trained function, potentially benefiting broader visual capabilities [36,37]. Meanwhile, a generalization of blindsight training to different visual functions has been documented several times, which would mean that one training fits several aspects of vision. On the other hand, small increases of the visual field have also been documented after short compensatory training, and if specifically documented, the increase in the visual field after blindsight training was mainly between 1 and 3 degrees (Fig. 4.8).

4.5.3 Challenges in blindsight rehabilitation and limitations

One of the major challenges in using blindsight-based rehabilitation is the high training demand, with some protocols requiring up to 300

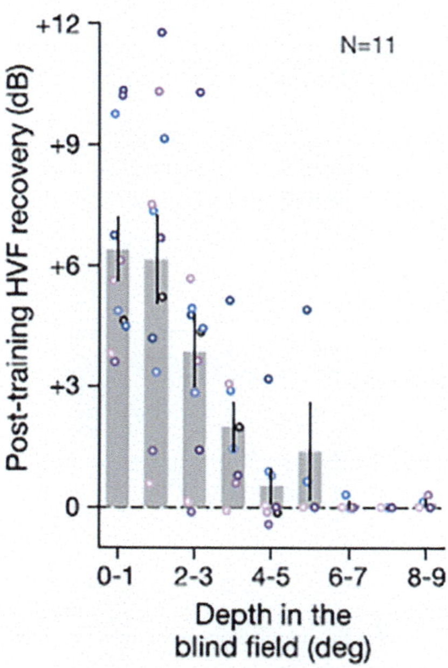

FIGURE 4.8 Training of visual perception are limited to the boarder of the field defect [29].

sessions. To date, there are no RCTs comparing blindsight-based training with an active control group or compensatory approaches. Most blindsight studies focus on chronic patients and rely on intragroup comparisons, limiting generalizability. Moreover, an improvement in task-specific performance—such as correctly guessing stimulus presence—does not necessarily translate into increased functioning in activities of daily living. In real-world settings, relying on guesses is often insufficient for safe navigation and visual orientation. As a result, the significance of blindsight training has still to be evaluated to produce meaningful changes in everyday behavior.

4.5.4 Audiovisual stimulation

Audiovisual stimulation uses simultaneously presented visual and auditory stimulation from spatially similar positions to remediate VFD [28,38,39]. The theoretical background lies in multisensory integration at the level of the superior colliculus, where spatial signals from different sensory modalities are merged subcortically. This is neurophysiologically similar to blindsight relying on preserved subcortical processing pathways, but differs in its neuropsychological rationale: here, auditory cues are used to guide visual orienting and elicit goal-directed saccades into the blind field, serving as a compensating mechanism.

Animal studies have shown that such cross-modal stimulation of visual and auditory spatial information at the level of the superior colliculus promotes functional recovery from artificially induced VFD, even in anaesthetized cats [40,41]. In humans with chronic VFD, audiovisual stimulation has been shown to train patients to initiate accurate saccades towards unseen targets [38]. The effect of the training generalized to visual search, reading, and the feeling of safety during everyday activities. These responses were not conscious, but systematically tied to stimulus presence, surpassing the more random scanning behavior typically observed in standard compensatory strategies. Interestingly, a more recent study on audiovisual stimulation initiated at the subacute poststroke stage also found a partial re-emergence of conscious visual perception [4,32].

Although these findings are promising, sample sizes remain small (often $n < 10$), and many are based on single-case series. Therefore this approach is not yet ready for clinical routine but holds potential—especially when conventional compensatory training reaches its limits. The firm neurobiological basis and promising effects in animal experiments suggest that audiovisual stimulation may become a more prominent strategy in future neurorehabilitation paradigms.

4.5.5 Practical implementations

The primary rehabilitative goal of blindsight-based training is not merely to increase the rate of correct guesses but to enhance stimulus awareness within the blind field. This implies that nature and timing of feedback may be more critical than the number of trials alone. Most current studies prioritize objective task performance, but from a clinical perspective, the crucial issue is how implicit perception can be made accessible to conscious experience—without inflating false-positive responses.

Garric, Sebaa, Caetta, Perez, Savatovsky, Sergent, and Chokron [42] showed that more patients exhibit above-chance sensitivity to subjective awareness scales, despite being unable to identify the stimulus during the forced-choice task. This highlights the importance of using awareness-sensitive methods to assess and enhance perceptual consciousness, rather than relying solely on accuracy metrics. Ideally, training should focus on whether these perceptual improvements translate into benefits for everyday life—such as navigation, reading, or hazard detection—rather than isolated laboratory gains.

References

[1] de Haan GA, Heutink J, Melis-Dankers BJ, Tucha O, Brouwer WH. Spontaneous recovery and treatment effects in patients with homonymous visual field defects: a meta-analysis of existing literature in terms of the icf framework. Surv Ophthalmol 2014;59:77–96.

[2] Rowe F, Brand D, Jackson CA, Price A, Walker L, Harrison S, et al. Visual impairment following stroke: do stroke patients require vision assessment? Age Ageing 2009;38:188–93.

[3] Pollock A, Hazelton C, Rowe FJ, Jonuscheit S, Kernohan A, Angilley J, et al. Interventions for visual field defects in people with stroke. Cochrane Database Syst Rev 2019;5. CD008388.

[4] Saionz EL, Busza A, Huxlin KR. Rehabilitation of visual perception in cortical blindness. Handb Clin Neurol 2022;184:357–73.

[5] Zhang X, Kedar S, Lynn MJ, Newman NJ, Biousse V. Natural history of homonymous hemianopia. Neurology 2006;66:901–5.

[6] Zhang X, Kedar S, Lynn MJ, Newman NJ, Biousse V. Homonymous hemianopia in stroke. J Neuroophthalmol 2006;26:180–3.

[7] Zeki S, Leff A. The striate cortex and hemianopia. Handb Clin Neurol 2021;178:115–29.

[8] Skorkovská K. Homonymous visual field defects. Springer International; 2017.

[9] Leff AP, Crewes H, Plant GT, Scott SK, Kennard C, Wise RJ. The functional anatomy of single-word reading in patients with hemianopic and pure alexia. Brain 2001;124:510–21.

[10] Zihl J. Eye movement patterns in hemianopic dyslexia. Brain 1995;118(Pt 4):891–912.

[11] Hanley JR, Kay J. Reading speed in pure alexia. Neuropsychologia 1996;34:1165–74.

[12] Nieuwenhuys RV, van Huijzen J. Chris the Human Central Nervous System. *Berlin: Springer*; 2008.

[13] Zhang X, Kedar S, Lynn MJ, Newman NJ, Biousse V. Homonymous hemianopias: clinical-anatomic correlations in 904 cases. Neurology 2006;66:906–10.

[14] Kerkhoff G, Rode G, Clarke S. Treating neurovisual deficits and spatial neglect. In: Platz T, ed. *Clinical pathways in stroke rehabilitation: Evidence-based clinical practice recommendations*. Cham (CH); 2021:191-217.
[15] Derrien D, Garric C, Sergent C, Chokron S. The nature of blindsight: implications for current theories of consciousness. Neurosci Conscious 2022;2022:niab043.
[16] Marzi CA, Tassinari G, Aglioti S, Lutzemberger L. Spatial summation across the vertical meridian in hemianopics: a test of blindsight. Neuropsychologia 1986;24:749–58.
[17] Weiskrantz L. Varieties of residual experience. Q J Exp Psychol 1980;32:365–86.
[18] Fang Q, Chou XL, Peng B, Zhong W, Zhang LI, Tao HW. A differential circuit via retino-colliculo-pulvinar pathway enhances feature selectivity in visual cortex through surround suppression. Neuron 2020;105:355–69. e356.
[19] Weiskrantz L, Weiskrantz L. Blindsight: a case study spanning 35 years and new developments. Oxford; New York: Oxford University Press; 2009.
[20] Kerkhoff G, Haaf MU, Eberle-Strauss E, Stogerer G. E. Rehabilitation of homonymous scotomata in patients with postgeniculate damage of the visual system: Saccadic compensation training. Restor Neurol Neurosci 1992;4:245–54.
[21] Pambakian AL, Mannan SK, Hodgson TL, Kennard C. Saccadic visual search training: a treatment for patients with homonymous hemianopia. J Neurol Neurosurg Psychiatry 2004;75:1443–8.
[22] Hayes A, Chen CS, Clarke G, Thompson A. Functional improvements following the use of the nvt vision rehabilitation program for patients with hemianopia following stroke. NeuroRehabilitation 2012;31:19–30.
[23] Nelles G, Pscherer A, de, Greiff A, Gerhard H, Forsting M, et al. Eye-movement training-induced changes of visual field representation in patients with post-stroke hemianopia. J Neurol 2010;257:1832–40.
[24] Postuma E, Heutink J, Tol S, Jansen JL, Koopman J, Cornelissen FW, et al. A systematic review on visual scanning behaviour in hemianopia considering task specificity, performance improvement, spontaneous and training-induced adaptations. Disabil Rehabil 2024;46:3221–42.
[25] Maeyama T, Okada H, Sakai S. The effects of rehabilitative interventions on reading disorders caused by homonymous visual field defects: A meta-analysis focusing on improvement in reading speed. Acta Neurol Belg 2024;124:123–40.
[26] Kerkhoff G, Kraft A. The effects of a novel treatment for hemianopic dyslexia on reading, symptom load, and return to work. Brain Sci 2024;14.
[27] Schuett S. The rehabilitation of hemianopic dyslexia. Nat Rev Neurol 2009;5:427–37.
[28] Casco C, Barollo M, Contemori G, Battaglini L. Neural restoration training improves visual functions and expands visual field of patients with homonymous visual field defects. Restor Neurol Neurosci 2018;36:275–91.
[29] Barbot A, Das A, Melnick MD, Cavanaugh MR, Merriam EP, Heeger DJ, et al. Spared perilesional v1 activity underlies training-induced recovery of luminance detection sensitivity in cortically-blind patients. Nat Commun 2021;12:6102.
[30] Elshout JA, Bergsma DP, van den Berg AV, Haak KV. Functional mri of visual cortex predicts training-induced recovery in stroke patients with homonymous visual field defects. Neuroimage Clin 2021;31:102703.
[31] Poggel DA, Treutwein B, Sabel BA, Strasburger H. A matter of time: improvement of visual temporal processing during training-induced restoration of light detection performance. Front Psychol 2015;6:22.
[32] Saionz EL, Tadin D, Melnick MD, Huxlin KR. Functional preservation and enhanced capacity for visual restoration in subacute occipital stroke. Brain 2020;143:1857–72.
[33] Zimmermann P. Testbatterie zur aufmerksamkeitsprüfung (tap). 1992.

[34] Modden C, Behrens M, Damke I, Eilers N, Kastrup A, Hildebrandt H. A randomized controlled trial comparing 2 interventions for visual field loss with standard occupational therapy during inpatient stroke rehabilitation. Neurorehabil Neural Repair 2012;26:463–9.

[35] Mazzi C, Bagattini C, Savazzi S. Blind-sight vs. Degraded-sight: different measures tell a different story. Front Psychol 2016;7:901.

[36] Melnick MD, Tadin D, Huxlin KR. Relearning to see in cortical blindness. Neuroscientist 2016;22:199–212.

[37] Willis HE, Caron B, Cavanaugh MR, Starling L, Ajina S, Pestilli F, et al. Rehabilitating homonymous visual field deficits: white matter markers of recovery-stage 2 registered report. Brain Commun 2024;6:fcae323.

[38] Alwashmi K, Meyer G, Rowe FJ. Audio-visual stimulation for visual compensatory functions in stroke survivors with visual field defect: a systematic review. Neurol Sci 2022;43:2299–321.

[39] Rowland BA, Bushnell CD, Duncan PW, Stein BE. Ameliorating hemianopia with multisensory training. J Neurosci 2023;43:1018–26.

[40] Jiang H, Rowland BA, Stein BE. Reversing hemianopia by multisensory training under anesthesia. Front Syst Neurosci 2020;14:4.

[41] Jiang H, Stein BE, McHaffie JG. Multisensory training reverses midbrain lesion-induced changes and ameliorates haemianopia. Nat Commun 2015;6:7263.

[42] Garric C, Sebaa A, Caetta F, Perez C, Savatovsky J, Sergent C, et al. Dissociation between objective and subjective perceptual experiences in a population of hemianopic patients: a new form of blindsight? Cortex 2019;117:299–310.

CHAPTER

5

Rehabilitation of unilateral visuospatial deficits

5.1 Introduction

Visuospatial neglect (VSN) is a common neuropsychological consequence of right-hemispheric stroke, most frequently following infarcts in the territory of the right middle cerebral artery (MCA). Patients with VSN typically fail to detect stimuli on the left side of space and often present with characteristic reading impairments, such as omitting or misreading the left portion of words or text [1,2].

Importantly, the presence of neglect is associated with longer durations of inpatient rehabilitation and more pronounced impairments in activities of daily living (ADLs), even when compared to stroke patients with comparable motor deficits [3]. Although spontaneous recovery is frequent, particularly within the first 6 to 12 weeks, visuospatial hemi-inattention persists in approximately 10% to 20% of right MCA stroke patients even 6 months poststroke. A recent metaanalytic review confirmed that the majority of recovery from neglect occurs within the first 3 months, with additional gains possible up to 6 months; nonetheless, over 40% of patients show persistent symptoms beyond this period [4]. An effective treatment of neglect during stroke rehabilitation is therefore of particular importance [2,3,5].

Numerous comprehensive reviews have addressed VSN, its diagnostic and clinical implications [2,4–7]. The present chapter provides a brief overview of its diagnostic and prognostic features, with a primary focus on evidence-based therapeutic interventions in early neurological rehabilitation.

5.2 Defining neglect syndromes

VSN is not a unitary condition but a syndrome comprising multiple distinct symptoms, which can vary depending on the affected branches of

Applied Neuropsychology of Cerebrovascular Diseases
DOI: https://doi.org/10.1016/B978-0-443-45450-9.00006-0

the MCA. Numerous subtypes of neglect have been described, including distinctions based on spatial domain (e.g., near vs far space) and sensory modality (e.g., visual, auditory, and tactile). However, for clinical purposes, particularly in the context of rehabilitation, it is often sufficient to differentiate between a few key forms of neglect. These distinctions are relevant either because they are associated with differential prognoses or because they require distinct therapeutic strategies.

5.2.1 (Pre)motor neglect

Isolated strokes affecting the premotor branches of the MCA can lead to contralateral gaze paresis and motor neglect (Fig. 5.1) [9]. Motor neglect refers to a patient's inattention to or failure to use the contralesional limb, even when doing so would clearly be more efficient. This phenomenon should be differentiated from premotor neglect, also referred to as *directional hypokinesia*, which involves a reduction or delay

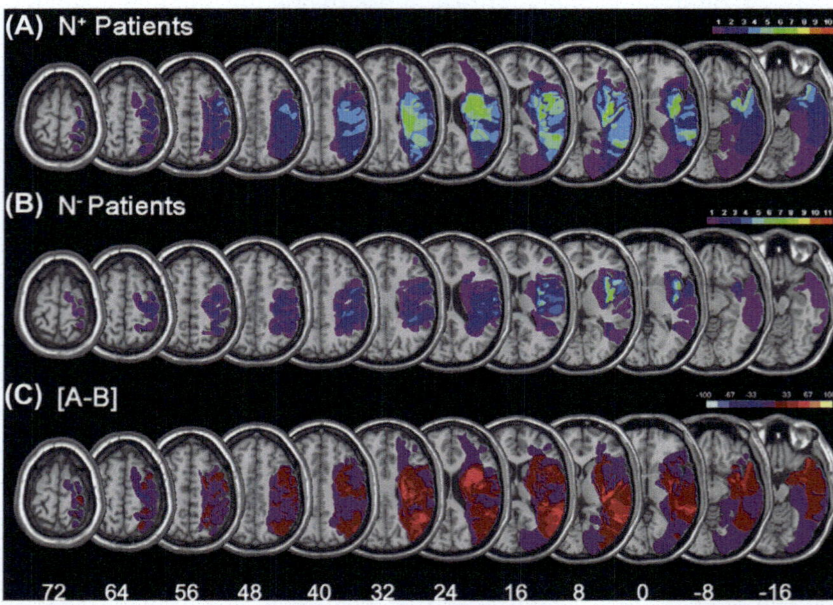

FIGURE 5.1 Major lesion locations related to neglect. *Note*. Lesion overlap maps in patients with neglect (N+) and without neglect (N−). (A) N+ patients show predominant right hemispheric fronto-parietal and subcortical lesions. (B) N− patients show smaller and less overlapping lesions. (C) Difference map (A–B) highlighting regions more frequently associated with neglect, particularly fronto-subcortical regions linked to motor neglect and parietal regions linked to visuospatial neglect. The figure also illustrates that stroke lesions commonly extend across cortical and subcortical territories following vascular anatomy rather than functional boundaries. Adapted from Grimsen et al. [8].

in initiating movements toward the contralesional side and reduced spatial exploration in that direction [10]. Premotor neglect can be restricted to eye movements or hand/arm movements, depending on the specific lesion localization [11]. Taken together, whereas patients with motor neglect typically ignore the presence of the contralesional limb, patients with premotor neglect may acknowledge the limb but fail to act in the contralesional space [9,12]. In clinical reality, however, motor and premotor neglect symptoms often overlap and are difficult to fully dissociate based on behavioral observation alone.

The prognosis of isolated motor or premotor neglect is generally favorable. In animal studies, most subjects show a near-complete resolution of behavioral symptoms within approximately 6 weeks of recovery. However, when premotor neglect results from anterior cerebral artery rather than MCA infarcts [12], recovery may be slower, and symptoms may involve a generalized loss of spontaneous movement, including severe akinesia that affects the entire body.

Premotor and motor neglect can also emerge after postacute basal ganglia strokes [13], with the basal ganglia receiving their blood supply from perforating arteries. While systematic data on the prevalence of (pre)motor versus VSN in this patient group is lacking, it is known that patients with large basal ganglia infarcts frequently exhibit VSN as well. Nonetheless, as for (pre)motor neglect following a frontal stroke, the recovery rate of VSN in patients with isolated basal ganglia strokes is generally favorable.

5.2.2 Visuospatial neglect

Strokes affecting the parietal and temporoparietal branches of the MCA frequently result in VSN (Fig. 5.1). VSN is characterized by a failure to spontaneously orient toward stimuli on the contralesional side (mostly the left) unless prompted by highly salient cues [1,2]. Although impaired visuospatial processing is the core symptom, this deficit is not restricted to a specific body part or sensory modality but rather encompasses multiple domains (e.g., visual, auditory, and proprioceptive).

The severity of VSN depends on attentional load: when patients are required to search for conjunctions of features, such as locating a red square among red circles and blue squares in a large and densely populated array, the severity of symptoms increases significantly [8,14]. In contrast, highly salient "pop-out" features, such as a red dot among green dots, are often detected much better, sometimes almost unimpaired. However, automatic attention is also impaired in neglect, which becomes evident when measuring the response times to left-sided targets. Using different cueing paradigms has consistently shown that, with or without valid cues, patients with neglect consistently respond more slowly to stimuli presented on the left.

The interpretation of these core features—slowed responses to contralesional targets and inattention to contralesional targets during visual search—remains a topic of scientific debate. The presence of these two symptoms is often referred to as *egocentric* VSN, but its underlying mechanism is still contested. One perspective argues that patients exhibit an attentional gradient across the entire environment, leading to reduced attentional allocation that extends even into the ipsilesional space. In contrast, another theory suggests that the attentional focus is shifted toward the ipsilesional side, effectively rotating the subjective midline, such that search behavior is unimpaired around the new, rightward-shifted center of space.

Beyond these theoretical considerations, clinical outcome is influenced by the extent and location of brain damage. Large parietal strokes are associated with limited recovery, both spontaneous and treatment-induced. In particular, strokes involving the ventral parts of the angular gyrus and dorsocaudal parts of the supramarginal gyrus limit recovery potential if the lesion exceeds a specific size [2,4,15,16].

5.2.3 Allocentric neglect

Lesions affecting the (inferior) temporal branches of the MCA can result in *allocentric* neglect (Fig. 5.2; for a detailed description of symptoms, see the final section of this chapter) [17,18]. In such cases, patients may be able to orient toward the contralesional side of space yet fail to recognize or process features located on the contralesional side of individual objects, regardless of where those objects are positioned in the environment. Thus even when an object is located far to the right, well within the patient's field of attention, the patient may omit or misidentify features on the object's left side, based on the object's own internal reference frame (i.e., its intrinsic axis), rather than the viewer's spatial

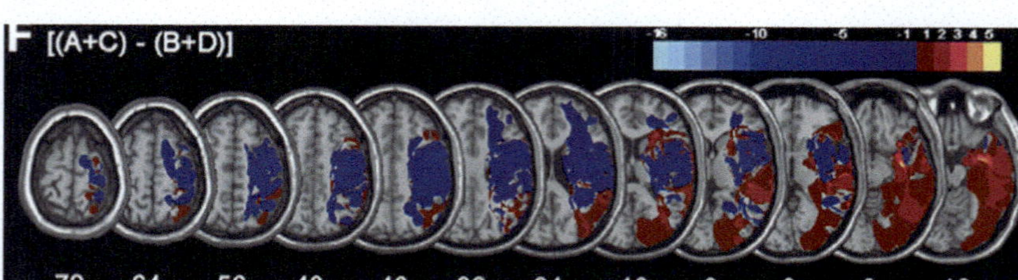

FIGURE 5.2 Lesion subtraction analysis: neural correlates of egocentric and allocentric neglect. *Note.* Lesion subtraction analysis comparing stroke patients with allocentric neglect to those with egocentric neglect or no neglect, Grimsen et al. [8].

orientation. Similarly, if an object is rotated or tilted, patients may still neglect its left side, even when that part appears on the right in viewer-centered space, since it is still on the contralesional side according to its intrinsic axis.

The recovery of allocentric neglect in right MCA patients shows more irregular and less predictable patterns of recovery. It has been argued that the prognosis is poorer for allocentric neglect than for egocentric neglect [16,19,20]. Moreover, widely used therapeutic interventions, such as cueing, prism adaptation (PA), or transcranial direct current stimulation that have shown efficacy in reducing egocentric neglect symptoms, appear to have little to no effect on allocentric neglect [21,22].

Despite growing interest in the condition, clinical understanding of allocentric neglect remains limited, and further research is needed to clarify its mechanisms, prognosis, and effective rehabilitation strategies.

5.2.4 Left-hemisphere versus right-hemisphere neglect

Although VSN following left-hemisphere MCA stroke is less common, it still occurs with notable frequency. In many cases, however, it is masked by cooccurring aphasia, which significantly limits behavioral assessment and the detection of neglect symptoms. Nevertheless, a recent meta-analytic review demonstrated that patients with left-hemispheric (LH) lesions generally exhibit more favorable recovery compared to those with right-sided damage, raising the question of whether there are significant differences in the cognitive structure of neglect depending on the lesion side [4].

In two earlier studies, we analyzed serial and parallel visual search performance in patients with left- and right-sided MCA strokes [8,23]. We observed that left MCA strokes produced a comparable visuospatial hemi-inattention (i.e., egocentric neglect) similar to that seen after right-hemisphere damage. In serial search tasks, these patients showed the characteristic increase in response times for contralesional targets. However, during parallel search tasks, no spatial search gradient was observed in patients with left-hemisphere lesions, meaning that they responded similarly to targets across different spatial positions.

Analysis of omission patterns revealed that allocentric neglect-like behavior (i.e., omissions based on features located on the left side of individual objects) was only present when visuospatial search deficits (i.e., egocentric neglect) were present as well. In other words, in left MCA stroke, allocentric errors appeared to be nested within broader visuospatial attention deficits. By contrast, right MCA stroke patients displayed a spatial gradient of inattention even during parallel search tasks, indicating more automatic attentional disruption. Importantly, in this group, the position of object features in allocentric coordinates independently influenced performance, suggesting a distinct feature-based component of neglect that was not dependent on egocentric deficits. Taken together, left-hemisphere lesions can produce milder forms of egocentric neglect, while pure allocentric neglect appears to occur exclusively in patients with right-hemisphere damage.

Although most clinical trials and intervention studies have focused on egocentric neglect following right-hemisphere stroke, some evidence indicates that similar treatment approaches can also benefit patients with left-hemisphere neglect [24]. Nevertheless, due to the overwhelming dominance of right MCA cases in the treatment literature, the present chapter approaches the rehabilitation of neglect primarily from the perspective of right-hemisphere lesions.

5.3 Treatment of neglect

The rehabilitation of VSN depends on recognizing its diverse symptoms, underlying mechanisms, and patterns of recovery. This section outlines a phased model of intervention, distinguishing between bottom-up and top-down strategies and highlighting their application across different stages of recovery. It begins with approaches suitable for patients in the immediate postacute phase and moves toward more structured, cognitively driven techniques as recovery progresses. Key topics include the use of spatial working memory (SWM), cueing techniques, motor activation, and sensory stimulation to reduce spatial bias and support functional engagement. The overarching aim is to provide practical guidance for selecting therapeutic strategies that can improve real-world functioning and long-term outcomes.

5.3.1 Treatment of early postacute severe neglect

Neglect in the early postacute state is often particularly severe. During this period, patients frequently show marked reduced alertness, a lack of sustained attention, and poor compliance with therapeutic demands. As a result, focused and structured treatment is usually not yet feasible. The primary goals at this stage include diagnostic clarification, particularly regarding cooccurring cognitive impairments, and determining whether the patient can respond to salient sensory cues, especially those that support orientation toward the midline or the left side of space.

5.3.1.1 Observational assessment of spatial working memory

In patients with severe neglect, traditional diagnostic paradigms like the Posner task are often impractical. Tasks involving complex visual scanning or digital interfaces, such as computerized cancellation tests, may overwhelm the patient's limited capacity for attention and sustained engagement. Even if repetition of such tasks is possible, fluctuations in alertness often make interpretation of the results unreliable. Thus, clinical observation remains essential in assessing whether SWM can be incorporated into treatment. Table 5.1 provides examples of sensory cueing strategies and simple clinical observations that can guide decisions about the patient's usable working memory capacity.

5.3.1.2 *Fall risks and the importance of early mobilization*

A common clinical issue in this phase is the high risk of falls [25]. Many patients with severe neglect lack awareness of their deficits and may not comprehend the extent to which their impairments affect motor abilities like standing and walking. Combined with restlessness and impulsivity commonly seen in these patients, this can result in attempts to stand or walk independently without calling for assistance. Falls in this stage are a major concern, frequently requiring physical restraint in beds or wheelchairs. Early mobilization, combined with clear, repeated discussions about safety and the necessity of supervision, is critical and remains important if neglect persists (Table 5.2).

5.3.1.3 *Orienting strategies using eyes, head, and hand*

In patients with severe neglect, the ability to look toward the left is often more impaired than the ability to reach with the left hand [11]. A helpful clinical technique is to prompt the patient to fixate on the therapist's eyes from a position on the left and then ask the patient to point to the same location. Many patients are more successful with pointing than with fixation, suggesting a dissociation between oculomotor and limb motor systems. In some cases, this may reflect additional damage to the frontal eye fields. Regardless, prompting patients to look toward the therapist's eyes, accompanied by verbal prompts such as "here," can be a powerful cue. If this is not sufficient, passive guidance of the hand toward the left and reintroducing the verbal cue may be enough to trigger reorientation.

Once eye contact is established, the therapist can gradually shift position further to the left, prompting the patient to maintain fixation. The same holds true for hand movements: if the patient can reliably reach leftward on command, the target location can be incrementally shifted leftward to expand spatial awareness.

TABLE 5.1 Sensory cueing and clinical assessment of working memory in patients with severe neglect.

	1	2	3	4
Sensory cueing	Ask: "Where are my eyes?"	Move the patient's right hand to midline	Sit on the patient's left and request to pass over objects	Use elongated, well-structured objects to guide attention leftward
Working memory	Observe whether the patient can re-fixate on the eyes after initially looking away to the right and being prompted again	Assess whether the patient can reposition the hand independently after it has been moved away	Monitor if the patient's ability to orient leftward improves gradually with repeated attempts	Determine whether the patient becomes more accurate at identifying or responding to left-sided features over time

Note. These observations support clinical judgment on whether spatial working memory (SWM) can be used in early therapy or if treatment should rely on external cues and passive guidance.

TABLE 5.2 Goals and interventions by stages of neglect recovery.

	Global task	Specific treatment
Early postacute, severe neglect	Preventing unsupervised mobility to avoid falls. Establishing reliable agreements to ask for assistance before standing up.	Increasing awareness of motor impairment and the need to wait for clinical improvement.
Postacute severe to moderate neglect	Cueing midline positions and facilitating orientation through coordinated movements of the eyes, head, and hand toward these targets.	Facilitating early self-care tasks (e.g., hygiene, dressing). Improving awareness of food residue in the left oral cavity.

Note. This table presents an overview of different stages of recovery in neglect and the global and specific goals of the treatment.

5.3.1.4 *Movement-based stimulation and functional engagement*

At this early stage of recovery, all interventions should include some form of movement to promote alertness. Large game boards (e.g., Solitaire) may be used to cue hand movements toward the midline. Sound cues (e.g., knocking) can help localize target positions. Although passive assistance is sometimes necessary, patients often resist and care should be taken to foster voluntary participation. Encouraging reaching movements of the hand to the left and right is a valuable intervention in the initial phase of recovery.

If SWM appears sufficiently preserved, it can be actively integrated into therapy. Two main strategies are recommended:

1. **Position-based working memory**: patients may be asked to remove Solitaire rods from the left side and return them to their storage box, reinforcing memory for left-sided spatial locations.
2. **Object knowledge-based strategies**: familiar objects, such as a ballpoint pen, can be placed on a page. Patients can be instructed to identify the pen tip, drawing on semantic memory to locate the left-sided starting point of a text line.

5.3.2 Major approaches to neglect rehabilitation in later recovery stages

Once patients show some degree of general recovery, such as increased alertness, improved compliance, and better orientation, more specialized treatments for VSN become feasible [2,26,27]. These can be broadly divided into two main therapeutic approaches: (1) compensation and (2) restitution.

The compensatory approach aims to help patients develop awareness of their neglect and consciously learn strategies to counteract it [28]. A central goal is to improve insight into the attentional deficit on the left side and to internalize routines of cue setting and cue re-finding on the left. Depending on the severity of neglect and the patient's level of alertness, different compensatory strategies can be introduced (Table 5.3). These may include systematic left-side checking routines, the use of spatial landmarks, and the practice of orienting behaviors that gradually become more automated. They can be manualized and used systematically. Although such behavior may eventually become habitual, its initial learning is cognitively mediated, making this a primarily *top-down* approach based on conscious effort and structured training.

The restitutive approach, by contrast, aims to restore the underlying balance of spatial attention that is believed to be disrupted in neglect. It assumes that VSN arises from a rotation, shift, or shrinkage of visuospatial attention to the detriment of the left. Consequently, interventions that stimulate the neglected side through bottom-up mechanisms are intended to rebalance this system, realign visuospatial attention, and promote recovery. Since spatial attention involves multiple sensory domains, including visual, auditory, tactile, and proprioceptive, diverse stimulation methods across these modalities have been employed to address the imbalance. Additionally, noninvasive brain stimulation techniques, such as transcranial magnetic or transcranial direct current stimulation, are increasingly used as part of this restitution-focused, bottom-up therapeutic strategy.

Table 5.3 gives an overview of the two different approaches and their possible application depending on the state of recovery.

5.3.3 Top-down approaches for neglect rehabilitation: internalisation of cues

Numerous experimental studies have shown that patients with neglect can attend to the left side of space when they are explicitly cued or instructed to do so [29–32]. These cues may be exogenous (stimulus-driven, bottom-up) or endogenous (intrinsic, top-down). Repeated trials using valid and invalid cues demonstrated that such directional prompts become incorporated into patients' visuospatial behavior, leading to measurable reductions in neglect symptoms [33]. Building on these insights, many rehabilitation approaches have incorporated left-sided visual cueing, which primarily engages top-down attentional processes, albeit with some contribution from stimulus-driven mechanisms [34–36].

TABLE 5.3 Two approaches to neglect rehabilitation.

	Approach for neglect rehabilitation	
Stage of recovery	Top-down (via cognition)	Bottom-up (via stimulation)
(Early) postacute severe neglect	– Eye fixation training – Guided movement of the right hand toward the midline – Single-word reading with leftward cueing and eye contact prompts ↓	– Acoustic cueing (right-left moving tones) – Passive optokinetic stimulation ↓
Postacute severe to moderate neglect	– Index finger cueing on the left – Flickering stimuli on the left of critical objects/words ↓	– Active following of optokinetic stimuli – Neck stimulation – Gamified prism adaptation (PA) – Acoustic cueing ↓
Moderate neglect	– Guided search for the first letter of a word at the beginning of a text line – Use of elongated objects with salient endpoints for searching toward the left ↓	– Active optokinetic tracking with tasks on the left – Neck stimulation, – Gamified PA ↓
Moderate to mild neglect	– Frequent spontaneous reminders to attend to the left side ↓	– Active optokinetic tracking with tasks on the left – Neck stimulation – Any form of PA ↓
Mild neglect	– Reactive reminders during search tasks ↓	– Active optokinetic tracking with tasks on the left – Neck stimulation – Any form of PA ↓
Very mild neglect	– Search tasks with adaptive attentional load using rehabilitation software	

Note. *tDCS*, transcranial direct current stimulation; *rTMS*, repetitive transcranial magnetic stimulation. Both approaches are only possible when there is no craniectomy, no signs of convulsion, and no electrical assistive apparatus.

These interventions rely on the patient's cognitive capacity to learn and eventually internalize compensatory strategies, which is particularly important for improving awareness and autonomy.

One example of this approach is a cueing procedure introduced by Weinberg et al. [36]. During a reading task, 22 patients received verbal instructions, visual anchors (e.g., a left-handed margin), and sequentially numbered lines of text [22]. Training was administered daily for one hour over 4 weeks, with cueing intensity gradually reduced as reading performance improved. The results showed significant gains not only in reading but also in copying and cancellation tasks.

Similarly, a study by Antonucci et al. [37] and Paolucci et al. [38] used a cross-over design to compare neglect treatment with an active control group. Their intervention involved large-screen visual scanning, reading and copying exercises, and scene description tasks. Visual cues were provided and gradually faded as performance improved. After 40 sessions, the treatment group showed enhanced outcomes on neglect-related tasks, as well as improved scores on the Barthel Index. However, despite these improvements, patients with neglect still showed a lower overall functional recovery compared to a control group without neglect who also received neuropsychological treatment and the same number of physiotherapeutic sessions.

A crucial component of cueing-based treatment should be the gradual fading of external cues to promote spontaneous, independent attention to the left side. While Weinberg et al. [36] reduced cueing intensity as performance improved, and Antonucci et al. [37,38] used progressively challenging tasks based on severity, neither study implemented a clearly structured, systematic cueing hierarchy. To achieve true fading-out, explicit criteria for neglect severity should be predefined, guiding the selection and progression of tasks and cues. This structured approach allows for a more individualized treatment plan that adapts both task complexity and cueing strategy to the patient's current level of impairment. To our knowledge, no previous study in neglect rehabilitation has explicitly operationalized severity levels in this way or systematically aligned cueing and task demands with those levels.

Therefore, we did a randomized controlled trial crossover study with cues requiring bottom-up and top-down attentional processing presented in a reading task, which were adapted to the severity of neglect of the patients [28].

Table 5.4 outlines our approach to severity grading, task adaptation, and cue manipulation, divided by exogenous (stimulus-driven, bottom-up) and endogenous (intrinsic, top-down) cues. It documents a hierarchy of different tasks, partly from existing rehabilitation software, which allows adaptation to the severity of mild to severe neglect. In very mild neglect cases, more sensitive measures, such as reaction time tasks, should be used. Table 5.5 also provides more detailed guidance for the implementation of cueing, working memory, reading, and search tasks.

TABLE 5.4 Cueing protocol.

Neglect severity	Task	Exogenous cue	Endogenous cue
1. Severe	Single-word reading on the computer	• Flickering light at the beginning of the word	• Therapist asks for eye contact
2. Severe-moderate	Reading a text on the computer or on paper	• Colored highlight on most of the first letter/first words of the line • Colored marking of the first letter of omitted words	• Therapist asks to search for the marked letter/word • Therapist asks to search her index finger, which is positioned at the beginning of the line • Asking for eye contact is reduced a little
3. Moderate	Reading a text on paper	• Colored highlight of the first letter of omitted words if necessary	• Therapist names the first letter of the omitted word and asks to search for it (if necessary, add colored marking) • Indirect request for eye contact
4. Moderate-mild	Reading a text on paper	• Colored highlight of the first letter of omitted words if necessary	• Therapist names the first letter of the omitted word and asks to search for it (less need for colored marking) • Therapist asks to search further to the left
5. Mild	Reading a text on paper		• If a word is omitted, the therapist asks to read the sentence again

Note. The cueing protocol aligns cue type and task complexity with defined levels of neglect severity. Exogenous cues provide external stimulation, while endogenous cues rely on the patient's internal attentional control. [28]

The results of this study indicated a significant reduction in all primary outcome measures, including word and text reading, as well as performance on the Catherine Bergego Scale, which reflects daily life activities. Patients improved by an average of 9 points—nearly one-third of the total scale, suggesting not only direct gains in trained tasks but also meaningful transfer to everyday functioning.

Our results [28] were in line with the findings of Weinberg et al. [36], who also used paragraph reading (51-word texts vs 58–63 words in our study) as a central task. However, while their intervention lasted 4 weeks,

TABLE 5.5 Hierarchical steps for intervention across domains.

Step	Sensory cueing	Working memory	Reading	Searching
1	Ask: "Where are my eyes?"	Move the right hand to midline, remove it, and ask for repositioning	Single words of increasing length	Large pop-out target search
2	Guide gaze orientation toward other spatial positions via hand movements	Sit on the left and ask the patient to pass objects	Words with ambiguous beginnings	Small nonpop-out target search
3	Use elongated, well-structured objects to guide attention leftward	Ask for repeated leftward eye movements	Multidigit numerical strings	Search for highly salient features among increasing distractors
4	Use pop-out, visual anchors (e.g., colored lines)	Ask for repeated fixation just left of the middle	Narrow paragraphs in large fonts	Feature conjunction search with increasing distractors
5	Use the patient's left hand as an attentional anchor	Copy the right-sided patterns on the left	Wide paragraphs in small fonts	Compare objects for salient features
6	Provide occasional verbal reminders to focus on the left	Observe and reinforce balanced eye movements	Scattered paragraph layouts	Compare patterns for nonsalient features

Note. The hierarchy presents structured interventions across sensory cueing, working memory, reading, and search domains. Each step builds on the previous, allowing task complexity and cueing demands to be adapted to the patient's current level of neglect severity and cognitive capacity.

our adaptive cueing protocol lasted three, suggesting greater efficiency, as seen in an economical advantage and progress in the development of neglect treatment. In contrast to Paolucci et al. [38], we did not find significant improvement on the Barthel Index, which may be attributable to our shorter treatment period (15 sessions vs 40). Supporting this, a smaller-scale trial using our cueing protocol in combination with rivastigmine showed improvements on neuropsychological tests, but no gains on the Barthel Index, possibly due to insufficient treatment intensity. Unfortunately, the Catherine Bergego Scale was not used in that study.

5.3.3.1 The relationship between spatial working memory and neglect

One important diagnostic question when selecting top-down interventions for treating VSN is whether the patient shows any signs of preserved visuospatial working memory (SWM), meaning the ability to reorient quickly toward the left or toward a previously cued left-sided target.

The conceptual and empirical relationship between SWM and VSN remains unresolved [39–42]. A strong theoretical position holds that all forms of neglect impair SWM, since neglect is fundamentally an attention disorder. Attending to spatial locations involves not only detecting stimuli but also maintaining mental representations of these locations in working memory. Therefore, spatial neglect should impair both perception and short-term memory of contralesional space [43].

However, other models of neglect argue that neglect arises from a shift or rotation of attentional coordinates, rather than a true loss of spatial representation [44–46]. In this framework, SWM might remain intact, but be biased or distorted by an altered frame of reference.

This gives rise to three theoretical models for how SWM functions in patients with neglect:

1. **Complete SWM impairment**: neglect disrupts the internal spatial framework entirely, making it impossible for the patient to mentally represent or recall positions on the left. In such cases, strategies relying on internal cues, such as mental visualization, are likely to fail, as the patient lacks cognitive access to contralesional space.
2. **Preserved SWM with shifted reference frame**: this model proposes that neglect does not impair SWM but instead alters the internal coordinate system in which spatial information is processed. Rather than a true loss of access to left-sided space (as, for instance, in hemianopia), patients experience a rightward shift in their attentional focus, leading them to encode and retrieve spatial relationships relative to this shifted frame of reference. As a result, SWM remains

functionally intact but is anchored to a distorted representation of space. In practical terms, patients may still remember left-sided positions, but do so based on their altered internal orientation, allowing SWM to support compensation when properly engaged.

3. **Partial SWM access with limited spontaneous use**: this view holds that SWM and neglect are separable components but interact with each other, with neglect typically exerting a greater influence on behavior than SWM.

Importantly, the validity of these three theoretical assumptions has significant implications for the treatment of patients with VSN.

If the first model holds true (complete impairment of SWM), then any attempt to internalize left-sided positions would be futile, as these positions cannot be mentally represented or accessed. Some patients, in fact, behave as though they have entirely lost their visuoSWM: when directed to the left using strong social or auditory cues, they immediately lose awareness of that position and are unable to initiate orientation. For these individuals, only noncognitive interventions, such as bottom-up stimulation or conditioning, may offer therapeutic benefit.

In contrast, the second model (preserved SWM with a shifted reference frame) suggests that patients may retain a functional representation of space, albeit within a shifted or distorted frame of reference. This would support the use of internal cues as a means of compensation. Clinical observations confirm this possibility: some patients can read entire paragraphs without omissions, even if slower than prestroke, though formal neuropsychological testing reveals VSN. These individuals seem to rely on internalized knowledge, such as the expectation that text lines begin on the left, which helps them initiate and guide visual scanning. This suggests that preserved SWM can support compensatory strategies, at least in structured contexts.

The third model (partial SWM access) finds support in patients who can locate left-sided targets only when repeatedly prompted. These individuals appear capable of mentally representing contralesional space but require ongoing external stimulation to activate or maintain access to it. In such cases, SWM is intact but not spontaneously accessible, indicating an interaction between preserved memory capacity and impaired attentional control.

Various experimental paradigms have been employed to investigate the relationship between SWM and neglect, with results reflecting the same heterogeneity observed clinically. One line of research uses visual search tasks that vary in how targets are marked or removed once identified [47–49]. Another approach involves the well-established Posner cueing task. In this paradigm, participants are instructed to orient their attention to a location indicated by a cue before a target appears.

By increasing the stimulus-onset-asynchrony, meaning the delay between the cue and the target, the cue must be held in SWM for longer periods of time. Comparing performance in valid versus invalid trials reveals whether the internally maintained spatial representation influences the severity of neglect.

The results of these studies argue that cueing does play a significant role in shaping behavior in neglect. Structured training with strategic and meaningful cues may help patients gradually regain improved spatial awareness and functional engagement with the neglected side of space. However, this approach may not be optimal for patients with severe SWM disorders.

5.3.4 Bottom-up approach for neglect rehabilitation

Top-down approaches rely on the patient's ability to use intact cognitive functions, such as insight, attention, and strategy use, to compensate for their deficits and gradually internalize adaptive behavior. Therefore, they will turn out to be ineffective or impractical for neglect patients if these compensatory mechanisms are also impaired. For these reasons, bottom-up approaches, which aim to stimulate neglected space directly without requiring cognitive insight, have become a major focus of research and clinical application over the past decades.

The first biologically grounded bottom-up approach to neglect rehabilitation was introduced by Sprague [50] through influential studies in cats. In these experiments, unilateral lesions were induced in the occipital and parietal lobes, resulting in behavior that closely resembled VSN. After a period of spontaneous recovery without improvement in the neglect-like symptoms, Sprague [50] performed a second lesion, this time targeting either the contralateral superior colliculus or, in later experiments, the commissures connecting the colliculi. Remarkably, these additional lesions led to a partial recovery of the neglect-like symptoms. Table 5.6 illustrates the cats' behavior after the first (left column) and second (right column) lesion.

These findings provided compelling evidence that subcortical structures, particularly the superior colliculi, play a critical role in the pathophysiology of neglect. They also introduced the idea that modulating activity in these structures, either through up- or downmodulation, could potentially alleviate neglect symptoms, with the specific approach depending on the affected hemisphere [51,52]. Figs. 5.3 and 5.4 illustrate the extensive afferent and efferent connections of the superior colliculi, emphasizing their integrative role in coordinating visuospatial attention through cortical, thalamic, and brainstem pathways.

TABLE 5.6 Recovery of neglect-like symptoms in cats following superior colliculus lesion.

Deficits after the first right cortical lesion	Deficits after the subsequent lesion in the left superior colliculus
Total hemianopia for the left field, however, normal right field	Response to stimuli in left fields (0 degrees to 1000 degrees) Response to stimuli in right fields 00 to 450 initially, improving slowly to 700, then to 1000
Following only to the right	Following only to the left initially, slowly appearing on the right, but left favored Blink to threat initially only on the left, slowly appearing on the right
Blink to the lateral threat only on the right	Blink to threat initially only on the left, slowly appearing on the right
Lateral visual placing only on the right	Placing initially on the left, slowly appearing on the right
Tendency to circle right	Marked initial circling to the left, slowly reduced to a tendency to circle left
Eye movements and pupils normal	Pupils normal; eye movements to the right initially absent, slowly improving to almost normal, slightly better to the left

Note. Derived from Sprague [50]. The left column shows deficits after a right cortical lesion in cats, resembling neglect. The right column shows functional improvements after an additional lesion to the left superior colliculus, demonstrating partial recovery.

5.3.4.1 *Bottom-up approach for neglect rehabilitation: sensory facilitation*

Based on these findings, a range of bottom-up interventions has been developed to directly stimulate neglected space and reduce attentional imbalance in patients with VSN.

5.3.4.1.1 Caloric stimulation

One of the earliest interventions developed from research on subcortical contributions to neglect was caloric stimulation of the vestibular system [54,55]. In this procedure, cold water infused into the left ear temporarily reduced neglect symptoms. Caloric stimulation activates the vestibular system and, therefore, the representation of the spatial orientation of the body. By inducing a systematic deviation of perceived body position toward the left, this method counteracts the rightward shift in the subjective body axis often seen in neglect. The effect is thought to involve modulation of midbrain structures, including the superior colliculus, as well as regions of the insular and parietal cortex responsible for automatic spatial orientation. One interpretation of the effects of

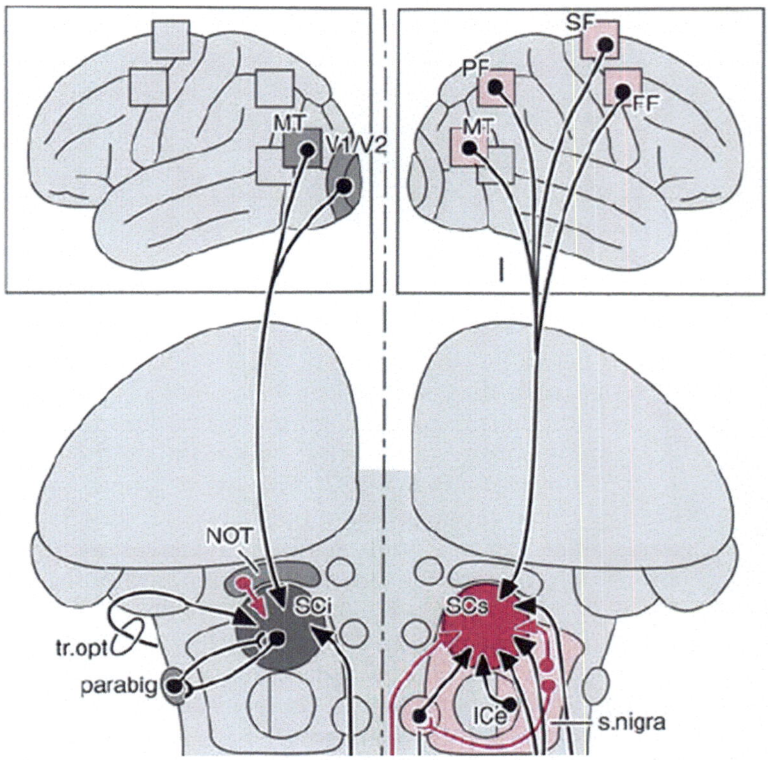

FIGURE 5.3 Efferent and afferent connections of the superior colliculi. *Note.* Schematic illustration of the major afferent and efferent connections of the superior colliculi, emphasizing their role in integrating cortical, thalamic, and brainstem pathways involved in visuospatial attention and orienting behavior. Adapted from Nieuwenhuys [53].

caloric stimulation is that it helps to rebalance collicular activity disrupted by a cortical lesion. However, despite its clinical relevance, caloric stimulation is not routinely used due to side effects such as dizziness and nausea. Table 5.7 illustrates additional bottom-up interventions that may similarly influence collicular activity and spatial reorientation.

5.3.4.1.2 Neck muscle stimulation

Another bottom-up intervention that has been explored in neglect rehabilitation is neck muscle stimulation, particularly targeting those on the left side of the back. This stimulation induces a sense of head rotation, which was proposed to compensate for the distorted spatial orientation that characterized neglect. The idea is that by altering proprioceptive

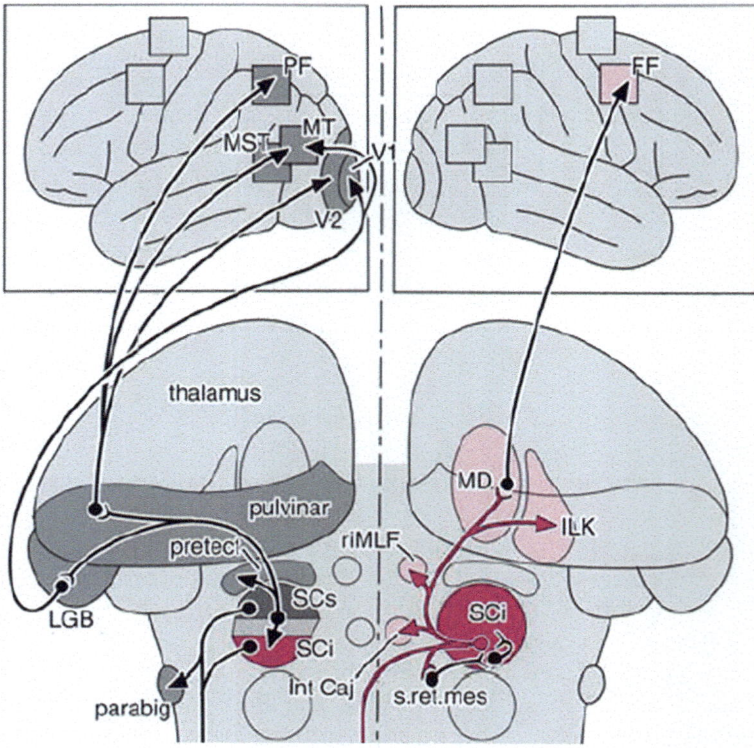

FIGURE 5.4 Efferent and afferent connections of the superior colliculi. *Note.* Schematic illustration of the afferent and efferent pathways linking the superior colliculi with visual cortical areas, thalamic nuclei, and brainstem structures involved in visuospatial attention, visual orienting, and oculomotor control. Adapted from Nieuwenhuys [53].

TABLE 5.7 Bottom-Up approaches to neglect rehabilitation via assumed inhibition of the contralesional colliculus.

- Neck vibration (realignment of head rotation and visual position)
- Prism adaptation (realignment of hand position and visual position)
- Auditory stimulation (realignment of auditory and visual position)
- Optokinetic stimulation, smooth pursuit
- Eye patching

input about head position, patients may recalibrate their internal representation of space.

Studies with healthy participants have shown that neck muscle stimulation can reliably shift spatial perception, supporting the hypothesis that the superior colliculi play a primary role in visual orientation [56]. Interestingly, a similar effect can be produced by transcranial magnetic stimulation above the left or right prefrontal cortex [57]. This connection is further supported by the fact that the head muscles are innervated by the accessory motor nuclei, located in the brainstem, which send afferent signals to the superior colliculus and contribute to the rapid computation of body orientation in space.

While early results using neck muscle stimulation in neglect patients were promising, no larger-scale studies have replicated them in recent years. Nonetheless, the intervention remains theoretically compelling, as it leverages proprioceptive feedback to influence spatial orientation—a core deficit in neglect.

5.3.4.1.3 Prism adaptation

PA is a bottom-up approach that involves retraining motor coordination after decoupling it from visuospatial input using prisms. In a typical PA task, patients wear prism glasses that laterally shift their visual field [58–60]. When reaching for a target (e.g., a small block or a target on a screen), the initial movements are typically misaligned due to the altered visual input. With repeated attempts, however, patients gradually adapt their motor responses and learn to compensate for the visual displacement. Notably, this recalibration persists even after the prisms are removed, resulting in so-called after-effects, prolonged reduction of neglect symptoms.

Consequently, PA was one of the most promising bottom-up treatments for neglect and was considered a game changer in neurorehabilitation for nearly a decade [7]. However, more recent metaanalytic reviews have raised questions about the overall effectiveness of PA in neglect [5,61–63]. While PA induces after-effects, the extent to which these translate into long-term functional improvements, especially in relation to neglect severity and its multimodal nature, remains under debate.

The mechanisms underlying PA are still not fully understood but are generally thought to involve two processes:

1. Rapid recalibration involves a fast cognitive adjustment of perceived visual positions to account for the shifted input.
2. Slow realignment of the motor learning process that re-establishes coordination between the visuospatial input and motor responses.

Activation in cerebellar, parietal, and midbrain regions contributes to these mechanisms. The superior colliculi may also play a role, because neurons in different layers of the superior colliculus, tuned to spatial orientation, interact to align visual and proprioceptive input and may contribute to motor learning and realignment. In contrast, recalibration appears to rely more heavily on parietal and frontal cortical regions, which are implicated in the rapid cognitive adjustment of spatial coordinates.

As a bottom-up approach, PA is typically assumed to improve VSN primarily through sensorimotor realignment. This view is supported by findings that the presence of after-effects, that is, motor biases persisting after prism removal, predicts treatment efficacy. However, several observations challenge this interpretation. The most compelling evidence stems from the comparison between PA with and without terminal exposure. In terminal exposure, patients only see their hand at the end of a movement (e.g., pointing or reaching), which engages cognitive recalibration of spatial coordinates. In contrast, when patients view the full movement trajectory from the beginning, recalibration is minimal, and only motor learning with realignment occurs. Studies show that PA without terminal exposure is less effective, suggesting that its therapeutic benefit may stem less from sensory realignment and more from a cognitive shift in attentional focus. One of the most integrative reviews of PA redefined it as a cognitively mediated process rather than a purely bottom-up restitution of visuospatial attention [59].

Despite these nuances, PA remains a practical and accessible intervention in clinical settings, particularly for patients with moderate neglect. It can be easily integrated into standard therapy routines and adapted to include more engaging tasks than simple pointing (the standard content of many studies on PA). For instance, we used activities such as reading, object identification, and screen-based information search, linking each task to numeric responses on a large keyboard [21,64]. This gamification enhances motivation and alertness, particularly when combined with performance-based feedback.

We also extended the action field beyond the typical 10-degree range used in many studies. This narrow field, approximately 10 cm to each side at a 50 cm distance, does not reflect the spatial demands of daily rehabilitation practice, where patients often need to operate within a broader range of 20 to 30 cm. In our view, expanding the action field better aligns with clinical goals and enhances functional relevance. Based on our findings, we argue that PA, despite recent meta-analyses questioning its efficacy, remains a valid and feasible option for treating neglect, especially in moderately affected patients. However, for those with milder symptoms, the benefits of PA may be limited, and alternative interventions should be considered.

5.3.4.1.4 Acoustic cueing

Acoustic cueing is a simple and low-demand intervention that can be applied even in severely impaired, early postacute neglect patients who are not yet able to participate in active therapy. Animal studies have shown that synchronized acoustic and visual stimulation can improve reorientation toward the contralesional side and reactivate silent neurons in the superior colliculi, even when these structures are not directly affected by the lesion. Remarkably, this effect was observed in anesthetized cats, suggesting that such interventions may be beneficial even in patients with very low compliance due to apathy or reduced consciousness.

Fig. 5.5 illustrates the effects of synchronized acoustic and visual stimulation in a cat model with cortical lesions, showing changes in spatial orientation behavior, collicular activity, and visual discrimination [65,66]. After the lesion, the ipsilesional colliculus showed reduced activity in neurons with contralesional receptive fields. Following multimodal stimulation, these neurons resumed activity, and behavioral responsiveness to contralesional stimuli improved. However, while these effects indicated a partial recovery from neglect, visual discrimination abilities remained impaired.

In clinical settings, acoustic cues can take the form of either static left-sided tones or voices, or dynamically moving sounds (e.g., music or speech shifting from right to left). Acoustic cueing has the advantage that it can easily be delivered through headphones, the treatment can be

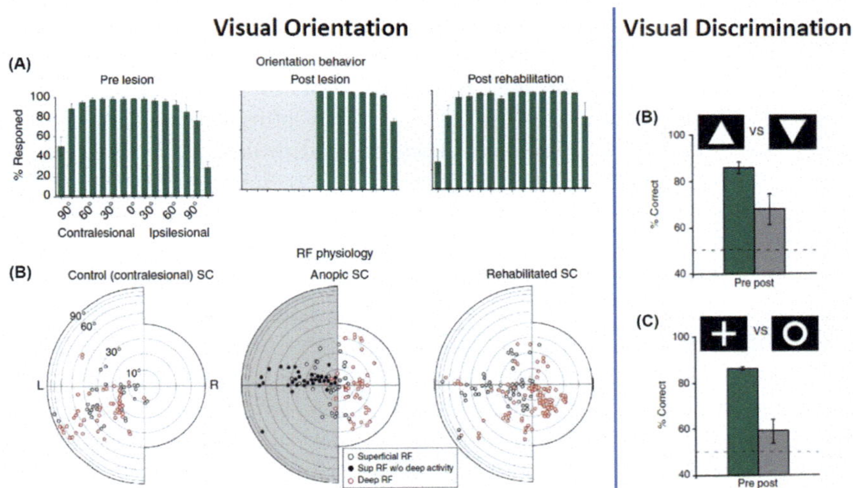

FIGURE 5.5 Multimodal stimulation effects on visual orientation and discrimination in neglect. *Note.* This figure illustrates behavioral and neural responses before and after synchronized visual and auditory stimulation in cats with cortical lesions with neglect-like deficits. Rehabilitation improved orienting responses to contralesional stimuli and altered superior colliculus receptive field organization, whereas visual discrimination deficits persisted. Adapted from Jiang et al. [65].

started early (for instance, on the stroke unit with the patient still lying in bed), and hearing music or podcasts can increase motivation and help alleviate the monotony of hospital routines.

Acoustic–spatial and visual–spatial information is integrated in the parietal lobe, but at a more basic level, in the superior colliculus. The superior colliculus consists of 7 layers: while the upper 3–4 layers are related to visual information and mapping the spatial location of such stimuli in the environment, the lower 3 layers are responsible for integrating and aligning auditory and proprioceptive inputs with visual space [53]. Interneuronal connections between these layers allow for a first multimodal spatial map of the environment. As such, auditory or proprioceptive cueing may modulate attention via collicular pathways, making acoustic cueing particularly promising in neglect rehabilitation.

We conducted two pilot studies investigating the impact of dynamic auditory cueing on egocentric neglect severity in a clinical-therapeutic setting [67]. In both studies, patients received 15 sessions of the intervention. In the first study, a double-blind trial with a historical control group, patients in the early postacute phase listened to music or audiobooks moving from right to left. Results showed a lasting reduction in egocentric neglect severity, which was not observed in the control group. In the second study, dynamic auditory cues were combined with optokinetic stimulation in a computer-based training. Both studies demonstrated a significant reduction in neglect severity.

Kaufmann et al. [68] also explored dynamic (i.e., sounds moving from right to left) auditory stimulation and its short-term effects on neglect behavior. Their results confirmed that such stimulation can reduce neglect symptoms for several minutes after stimulation. In their most recent studies [69,70], four conditions were compared: (1) unimodal acoustic, (2) unimodal visual, (3) bimodal acoustic, and (4) visual stimulation with no stimulation. All interventions were effective, but none outperformed the others (Kaufmann et al. [68]), a contrast to the earlier cat studies where bimodal stimulation had a superior effect.

Several factors may explain this discrepancy: first, the animal study used repeated stimulation sessions, whereas Geiser et al. [69,70] assessed after-effects of only a single intervention. Second, the nature of the visual stimulation differed: while Geiser et al. [69,70] used moving visual targets, Jiang et al. [65] used sudden-onset stimuli, which may be more effective at triggering spatial reorientation. The results of Geiser et al. [70] may also suggest that *motion* in any modality (auditory, tactile, or visual) is sufficient to activate a supramodal spatial representation, therefore, reducing the need for multisensory stimulation. On the other hand, the short duration of a single intervention may limit its effect, and the added benefits of a single intervention may be short-lived, and the advantage of bimodal stimulation might only become apparent with more sustained or repeated application.

Despite these uncertainties, the results of Schenke et al. [67] and Kaufmann et al. [68] support the clinical utility of acoustic cueing. It is a simple method for neglect rehabilitation, suitable across various stages of neglect severity. However, the effects may be limited, as long-term recovery requires active, physical interaction with the environment, which acoustic stimulation does not provide.

5.3.4.1.5 Optokinetic stimulation

Optokinetic pursuit from right to left is another intervention that may help reintegrate spatial representations at the level of the superior colliculus [71–73]. It involves visually tracking stimuli moving slowly from right to left, to trigger optokinetic nystagmus. While visual pursuit is a function rooted in midbrain structures, it also recruits frontal and parietal cortical areas. Although often classified as a bottom-up technique, optokinetic stimulation may also facilitate awareness of neglected space. In such cases, patients may gain insight into their neglect, which suggests a partial top-down component.

Numerous studies have demonstrated that optokinetic pursuit can effectively reduce neglect symptoms. Even beyond neuropsychological assessments, it is an impressive clinical experience that many of the patients who sit initially tilted toward the right in their wheelchairs before stimulation change their sitting position during treatment (although such clinical impressions do not indicate how long this postural change persists).

Optokinetic pursuit can be applied in different therapeutic settings. The most common approach, often used in research, involves the patient simply tracking moving stimuli from right to left. While effective, this method can be repetitive and unengaging. In another approach, patients are instructed to focus on the center of the screen (e.g., reading a sentence) while objects move from right to left. The assumption is that optokinetic pursuit helps generalize spatial attention from the "background" of attention into the focus of attention. Alternatively, optokinetic pursuit can be used as a permanent process of cueing: patients may be instructed to track moving objects and respond when a target reaches a specific position on the left (e.g., via a button press when a color changes).

From a cognitive perspective, these variants differ significantly, and it remains uncertain which is most effective. However, in early-stage patients with severe neglect, only the most basic approach is likely to be effective, as these individuals are typically unable to engage with tasks presented on the left side or to read content located in the center of the screen. As such, simplified pursuit tasks, though monotonous, may be the only viable option in this phase. Correspondingly, one study demonstrated that even this basic version can be effective in patients still bedridden with severe neglect. Although many of these patients cannot sustain prolonged fixation on a leftward-moving stimulus, short intervals of engagement with rest breaks appear sufficient to produce significant improvements in neglect.

5.3.4.2 Bottom-up approach for neglect rehabilitation: neurophysiological facilitation

The previously discussed interventions are primarily behavioral and aim to influence spatial attention through sensorimotor engagement. In contrast, a subset of strategies targets neurophysiological mechanisms more directly, with the intention of modulating specific patterns of brain activity to promote recovery from neglect.

5.3.4.2.1 Colliculi imbalance

Sprague's original theory that neglect results from an imbalance between the two superior colliculi has since found some support in humans. Case studies have shown that neglect symptoms resulting from a lesion in one hemisphere can be reversed by a second lesion in the contralateral hemisphere [74], or specifically in the contralateral superior colliculus [75]. As in other primates and cats, humans show contralateral dominance in the retinocollicular projection [53,76]. Most visual input from each retina crosses at the optic chiasm and is transmitted to the superior colliculus on the opposite side of the brain, while a smaller portion projects to the superior colliculus on the same side. Accordingly, it has been proposed that monocular occlusion (e.g., eye patching) may modulate visual input and help rebalance superior colliculus activity and serve as a therapeutic intervention in neglect (Figs. 5.5 and 5.6).

5.3.4.2.2 Monocular occlusion through eye patching

Posner and Rafal [77] were the first to postulate that covering the ipsilesional eye in neglect patients could help restore attentional balance. Their rationale was that monocular occlusion would reduce overstimulation of the contralesional superior colliculus, thereby disinhibiting the underactive ipsilesional superior colliculus. Consequently, this rebalancing was expected to improve attention to the contralesional side of space. Given the superior colliculi's key role in generating contralateral saccades [78,79], Swan [80] further suggested that patching the ipsilesional eye might directly facilitate contralesional saccadic eye movements. Despite this convincing neuroanatomical rationale, however, the clinical effectiveness of ipsilesional monocular eye patching in treating neglect has remained uncertain.

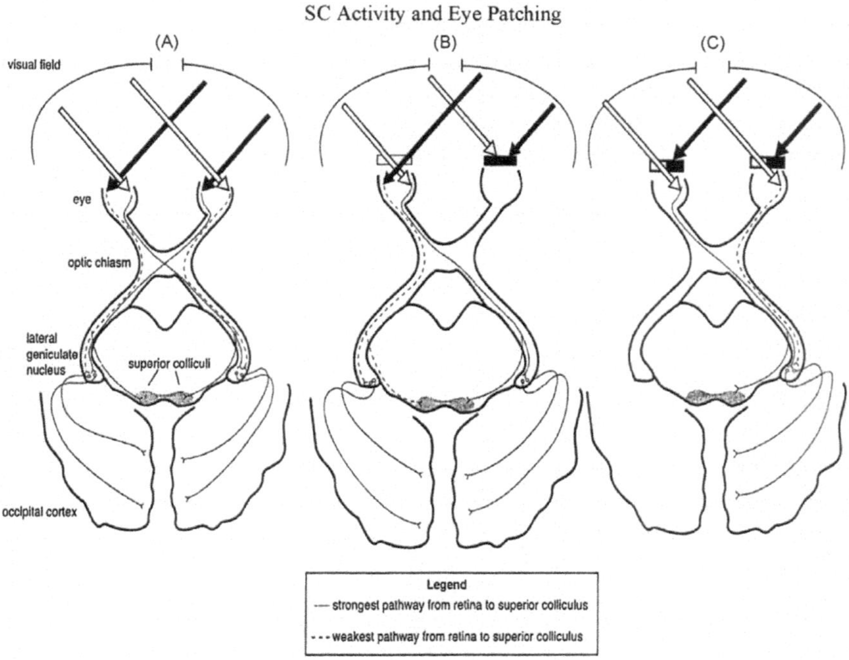

FIGURE 5.6 Superior colliculus activity and monocular occlusion in neglect rehabilitation. Schematic illustration of visual pathways linking the retina, superior colliculus, lateral geniculate nucleus, and occipital cortex under conditions of normal binocular vision and monocular occlusion. The figure demonstrates how eye patching may alter superior colliculus activation and visuospatial orienting in neglect rehabilitation. Adapted from Ogourtsova et al. [52].

Smania et al. [81] reviewed eight studies investigating the efficacy of monocular eye patching in patients with left-sided neglect following right-hemispheric stroke. Four studies reported positive effects of patching the ipsilesional eye, while one found no beneficial effect. Two studies reported no superiority of right-over left-eye patching, and one unexpectedly observed improvements following left eye patching. Based on these mixed results, the authors concluded that evidence supporting ipsilesional eye patching remains insufficient. However, several methodological limitations can be found across the reviewed studies: most employed single-case or case-series designs, and seven of the eight studies included patients in the late subacute or chronic stage poststroke. Only one study assessed patients with a stroke onset of less than a month. More critically, the reviewed studies primarily measured neglect using visual search, reading, drawing, and bisection tasks. Performance on these tasks relies on both bottom-up and top-down processes, meaning cognitive control, and involves strategic decisions. This introduces substantial variability and may obscure subtle improvements in neglect symptoms. In other words, the complexity and cognitive demands of these tasks can mask minor, yet clinically meaningful, changes in attentional performance.

Given these considerations, it is important to explore more direct indicators of attentional modulation. Specifically, neglect also affects more basic visuomotor functions, such as the ability to plan and execute eye movements. Patients often show impairments in generating saccades and in smoothly tracking moving targets [47,82], a process mediated by the superior colliculus [78,83]. Because monocular eye patching may influence activity in the superior colliculus, its effects are likely to be more accurately captured through oculomotor assessments, such as comparing the functional performance of both eyes, rather than through complex behavioral tasks alone. However, to date, no study has investigated the efficacy of monocular eye patching in patients with right-sided neglect after a LH stroke.

To address this gap, we conducted a video-oculographic study on the effects of monocular eye patching in patients with right-brain (RH) stroke [84,85]. Our findings revealed that eye patching modulated the performance of eye movements in the RH group, both in reactive saccades and smooth pursuit tasks. In both tasks, RH patients made fewer rightward saccades during right (ipsilesional) than left (contralesional) patching. In contrast, leftward saccades did not differ significantly between the two eye patch positions. Notably, in the reactive saccade task, this reduction in rightward saccades was observed only during right-eye patching, suggesting a lateralized effect.

This finding suggests that right-eye patching may enhance activation of the right superior colliculus, thereby modulating rightward saccade behavior. In this sense, our results confirm that ipsilesional monocular eye patching can influence attentional performance. However, the effect was specific to rightward saccades; no significant changes were observed in leftward saccades. This indicates that the observed small effect does not restore underactivation of the right superior colliculus but rather helps to counterbalance the overactivation of the contralesional (left) side.

5.3.4.3 *Bottom-up approach for neglect rehabilitation: brain stimulation*

Neuromodulatory interventions such as repetitive transcranial magnetic stimulation (rTMS) and theta burst stimulation have been used to inhibit activity in the nonlesioned frontal cortex. This approach aligns with the findings of Sprague [50], which showed that lesioning the contralateral superior colliculus can compensate for the overexcitation of the nonlesioned hemisphere. Such hemispheric imbalance is thought to contribute to a shift or rotation of the attentional focus.

Interventions using rTMS have produced robust effects in the treatment of neglect symptoms or related functions, even in the absence of concurrent behavioral training [51,86]. While rTMS appears to be effective, its application in neurorehabilitation settings is limited because it is more technically demanding and associated with risks, including the potential for seizures, interactions with pacemakers, and contraindications in patients with craniectomy.

5.3.4.4 Bottom-up approach for neglect rehabilitation: pharmacological intervention

Pharmacological interventions are based on the assumption that enhancing attention and motivation may support recovery from neglect. Various substances have been tested, including acetylcholinesterase inhibitors and different dopaminergic agonizts. While some uncontrolled studies have reported positive effects, randomized controlled trials have not demonstrated significant benefits, leaving the overall efficacy of these pharmacological approaches unproven.

5.3.4.5 Top-down and bottom-up approaches: which might be used when and for which patient?

Even when excluding pharmacological and direct brain-stimulating methods, this chapter has introduced a range of bottom-up treatments for VSN. However, only a few studies have directly compared these interventions, making it difficult to identify which approach is most effective and should be prioritized in clinical practice.

Despite compelling theoretical models underlying these interventions, several limitations remain. First, it is important to recognize that pure external stimulation—without engaging the patient´s internal processes—cannot be considered an effective treatment. At its most extreme, such stimulation merely serves as an external compensation for a lacking excitation. A successful treatment would mean that the compensatory external stimulation is generated by the body or brain again. Second, most (or all?) bottom-up treatments in fact incorporate top-down components. For example, optokinetic drift may involve voluntary tracking of visual stimuli. PA requires recalibration and conscious adjustment during the doffing and donning phases. Neck vibration involves sensory input but also demands some degree of cognitive calibration or engagement. It remains unclear which components—sensory stimulation or the cognitive response to it—are primarily responsible for the therapeutic effects observed. A similar issue arises with compensatory strategies: motor learning and voluntary movement may contribute significantly to observed improvements, blurring the line between bottom-up and top-down mechanisms.

This leads to the conclusion that both approaches are theoretically distinct but practically not exclusive. Still, during routine practice, it is necessary to answer the question of what treatment should be offered. Table 5.3 offers an overview of how the two approaches can be adapted to the different recovery phases. Based on our clinical experience, without having firm data for it, we propose the following:

- In the early postacute phase, passive stimulation using acoustic cues may be preferred. These interventions are minimally demanding and can be well tolerated by patients in a reduced general state.
- For patients with severe SWM impairments, bottom-up methods such as optokinetic drift and PA are recommended. These interventions directly address deficits in spatial attention and require less volitional engagement.
- In contrast, patients who demonstrate some insight and residual SWM capacity may benefit more from structured top-down interventions. These methods rely on preserved cognitive resources and promote compensatory strategy use.

5.4 The problem of allocentric neglect and its treatment

As previously mentioned, VSN includes both egocentric and allocentric neglect, which often occur together but are distinct phenomena. Egocentric neglect is space-based and causes patients to ignore stimuli on their contralesional side. This can result in a deviation of the eyes, head, and trunk toward the right. It is more common and generally much more evident than allocentric neglect. In contrast, allocentric neglect is object-based and causes patients to ignore the contralesional side of an object, regardless of its position in space [87].

Fig. 5.7 illustrates the concept of allocentric neglect [88]. They are taken from the case of a woman who suffered a traumatic brain injury (TBI) with contusional bleeding in the right hemisphere. The resulting lesion, as far as it is possible to localize a lesion after severe TBI, involved the right insular cortex, the caudate tail and body, and right mediobasal temporal structures (Fig. 5.7, upper right). While the patient was able to copy the overall shape (global gestalt) of objects, she consistently neglected the left-side details (Fig. 5.7, upper left and lower portion).

5.4.1 Assessing egocentric and allocentric neglect

In clinical practice, egocentric neglect is commonly assessed using visual search tasks and line bisection tests [89]. In contrast, allocentric

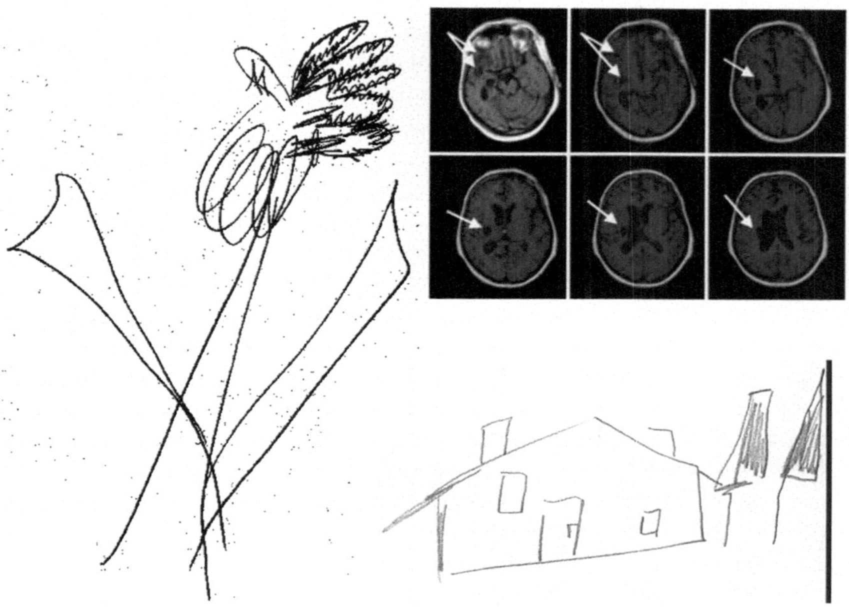

FIGURE 5.7 Manifestation of allocentric neglect following right-hemisphere traumatic brain injury. *Note*. Manifestation of allocentric neglect following right-hemisphere traumatic brain injury. **Note.** The patient reproduced the global shape of objects but consistently omitted or distorted details on the left side of individual objects, consistent with allocentric neglect. The MRI scans show right-hemispheric lesions involving the insular cortex, caudate nucleus, and mediobasal temporal regions. Adapted from Hildebrandt and Ebke [88].

neglect is typically evaluated through a visual search task in which small targets are defined by left- or right-sided features, defining them as hits or distractors. Such tasks additionally allow for assessment of both neglect types: egocentric neglect is reflected by the number of omissions on the left side of the search array, while allocentric neglect is indicated by misses of targets with a critical feature located on the left side of the object (for a review, Lee et al. [6]).

Apple's Cancellation Test is one of the most widely used neuropsychological tests following this approach [90]. It has been demonstrated that egocentric and allocentric neglect commonly cooccur [91,92], though some patients may present with only one subtype [16,90]. Notably, one known limitation of Apple's Cancellation Test is reduced sensitivity in detecting mild stages of neglect. In such milder cases, measuring response time or processing speed offers additional insights into side-specific differences not visible on cancellation tasks.

To further investigate this, we developed an experimental paradigm to study the effects of parallel and serial search tasks on allocentric neglect [8,23]. This allowed for a separate analysis of pop-out effects at both the item and spatial position level. Using this paradigm, we tested two patients: one with a lesion in the right premotor cortex, and another with a combined MCA and posterior cerebral artery stroke. Both performed similarly in the parallel search condition; however, their performance diverged in the serial search condition. The patient with the premotor MCA lesion exhibited pure egocentric neglect, with deficits restricted to features on the left side of the display, regardless of the object's internal structure. In contrast, the patient with the postcentral lesion demonstrated allocentric neglect. His performance was strongly affected by the side of the feature within the object: when the feature was on the right, performance was intact regardless of spatial position; when the feature was on the left side of the object, performance declined significantly, even when the object was on the right side of the screen. We were able to replicate these findings in larger group studies involving both left- and right-hemisphere patients (Figs. 5.8 and 5.9).

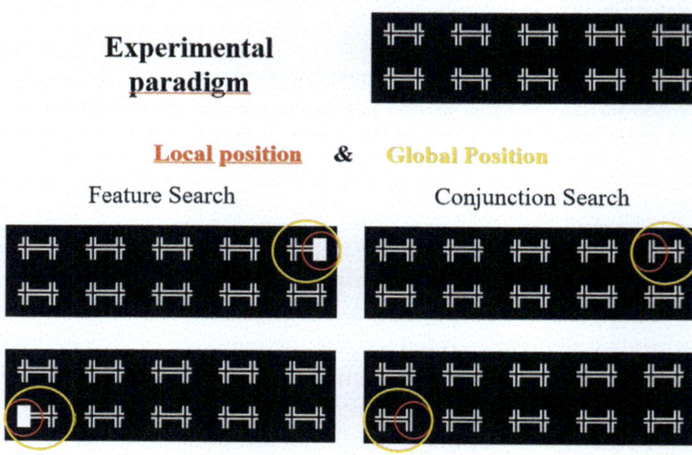

FIGURE 5.8 Experimental paradigm for differentiating egocentric and allocentric neglect. *Note.* This visual search paradigm distinguishes allocentric (within-object/local) from egocentric (viewer-centered/global) spatial deficits. In the feature search task (*left*), targets differ from distractors by a single feature located on the left- or right-sided position within the object. In the conjunction search task (right), targets are defined by a single feature located on the left or right side of the object. Red circles indicate allocentric (within-object) position, whereas yellow circles indicate egocentric (array-based) position. In the conjunction search task (*right*), targets are defined by a combination of features and their spatial position within the overall array. Red circles indicate allocentric (within-object) position, whereas yellow circles indicate egocentric (array-based) position.

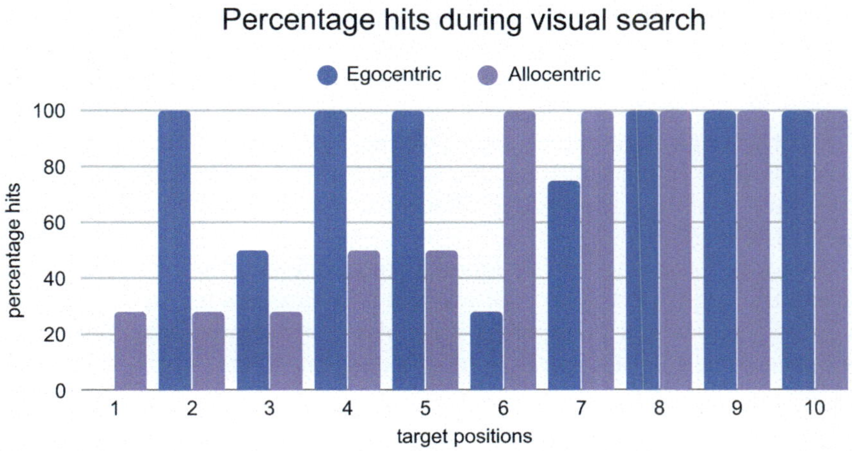

FIGURE 5.9 Visual search performance in two patients with neglect. *Note.* For understanding the task, compare Fig. 5.8 directly above. *Blue bars* represent a patient with egocentric neglect, showing reduced detection of targets in left-sided global positions, largely independent of the local position of the target feature. Performance improves progressively from left to right across the visual array. *Purple bars* represent a patient with allocentric neglect, showing impaired detection of targets with left-sided local features, regardless of their global position within the array.

5.4.2 Functional impairments following allocentric and egocentric neglect

Research has shown that egocentric and allocentric neglect are functionally independent, with no consistent interaction between the two [4]. Clinical studies have also documented that the two neglect subtypes may differ concerning their impact on functional impairments. For instance, Bickerton et al. [90] reported that patients with pure allocentric neglect exhibited greater impairments in ADLs (assessed via the BarthelIndex) compared to those with only egocentric neglect.

The recovery rate of these two subtypes appears to be different too. Moore et al. [16] assessed stroke survivors 6 months poststroke. They found that egocentric neglect followed a proportional recovery trajectory, meaning the extent of recovery was aligned with initial severity: patients with severe egocentric neglect in the acute phase tended to show more residual symptoms chronically. In contrast, allocentric neglect followed a nonproportional recovery pattern: recovery varied considerably among patients, with some showing no improvements, or even deterioration, regardless of initial severity, or even a worsening. Importantly, acute severity of allocentric neglect did not predict long-term outcome, making its progression more difficult to anticipate.

Lastly, there are differences between egocentric and allocentric neglect in terms of treatment effectiveness. While several interventions improve egocentric neglect, they have been ineffective in treating allocentric neglect [21,22,93]. Moreover, treatment strategies that specifically target allocentric neglect remain sparse [16], and no clear clinical consensus exists on how best to address this subtype [6]. Additionally, it remains uncertain whether improving allocentric neglect might also reduce egocentric neglect.

To address this gap, we designed a study to create an intervention for allocentric neglect [94]. Our goal was not only to assess its effectiveness in reducing allocentric symptoms but also to examine whether such improvements might generalize to egocentric neglect.

5.4.3 Development, implementation, and outcome of treatment study on allocentric neglect

The treatment approach was designed based on the conceptual framework presented in Table 5.8 and Fig. 5.10, distinguishing two task dimensions intended to manipulate attentional demands in allocentric neglect: copying versus constructing, and working with same-size elements versus scaling spatially undefined elements.

The theoretical background for the treatment scheme was the hypothesis that allocentric neglect arises from a failure to adapt the attentional window to the complete extent of the target object. Heinke and Humphreys [40] developed a computational model for visuospatial and

TABLE 5.8 Intervention matrix for allocentric neglect training.

Intervention level		
Drawing	Constructing	Segmentation
Copying of geometrical figures or objects	Reconstructing objects by matching parts	Segmenting of areas by simple spatial symmetries (e.g., line bisection)
Mirror simple geometrical objects towards the left	Constructing figures by parts of different sizes, with frontoplanar rotation of the parts	Segmenting limited parts of geometrical figures by size and orientation
Mirror real figures toward the left	Constructing figures by parts that must be rotated in the frontoplanar and in frontocoronar planes	Segmentation of plane areas without any indications in various parts violates the visible structure of the area.

Note. The table presents three intervention domains, drawing, constructing, and segmentation, each increasing in complexity. Tasks range from simple copying and mirroring to more advanced spatial constructions and segmentation without clear visual boundaries. The structure supports stepwise adaptation of object-centered attention in patients with allocentric neglect.

Task		Description
Copying Task	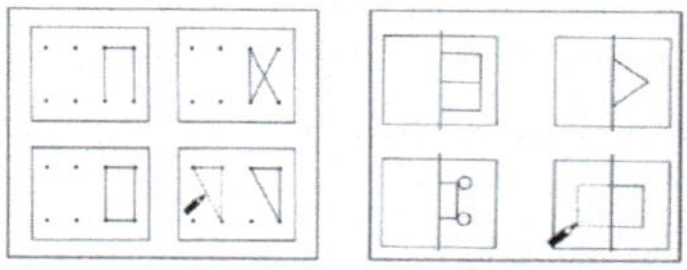	Left half: copying task for treatment of egocentric neglect Right half: copying task for treatment of allocentric neglect
Construction Task	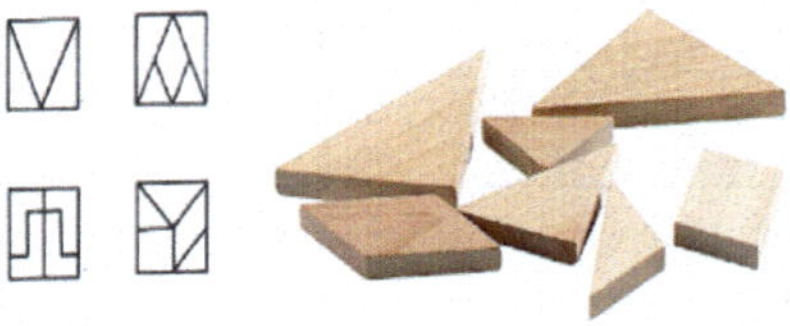	Upper left: simple reconstruction, no frontocoronar rotation required, but correct, object sizing may be needed. Upper right: increased difficulty due to more parts. Lower left: may require frontoplanar and frontocoronar rotation Lower right: requires multiple rotations and accurate size estimation of parts
Segmentation of Figures into Parts	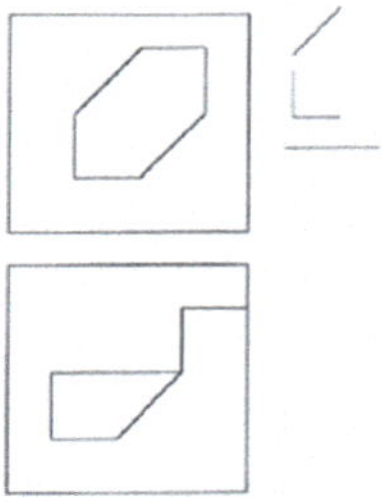	The geometrical figure on the left should be segmented into exactly four parts that fit the predefined elements on the right. For the upper geometrical figure the solution is two corners and two diagonal lines.
Segmentation and Reconstruction of Areas	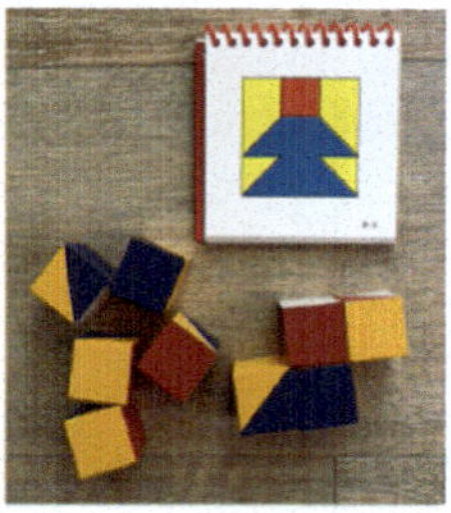	The Nikitin blocks that should be composed fitting the picture in the upper part.
Handling Everyday Objects	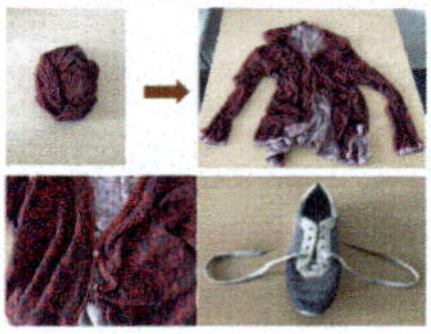	Everyday life tasks: Putting down a blouse to wear. Lacing up the shoes.

FIGURE 5.10 Tasks for allocentric neglect training. **Note.** The figure illustrates different training tasks targeting allocentric visuospatial processing and visuoconstructive abilities, including copying tasks, geometric construction, figure segmentation, reconstruction of spatial patterns, and the handling of everyday objects. Task complexity increases from simple copying and object assembly to spatial transformations and functional everyday activities. Adapted from Hildebrandt et al. [94].

object selection that supports this idea. According to their model, egocentric neglect results from a failure of spatial selection, whereas allocentric neglect is caused by incomplete retrieval of object information, which impairs global adjustment of attention to overall object extent. Consequently, left-sided aspects of objects are systematically ignored.

A related distinction was proposed by Halligan and Marshall [95]. They argued that egocentric neglect reflects a disorder in *global* attention, whereas allocentric neglect represents a deficit of *local* attention to left-sided features as parts of objects. They further demonstrated that enhancing global attention led to a reduction of VSN in their patient. Based on these theoretical considerations, we predicted that training patients to voluntarily adapt their attentional window to the scale of increasingly undefined object dimensions would remediate allocentric neglect [94].

To test this, 13 patients underwent a 3-week intervention program, which included both structured tasks (copying, constructing, segmenting) and handling everyday objects (e.g., shoes, T-shirts) to improve allocentric neglect symptoms. Following treatment, patients showed improvements in tests of egocentric neglect measures and functional outcome scores, including the Functional Independence Measure (FIM) and the Early Rehabilitation Barthel Index (ERBI), while the active control group only improved on the FIM. However, within the treatment group, no significant improvement was observed in allocentric neglect scores. Moreover, direct statistical comparisons with the control group showed no superiority of the treatment, even for secondary measures such as the ERBI or egocentric neglect tests. Therefore, the intervention did not produce significant improvements in allocentric neglect and only provided limited, indirect evidence for a weak improvement in egocentric neglect.

Excluding context-specific influences, such as disruptions related to the COVID-19 pandemic, comparison with previous control groups suggests two main explanations for the treatment's limited success. First, to our knowledge, this is the first study explicitly aiming to treat allocentric neglect and to investigate possible generalization to egocentric symptoms. It is therefore possible that the conceptualization and design of the tasks were incorrect. Our intervention was based on the model proposing that allocentric neglect results from an insufficient centering of local attention ("attentional window") on objects [40,95]. Consequently, the training focused on adapting the attentional window to varying object sizes. If this model is incorrect, however, the intervention would not have addressed the true underlying mechanism of allocentric neglect.

Second, the independence of egocentric and allocentric neglect may be less clear-cut than previously assumed. Although often treated as distinct syndromes, empirical evidence regarding their separation remains controversial [91,96]. Some authors argue that allocentric neglect is based on object coding in the ventral visual stream combined with hemi-inattention due to a lesion of dorsal visuospatial processing. In this framework, allocentric aspects play a role, but their specific meaning depends on the egocentric distribution of attention [91,97]. Allocentric coding representations would always be nested within egocentric coding, whereas egocentric attention operates independently of allocentric coding, but egocentric coding cannot be nested within allocentric. If this hierarchical model for allocentric neglect is accurate, then our intervention may have induced only a restricted partial reorientation of egocentric attention, insufficient to produce meaningful improvements at the allocentric level. Importantly, evidence from other studies showing that egocentric treatments do not improve allocentric neglect does not contradict this interpretation. Rather, interventions targeting only one spatial reference frame may produce domain-limited effects. In other words, meaningful improvements across both domains may require combined treatments addressing both the egocentric and allocentric components.

5.4.4 Allocentric neglect: conclusions

While egocentric and allocentric neglect often cooccur, accumulating evidence highlights their distinct neural bases, behavioral manifestations, and prognostic implications. Egocentric neglect primarily reflects deficits in spatial attention toward the contralesional side of space, whereas allocentric neglect involves object-centered omissions, independent of spatial location. Despite advances in diagnostic tools—including refined visual search paradigms and specialized cancellation tasks—the effective treatment of allocentric neglect remains challenging and, to date, has not yielded consistent improvements. Bottom-up interventions such as PA, visual scanning training, and neuromodulatory stimulation primary improve egocentric neglect.

Our intervention study, grounded in attentional window theory, aimed to address this gap by training patients to flexibly adapt their attentional window to varying object dimensions. No significant effects were found for allocentric neglect. These results suggest that current models incompletely capture the neural mechanisms underlying allocentric neglect. Furthermore, they underline the possibility that effective remediation may require simultaneous targeting of both egocentric and allocentric components of spatial processing.

In sum, further research is needed to refine the theoretical understanding of allocentric neglect, develop tailored intervention strategies, and explore combined treatment approaches that address the full spectrum of spatial attention deficits. Future studies should also consider the dynamic interplay between dorsal and ventral visual streams to clarify the interaction between space-based and object-based attention deficits in neglect.

References

[1] Heilman KM, Valenstein E, Watson RT. Neglect and related disorders. Semin Neurol 2000;20:463–70.
[2] Kerkhoff G, Schenk T. Rehabilitation of neglect: an update. Neuropsychologia 2012;50:1072–9.
[3] Bowen A, Hazelton C, Pollock A, Lincoln NB. Cognitive rehabilitation for spatial neglect following stroke. Cochrane Database Syst Rev 2013:CD003586.
[4] Overman MJ, Binns E, Milosevich ET, Demeyere N. Recovery of visuospatial neglect with standard treatment: a systematic review and meta-analysis. Stroke 2024;55:2325–39.
[5] Longley V, Hazelton C, Heal C, Pollock A, Woodward-Nutt K, Mitchell C, et al. Non-pharmacological interventions for spatial neglect or inattention following stroke and other non-progressive brain injury. Cochrane Database Syst Rev 2021(7):CD003586.
[6] Lee SH, Lim BC, Jeong CY, Kim JH, Jang WH. Assessment tools for differential diagnosis of neglect: focusing on egocentric neglect and allocentric neglect. World J Clin Cases 2022;10:8625–33.
[7] Luaute J, Halligan P, Rode G, Rossetti Y, Boisson D. Visuo-spatial neglect: a systematic review of current interventions and their effectiveness. Neurosci Biobehav Rev 2006;30:961–82.
[8] Grimsen C, Hildebrandt H, Fahle M. Dissociation of egocentric and allocentric coding of space in visual search after right middle cerebral artery stroke. Neuropsychologia 2008;46:902–14.
[9] Bisiach E, Geminiani G, Berti A, Rusconi ML. Perceptual and premotor factors of unilateral neglect. Neurology 1990;40:1278–81.
[10] Heilman KM. Intentional neglect. Front Biosci 2004;9:694–705.
[11] Himmelbach M, Karnath HO. Goal-directed hand movements are not affected by the biased space representation in spatial neglect. J Cogn Neurosci 2003;15:972–80.
[12] Migliaccio R, Bouhali F, Rastelli F, Ferrieux S, Arbizu C, Vincent S, et al. Damage to the medial motor system in stroke patients with motor neglect. Front Hum Neurosci 2014;8:408.
[13] Sapir A, Kaplan JB, He BJ, Corbetta M. Anatomical correlates of directional hypokinesia in patients with hemispatial neglect. J Neurosci 2007;27:4045–51.
[14] Treisman A, Sato S. Conjunction search revisited. J Exp Psychol Hum Percept Perform 1990;16:459–78.
[15] Lunven M, Rode G, Bourlon C, Duret C, Migliaccio R, Chevrillon E, et al. Anatomical predictors of successful prism adaptation in chronic visual neglect. Cortex 2019;120:629–41.
[16] Moore MJ, Vancleef K, Riddoch MJ, Gillebert CR, Demeyere N. Recovery of visuospatial neglect subtypes and relationship to functional outcome six months after stroke. Neurorehabil Neural Repair 2021;35:823–35.
[17] Kenzie JM, Girgulis KA, Semrau JA, Findlater SE, Desai JA, Dukelow SP. Lesion sites associated with allocentric and egocentric visuospatial neglect in acute stroke. Brain Connect 2015;5:413–22.

[18] Riddoch MJ, Chechlacz M, Mevorach C, Mavritsaki E, Allen H, Humphreys GW. The neural mechanisms of visual selection: the view from neuropsychology. Ann N Y Acad Sci 2010;1191:156–81.
[19] Chechlacz M, Rotshtein P, Roberts KL, Bickerton WL, Lau JK, Humphreys GW. The prognosis of allocentric and egocentric neglect: evidence from clinical scans. PLoS One 2012;7:e47821.
[20] Demeyere N, Gillebert CR. Ego- and allocentric visuospatial neglect: dissociations, prevalence, and laterality in acute stroke. Neuropsychology 2019;33:490–8.
[21] Gossmann A, Kastrup A, Kerkhoff G, Lopez-Herrero C, Hildebrandt H. Prism adaptation improves ego-centered but not allocentric neglect in early rehabilitation patients. Neurorehabil Neural Repair 2013;27:534–41.
[22] Mancuso M, Damora A, Abbruzzese L, Zoccolotti P. Prism adaptation improves egocentric but not allocentric unilateral neglect: a case study. Eur J Phys Rehabil Med 2018;54:85–9.
[23] Hildebrandt H, Schutze C, Ebke M, Brunner-Beeg F, Eling P. Visual search for item- and array-centered locations in patients with left middle cerebral artery stroke. Neurocase 2005;11:416–26.
[24] Turgut N, Miranda M, Kastrup A, Eling P, Hildebrandt H. Tdcs combined with optokinetic drift reduces egocentric neglect in severely impaired post-acute patients. Neuropsychol Rehabil 2018;28:515–26.
[25] Czernuszenko A, Czlonkowska A. Risk factors for falls in stroke patients during inpatient rehabilitation. Clin Rehabil 2009;23:176–88.
[26] Diamond PT. Rehabilitative management of post-stroke visuospatial inattention. Disabil Rehabil 2001;23:407–12.
[27] Lisa LP, Jughters A, Kerckhofs E. The effectiveness of different treatment modalities for the rehabilitation of unilateral neglect in stroke patients: a systematic review. NeuroRehabilitation 2013;33:611–20.
[28] Turgut N, Moller L, Dengler K, Steinberg K, Sprenger A, Eling P, et al. Adaptive cueing treatment of neglect in stroke patients leads to improvements in activities of daily living: a randomized controlled, crossover trial. Neurorehabil Neural Repair 2018;32:988–98.
[29] Bartolomeo P, Chokron S. Orienting of attention in left unilateral neglect. Neurosci Biobehav Rev 2002;26:217–34.
[30] Bartolomeo P, Thiebaut de Schotten M, Chica AB. Brain networks of visuospatial attention and their disruption in visual neglect. Front Hum Neurosci 2012;6:110.
[31] Losier BJ, Klein RM. A review of the evidence for a disengage deficit following parietal lobe damage. Neurosci Biobehav Rev 2001;25:1–13.
[32] Olk B, Hildebrandt H, Kingstone A. Involuntary but not voluntary orienting contributes to a disengage deficit in visual neglect. Cortex 2010;46:1149–64.
[33] Turgut N, Jansen AL, Nielsen J, Heber I, Eling P, Hildebrandt H. Repeated application of the covert shift of attention task improves endogenous but not exogenous attention in patients with unilateral visuospatial inattention. Brain Cogn 2021;151:105732.
[34] Diller L, Weinberg J. Hemi-inattention in rehabilitation: the evolution of a rational remediation program. Adv Neurol 1977;18:63–82.
[35] Riddoch MJ, Humphreys GW. The effect of cueing on unilateral neglect. Neuropsychologia 1983;21:589–99.
[36] Weinberg J, Diller L, Gordon WA, Gerstman LJ, Lieberman A, Lakin P, et al. Visual scanning training effect on reading-related tasks in acquired right brain damage. Arch Phys Med Rehabil 1977;58:479–86.
[37] Antonucci G, Guariglia C, Judica A, Magnotti L, Paolucci S, Pizzamiglio L, et al. Effectiveness of neglect rehabilitation in a randomized group study. J Clin Exp Neuropsychol 1995;17:383–9.

[38] Paolucci S, Antonucci G, Guariglia C, Magnotti L, Pizzamiglio L, Zoccolotti P. Facilitatory effect of neglect rehabilitation on the recovery of left hemiplegic stroke patients: a cross-over study. J Neurol 1996;243:308–14.
[39] De Nigris A, Piccardi L, Bianchini F, Palermo L, Incoccia C, Guariglia C. Role of visuo-spatial working memory in path integration disorders in neglect. Cortex 2013;49:920–30.
[40] Heinke D, Humphreys GW. Attention, spatial representation, and visual neglect: simulating emergent attention and spatial memory in the selective attention for identification model (SAIM). Psychol Rev 2003;110:29–87.
[41] Moreh E, Malkinson TS, Zohary E, Soroker N. Visual memory in unilateral spatial neglect: immediate recall versus delayed recognition. J Cogn Neurosci 2014;26:2155–70.
[42] Toba MN, Rabuffetti M, Duret C, Pradat-Diehl P, Gainotti G, Bartolomeo P. Component deficits of visual neglect: "Magnetic" attraction of attention vs. Impaired spatial working memory. Neuropsychologia 2018;109:52–62.
[43] Bisiach E, Luzzatti C. Unilateral neglect of representational space. Cortex 1978;14:129–33.
[44] Karnath HO. Spatial attention systems in spatial neglect. Neuropsychologia 2015;75:61–73.
[45] Karnath HO, Ferber S. Is space representation distorted in neglect? Neuropsychologia 1999;37:7–15.
[46] Karnath HO, Niemeier M, Dichgans J. Space exploration in neglect. Brain 1998;121(Pt 12):2357–67.
[47] Cox JA, Aimola Davies AM. Keeping an eye on visual search patterns in visuospatial neglect: a systematic review. Neuropsychologia 2020;146:107547.
[48] Fabius J, Ten Brink AF, Van der Stigchel S, Nijboer TCW. The relationship between visuospatial neglect, spatial working memory and search behavior. J Clin Exp Neuropsychol 2020;42:251–62.
[49] Ten Brink AF, Visser-Meily JMA, Nijboer TCW. What does it take to search organized? The cognitive correlates of search organization during cancellation after stroke. J Int Neuropsychol Soc 2018;24:424–36.
[50] Sprague JM. Interaction of cortex and superior colliculus in mediation of visually guided behavior in the cat. Science 1966;153:1544–7.
[51] Valero-Cabre A, Toba MN, Hilgetag CC, Rushmore RJ. Perturbation-driven paradoxical facilitation of visuo-spatial function: revisiting the 'sprague effect. Cortex 2020;122:10–39.
[52] Ogourtsova T, Korner-Bitensky N, Ptito A. Contribution of the superior colliculi to post-stroke unilateral spatial neglect and recovery. Neuropsychologia 2010;48:2407–16.
[53] Nieuwenhuys R, Voogd J, Huijzen Cvan. The Human Central Nervous System. 4th ed. Berlin: Springer-Verlag; 1998.
[54] Moon S, Lee B, Na D. Therapeutic effects of caloric stimulation and optokinetic stimulation on hemispatial neglect. J Clin Neurol 2006;2:12–28.
[55] Oppenlander K, Keller I, Karbach J, Schindler I, Kerkhoff G, Reinhart S. Subliminal galvanic-vestibular stimulation influences ego- and object-centred components of visual neglect. Neuropsychologia 2015;74:170–7.
[56] Corneil BD, Munoz DP, Chapman BB, Admans T, Cushing SL. Neuromuscular consequences of reflexive covert orienting. Nat Neurosci 2008;11:13–5.
[57] Gu C, Corneil BD. Transcranial magnetic stimulation of the prefrontal cortex in awake nonhuman primates evokes a polysynaptic neck muscle response that reflects oculomotor activity at the time of stimulation. J Neurosci 2014;34:14803–15.
[58] Farne A, Rossetti Y, Toniolo S, Ladavas E. Ameliorating neglect with prism adaptation: visuo-manual and visuo-verbal measures. Neuropsychologia 2002;40:718–29.

[59] Redding GM, Wallace B. Prism adaptation and unilateral neglect: review and analysis. Neuropsychologia 2006;44:1–20.
[60] Rossetti Y, Rode G, Pisella L, Farne A, Li L, Boisson D, et al. Prism adaptation to a rightward optical deviation rehabilitates left hemispatial neglect. Nature 1998;395:166–9.
[61] Li J, Li L, Yang Y, Chen S. Effects of prism adaptation for unilateral spatial neglect after stroke: a systematic review and meta-analysis. Am J Phys Med Rehabil 2021;100:584–91.
[62] Qiu H, Wang J, Yi W, Yin Z, Wang H, Li J. Effects of prism adaptation on unilateral neglect after stroke: an updated meta-analysis of randomized controlled trials. Am J Phys Med Rehabil 2021;100:259–65.
[63] Hildebrandt HL, et al. Non-pharmacological interventions for spatial neglect or inattention following stroke and other non-progressive brain injury. Cochrane database Syst Rev 2021;32:2673–8. *Neuropsychol Rehabil*. 2022.
[64] Scheffels JF, Korabova S, Eling P, Kastrup A, Hildebrandt H. The effects of continuous vs. Intermittent prism adaptation protocols for treating visuospatial neglect: a randomized controlled trial. Front Neurol 2021;12:742727.
[65] Jiang H, Stein BE, McHaffie JG. Multisensory training reverses midbrain lesion-induced changes and ameliorates haemianopia. Nat Commun 2015;6:7263.
[66] Jiang H, Rowland BA, Stein BE. Reversing hemianopia by multisensory training under anesthesia. Front Syst Neurosci 2020;14:4.
[67] Schenke N, Franke R, Puschmann S, Turgut N, Kastrup A, Thiel CM, et al. Can auditory cues improve visuo-spatial neglect? Results of two pilot studies. Neuropsychol Rehabil 2021;31:710–30.
[68] Kaufmann BC, Cazzoli D, Bartolomeo P, Frey J, Pflugshaupt T, Knobel SEJ, et al. Auditory spatial cueing reduces neglect after right-hemispheric stroke: a proof of concept study. Cortex 2022;148:152–67.
[69] Geiser N, Kaufmann BC, Cazzoli D, Nef T, Nyffeler T. Auditory motion stimulation as an add-on therapeutical approach is feasible, enjoyable, and associated with a significant improvement of neglect outcome: a non-randomized, controlled group-matched study. Neuropsychol Rehabil 2025:1–15.
[70] Geiser N, Kaufmann BC, Knobel SEJ, Cazzoli D, Nef T, Nyffeler T. Comparison of uni- and multimodal motion stimulation on visual neglect: a proof-of-concept study. Cortex 2024;171:194–203.
[71] Keller I, Lefin-Rank G, Losch J, Kerkhoff G. Combination of pursuit eye movement training with prism adaptation and arm movements in neglect therapy: a pilot study. Neurorehabil Neural Repair 2009;23:58–66.
[72] Kerkhoff G, Keller I, Artinger F, Hildebrandt H, Marquardt C, Reinhart S, et al. Recovery from auditory and visual neglect after optokinetic stimulation with pursuit eye movements–transient modulation and enduring treatment effects. Neuropsychologia 2012;50:1164–77.
[73] Pizzamiglio L, Fasotti L, Jehkonen M, Antonucci G, Magnotti L, Boelen D, et al. The use of optokinetic stimulation in rehabilitation of the hemineglect disorder. Cortex 2004;40:441–50.
[74] Vuilleumier P, Hester D, Assal G, Regli F. Unilateral spatial neglect recovery after sequential strokes. Neurology 1996;46:184–9.
[75] Weddell RA. Subcortical modulation of spatial attention including evidence that the sprague effect extends to man. Brain Cogn 2004;55:497–506.
[76] Sterling P. Quantitative mapping with the electron microscope: retinal terminals in the superior colliculus. Brain Res 1973;54:347–54.
[77] Posner MI, Rafal RD. Cognitive theories of attention and the rehabilitation of attentional deficits. In: Meier MJ, Benton AL, Diller L, editors. Neuropsychological Rehabilitation. The Guilford Press; 1987. p. 182–201.

[78] Basso MA, May PJ. Circuits for action and cognition: a view from the superior colliculus. Annu Rev Vis Sci 2017;3:197–226.
[79] King AJ. The superior colliculus. Curr Biol 2004;14:R335–8.
[80] Swan L. Unilateral spatial neglect. Phys Ther 2001;81:1572–80.
[81] Smania N, Fonte C, Picelli A, Gandolfi M, Varalta V. Effect of eye patching in rehabilitation of hemispatial neglect. Front Hum Neurosci 2013;7:527.
[82] Kudo Y, Takahashi K, Sugawara E, Nakamizo T, Kuroki M, Higashiyama Y, et al. Bedside video-oculographic evaluation of eye movements in acute supratentorial stroke patients: a potential biomarker for hemispatial neglect. J Neurol Sci 2021;425:117442.
[83] Krauzlis R, Dill N. Neural correlates of target choice for pursuit and saccades in the primate superior colliculus. Neuron 2002;35:355–63.
[84] Schenke N, Diestel E, Kastrup A, Eling P, Hildebrandt H. Monocular eye patching modulates reorienting of covert attention in patients with unilateral middle cerebral artery stroke. Brain Cogn 2023;169:106000.
[85] Schenke N, Eling P, Duning T, Hildebrandt H. Monocular eye patching modulates ipsilesional reactive saccades and smooth pursuit in patients with left hemispatial neglect. Brain Cogn 2023;173:106101.
[86] Elsner B, Kugler J, Pohl M, Mehrholz J. Transcranial direct current stimulation (tdcs) for improving activities of daily living, and physical and cognitive functioning, in people after stroke. Cochrane Database Syst Rev 2020;11:CD009645.
[87] Leyland LA, Godwin HJ, Benson V, Liversedge SP. Neglect patients exhibit egocentric or allocentric neglect for the same stimulus contingent upon task demands. Sci Rep 2017;7:1941.
[88] Hildebrandt H, Ebke M. neglect dyslexia owing to traumatic fronto-temporal right hemisphere bleeding]. Fortschr Neurol Psychiatr 2003;71:8–16.
[89] Sprenger A, Kompf D, Heide W. Visual search in patients with left visual hemineglect. Prog Brain Res 2002;140:395–416.
[90] Bickerton WL, Samson D, Williamson J, Humphreys GW. Separating forms of neglect using the apples test: validation and functional prediction in chronic and acute stroke. Neuropsychology 2011;25:567–80.
[91] Li D, Karnath HO, Rorden C. Egocentric representations of space co-exist with allocentric representations: evidence from spatial neglect. Cortex 2014;58:161–9.
[92] Rorden C, Hjaltason H, Fillmore P, Fridriksson J, Kjartansson O, Magnusdottir S, et al. Allocentric neglect strongly associated with egocentric neglect. Neuropsychologia 2012;50:1151–7.
[93] Abbruzzese L, Damora A, Antonucci G, Zoccolotti P, Mancuso M. Effects of prism adaptation on reference systems for extrapersonal space in neglect patients. Brain Sci 2019;9.
[94] Hildebrandt H, Meißner K, Stahl C, Duning T, Eling P. Can allocentric neglect be treated by functional training and by stimulating bottom-up neuroplasticity? A randomized cross-over trial. Neurol Rehabil 2025;31:87–94.
[95] Halligan PW, Marshall JC. Focal and global attention modulate the expression of visuo-spatial neglect: a case study. Neuropsychologia 1994;32:13–21.
[96] Turgut N, Modden C, Brumund T, Eling P, Hildebrandt H. A study on the independence of egocentric and allocentric neglect. Cortex 2017;96:95–104.
[97] Chen Q, Weidner R, Weiss PH, Marshall JC, Fink GR. Neural interaction between spatial domain and spatial reference frame in parietal-occipital junction. J Cogn Neurosci 2012;24:2223–36.

CHAPTER

6

Rehabilitation of language disorders after stroke ("aphasia")

6.1 Introduction

6.1.1 Stroke, aphasia, and functional treatment

Aphasia, a language disorder affecting comprehension and/or production of speech, and apraxia of speech, a motor planning deficit impairing voluntary speech movements, are frequent acute consequences of a left arteria cerebri media (ACM) stroke, affecting 21%–40% of poststroke patients [1–3]. As in neglect, spontaneous recovery of the aphasia is high during the first 6 to 12 weeks. Still, up to one-third of left ACM stroke patients suffer from residual aphasic symptoms even half a year after the event. A large metaanalytic analysis demonstrated that across all language domains, when a significant change from baseline was evident, the greatest change in language performance from baseline was among participants enrolled within 1 month of stroke [4]. This fits the results from artificial stroke in rodents (Chapter 3), especially to start early but not too early with rehabilitation [5].

Language disorders following right ACM stroke are also frequent ("speech arrest"), however, less than after left ACM stroke, and with recovery in minutes to hours. Persisting deficits due to right ACM stroke may concern prosody, comprehension of complex messages, and social interaction in right-handers, which are higher-order features of verbal communication. Therefore we will concentrate on the treatment of aphasia restricted to lesions of the left hemisphere.

Aphasia is a term for different syndromes, and the branches of the ACM occluded by the stroke are related to the prevailing symptoms. Isolated strokes of the insular and ventral premotor branches lead to *apraxia of speech*, a motor speech disorder that is characterized by slowed speech rate, articulatory imprecision, visible/audible groping for articulatory postures, and dysprosody [3,6]. Thus the correct timing and

Applied Neuropsychology of Cerebrovascular Diseases
DOI: https://doi.org/10.1016/B978-0-443-45450-9.00010-2

sequencing of movements for fluent speech are impaired, and the impairment cannot be explained by dysarthria. Strokes of more dorsal and premotor ACM branches and branches that supply the adjacent rostral brain areas are associated with *Broca's aphasia* [7]. Patients with Broca's aphasia may produce primarily nouns while omitting verbs. Prepositions and articles of sentences show errors in tense, number, and gender. Comprehension of short and standard sentences is intact, however, understanding of sentences (and even more producing) in noncanonical order is impaired. Speech production sounds nonfluent.

Strokes in the posterior temporoparietal branches of the ACM most frequently impair the understanding of sentences [7]. This is due to an inability to convert the phonological structure of the sequences of words into semantics, which corresponds to the word messages. Speech production is often fluent but accompanied by word-finding problems. Produced distortions in language production often remain unnoticed and therefore without any correction. If the anterior temporal lobe is involved, understanding of single words is the dominant problem. If the stroke spares the posterior temporal branches (which is rarely the case), the understanding of sentences is better than that of words [7]. Both syndromes are termed Wernicke's aphasia; however, due to two different impairments: parsing phonological sounds and accessing meaning versus losing the stored semantic representation of words.

While traditional models emphasize specific cortical loci, such as Broca's and Wernicke's areas, effective language function depends equally on the integrity of the connections between these regions [8]. If the stroke involves multiple brain regions or a key area along with its connecting fiber pathways, the resulting symptom may not be due to direct damage alone. Instead, they could be caused by diaschisis, a phenomenon where one brain region becomes functionally impaired because it loses input from another damaged area. Subcortical white matter tracts, which mediate communication within the language network, can be critically involved. Damage to these connecting pathways may disrupt network dynamics and produce language deficits, even when cortical regions themselves are partially spared. This means that aphasia symptoms may arise from different underlying causes, because language processing relies on distributed neural networks rather than isolated cortical regions.

However, this is not the only problem for clinical symptom-lesion mapping. Similar symptoms may also have different causes. For example, anomic aphasia, characterized primarily by word-finding difficulties, is a very common consequence of left ACM stroke. It can result from difficulties in retrieving the phonological word form or impairments in the search mechanism that lead to word retrieval. In the case of large

ACM strokes, the damage can be so extensive that it leads to global aphasia, where both language comprehension and production are severely impaired. This occurs because large strokes affect multiple areas involved in different aspects of language, causing an overlap of symptoms from various aphasia syndromes. Thus while stroke localization is crucial for understanding aphasia, there is no simple one-to-one correspondence between lesion sites and specific aphasic syndromes.

The chance for recovery from aphasia differs according to the extension of stroke, age, and brain reserve of the patients. Older age and larger extension of the stroke reduce the chance for recovery, whereas brain reserve is associated with the opposite [4,9]. Aphasia due to left thalamic strokes is a rare event and recovery usually occurs very fast. In the case of basal ganglia stroke, recovery depends on the number of nuclei involved. If the lesion is restricted to only one of the major basal ganglia nuclei—caudatum, putamen, or globus pallidus—recovery will be fast and almost complete. If two or three nuclei are involved or if the anterior capsula interna adjacent to the basal ganglia is also hit by the stroke, symptoms and recovery are slow and possibly not unrestricted.

Recovery is also associated with the syndrome status [3]. Older case series argue that patients with global aphasia for 4 months will show no relevant further recovery during the next 3 months. However, patients with Broca's aphasia still have a good chance of considerable recovery (more than 42% show such a recovery). Only one-fourth of patients with Wernicke's aphasia show clear recovery after an additional 3 months. However, during an even later, chronic stage, treatment of Wernicke's aphasia patients might reveal better results than those with Broca's aphasia [9]. These are important information for communicating the prognosis to the patients and their relatives during the 1st weeks after the stroke.

6.1.2 A model for understanding and treating aphasic disorders

There are several excellent reviews of the classical framework to understand language processing and explain aphasic syndromes [3,7,10–12]. This framework is also the theoretical background for many existing approaches to treat aphasic syndromes, as mentioned below. In the following, we will deviate from this framework and focus on Levelt's [13] action theory of language production, assuming two major and different levels in developing spontaneous or reactive speech (Fig. 6.1, dark shadowed rectangles). The major advantage of Levelt's model [13–15] is that it allows us to define a common background for the patients and the neuropsychologist during the treatment, and we will use

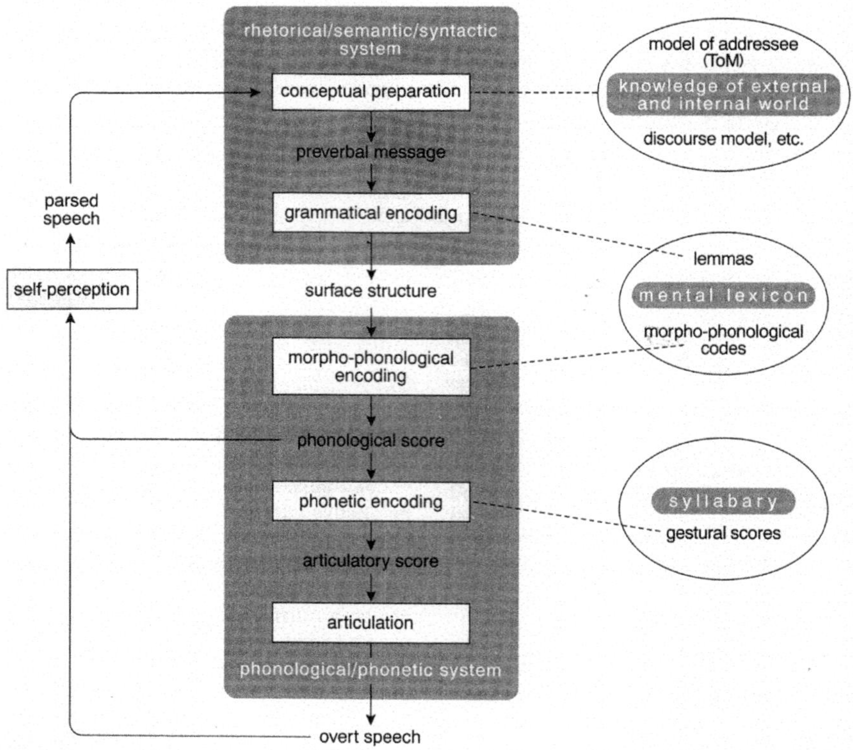

FIGURE 6.1 Levelt's model of speech production. *From Levelt W.J. Models of word production. Trends Cogn Sci 1999;3:223–232.*

the components of the model to distinguish between interventions according to the severity of aphasic syndromes and the level of interaction remaining possible.

Levelt's model [13–15] starts with the process of conceptual preparation, encompassing a global conception of the content to be communicated (which may entail different statements and therefore a sequence of sentences) and about the knowledge and interest of the recipients of that message. It seems to be necessary to assume that conceptual preparation not only takes place during the production of language but also during perception, starting with some basic assumptions, what the theme of the message will be, and then building up a more and more sophisticated representation of the message received. Successful communication presupposes that the conceptual preparation of the produced and perceived message become increasingly aligned. This means that the level of verbal communication is not the understanding of words, but the understanding of sentences in the context of perspectives of mental or

TABLE 6.1 Semantic feature analysis of animals.

	Teeth	Feathers	Legs	Beaks	Able to swim	Able to fly
Fish	Yes	No	No	No	Yes	No
Birds	No	Yes	Yes	Yes	Some	Most
Reptiles	Yes	No	Yes	No	Some	No
Mammals	Yes	No	Yes	No	Yes	No

physical spaces. Such a fit between perspectives can only be achieved with the help of working memory, the holding and working with the already present memory to adapt the representation to the whole message.

Framed as a working memory task, conceptual preparation for understanding language will use the already decoded meaning of phonological word representation and therefore will not be identical with the phonological working memory. Decades ago, Alan Baddeley proposed that there is a WM system for something such as meaningful scripts, which he called the episodic buffer [16]. The episodic buffer reorganizes the meaning of aspects of an episode into a coherent script for better understanding and storage. This is done according to the context of the different information experienced during that episode. Therefore conceptual binding along plausible relations between different aspects is one of the major tasks of the episodic buffer (and binding is one major topic of research on the episodic buffer and its relation to aphasia [17]). It should be noted that the episodic buffer is not the prototypical "conceptual space" of semantic feature analysis (Table 6.1), because the episodic buffer will be organized according to themes, possible scripts and contextual expectations about perspectives of the other person, whereas semantic feature analysis includes aspects of the episodic buffer but also arbitrary similarities or dissimilarities of words [17].

Conceptual preparation [13] plays an important role in the language comprehension of severely aphasic patients. Clinical routine interactions with such patients inform that there is a "situational" understanding in many of them, even if being severely impaired. Situational understanding is also one of the first recovery steps noted in reports on these patients. However, if the understanding of questions concerns any objectives not evidently present in the situation, the patients will fail to understand and respond to them. Discussed in the framework of Levelt's model [13–15,18], this means that if conceptual preparation for word finding and word understanding is minimal, aphasic patients are able to understand and respond to questions related to exactly that state. Comprehension and word production become a problem for such patients as soon as they have to adopt an "abstract" or, as called by the old-fashioned neuropsychologist, a "symbolic" attitude [19,20], including verbal elements, association, or drawing not immediately present (or being not directly picked up from) in the situation.

For a better understanding of the conceptual preparation level of Levelt [13] and its meaning for aphasia, compare such an understanding with the situation, where the patient reads aloud sentences and looks for the last word completing the sentence. In this case, the conceptual preparation involves a common definition of the task ("to complete sentences"), but also the meaning of the sentence, which is not part of the situation. It implies the understanding of sentences not anchored in the situation but defined by a common knowledge of the world—that is, the content of the sentence—which must be shared for finishing an incomplete sentence with a final word. The amount of the conceptual preparation's burden to read the sentence and find the missing word varies: it depends on the difficulty of the sentences (I am playing with the ... [table/ball] versus democracy is based on [humans/representation]) and on using sentences varying in length and scripts (sentences with different adjectives or clauses; sentences related to one topic, e.g., the kitchen and to cooking, vs sentences about various situations). The goal of aphasic treatment is to achieve a shift from simple, unidimensional conceptual representations to symbolic interactions able to define mental spaces for verbal interactions independent from any concrete environment, either for understanding or for communicating the message. This leads back to the question of working memory for the treatment of aphasic patients. Depending on the specific aphasic syndrome, it can be stated that an "episodic buffer" serving as a module for the conceptual preparation is part of the treatment. It will be used unconsciously by any person interacting with the patients in reducing the complexity of speech spontaneously to a level where communication becomes possible. And it is the starting point for any attempts to increase the complexity of verbal comprehension and production of the aphasic patient.

According to Levelt's model [13–15,18], the next step in producing and understanding language is a second linearization, developing the grammatical frame of the sentence and first semantic lemmas for the words to be used. This second linearization starts in parallel with the conceptual preparation (Fig. 6.1) and helps to refine the working representation of the content of the message. Two of the mentioned treatments for aphasia can be related to these aspects of Levelt's model: [13–15,18] the treatment of underlying forms (TUF) (see below) tries to remediate impairments in grammatical encoding, starting with simple canonical sentences and increasing the level of sentences into those with relative clauses and in a noncanonical order. This ability allows a flexible adaptation of speech in the case that the second linearization was not specific enough, starting to speak the sentence. In such cases, the structure of the sentence must be adapted "on the fly" for a correct expression of the content. For the treatment of an aphasic patient, the more concrete or direct canonical stance can be used to come up with the specific word. Semantic feature analysis intends to increase the ability to fill lemmas with concrete words. Sticking to word finding tasks in a similar conceptual domain and focusing on the most distinguished exemplars are important tools in the treatment of aphasia.

Levelt's model [13–15,18] proposes a second module for language production which gets activated along with the intention to speak and the selection of the specific word and this module concerns morphological and phonological components of the words (Fig. 6.1). In terms of the working memory systems, this module concerns the phonological representation of words, not the meaning of the message. Now, the phonological representation of words is essential for understanding the meaning and also for producing the phonological codes, and therefore its manipulation should be possible or an essential part of any treatment, depending on the specific aphasic impairment. The to be produced phonological structure may be difficult to pronounce, just like the German word "Quelle," or as easy as the German word "Hand." Similarly, the length and complexity of word pronunciation are important negative factors for the effectiveness of verbal working memory representation (phonological loop). Production of words on a phonological level can also be endorsed by imitating mouth movements or by reading based on grapheme–phoneme regularities, which are both independent of any word meaning. Moreover, the therapist can help the patient to read by choral shadowing, a technique where the patient repeats or mimics the speech of the therapist. Thus the phonological module interpreted as phonological working memory also offers aspects, that are important for treating aphasic patients. The morphological level of word production can be used by initiating the phonological representations by using the correct grammatical gender of the word, which is possible for the German language, because of its three different genders. It can also be endorsed by varying the frequency and abstractness of accompanying adjectives.

6.2 How to treat aphasic disorders?

Functional treatment of aphasia is the task of speech therapists. In the following, classical training used to treat aphasic patients will be introduced shortly. However, detailed discussion of these methods, as well as interventions targeting the chronic phase or the use of nonverbal tools, will not be addressed here, as this is beyond the scope of neuropsychological responsibility.

Still, in the context of in-hospital postacute rehabilitation, the number of aphasic patients is high, and neuropsychologists are involved in their assessment and treatment. The focus of the second part of this section is on this stage of recovery (postacute) and on severe patients suffering from global aphasia, severe Broca's or Wernicke's aphasia, or severe word-finding problems. The approach, which will be proposed, is therefore not based on data from large randomized controlled trials (RCTs), but rather a clinical framework. However, before moving on, we shortly introduce standard treatments for aphasic patients.

6.2.1 Classical approaches for treating aphasic patients

There are various treatment options for aphasic patients that target different aspects of language impairments and are based on different models of language processing [5].

6.2.1.1 Semantic feature analysis

The most widely followed intervention, namely Semantic Feature Analysis (SFA), aims to decrease word-finding problems. It assumes that our semantic system is organized as a network of concepts [21]. Semantic features are associated not only with one concept but may be associated with several other concepts. Such common features may be, among others, the superordinate category (e.g., animal), the habitat (e.g., continent and sea), being a predator or not, or being able to fly (Table 6.1). These features together define the specific exemplar and activate its verbal representation. However, if the features are not very specific or incomplete, they may also activate different concepts, which may result in the production of false words or indecisiveness and, therefore in word-finding problems. SFA attempts to address this problem by strengthening the semantic representations associated with target words.

The approach assumes that stroke-related damage has impaired the conceptual-semantic networks and, thus the automaticity of word finding. The main strategy of SFA therefore is to teach the patients the different specifying features of the concepts corresponding to the words that cannot be reproduced anymore. To achieve that goal, lists of features are written down for each concept related to their superordinate category, their properties and appearance, and the patient's individual experience with it. Such a re-enrichment of the semantic structure of concepts is assumed to increase their uniqueness and therefore the chance that the corresponding word is being activated. Various studies have shown that after treatment, the trained word can be produced better and that there may be some generalization toward other words [22]. It should be clear that such a treatment strategy only works in patients with mild aphasia, at least if the patient can find and name the features themselves.

SFA is a mixture of a bottom-up training approach with a strategic component for improving word access. The training involves a rebuilding of the links between the semantic representation of a concept and the word form, and the strategy for improving the search for such a retrieval (using the different aspects during search for the word). In these aspects, it shares similarity with the transfer appropriate process model for rehabilitating verbal memory performance. SFA may be criticized for oversimplifying the organization of conceptual-semantic networks. It is not very important that elephants and trucks may have a similar height, weight, and color and can be used for transport, although they share these common features. There are strong arguments that human conceptual networks are organized in scripts for action and possibilities, and this aspect is only one of several in SFA (compare Table 6.1). Moreover, even in "simple" cognitive language models, four different pure word finding deficits may be distinguished: (1) a loss of the meaning of the words (semantic aphasia), (2) a deficit in accessing the meaning of the sentences , (3) a deficit in accessing the phonological representation (tip of the tongue phenomenon), and (4) a loss of an adequate linearization of the sentence structure. Word-finding problems may also be due to losing the conceptual representation of the communication content. Therefore SFA may not target the most central deficits explaining the word-findings problems. Still, intensive SFA-based training is one of the most extensively studied evaluated functional treatments and supported by a comparatively strong empirical evidence base.

6.2.1.2 Phonomotor treatment/output-oriented treatment

Cognitive models for language production argue that word-finding problems and hesitating speech may be caused, for example, by unsuccessful retrieval of articulatory-kinematic routines. Phonomotor treatment starts on the opposite, output-related level of speech production by training phonemes (sounds) and phoneme sequences [21]. Access to phonology and/or phonological sequencing may be disturbed, isolated and on its own, which would be identical to apraxia of speech [22]. In patients with word-finding problems due to apraxia-of-speech-like impairments, other treatments have been shown to be effective, including speech entrainment, in which the clinician and patient read aloud a passage simultaneously, with both visual and auditory mirroring [22].

Linearization of messages in or by sentences may also be a reason for word-finding problems. Each sentence has a structure with an agent, a verb, and an object relation for the verb. If the structure to linearize the sentence gets lost, speech would become hesitant and reduced to the global theme, whereas verbs will not be used anymore, because their specific characteristics presuppose additional grammatical relationships to be implemented in messages. Such a deficit may be due to a loss of verbs or to a loss of grammar.

6.2.1.3 Treatment of underlying forms

TUF is a treatment approach, which trains the comprehension and production of complex sentences by addressing the sentence syntax level and the morphological level of word generation [21,23,24]. In simple terms, it focuses on how different parts of a sentence are combined, thereby rebuilding grammatical sentence structure. The components of sentences (agent, verb, and object relation of action) are written on cards and paired with an action picture. Patients should identify the verb of the picture-related sentence, and are then taught to physically move the cards to reorder the components of the simple sentence to construct a more complex sentence. During training, the therapists provide explicit information if the movement of the cards position in the sentence is correct, about the grammatical roles of the words on the cards, and how it influences the meaning of the sentence (Fig. 6.2). Moreover, information about the morphological changes is given related to the word's role in the sentence, such as the gender of nouns or the tense of verbs (e.g., present or past tense). As for the other approaches for rehabilitation of poststroke

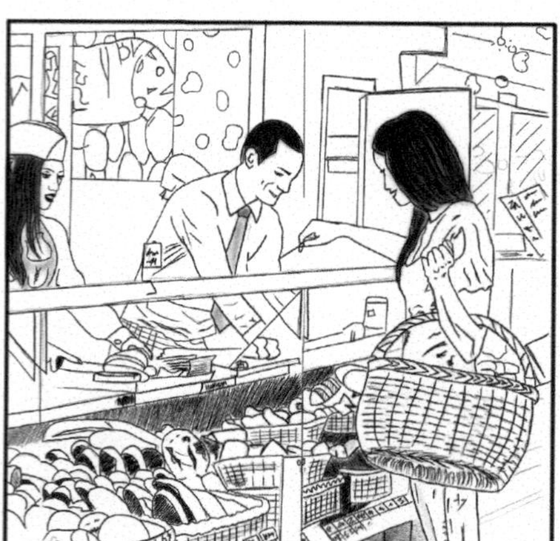
Please, arrange the following words that they fit what you see on the picture:
THE BREAD
BOUGHT
NANCY
WHO
IT WAS

FIGURE 6.2 Treatment of underlying forms.

aphasia, there are several studies showing that the TUF is effective, for example, in increasing the complexity of verbal messages of the patients. One advantage of this approach for treating aphasic patients is that the authors directly address the question of which condition the patients should fulfill to benefit from the intervention. As in semantic feature analysis, the focus is on moderate to mild impaired patients, who are able to read and understand words and phrases.

TUF focuses on increasing the grammatical complexity of sentences during recovery. The likelihood of an association between the agent and the verb read aloud in sentences with missing final words determines whether the sentence can be successfully completed. If the missing word is common and used broadly, patients tend to succeed. If it's rare or highly specific, word finding is harder. Semantic feature analysis assumes that word finding improves when patients activate semantic associations between words. Yet, in TUF, the associated meaning of objects and words differs along the function for common or cooperative use, at least within the frame of the episodic buffer model. Therefore even if both approaches share a common element (activation of words by semantic associations) in terms of TUF, it seems to be somewhat odd to classify objects schematically for arbitrary features as proposed in semantic feature analysis.

Having discussed three very different approaches for the treatment of aphasic disorders, it should be kept in mind that the motor and syntactical deficits might be impaired in addition to semantic access (and vice versa), which would mean that concept representations (semantics), articulatory motor representations, and syntactic linearization together enable fast and automatic word retrieval. Thus treatment on only one level might not be enough to deal with the multifaceted problems of the patients, at least if the stroke affected different regions of the brain.

6.2.2 A short guide on how to treat postacute patients with severe aphasia

In this section, only the treatment of patients in a postacute stage and with severe language impairments will be discussed. As in visuospatial hemi-inattention (neglect), the treatment of aphasia is based on cueing (or "facilitation" to use an older term), that is, defining a situation by interventions that enable the patients to speak (as in visuospatial neglect to turn attention toward the left). Levelt's model [13–15,18] (Fig. 6.1) and its relation to verbal working memory allows to conceptualize the major levels of cueing for severely aphasic patients. Tables 6.2–6.4 provides an overview of the quality and severity of the impairment and the proposed

TABLE 6.2 Impairment in the production of speech.

	Conceptual representations	Phonological representations
Massive motor aphasia (not speaking any words)	Speaking in series: prescribing the numbers when naming loudly, reading aloud (twice with a delay per number the second time), starting the third time, waiting for the initiative of the patients, speaking along quietly when the patient starts. Working through a hierarchical sequence of cueing from showing, semantic cues to initiate speaking of the word "hand."	Read numbers one to nine, use of first letter cueing, and imitation mouth movement. Choir shadowing with decreased loudness. If reasonably confident in counting, transition to simple object naming. Use writing down, phonological first letter cueing, or mouth movement imitation to achieve work speaking.
Moderate motor aphasia (individual words can be cleared safely, but rather as a series of words or after a combination of different cues)	Conceptual preparation for simple but changing meanings. Semantic: different body parts or distinguished pictures from similar categories. Search for a single number between distractors that must be found and named. Facilitation by counting starting from two numbers before.	Read written body parts, use of first letter cueing, imitation mouth movement, and choir intonation. Use of first letter cueing, if necessary.
Mild motor aphasia, amnestic aphasia (in interaction about simple facts, the telegram style, and a word-finding disorder dominate)	Formulate a sentence to describe actions on pictures (i.e., "x is doing y"). Sentences as cues (read aloud and then passively complete). Words first with, then without visible images from memory with increasing delay, using visuospatial cues ("which picture was here and which here?").	Writing down the sentence. Use the agent as a cue for verb produced by the patient. Sentence completion tasks (shadow reading of the patient, pronounce phonological cues).
Amnestic aphasia (the word-finding disorder occurs in the context of	Formulate stories displayed on four to six action pictures.	Write down a word with the most important information for the single picture, and point to that

(Continued)

TABLE 6.2 (Continued)

	Conceptual representations	Phonological representations
sentences that have been started)	Position of the individual images as a cue for keeping track of the story. Cover picture to formulate from working memory with a growing delay from the last seeing. Introduce a distraction between picture viewing and storytelling. Repetition of fictitious, recurring everyday situations.	word in the case of hesitating speech.

intervention. It also shows how to proceed through these levels, adapted to the severity of disturbances.

Patients with large left ACM strokes in a postacute stage are often unable to speak any words, and they may even be unable to verbalize any sounds. Concerning Levelt's model [13–15,18], on the conceptual level, the situation should completely define the topic of the verbal message. The grammatical structure should be as simple as possible, and the meaning of the word produced as a result of the situation and the grammar. Moreover, the intended word should be easy to pronounce. Counting from one to eight, if prepared as proposed in Tables 6.2–6.4 often allows patients to speak a first word after stroke, even in a state of global aphasia and apraxia of speech. It should be noted that meaning and grammar do not really play a role in counting, because counting is an automatized action. Thus while the spoken word is triggered, it is not really a message on a symbolic level (it does not refer to something else). Triggering is maximal if the therapist starts with writing and reading the sequence of numbers, then reading them at normal speed, and then again with delays between the numbers to allow for anticipation of the coming number by the patients. Pointing to the pronounced numbers should also be part of the intervention. Often, the "three" or the "eight" are the first words, which the patients will be able to speak, because in German, the pronunciation of these numbers is easiest. Therefore extended delays with gestural hints to speak the following numbers should be introduced, especially after the "2" or the "7."

If the first numbers are triggered, the complexity of the communicative stance can be increased to tasks producing the appropriate word for one

TABLE 6.3 Impairment in comprehension of speech.

1. Receptive aphasia	Conceptual preparation	Phonological preparation
Severe speech comprehension disorder without excessive speech production (patient understands max. simplest prompts)	Sorting objects by semantic categories (excluding visual agnosia!). Assigning semantically different, frequent, and well-known images/objects to written words. Expand this training to infrequent and more similar objects.	Read the words for the patients. Encourage the patient to repeat the word phonologically (if possible) or to copy the word.
Moderate sensory aphasia or speech comprehension disorder without excessive speech production (simple tasks are understood situationally, without situational context, little language understanding)	Ask for labels for images or words for semantic relationships between objects. Selection of action statements or descriptions for action representations. Introduce delay and distraction before naming. Play the game that everybody gets a mix of images and should take turns requesting without using the direct name of the picture.	Propose written exemplars of labels or for semantic relationships, which should be read aloud and chosen afterwards. Introduce synonyms for the same objects.
Mild speech comprehension disorder (understanding becomes difficult when the situation or context does not guide understanding or when the facts become complex or abstract)	Sentence completion tasks: **1.** Used the same conceptual space for consecutive sentences **2.** Use more and more changing conceptual space for different sentences **3.** Increase sentence length and grammatical complexity Ask for term definitions and headings for different abstract terms. Deducing the meaning of words from complex stories.	Write down the underlying word forms components and ask to sort them in the necessary order for noncanonical sentences or sentences with relative clauses. Use anagrams as games to find the semantical meaning of words.
Mild comprehension deficit (speech comprehension fails with somewhat longer sentences)	Responding to requests of increasing complexity. Relative clauses, such as "Give me the small square that lies next to the rectangle."	Addition problems with two then three terms, alternation of addition and subtraction at three terms. Keeping results and further calculating others.

(Continued)

TABLE 6.3 (Continued)

2. "Wernicke's" aphasia	Conceptual preparation	Phonological preparation
Sensory aphasia with excessive speech production that is not intelligible.	1. Introduce stop signal 2. Gaining insight into the incomprehensibility of speech production 3. Gain insight into the cause of the malfunction Plus, the same therapy as for a simple speech comprehension disorder.	Individual words instead of sentences. For stopping speech showing of hands. Record patient's speech and play it back. Introduce a timer to decrease speech production.

simple picture or object (compare Tables 6.2–6.4, first and second line, e.g.,). The triggered word should be frequent, concrete, and easy to pronounce. Still, the patients do not need to represent what the focus of the interaction is, except for the relation between the object and the word. The target word should always be embedded in a canonical sentence, with a high frequency for common use of agent, verb, and object (compare Fig. 6.6 A–D for cueing the word "hand," which is a frequent and easily pronounced word. Moreover, the word production can be triggered by specific real action). If it is possible for the patient to speak a single word after cueing, the number of words and meanings can be increased, and the number of canonical sentences per word decreased. The presented examples of Fig. 6.6 A–C illustrate how to use the starting point of the sentence to serve as a simple trigger for triggering word production.

On the next level of recovery (Tables 6.2–6.4), the complexity of grammar to be produced can be increased. Picture showing a single person performing a simple action can be used as treatment material (Fig. 6.3), and the task for the patient is to complete sentences. It should be tested out, whether the patients are able to read (at least phonologically) the sentences describing the actions. If that is the case, completion of simple sentences can be defined as the next intervention level. This would be for the first time that conceptual representation comes into play, whereas the difficulty of grammatical construction is reduced again (Table 6.5, showing a list of sentences on different scripts).

Now the sentences must be interpreted as episodes, and the missing word is something which completes the episode, but which is not part ("invisible") of the concrete situation of the patient and the therapist. Clearly, this is a major step towards using language to communicate meaning independent of a concrete situation (which may be subsumed to

TABLE 6.4 Add-on and associated treatments.

1. Treatment of affect		
Catastrophic emotional behavior related to aphasia	Achieving affective transference by coping with everyday content and establishing everyday normality (as far as possible)	Use selective serotonin reuptake inhibitors?
No improvement after systematic cueing for 3 weeks	Changing the therapy content to the nonlinguistic area to increase self-confidence again	Playing simple visuospatial games as common enterprise with relatives
2. Add-on stimulation		
Direct neuromodulation	Use transcranial direct current stimulation in addition to functional treatment (2 mA, for 20 minutes in the beginning of the session). repetitive transcranial magnetic stimulation either on the left hemisphere for increasing neuroplasticity or for inhibiting the hyperactive right hemisphere?	Left frontal and cathodal right frontal stimulation for improving naming. Left supramarginal, posterior temporal stimulation for improving comprehension?
Pharmacological recommendations	Try acetylcholine esterase inhibitors in addition to functional treatment	Alternatively, piracetam?

symbolic behavior in the terminology of Kurt Goldstein [19,20]). Often, sentence completion is only possible with the help of shadow reading, because the patients are unable to pronounce specific words and lose the meaning of the sentences consequently. Intervening with shadow reading allows a more or less fluent reading.

Sentence completion varies in difficulty related to shifts in scripts used for formulating the sentences. A single script as a starting point for different sentences (sentences about the script to prepare a meal or for mowing in the garden) is much easier than a list of unpredictable sentences, which presupposes various conceptual preparations to simulate the episode and to find the correct word. Training elements based on the TUF can be added at this point, which shifts the topic of the intervention from meaning (which is the correct last word, making the

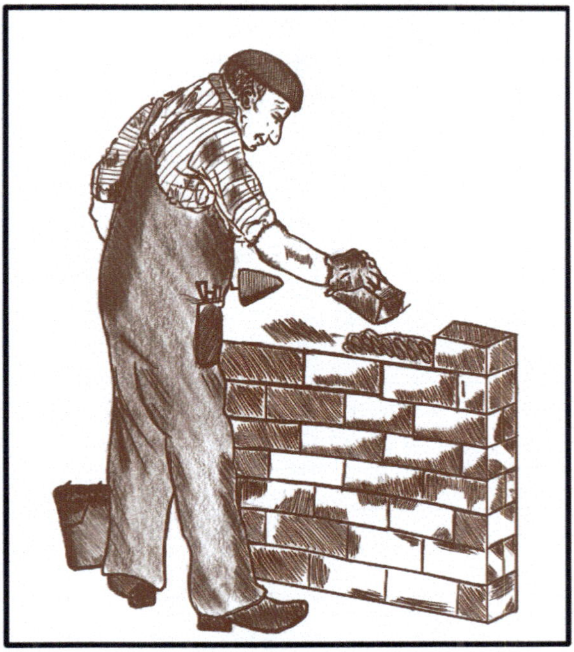

FIGURE 6.3 Drawing of actions for cueing words.

sentence understandable) to what kind of grammatical construction is possible to express the meaning (Fig. 6.4).

On an even higher level, picture stories can be used for the treatment. The patient has to integrate the different actions and situations of the picture into a coherent episode to select for the event the most important features of the single pictures. This presupposes to have representation of the story and the knowledge of what aspects of the information are necessary for the other person to understand it, which is the first step in conceptual preparation during flexible intercourse.

Up to now, the main topic was how to treat global aphasic and Broca's aphasia patients. However, patients may also suffer from Wernicke's aphasia. Tables 6.2–6.4 also inform how to treat patients with primarily comprehension problems. Two different patient groups can be distinguished: one with reduced speech and reactive responding because of impaired semantic storage (semantic aphasia), the other group with increased but seemingly meaningless speech (classical Wernicke's aphasia). The main task for the first group is to retrain semantic associations, concepts, and relate them to words. This can be done in many respects on a preverbal level and then by assigning the word to the reconstructed semantic meaning (Tables 6.2–6.4). Often, loss of meaning

TABLE 6.5 Scripts for cueing word production.

Read the sentence aloud and complete the correct word!

Words:
Bed, Tree, Head, Stove, Lawn Mower, Breakfast, Food, Birthday, Water, Blanket, Table, Tower

In the morning I sit down and eat	
When it gets cold, I throw new wood into the	
To look into the distance, I climb the	
The apple hangs high on the	
Before the grass gets too high I get the	
To eat, you sit down at the	
I'll give the flowers as a gift	
You can take the boat to the	
Because he is exhausted, he lies down on the	
Before he goes outside, he puts his hat on the	
For sleeping you need a pillow and a	
Many people brush their teeth after each	

representations concerns specific concepts, not more abstract categorization. Therefore the definition of the specific features of exemplars in contrast to similar objects and concepts should be trained. Semantic feature analysis plays a major role in treating such patients, but only if complemented with features dimensions that are directly visible. Because these patients often perform better on the level of sentences compared to single words, the meaning of words can be re-activated or re-constructed, embedded in different sentences, referring to the same word.

It is important to test if these patients suffer from central dyslexia, and, if so, whether in the form of surface or phonological dyslexia. If they do not suffer from dyslexia, they will be able to read words (however, some of them only on a phonological level without semantic understanding). In this case, writing the correct word below the picture to be named may help, and copying the word by the patient, too. After having established the naming of the objects during presentation and in front of the written word, the written word should be canceled. Afterwards, a short delay

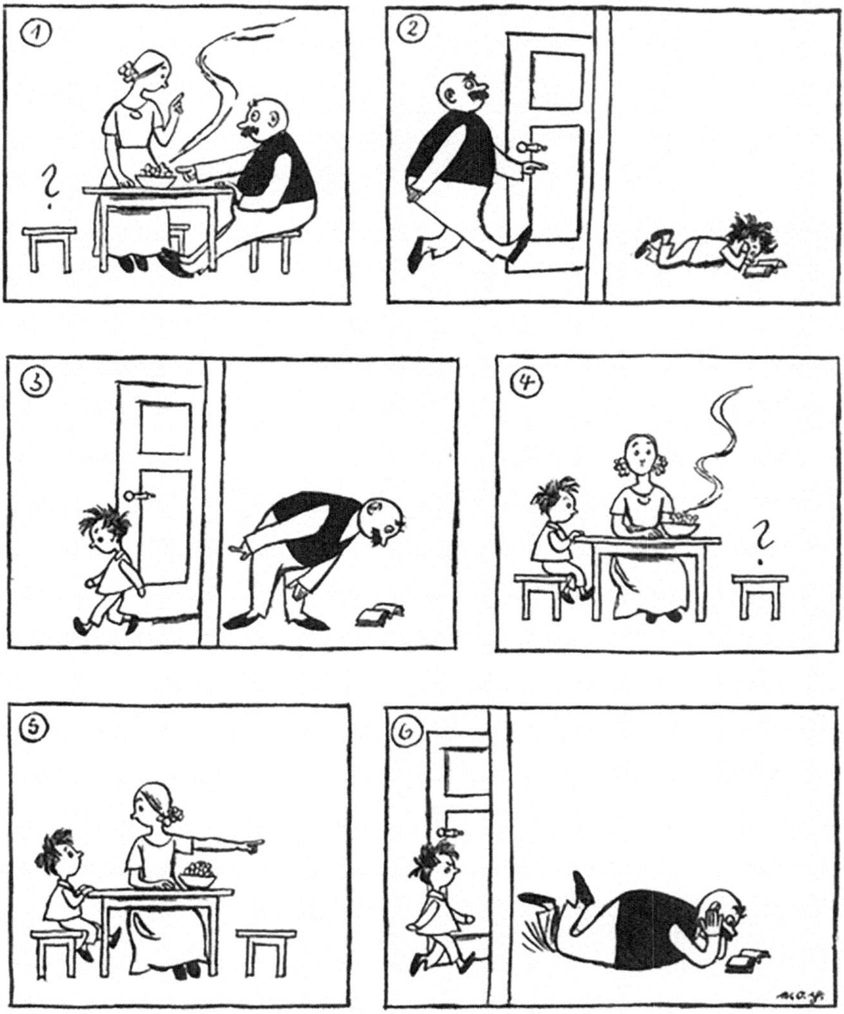

FIGURE 6.4 Four pictures from the "Vater und Sohn" picture stories. *Datei:Vater und Sohn - Der Schmoeker.png – Wikipedia.*

should be introduced, where the patient is getting distracted, before another naming trial. If naming after a delay (from working memory) is possible, the pictures should be covered and named just by pointing to the previous position. This step of increasing the load on naming from memory and working memory extends the ability to use language on a more abstract level without a concrete reference from the immediate visible situation.

The second group of patients with primarily understanding problems is those with the classical Wernicke's aphasia syndrome. These patients produce too many phrases, without becoming aware of the fact that other people are unable to understand what they are saying. Related to Levelt's model [13–15,18], self-perception of language production is disturbed, and this impairment not only concerns the perception of speech of others but also that of one's own speech production. The interruption of self-perception takes place on different levels: there is no internal correction for incorrect morpho-phonological encoding, which leads to paragrammatism. The sentence constructions sound as if they have some structure, but the phonological sound includes many semantic paraphasias and wrong inflections of words. Consequently, the final output results in sentences that cannot be understood, with the patient seeming unaware of that, as seen by them not showing any signs of hesitating speech related to a lack of understanding of their own language output, or by asking no questions, as one would do if one does not understand what the other person is telling. In these patients, understanding single words is often better preserved than understanding sentences. Motivation to communicate verbally in these patients is often high, which might be an argument that conceptual preparation of communication content is present. The most important topic for the treatment of these patients is to gain insight into the impairment and to reduce speech production. Tables 6.2–6.4 give an overview of possible interventions in this, but also in the other patient groups with speech comprehension deficits. We would like to mention in this respect that two aphasia-like symptoms or syndromes are discussed in different chapters: akinetic mutism in the chapter on early rehabilitation, and agraphia of one's own name in the chapter on memory rehabilitation. However, in the following section, the different aspects of the table will be described in more detail.

Patients with aphasia may show strong affective reactions which prevent any kind of aphasic treatment, especially if they do not have insight into their situation and deficit. These patients start to become severely depressed and may reject all therapeutic offers, with the exception of physiotherapeutic trainings such as standing or walking, which often allows for nonverbal participation and often more visible progress. In such a case, a pharmacological treatment to reduce depressive moods should be initiated, and because of the agitated status, selective serotonergic re-uptake inhibitors seem to be the first choice, if there is no severe sleep disorder, which otherwise should be the primary symptom to be impacted by antidepressant medication. In this case, if the specific treatment for improving language does not show any effect, the treatment goal should be changed. To enable further positive interactions, it should be tested which kinds of nonverbal games or activities are possible for the patient. Many of them also suffer from severe apraxia or executive deficits, and it is not easy to single out such activities. However, finding such activities or games is extremely helpful for relatives and friends to spend time together with the patient.

6.2.3 How to organize the treatment in microsteps: two additional principles from cognitive neuropsychology

6.2.3.1 Verbal working memory

Up to now, the topic was to provoke the production and understanding of language by varying the complexity of conceptual representation, grammatical structure, associations between terms, and complexity of phonological pronunciation. However, the meaning of sentences unfolds during speaking and reading—it can be undetermined until the last word has been spoken. This argues that verbal working memory plays a major role in comprehension. The role of verbal working memory for comprehension can be conceptualized on two different levels. First, there is the phonological level. Without an ongoing inner representation of the words, it is impossible to disentangle the relationship between the words of a sentence and its meaning. Impairments in this representation can be studied in Wernicke's aphasia, but even more clearly in patients with a logopenic variant of Alzheimer's disease. However, working memory representation of words is time-limited if rehearsal cannot be used because hearing a longer series of sentences makes rehearsal impossible. Therefore WM representation on a phonological level has to be complemented by an expectation of what the global message will be and how different features of a complex message fit into their specific roles during the development of the message.

Integrating verbal working memory as a central aspect of aphasic treatment also allows us to formulate a first but systematic step into the direction of a *spontaneous* production of language, irrespective of the concrete features of the present situation. Spontaneous production and understanding of language are central features of higher-order human verbal communication. Using working memory for treating aphasic patients means that the time between the stimuli (the question or the presentation of a picture) and the production of words can be varied by introducing a delay. Any delay between a stimulus and an action means that working or episodic memory comes into play, and spontaneous speech can also be defined as language based on episodic constructions without specific external occasions. Using working memory for delaying word production is a first step in this direction, other steps are if the words have to be produced without the presence of the stimuli (with covered pictures to be named or to be described) or even after a short active distraction. Therefore the introduction, the variation of the length, and the filling of the delay between eliciting and executing a verbal message are a central part of the treatment.

6.2.3.2 *Massed practice versus spaced retrieval*

Using pictures of an acting person as a starting point for provoking word productions in aphasic patients can be structured quite differently, depending on the explicit or implicit models for increasing recovery. If the assumption is that re-learning to access the (uninvolved) word lexicon is the major problem, many different pictures should be shown to increase the automaticity of access. If the assumption is that the word lexicon is also involved (no "simple" disconnection syndrome), rebuilding the lexicon is the major starting point. And if the assumption is that the automaticity of accessing specific words is disturbed, the goal for the treatment differs from both other conceptualization of the primary cognitive disturbance explaining the aphasic disorders.

Because the main goal of the treatment is to enable the patients to speak (more and more spontaneously and independently), it is important to know which learning approach will produce the most efficient, long-lasting results. In the chapter on memory rehabilitation, the method of spaced retrieval was introduced to allow patients to remember relevant information. This method can also be used in aphasia. Spaced retrieval means that pieces of information are

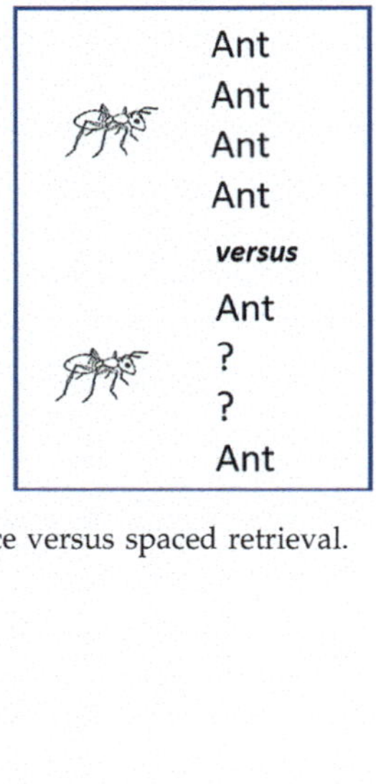

FIGURE 6.5 Massed practice versus spaced retrieval.

repeated with increasing time intervals between the repetitions. It is effective in protecting information from interference and from being wiped out by new information. Fig. 6.5 shows the difference between massed practice and spaced retrieval. It should be noted that the efficacy of spaced retrieval is dependent on what the task is during the period of not repeating the information (as mentioned in the chapter on memory and on the method of wakeful rest).

Several studies have shown that spaced retrieval outperforms massed practice in treating word finding problems of aphasic patients (for a review: Middleton and Schwartz [25]) [26,27]. This also argues that recovery is not based on simply accessing the relation between object recognition and word production. The following different aspects can be concluded from the studies on spaced retrieval versus massed practice for the treatment of aphasic patients. First, restrict the number of words to be learnt to be accessed per session. Try to find the correct complexity and timely extension for the period before the first and the following retrieval attempts are started, so that the word can be produced with a high probability. This will depend on the severity and quality of the word-finding problems. If the patient is able to reproduce the word after a longer period of time, reduce the trigger for the repetition, that is, try to base the repetitions on memory and on agreed conceptual preparation. Only the last step allows for spontaneous and voluntary verbal interaction, which is the ultimate goal of language use.

6.2.4 Pharmacological treatment

There is no clear-cut evidence for an effect of pharmacological treatment on recovery from aphasia. Some early and small studies found that piracetam in a dosage of 4.8 g/day increased the effectiveness of the treatment of aphasic disorders. However, a recent metaanalytic review argued that piracetam affected only benefits in written language ability, not in spoken language [28]. Other smaller studies also showed add-on training effects with acetylcholinesterase inhibitors, amphetamine, and, in some cases, dopamine agonizts (the latter only for nonfluent aphasias, probably with some aspects of akinetic mutism). These studies need replication in larger RCT trials. A large metaanalysis of fluoxetine revealed no effect on recovery from aphasia [29]. (Fig. 6.6 A–C, A–D) (Fig. 6.7)

(A)

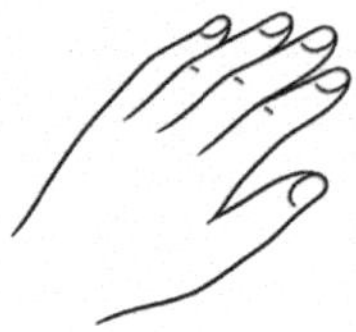

This is my hand

This is my (short delay, then)
Hand

This is my (long delay, then)
Hand

This is my hand (waiting for response)

If no correct response move on to

Five Finger has the hand

(B)

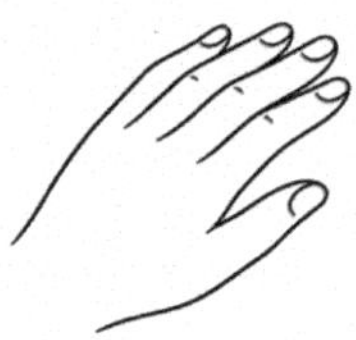

Five Finger has the (short delay, then)
Hand

Five Finger has the (long delay, then)
Hand

Five finger has the hand (waiting for response)

If no correct response move on to

For greeting we shake our hands (doing that symbolically without touching the patients)

(C)

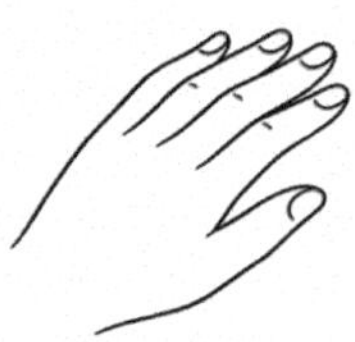

For greeting we shake our (short delay, then)
Hand

For greeting we shake our (long delay, then)
Hand

For greeting we shake our (waiting for response)

If no correct response move on to

Take the hand of the patients and press it

(D)

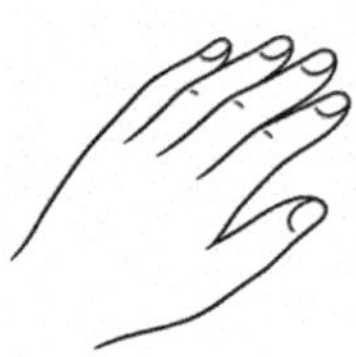

We are pressing our hands

We are pressing our (short delay, then)
hands

We are pressing our (long delay, then)
hands

We are pressing our (waiting for response)

If no correct response, repeat whole sequence up to three times

FIGURE 6.6 A–D: sequence for cueing the word "hand." A–C: sequence for cueing the word "hand."

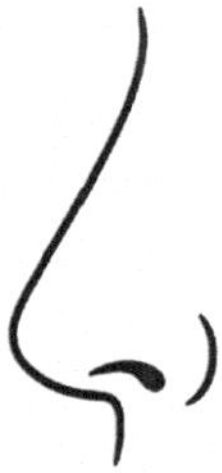

Don't fall on your nose

Don't fall on your (short delay, then)

nose

Don't fall on your (long delay, then)

nose

Don't fall on your (waiting for response)

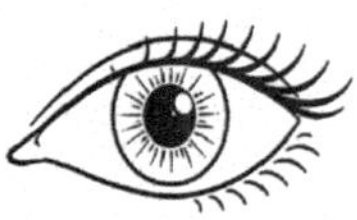

The woman has blue eyes

The woman has blue (short delay, then)

eyes

The woman has blue (long delay, then)

eyes

The woman has blue (waiting for response)

FIGURE 6.7 (A) and (B): two further examples for facilitating word production.

References

[1] Cichon N, Wlodarczyk L, Saluk-Bijak J, Bijak M, Redlicka J, Gorniak L, et al. Novel advances to post-stroke aphasia pharmacology and rehabilitation. J Clin Med 2021;10.

[2] Stipancic KL, Borders JC, Brates D, Thibeault SL. Prospective investigation of incidence and co-occurrence of dysphagia, dysarthria, and aphasia following ischemic stroke. Am J Speech Lang Pathol 2019;28:188–94.

[3] Huber W, Poeck K, Weniger D. Aphasie. In: Hartje Wolfgang, Poeck Klaus, editors. Klinische neuropsychologie. Stuttgart - New York: Thieme Verlag; 2002. p. 93–173.

[4] Brady M.C., Ali M., VandenBerg K., Williams L.J., Williams L.R., Abo M., et al. Complex speech-language therapy interventions for stroke-related aphasia: the release study incorporating a systematic review and individual participant data network meta-analysis. Southampton (UK); 2022.

[5] Burton B, Isaacs M, Brogan E, Shrubsole K, Kilkenny MF, Power E, et al. An updated systematic review of stroke clinical practice guidelines to inform aphasia management. Int J Stroke 2023;18:1029–39.

[6] Basilakos A. Contemporary approaches to the management of post-stroke apraxia of speech. Semin Speech Lang 2018;39:25–36.

[7] Bunker LD, Hillis AE. Vascular syndromes: revisiting classification of poststroke aphasia. Handb Clin Neurol 2022;185:37–55.

[8] Gill DJ, Damann KM. Language dysfunction. Contin (Minneap Minn) 2015;21:627–45.

[9] Kristinsson S, den Ouden DB, Rorden C, Newman-Norlund R, Neils-Strunjas J, Fridriksson J. Predictors of therapy response in chronic aphasia: building a foundation for personalized aphasia therapy. J Stroke 2022;24:189–206.

[10] Heilman KM. Aphasia and the diagram makers revisited: an update of information processing models. J Clin Neurol 2006;2:149–62.

[11] Mesulam MM, Thompson CK, Weintraub S, Rogalski EJ. The wernicke conundrum and the anatomy of language comprehension in primary progressive aphasia. Brain 2015;138:2423–37.

[12] Antony K, Bengough T, Laschkolnig A. Sprachtherapie bei aphasie. Schriftenreihe Health Technol Assess 2021;143. IBfArM, Köln 2021.

[13] Levelt WJ. Models of word production. Trends Cogn Sci 1999;3:223–32.

[14] Levelt WJ. Spoken word production: a theory of lexical access. Proc Natl Acad Sci U S A 2001;98:13464–71.

[15] Levelt WJ, Roelofs A, Meyer AS. A theory of lexical access in speech production. Behav Brain Sci 1999;22:1–38. discussion 38-75.

[16] Baddeley A, Wilson BA. Prose recall and amnesia: implications for the structure of working memory. Neuropsychologia 2002;40:1737–43.

[17] Henderson A, Kim H, Kintz S, Frisco N, Wright HH. Working memory in aphasia: considering discourse processing and treatment implications. Semin Speech Lang 2017;38:40–51.

[18] Maess B, Friederici AD, Damian M, Meyer AS, Levelt WJ. Semantic category interference in overt picture naming: sharpening current density localization by PCA. J Cogn Neurosci 2002;14:455–62.

[19] Hoffmann T. Kurt goldstein und das programm einer konkreten humanwissenschaft. In: Lanwer W, Jantzen W, editors. Jahrbuch der Luria-Gesellschaft 2016. Berlin: Lehmanns Media; 2017. p. 12–39.

[20] Stahnisch FW. Assessing Kurt Goldstein's lasting influence in the neuropsychology of language versus his use of aphasic symptoms as diagnostic insights into brain injuries. Front Psychol 2024;15:1356824.

[21] Cherney LR, Carpenter J. Behavioral interventions for poststroke aphasia. Handb Clin Neurol 2022;185:197–220.

[22] Vitti E, Hillis AE. Treatment of post-stroke aphasia: a narrative review for stroke neurologists. Int J Stroke 2021;16:1002–8.

[23] Thompson CK, Shapiro LP. Treating agrammatic aphasia within a linguistic framework: treatment of underlying forms. Aphasiology 2005;19:1021–36.

[24] Thompson CK. Neurocognitive recovery of sentence processing in aphasia. J Speech Lang Hear Res 2019;62:3947–72.

[25] Middleton EL, Schwartz MF. Errorless learning in cognitive rehabilitation: a critical review. Neuropsychol Rehabil 2012;22:138–68.

[26] Middleton EL, Rawson KA, Verkuilen J. Retrieval practice and spacing effects in multisession treatment of naming impairment in aphasia. Cortex 2019;119:386–400.

[27] Middleton EL, Schwartz MF, Rawson KA, Garvey K. Test-enhanced learning versus errorless learning in aphasia rehabilitation: testing competing psychological principles. J Exp Psychol Learn Mem Cogn 2015;41:1253–61.

[28] Zhang J, Wei R, Chen Z, Luo B. Piracetam for aphasia in post-stroke patients: a systematic review and meta-analysis of randomized controlled trials. CNS Drugs 2016;30:575–87.

[29] Mead G, Graham C, Lundstrom E, Hankey GJ, Hackett ML, Billot L, et al. Individual patient data meta-analysis of the effects of fluoxetine on functional outcomes after acute stroke. Int J Stroke 2024;19:798–808.

CHAPTER

7

Rehabilitation of orientation disorders and memory deficits

7.1 Introduction

7.1.1 Incidence and clinical significance

The incidence of memory disorders following acquired brain injury varies widely. According to a review by Snaphaan and de Leeuw [1] the prevalence of memory impairment in the first month after stroke ranges between 13% and 50%. These rates tend to decrease over the first year, depending on the severity of the impairment. Mild to moderate memory impairments after stroke often show good recovery, whereas severe memory disorders have a poor prognosis and is more likely to lead to dementia.

In acute settings, about one-fourth of the patients suffer from *poststroke delirium*—an acute severe impairment of attention and memory—with higher prevalence in older age groups (20%, 25%, and 34% for ages 60–64, 65–74, and 75–79). The frequency of delirous states is even higher after intracerebral or subarachnoid bleeding. However, all these figures apply specifically to delirium—not to orientation disorders in the broader sense, which will be introduced below.

The clinical significance of memory disorders on everyday functioning, as diagnosed by neuropsychological tests, depends on both etiology and age. For example, in younger patients with neurological conditions such as multiple sclerosis (MS) or traumatic brain injury (TBI), memory performance on the California Verbal Learning Test (CVLT) has been shown to be a reliable predictor of their ability to return to work. This relationship remains significant even after controlling for factors such as depression, age, and other variables [2–5]. Similarly, test performance in the Rivermead Behavioral Memory Test can also predict whether a person will be able to live independently again after brain injury [6,7].

Applied Neuropsychology of Cerebrovascular Diseases
DOI: https://doi.org/10.1016/B978-0-443-45450-9.00002-3

In older individuals with suspected neurodegenerative disease, memory test performance has been linked to their ability to perform instrumental activities of daily living. Large-scale studies show that memory deficits correlate with impairments in telephone usage, mobility, and managing finances [8,9]. However, for basic everyday activities such as washing or dressing, neuropsychological examination of memory performance does not provide predictive information. Basic activities of daily living do not depend on episodic memory; they are automatized skills and therefore rather resilient to stroke and other brain injuries.

7.1.2 Treatments of memory disorders should distinguish between severity and stage of recovery

Several extended reviews exist on neuropsychological assessments of memory disorders, as well as some on their treatment [10–13]. This chapter therefore will focus on rehabilitation strategies.

Most of the existing reviews and guidelines on memory rehabilitation do not distinguish between patients based on etiology, severity, and different phases of recovery [10,11]. Most studies have focused on patients with TBI or MS, or have included mixed etiological groups, making it impossible to analyze the effect of interventions exclusively on stroke. TBI and MS lesions are typically associated with multifocal pathology, whereas stroke more often produces focal lesions. However, animal studies suggest that the effectiveness of treatment may depend on the involvement of focal memory structures, on the associated severity, and when the intervention starts (Chapter 3). Unfortunately, there are no comparative studies distinguishing between these aspects in human patients.

As a first step, this chapter follows the German guideline for memory rehabilitation, distinguishing between individuals with severe amnesia and those with mild or moderate memory impairment (see Fig. 7.1) [14]. This guideline argues that compensation for memory impairment should be promoted through adaptation of the environment, including assistive technologies, especially when memory impairments significantly interfere with daily life. For patients with severe memory impairment, where little to no information is retained after delay, the guideline recommends the use of implicit learning techniques to facilitate rehabilitation, and for less impaired patients, the training of internal strategies [14].

However, these recommendations ignore the relation between the stage of recovery (acute, postacute, and chronic) and the severity of memory impairment. For example, severe memory impairment can occur even without structural brain damage. The same severity of memory impairment may have very different implications depending on the

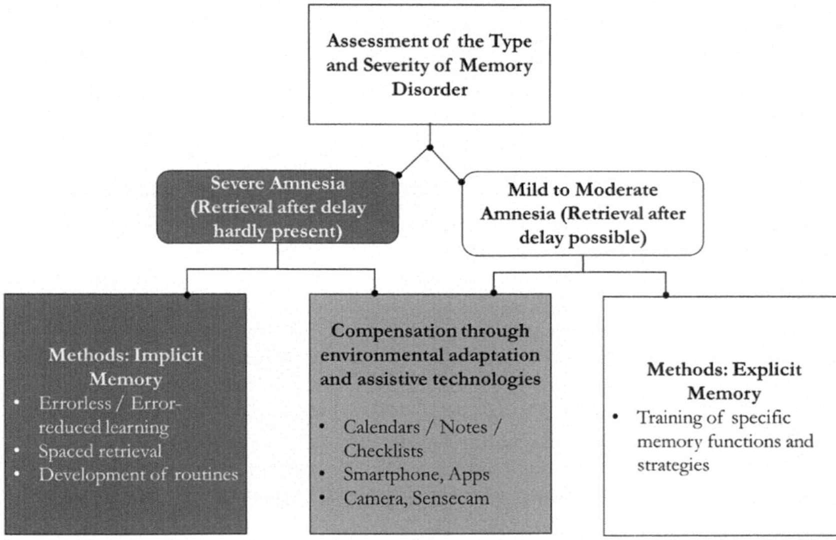

FIGURE 7.1 German guideline for memory rehabilitation. *Customized from "Summary of the S2e guideline ""Diagnosis and therapy of memory disorders in neurological diseases (AWMF-030/124)" by Thöne-Otto et al. (2020).* Journal of Neuropsychology, *31(3), 107–128 https://doi.org/10.1024/1016-264X/a000298 © 2020 Hogrefe.*

timing and course of the condition. For example, acute memory impairments may occur after anesthesia, where patients experience a delirium-like state with profound memory deficits lasting several days or even weeks. Similarly, postacute cerebral edema following a large stroke can lead to a severe but only temporary decline in memory performance. In such cases, it is often too early to determine the long-term prognosis. Therapeutic goals for these patients should therefore differ from those for individuals with enduring memory disorders.

In contrast, *chronic* severe memory impairment presents a different set of challenges. Patients typically return to a stable environment with repetitive daily demands. Chronic patients often have gained insight into the consequences of cognitive deficits on their daily lives. For such patients, a key question is whether rehabilitation should focus on acquiring specific essential information or whether the primary goal should be to reduce more global, limitations affecting personal identity and autonomy.

Therefore, the recommended interventions must be further refined based on both the stage of recovery and the specific therapeutic goals. Table 7.1 outlines this distinction for severe memory disorders. Table 7.5, introduced later in this chapter, offers similar information for the treatment of patients with mild to moderate memory impairments, and

TABLE 7.1 Interventions for *severe* memory disorders depend on the recovery stage.

Stage	Goals	Specific contents and interventional approaches
Early postacute	Reducing orientation disorder and managing affective stress.	Reestablishing wake–sleep pattern. Supportive interactions and providing relevant information.
Postacute	Focus on external memory aids if the prognosis argues for enduring severe deficits. Source memory training for the treatment of confabulation.	Spaced retrieval of orientation-relevant information. Errorless learning depends on whether the error stems from impaired memory consolidation or a storage-related deficit.
Chronic state	Establishment of external memory aids: depending on the additional cognitive disorders, as an exercise in external memory aids, or the use of a memory aid for a specific purpose.	Self-preservation therapy (external memory aid for maintaining a certain self-identity).

Fig. 7.13 at the end of the chapter provides a conceptual overview of different treatment strategies for mild to moderate memory disorders. It should be noted, however, that many of the recommendations presented in this chapter are derived from clinical experience and theoretical models of memory, as randomized controlled trials directly comparing interventions across levels of severity and stages of recovery are lacking.

We will start with acute memory disorders, then discuss interventions for chronic memory disorders, and finally for patients with mild to moderate impairments [12,15].

7.2 Orientation disorders during the early postacute stage

7.2.1 The difference between orientation disorders and delirium

In this section, the term "orientation disorder" will refer to cognitive and affective disturbances affecting a person's ability to recognize their location, time, situation, and/or personal identity. The term denotes a temporary cognitive, affective, or behavioral impairment that cannot be fully explained by the brain lesion (in this case, the correct term would be organic memory disorder or dementia). Orientation disorders may have a somatic background (e.g., an acute response of the brain to anesthesia).

It may also arise from the individual's adaptation to a new situation, such as hospitalization. For instance, if preexisting amnesia is present, it may prevent patients from remembering why they are in the hospital, leading to repeated confusion over weeks. In this respect, orientation disorders encompass a broad range of behavioral symptoms that reflect disrupted interactions between the patient and the environment.

According to this definition, a delirium, a term which is often used in clinical routine practice for the classification of such behavior or state, is a subcategory of orientation disorders. The two conditions differ in three key ways: (1) the term delirium focuses on acute, reversible metabolic or immunologically triggered orientation disorders. The term orientation disorder, on the other hand, applies to patients with structural brain injury confirmed by neuroimaging. The differential diagnostic question of whether a structural (or neurodegenerative) disease is also present, as it plays a central role in delirium diagnosis, is therefore irrelevant. The main question is whether the existing lesion accounts for the observed symptomatology. (2) Both concern amnesia and circadian disorder, but orientation disorders have a focus on acute anterograde and retrograde amnesia and primarily affective states (complete loss of locus of control, severe apathy, and stupor) (see Table 7.2). The term delirium focuses primarily on attention (see Table 7.2, columns 3 and 5), and even if the distinction between hyperactive and hypoactive delirious states is common, the assessment is based mainly on attention disturbance [18–26]. (3) The term delirium is a purely behavioral description of the patient's state, whereas the term orientation disorder allows for causative interpretations (see below).

Orientation disorders pose a significant challenge in neurological rehabilitation, as they lead to self-endangering or socially disruptive behavior, influencing the practical organization of rehabilitation and its outcome. Orientation disorders with a focus on cognitive functions, including classic hyperactive delirium (see Table 7.2), require constant monitoring due to an increased risk of wandering, falls, or self-harm (for instance, active and passive risk of leaving the rehabilitation unit and getting lost). Additionally, disruptive behaviors, such as shouting or interacting inappropriately with other patients, may pose challenges for both caregivers and fellow patients. Orientation disorders may also interfere with the spontaneous remission and the rehabilitation process, as these patients may fail to engage in treatment through a lack of drive or active counteraction (see Table 7.2, right half). This is problematic because the first few months of recovery are critical for therapeutic success. In this respect, the diagnosis of orientation disorders should always prompt the rapid implementation of an appropriate treatment strategy (see below).

TABLE 7.2 Taxonomy of orientation disorders.

Neuropsychological cause, primary presentation, and therapy complication							
Cognition				**Emotion**			
Memory		**Attention/perception**		**Hyperactivity**		**Hypoactivity**	
Place, time	Situation	Daytime	Environment	Person	Self	Person	Self
	Confusion	(Fluctuating) twilight states	Perceptual disorder	Delirious	internally agitated	Pseudo-neurasthenic	
Amnesia	Confabulation	Sleep/wake rhythm	Hallucinations	Anxiety/inner restlessness	Self-reproach, guilt	Apathy	Stupor
Passive risk of running away	Active risk of running away	Restless on the ward or somnolence	Frequent calls for nursing staff	Perseveration, motor restlessness	Reactive turning away, active refusal of therapy	Lack of exercise, akinesia, passive refusal of therapy	Motion rigidity
Common etiology							
Herpes encephalitis, hypoxia, TBI, posterior stroke	Acoa aneurysm, RH media stroke	For example, TBI, nontraumatic subarachnoid haemorrhage (SAH), large ICB, *for other causes, see the LL delirium* [16]	For example, cortical Lewy bodies	For example, TBI, hypoxia, media stroke, *for other causes, see the LL delirium* [16]	For example, LH media stroke	For example, SAH media on the right, *for other causes, see the LL delirium* [16]	For example, ICB with ventricular rupture

TABLE 7.2 (Continued)

Neuropsychological cause, primary presentation, and therapy complication							
Cognition				**Emotion**			
Memory		**Attention/perception**		**Hyperactivity**		**Hypoactivity**	
Possible biological and psychological causes							
Limbic system disorder	Disruption of the right ventrolateral cortex or medial orbitofrontal cortex	Circadian hypothalamic pattern generators, melatonin, cortisol, orexin, histamine dysregu-lation?	Sensory disorders, neuronal deafferentation of secondary somatosensory cortices	Autonomous-vegetative, noradre-nergic-dopaminergic hyper-function?	Overactivation of the basal ganglia? Serotonergic deficit?	Basal ganglia, dorsomedial-frontal cortex-dopaminergic deficiency?	Amygdala, ventral caudatum? GABAergic hyper-function?
Anxiety	Self-protection against loss of importance?	Helplessness syndrome? Experiencing loss of control?	Deprivation?	Deprivation, experiencing loss of control	Helplessness syndrome?	Loss of affective attribution?	Helplessness syndrome? State of shock

Abbreviations: TBI = traumatic brain injury, SAH = subarachnoid hemorrhage, ICB = intracerebral hemorrhage, LH = left-brain, RH = right-brain, LL = guideline. The existence of "?" indicates that the evidence for the assumption is highly speculative.

Based on Schenke N., Korabova S.D., Thomas, Hildebrandt H. Orientierungsstörungen in der neurologischen rehabilitation. In: Mokrusch T., Gorsler A., Dohle C., Liepert J., Rollnik (Hg.) J., editors. Curriculum Neurorehabilitation der Deutschen Gesellschaft für Neurorehabilitation e.V. (DGNR). 2023. pp. 289–304.

Table 7.2 offers an overview of different aspects of orientation disorders (as defined here) according to disorders of place, time, situation, and person, including their interaction with the environment. It allows a relatively accurate representation of aspects that are discussed for the description of delirium (see Table 7.2, lines one to six). The advantage of Table 7.2 is that the introduced aspects are clinically important in their treatment, as rehabilitation strategies differ depending on whether a patient's disorientation is primarily cognitive, affective, or behavioral.

Orientation disorders are often accompanied by strong emotional responses. Severe amnesia may trigger increased anxiety as the patients repeatedly forget their present circumstances. The risk of escaping rehabilitation is particularly high if the affected person has a strongly self-determined job and becomes restless to continue previous activities. An affective reaction is also assumed for the content of confabulations, as they often focus on the social significance of the patient and thus help to compensate for the enforced insignificance and the experienced loss of control in the rehabilitation facility [27–30].

Various studies have shown that psychological aspects are important for the severity of orientation disorders [18,31]. Severe pain perception impairs orientation, affects cognitive disorganization, and should be treated pharmacologically [32]. Increased anxiety and autonomic vegetative hyperarousal are associated with fluctuating circadian states and hyperactive delirium. The investigation of Sandberg, Gustafson, Brannstrom, and Bucht [20] compared the incidence of mood disorders in the elderly in different treatment facilities between delirious and nondelirious individuals (see Table 7.3). It showed a high prevalence of affective dysregulation in orientation disorders, a finding that, unfortunately, has received limited attention in assessment and treatment approaches.

The definition of delirium does not primarily contain any affective criteria, because it is meant as a purely behavioral description [16,25], and therefore nonobservable affective states causing that behavior are beyond the scope of the assessment. The distinction between hyperactive and hypoactive delirium corresponds most closely to a consideration of affective aspects (see the columns of Table 7.2 on the right), but the terminology still focuses only on observable behavior. This is a sound conceptual basis for classifying patients and, in many cases, an explanatory attempt may not be needed, because of a quick and complete recovery from delirious symptoms. However, in patients with enduring brain lesions, which seemingly do not explain the severity of the affective and cognitive symptoms, a more neuropsychological, explanatory approach seems to be reasonable and is helpful to structure the interventions.

TABLE 7.3 Affective disorders in comparable elderly patients with and without delirium.

Affective disorder like	Nondelirious patients (%)	Delirious patients (%)
Depression	31,8	52,4
Affect lability	23,6	31,4
Fear	44	59,7
Unrest and agitation	14,9	32,1
Irritability	31,7	50,2
Aggressiveness	7,5	18,5
Euphoria	6,7	14,0
Delusions	7,2	20,4
Hallucinations	3,7	21,9
Delayed replying	18,7	40,0
Psychomotor slowing	34,2	59,7
Persecution complex	16,4	29,2

From Sandberg O., Gustafson Y., Brannstrom B., Bucht G. Clinical profile of delirium in older patients. J Am Geriatr Soc 1999;47:1300–1306.

Affective aspects of orientation disorder can be additional signs of organic noxious agents (such as attention and memory disorder), and they can also have a reinforcing effect on them. The latter consideration is supported by the increased risk of suffering delirium if there are preexisting mental illnesses. Older studies have also documented a relation between hyperactive delirium and personality variants of the patients, but this has not been investigated in further studies to our knowledge [33]. Increased anxiety before surgery appears to increase the risk of delirium, although not always replicated [32,34]. A preexisting depression represents an additional increase in risk factor for delirium [35,36]. More specifically, Stransky, Schmidt, Ganslmeier, Grossmann, Haneya, Moritz, Raffer, Schmid, Graf, and Trabold [37] showed that a history of depression is a risk factor for the development of hypoactive delirium.

Orientation disorders are associated with a profound loss of perceived control, and it is known from animal research that such states of experienced helplessness [38] can result in an apathetic behavioral pattern that shares features with stupor (Chapter 9), which also lasts longer than the circumstances that lead to helplessness [39]. Neurological rehabilitation patients often experience long periods of sensory deprivation or uncontrollable stimulation in the intensive care unit. Deprivation and overstimulation can both be experienced as helplessness and can also lead to hallucinations, although studies to prove such an effect have not really been successful [18,31,40]. However, reduced sensory stimulus absorption, such as untreated visual impairment and hypoacusis, increases the risk of developing delirium in the intensive care unit, as documented by the studies of Ferrante, Pisani, Murphy, Gahbauer, Leo-Summers, and Gill [41], and Inouye, Viscoli, Horwitz, Hurst, and Tinetti [42].

7.2.2 Treatment of orientation disorders in the early postacute stage

Table 7.4 provides an overview of the proposed interventions for disorientation disorders and will be used to structure the following section [17].

7.2.2.1 Orientation training

Surprisingly, few studies have systematically evaluated orientation training in the postacute phase [43]. De Guise, Leblanc, Feyz, Thomas, and Gosselin [44] investigated in a two-center study the effect of orientation training on the duration of posttraumatic amnesia, which is known to be a major predictor of the consequences of TBI. The methodological problems, such as age differences between groups and lack of randomization, limit conclusions. Although orientation training resulted in a 4.5-day reduction in the duration of posttraumatic amnesia, the result was not statistically significant due to the high variance.

Langhorn, Holdgaard, Worning, Sorensen, and Pedersen [45] investigated the effect of orientation training on the extended Glasgow outcome scale and compared patients at 12 months. This study was also not randomized, and the two groups differed significantly in the duration of posttraumatic amnesia. The difference in the extended Glasgow outcome scale was not significant; however, in absolute values, the values of the treated group were in a better range than those of the untreated group, although the former had a significantly longer period of posttraumatic amnesia.

Hshieh, Yue, Oh, Puelle, Dowal, Travison, and Inouye [46] reviewed the effectiveness of multidimensional interventions in delirium of nonspecific cause on fall frequency. The orientation training was only one measure among several, such as physiotherapy, which corresponds to treatment as usual in early rehabilitation facilities. Four randomized trials were included in the review analysis. Across four randomized trials, orientation and physiotherapy together significantly reduced fall risk, with an average odds ratio of 0.38.

Table 7.4 argues that different approaches of treatment are indicated, depending on severity and the leading impairment. For disorientation

TABLE 7.4 Functional treatment of orientation disorder symptoms

Functional treatment of orientation disorders							
Cognition				**Emotion**			
Memory		**Perception and attention**		**Hyperactive**		**Hypoactive**	
Design of the hospital ward, external memory aids, orientation training	Source memory training, cerebrospinal fluid (CSF) relief puncture, or shunt implantation?	Sleep hygiene, physical strain, daylight lighting	Sensory training, passive relaxation	Passive relaxation, music therapy, physical exertion, calming conversations	Positive biographical cues, conversations, music therapy, aromatherapy	Passively guided forced use, gait trainer, positive reinforcement	Passive relaxati-on

Based on Schenke N., Korabova S.D., Thomas, Hildebrandt H. Orientierungsstörungen in der neurologischen rehabilitation. In: Mokrusch T., Gorsler A., Dohle C., Liepert J., Rollnik (Hg.) J., editors. Curriculum Neurorehabilitation der Deutschen Gesellschaft für Neurorehabilitation e.V. (DGNR). 2023. pp. 289–304.

disorder in the narrow sense, these can be differentiated as external orientation aids and face-to-face therapy.

External orientation aids: An essential component of the treatment of orientation disorders is the appropriate design of the (hospital ward) environment. Clear signage and a consistent color scheme help with spatial orientation at both room and ward levels. A large wall clock and a wall calendar are essential basic components of temporal orientation. Information such as the reason for hospitalization, current location, and duration of stay should be clearly visible. Additional person-oriented aids include, for example, family photos, photo albums, or the drawing of a family tree. This material should be integrated into daily therapy routines, with all therapeutic and nursing staff referencing it regularly.

Alongside passive cues, patients benefit from actively used external aids, such as a memory book. A basic version includes a paper calendar in which appointments (e.g., treatment sessions), necessary errands, and events that have taken place (e.g., time, duration, and content of the therapies) are recorded daily. The key to effectiveness lies in consistent integration into the patient's daily routine, reinforced by repeated reminders from staff.

Face-to-face therapy: Orientation disorders should also be treated therapeutically. For this purpose, information about the person, the date, the location, and the current situation is written on a piece of paper, preferably by the patients themselves. This is followed by an immediate free recall, which can be supported by cueing if necessary. If information is not retained, it is reviewed and tested again after a distraction task. After an interference phase, in which another, preferably nonlinguistic task is processed, a delayed retrieval of the information follows, in which cueing can be used again. If all information has been named correctly, a new, longer interference phase can take place with subsequent delayed retrieval to support consolidation.

For spatial training, backward chaining combined with the method of vanishing cues (for an explanation, see below) can be used. For instance, a patient learning the route from the therapy room to their own room begins near the destination. Once this segment is mastered, the start point is extended. Prominent visual cues (e.g., pictures on the wall) on the route can help to make it easier to find the correct route.

7.2.3 Treatment of confabulations and hallucinations

Severe memory disorders can be accompanied by confabulations and then pose a special challenge to neurological rehabilitation. Confabulations are statements about the current situation or past events that are demonstrably false but are experienced by the patient as subjectively convincing (compare Chapter 1 for a cognitive explanation of confabulations) [12]. They can appear provoked as erroneous answers to questions or spontaneous, without a clear reason for the situation. Spontaneous confabulation patients are therefore at increased risk of leaving the rehabilitation setting unsupervised and becoming lost and often have to be accommodated in closed facilities. Confabulations meet many conditions of delirium and often occur during hyperactive delirium. Even outside of hyperactive delirium, they are usually of a temporary nature (rarely last longer than 3 months) and fluctuate depending on the situation [47]. Confabulations can be the result of cerebrospinal fluid build-up, for example, after a traumatic or nontraumatic subarachnoid hemorrhage, so that appropriate imaging should be carried out if the onset of confabulation tendency is delayed [47,48].

To date, very few studies have examined on the functional treatment of confabulations, with the exception of Trivino, Rodenas, Lupianez, and Arnedo [49], who developed a neuropsychological treatment program for patients with nondelirious confabulations. The theoretical background for this program was the assumption that these patients have a severe form of "source amnesia," that is, they cannot retain the context of the information; consequently, correct knowledge is activated at the wrong time and is wrongly assumed to be relevant and correct. For the treatment of patients, a system of documentation was developed to make sure what information comes from whom and when (from therapists or patients, from just now or from the past). When checking the memory performance with the patient, so-called source errors (assignment of the information to a wrong source or a wrong person) were then confronted with the contents of the documentation system. The documentation system ensured that patients increasingly perceived the erroneous nature of their memory and better controlled memory occurrences with regard to their plausibility. After 3 weeks of training (a total of 9 hours of therapy time), there was a significant reduction in the number of memory errors in the treated patients, while there was practically no change in the untreated patients. So, the training was highly effective. Critically, it should be noted that the control group consisted of a passive waiting group, and there is still no replication of this clinically highly relevant study by another group.

The study of Trivino, Rodenas, Lupianez, and Arnedo [49] used the documentation system to avoid conflicts with the patients on the question, if their memories are correct or incorrect. This is only possible in a specific therapeutic situation. A positive therapeutic alliance is necessary for proper treatment, so that the relationship of trust can be used to confront the false assumptions of the confabulations with the real state of affairs [47]. Ideally, this would require the involvement of people who are familiar with the patient. In addition, keeping a diary together can be used to regain an anchoring in reality when confabulations occur, without a direct confrontation between patient and staff. Furthermore, with initial neutrality towards the accuracy of the confabulations, a more cautious and direct confrontation with the correct point of view should take place step by step [47].

Hallucinations, such as confabulations, can be understood as disruptions in the integration of perception and memory, particularly in the context of impaired reality monitoring. The association between sensory deprivation, such as in hemianopia, and hallucinations is well documented (for instance, by the Charles Bonnet syndrome or visuoperceptive deficits in hallucinating Lewy body dementia). Based on this, one may assume that any intervention reducing sensory deprivation (as developed in Chapter 9) and increasing perceptual discrimination performance should reduce hallucinations. However, to our knowledge, no treatment study has specifically examined interventions aimed at reducing visual misperception or hallucination.

7.2.4 Treatment of circadian dysregulation

Disturbances of the sleep–wake rhythm often occur in neurological patients in a subacute state (see the review by Howell and Griesbach [50]), and sleep disorders increase the risk of developing a delirium. Physical activity and disturbances of the sleep–wake rhythm are closely associated. In patients with hyperactive delirium, there is increased and more irregular physical activity throughout the day, as shown by Davoudi, Manini, Bihorac, and Rashidi [51] in a review on the use of accelerometers in delirious patients.

Structuring the daily routine: Functional measures to regain a normal sleep–wake cycle include a number of dietary adjustments (limiting caffeine intake, especially in the late afternoon), restriction of sensory stimulation at night (sufficient darkening of the room or alternatively the use of a sleep mask), and maintaining a consistent daily routine such as fixed dinner and bedtime schedules. It is important to note that while darkening the room helps sleep, darkening the room may increase the risk of falls. In order to understand the premorbid sleep–wake rhythm, sleep times and quality should be recorded and documented in order to take them into account when planning sleep times (see the review [52]).

Patients may have insufficient exposure to natural daylight due to the long length of stay in the hospital. As a result, a melatonin deficit can occur. The length of daylight exposure is a significant factor in the risk of developing delirium [53]. The melatonin concentration throughout the day plays an essential role in the amount and quality of sleep. A melatonin deficit was observed in hypoactive delirium, while a reduced concentration of melatonin in the urine was measured in hyperactive delirium [21]. A simple method for the treatment of sleep–wake arrhythmias would therefore be to implement lighting in patient rooms similar to the natural light spectrum. However, in two recent studies on patients with TBI [54] or stroke [55], no significant effect on the sleep–wake rhythm was found. The study situation on the prevention of delirium through appropriate lighting is also contradictory [56].

Face-to-face therapy: The lack of clarity about the further course of the disease is a stress factor for healthy sleep. Appropriate information and prognosis of the disease are therefore an essential part of sleep hygiene. Therapeutically, bedtime and bedtime rituals, as well as the use of relaxation techniques, continue to form the contents of psychological therapy for sleep disorders.

In a study by Zhang, Su, Wang, Tang, Hu, Mao, Ren, Liu, and Yu [57] the effectiveness of zopiclone versus zopiclone plus cognitive behavioral therapy for sleep disorders after intensive care was compared. Functional treatment included psychoeducation, sleep hygiene, time restriction in bed, stimulus control, cognitive therapy, and relaxation techniques, all of which are elements that are easily realized in the context of neurological rehabilitation. It turned out that the combination of behavioral therapy and pharmacological treatment was superior to mere pharmacological treatment. A recent systematic review of Li, Feng, Xia, Zhou, Chen, Chen, Fan, Wang, Ding, and Du [58] documents positive effects of cognitive behavioral therapy on the sleep quality of patients with TBI. The systematic review of Pilon, Frankenmolen, and Bertens [59] concludes that cognitive behavioral therapy is the method of choice for the treatment of sleep disorders following acquired brain damage. However, the vast majority of studies were based on self-assessments in their outcome measurement. It is therefore unclear whether the objectively measurable amount and rhythm of sleep can also be influenced by face-to-face therapy.

7.2.5 Treatment of disorders related to the self

Chapter 9 provides how to treat affective disorders of consciousness, such as apathy and stupor.

7.2.6 Pharmacological treatment

Acute hyperactive delirium is often treated with neuroleptics or adrenoceptor agonists (e.g., clonidine). A recent study with over 1600 patients by Smit, Dijkstra-Kersten, Zaal, van der Jagt, and Slooter [60] shows that the administration of both drugs did not reduce delirium duration and was associated with poorer clinical outcome. The negative effect was mainly related to haloperidol and depended on the duration of administration. Short-term applications seem not to harm the rehabilitation process. Although the study did not include explicitly and exclusively neurologically affected people, it provides a valuable indication that, in early neurological rehabilitation, neuroleptics or adrenoceptor agonists should only be used to manage motor restlessness when absolutely necessary—for example, when nursing care is heavily strained—and only for brief periods.

Based on the assumption that *confabulations* are related to a lack of cholinergic modulation of memory-relevant brain structures, a treatment with an acetylcholinesterase inhibitor would be obvious [61], but there is no scientific evidence for an effect on the confabulation tendency [62].

The guideline from the German Neurological Society (DGN) recommends melatonin, mirtazapine, long-acting low-potency neuroleptics, but no benzodiazepines and no Z-substances for treating delirium-related *sleep disorders* [16]. Several recent reviews come to the conclusion that the effectiveness of melatonin for the prophylaxis and treatment of delirium still has to be shown in large studies, but can at least be assumed to be likely [55,63–65]. Melatonin is also recommended, especially for patients with disturbances of the sleep–wake rhythm after TBI [63,65]. On the other hand, there is some evidence that Z-substances should be avoided in the case of sleep–wake rhythm disorders because of the significant side effects [66]. In general, neuroleptic medication has a negative effect on learning performance and neuroplasticity after acute brain lesions (Goldstein, 2003), so that they should be avoided as part of neurological rehabilitation if possible.

7.3 Treatment of patients with enduring severe amnesia

The treatment of patients with enduring or chronic severe amnesia is based on two different interventions—the use of external memory aids and the principles of errorless or implicit learning. We will start with the use of external memory aids.

7.3.1 External memory aids

The introduction and use of external aids is an essential aspect of neuropsychological memory rehabilitation that should be used for both moderate and severe memory disorders. Memory aids can be divided into two different groups: those that are actively or passively used by the patients.

For those affected with moderate memory impairment, actively and independently guided memory aids should be considered [12,15]. These aim to compensate for memory as such (i.e., absorption, consolidation, and retrieval of information). In the case of patients with severe and enduring amnesia, the patient's condition and biography play a role in deciding which memory aid should be introduced. In the case of an amnestic syndrome, where there is hardly any retrieval capacity, an actively guided memory aid should only be introduced therapeutically if two conditions are fulfilled: (1) the patient should be purely amnestic and not suffer from additional severe cognitive disorders (concerning attention, executive functions, etc.), and (2) the patient should be used to working with calendars. If such aids have not played a role in life so far, it is unlikely that they will be used even after effective training [12].

The patient's biography also plays an essential role in the therapy decision, which memory aid should be introduced: if the use of electronic devices such as smartphones and tablets is known and the calendar function was already used accordingly before the event, then such devices should be used due to their easy accessibility and the many additional functions. If these devices were used rather rarely or not at all before, then it should be weighed up how much additional learning effort will have to be spent in order to be able to handle them safely, and, if necessary, low-tech variants (notes and diary) should be chosen.

If the patient has not relied on memory aids before and/or suffers from additional cognitive disorders, it is better to think of a caregiver-managed memory aid, that is, one that is filled with content by other people. Such memory aids are used and controlled by caregivers, not by the patients. Used as "reminders," they cue the patients to take one action or, at most, a very small number of actions per day (e.g., taking medication). Still giving the patients at least some additional independence, effective use of reminders is important for the self-maintenance of patients and allows relatives to spend longer time periods outside the house (go to work). There are several well-validated studies that passive reminder systems can also be helpful for severely affected individuals, as long as there are no additional severe impairments of executive functions [67–70]. If such an increase in independence is not a reasonable goal, but the maintenance of something such as a biographical identity, which has been endangered since the onset of anterograde amnesia, passively used memory aids, such as diaries or electronic documentation systems, can be considered.

7.3.2 Errorless learning in severe amnesia

In the treatment of patients with severe memory disorders, the method of implicit learning is the intervention of choice. The method of *errorless learning*, specifically the *backward chaining* with *vanishing cues*, enables therapeutic progress even in severe memory disorders [12]. The application of the combination of *backward chaining* and *vanishing cues* always starts with the final state of an action. Fig. 7.2 shows two examples using errorless learning for teaching two specific tasks: learning the name of a person and learning to find a way in a new environment. For learning the name of a person, the method starts with copying the last letter of the name. If this succeeds without directly presenting the last letter, the name is prescribed, and in the next step, the last two letters are to be completed by the patients. The therapist makes sure that the patients do not make any mistakes when inserting these letters. In this way, the writing of one's own name is systematically built up by cues until it succeeds independently again. For the second example, compare our description of how to proceed in the paragraphs on orientation disorders.

Errorless learning may be interpreted as nondeclarative, non-Papez-circuit-based procedural learning. It avoids trial-and-error-based consolidation, and proceeds only through correct answers, for example, brought about by vanishing cues. The avoidance of wrong instances makes the still very slow learning process somewhat faster.

Being essentially based on implicit memory performance, errorless learning can be considered motor learning or conditioning. On the one hand, this implies that the development of knowledge takes much longer with this form of learning and that the retrieval is context sensitive. Even slight changes in the context can lead to a significant disruption of recall (hyperspecificity of learning). On the other hand, errorless learning allows for helping severely declarative memory-impaired patients to

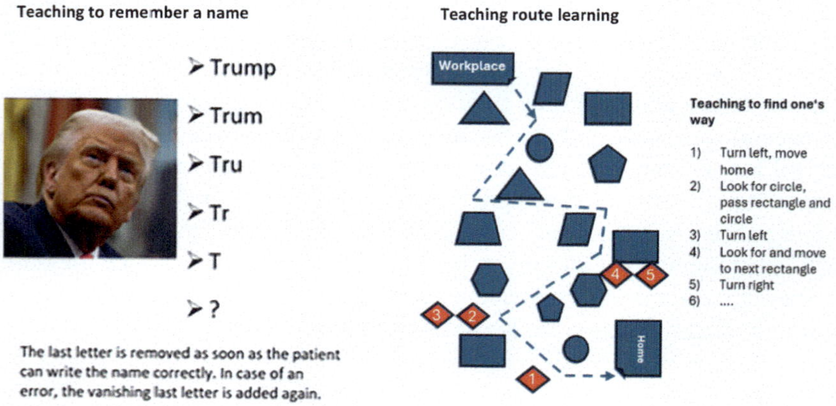

FIGURE 7.2 Errorless learning, vanishing cues, backward chaining, teaching to remember a name, and teaching to remember a path.

acquire new behavior in response to specific environmental conditions, and it is a powerful tool to help this patient group.

If the patient fulfills the essential criteria (see above), the use of an actively guided memory aid can be learned with this method, which then would enable the greatest possible independence in everyday life. Sohlberg and Mateer [71] showed in a densely amnesic patient that this is possible. Three stages in dealing with the memory book were defined for the treatment: (1) becoming familiar with the book and its functions, (2) its application during the treatment sessions, and (3) its application in situations outside the therapy session (transfer into everyday life). An example of one page of the memory book can be seen in Fig. 7.3.

In the first step, the purpose of the memory book was clarified with the patient, and its structure was explained, which took place exclusively in the context of neuropsychological therapy sessions. After the patient had gained an overview of the essential components of the memory book and its use and was able to name and classify all features with almost 100% certainty, the active use of the memory book was practiced in the second step (still only within the therapy session). With the help of role plays, the use of the memory book was practiced. The main task of the therapist was to give the patient cues as early as possible when difficulties arose, so that few mistakes were made. When the patient was able to use the memory book throughout the therapy sessions without further cues, the third step was to practice using it in everyday life. Successful action of the patient at a given stage of treatment was initially only possible with

Monday¤	Monday, 24.6.2002¤
What needs to be done today?¤	What have I done/experienced?¤
¤	Time:¤
¤	¤
¤	¤
¤	¤
Daily schedule¤	¤
Time:¤	¤
¤	¤
¤	¤
¤	¤
¤	¤
¤	¤
¤	¤
¤	¤

FIGURE 7.3 One example page for a memory book.

the maximum participation of the therapists, whose intervention was then systematically withdrawn until the next stage was reached. In fact, after about 100 treatment sessions and 1 year of therapy, also with intensive support from the family, the patient was able to live a largely independent everyday life by noting down the essential tasks of the day, ticking off their completion, and noting down and transmitting essential information that was relevant for the following days. One hundred treatment sessions may sound highly unrealistic for one patient, but adding the number of treatment sessions during early rehabilitation, additional inpatient rehabilitation after finishing early rehabilitation, and the possible number of ambulatory sessions, it should be possible to realize such a high intensity of treatment, if the decision to focus on this treatment approach is made very early.

Teaching intellectually disabled persons new skills to participate in sheltered working processes has some similarities with teaching memory-impaired patient the use of a memory book. In both instances, there is a workflow, and the patient or person should learn to follow it. We compared in an Randomized Controlled Trial with cross-over design goal management training, and app-assisted use of errorless learning to teach intellectually disabled persons new skills for their working place [72]. The difference between goal management training and errorless learning is that goal management training is based on explicit learning with (many) repetitions, whereas errorless learning is a purely implicit learning strategy. Both approaches were equally effective during the first phase of the cross-over design, whereas a passive control group did not show any improvement in learning the new task (see Fig. 7.4).

However, the efficacy differed after crossing the approaches. If goal management training was the first learning method, errorless learning was still effective, but significantly less compared to the opposite sequence with errorless learning before goal management training. On the other hand, retroactive interference on the already learnt new skill did not happen. In our view, this argues that a similar context (learning a new skill) interferes with procedural learning of another additional skill for errorless learning, but this is not the case with goal management training. One reason for this difference might be that the context sensitivity of learning in goal management training is smaller, being based also on declarative memory. However, unfortunately, there were no additional conditions using the same learning method sequentially for two different action skills. Without the results for such a condition, the effect of previous attempts of errorless learning on learning new and additional skills remains unclear.

The common background of the two mentioned studies is that the loss of episodic memory can be compensated for by procedural learning. In

The GAS (goal attainment scale)
is ranging from +2 to −2,

"much better than expected" (+2),
"better than expected" (+1),
"expected (0),
"less than expected" (−1),
"much less than expected" (−2).

Errorless learning might suffer from proactive interference if used as second learning method (but still being effective). No retroactive interference on the already learned task!

Goal Attainment Scaling

Time	Task	Groups		
		mGMTfirst	App+EL first	Control
		M (SD)	M (SD)	M (SD)
T1				
	Task 1	-.62 (1.20)	-.93 (1.16)	-.80 (1.42)
	Task 2¤	-.94 (.99)	-1.00 (1.06)	-.67 (.97)
T2	Training:	mGMT	RehaGoal App with EL	No Training
	"practised" task	1.44 (.89)	1.40 (1.24)	-.53 (1.35)
	"non practised" task	-.60 (1.45)	-.56 (1.20)	-.53 (1.18)
T3	Training:	RehaGoal App with EL	mGMT	No Training
	"practised" task	.40 (1.35)	1.62 (.80)	-.87 (1.30)
	"previously practised" task	1.25 (1.06)	1.33 (1.11)	-.33 (.72)

*note: Raw Score

FIGURE 7.4 Effects of modified Goal management training and App use plus errorless learning on practical skill learning in intellectual disabled persons.

patients with global aphasia because of a large left acm stroke, relearning of writing one's own name is of great importance. It is a prerequisite for signing documents, and even more importantly, it is essential for communicating who you are, for example, if you are lost in a new environment and suffer from a global aphasia. Is it possible to regain this ability using errorless learning? Please note that this is not the same situation as for patients with episodic memory loss. Patients with global aphasia are not completely amnesic. Even if they show verbal memory disorder, being unable to write one's own name is due to a loss of the *storage* specialized to store verbal information; it is not due to an inability to *consolidate* information. From a theoretical perspective, it is therefore unclear whether it is possible to transfer the principles of errorless learning from a consolidation deficit to a loss of memory storage for specific information.

The following Fig. 7.5 shows the learning process in two severely aphasic patients, whereby *massed practice* is to be understood as the frequent copying of one's own name, *errorless learning* as the combination of *backward chaining* and *vanishing cues*. While frequent copying of the name, which is called in memory research, massed practice did not show any significant effect (blue lines), the method of *errorless learning* was efficient enough to retrain the patients to write the name independently in the course of a week (red lines). Even if we did not evaluate that in a formal clinical study, we are quite convinced that this method works in these patient groups, and we have implemented it in our routine practice.

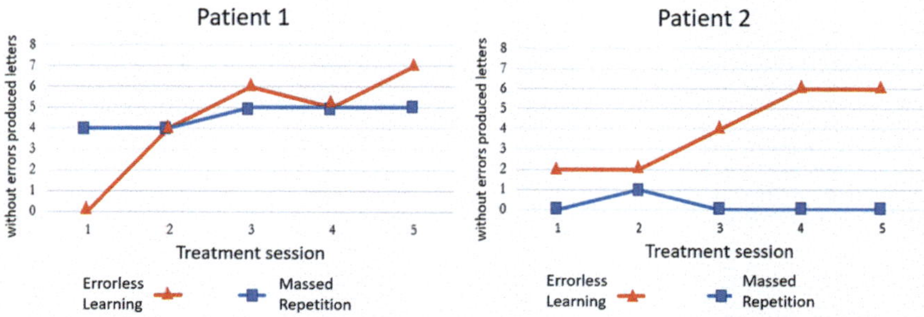

FIGURE 7.5 Effect of errorless learning versus massed practice relearning in two patients. Note: Examples of two global aphasic patients, who learnt to write their own names using the method of errorless learning, but not by massed practice. *From Turgut N., Hildebrandt H. Rehabilitation organisch bedingter gedächtnisstörungen: was, wann, für welche betroffenen?. Neurol Rehabil 2021;27:239–254.*

It is working in most of the global aphasic patients, with the prerequisite that they are able to write (not only to copy) letters, which is unfortunately not always the case.

These results argue that the method can be transferred to a wide variety of impairments and could be used in therapy for many persistent functional deficits in the rehabilitation sector. For example, patients with severe neglect or apraxia are often unable to learn to put on their T-shirt on their own. Even after weeks of usual occupational treatment, less than one-third of the patients with severe neglect show some improvement in the skill of dressing, and the percentage of patients being able to put on a T-shirt independently was very low. On the other hand, being able to dress oneself independently has a high meaning for the quality of life for the patients and their relatives. Therefore it is important to analyze whether the action steps to dress a T-shirt could be conveyed via vanishing cues and backward chaining (see Fig. 7.6). However, our pilot study in patients with severe neglect showed no added benefit from errorless learning over standard therapy [73].

The insignificant results of the study may be related to two factors: (1) the complexity of the task (17 action steps proved too long for procedural learning), and (2) limited training time (only 7 hours). A theoretical explanation may also apply: while global aphasia often results from cortical lesions, neglect can result from subcortical basal ganglia lesions. The basal ganglia lesions seem to play a major role in scheduling and learning of sequences and actions [74]. They are involved in the retrieval of genetic species-specific movement patterns (e.g., singing of birds), but also in the automatization of voluntary actions (Chapter 1). Lesions in the right hemisphere basal ganglia are associated with neglect, which may have acted as a negative selection bias for the included patients.

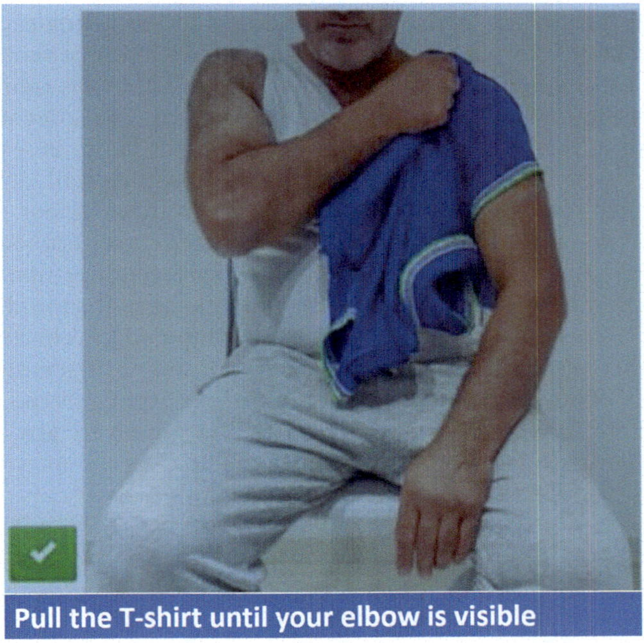

FIGURE 7.6 APP frontend view of one step treating patients with severe neglect to learn how to dress in a T-shirt. *From Ertas-Spantgar F., Muller S.V., Korabova S., Gabel A., Schiering I., Pape A.E. et al. Errorless learning and assistive technology did not improve the negative prognosis for severe dressing impairment after stroke if persisting for two weeks: a randomized controlled trial. Appl Neuropsychol Adult 2024;31:939–947.*

Unfortunately, large-scale investigations into the role of the basal ganglia in procedural learning and rehabilitation outcomes are still lacking.

7.4 A guideline for treating mildly to moderately impaired patients

Up to now, this chapter has dealt with severe memory or orientation disorders with one exception. The exception was that external memory aids should be offered and introduced in memory-impaired patients, irrespective of the severity of the impairment. In the following, the treatment of patients with mild to moderate memory impairment will be discussed. The German guideline for memory rehabilitation suggests that different interventions could be offered to these patients compared to severely affected ones [14]. We will argue that further treatment distinctions are useful within the mild to moderate patient group, which are mentioned but do not play a systematic role in the German guideline. These additional considerations concern the question if patients are in a postacute or in a rather chronic condition and whether the training aims to compensate for or restore memory performance. The latter will rarely be a useful goal in the chronic state. On the other hand, in a postacute condition, it is difficult to predict how the disorder will develop. In addition, the patient's desire for restoration may hinder an early transition to a purely compensatory therapeutic approach [75]. Table 7.5 gives an overview of the different interventions that could be used depending on the condition or therapeutic goal. It should be noted that there are no studies that systematically compared the effectiveness of different memory treatments, taking the localization of the stroke lesion, the severity of the impairment, and the status of the patients (postacute vs chronic) into account. Therefore the following sections are based on indirect comparisons and on clinical expertise.

7.4.1 Restorative, bottom-up interventions

Restoration of previous memory performance is the ultimate goal of any treatment, even when knowing that this goal is not achievable in many or most impaired patients. Restorative training is based on

TABLE 7.5 Rehabilitation of postacute and chronic moderate to mild memory disorders.

Stage	Compensatory interventions	Restorative interventions
Postacute	Mild impairment: modified story memory technique. Moderate impairment: transfer appropriate processing.	Mild impairment: combined PC training for attentional and memory functions. The repetition lag procedure is a theoretically sound method for restitutive training; however, the existing evidence is rather limited, with only training-specific improvement.
Chronic	Mild impairment: modified story memory technique. Mild to moderate impairment: transfer appropriate processing. If the major problem is remembering the text, the preview, question, read; state, test (PQRST) method should be introduced.	Mild impairment: combined PC training for attentional and memory functions.

Based on Turgut N., Hildebrandt H. Rehabilitation organisch bedingter gedächtnisstörungen: was, wann, für welche betroffenen?. Neurol Rehabil 2021;27:239–254.

intensive execution of the function that should be recovered, therefore computer training seems to be the intervention of choice. Whether PC training is effective in improving memory performance has been extensively researched in MS patients. One major advantage of neuropsychological studies on MS is that there is a common set of tests that are used, and therefore the effect of different studies can be averaged. A number of studies showed that in patients with MS, training with appropriate PC software has an effect on the measured memory performance [76]. Improvement in CVLT total number of learned words is about 3.5 words after the training, and for short-term free recall, two words. The following boundary conditions should be considered when evaluating these studies. A positive result has been achieved if the number of therapies equaled at least 20 units of 1 hour. Slightly higher training units hardly had an additional effect, but the effect is smaller if the patients practice for fewer time units. For a more recent study, Brissart, Omorou, Forthoffer, Berger, Moreau, De Seze, Morele, and Debouverie [77] investigated the effect of PC training with additional psychoeducational therapy components on language learning performance in a large study with 101 MS patients. The age of the patients was 46 years, the study was randomized and one-sided blinded, the therapy consisted of 13 therapy units with a 2 hour session each and was spread over a total period of 6 months. The control group received nonspecific stimulation with texts and conversations. The tasks used in all these studies were mixed and not exclusively related to memory performance. The verum group improved in learning performance and working memory performance, but not in other neuropsychological tests or concerning mood state. Still, the training effect could also have been achieved through an improvement in attention and not necessarily express a restitution effect of memory performance.

In the studies on memory rehabilitation of MS patients, the average age was lower than that of stroke patients. Computerized training for stroke patients also showed effects on attention and word fluency. However, the impact of computerized training on restoring memory performance was low or unclear, as two systematic reviews show [78,79].

The *repetition lag procedure* or the *recollection training* represents a genuine cognitive restitution training of memory and is most comparable to intensive treadmill training [80]. Patients are first presented with a list of words that they should remember. They are then shown a sequence of individual words, which must be answered by pressing a "yes" button if they were present in the list they learned first. However, during the recognition phase, words are also repeated that were not learned at the beginning (i.e., were not part of the first list). These words must be answered with a "no" answer, along with the words that only appear once in the recognition list. If this is achieved with 80% certainty, the distance between the words repeated only in the recognition list was increased, which means that the training automatically adapts to the achieved performance of the patients, which is a central aspect of restitutive treatments. By extending the number of words between the repetition presented twice only during the test phase, the feeling for the temporal distance ("I just saw the word") no longer helps to reject the "yes" response. Thus success becomes more and more dependent on the conscious memory of the context (this word was repeated during testing and this one stems from the study list), that is, the "*Recollection,*" while the mere feeling of familiarity is no longer sufficient for correctly answering [81]. Several studies have used the *repetition lag* method to treat people with memory deficits [80,82,83]. The study of Stamenova, Jennings, Cook, Gao, Walker, Smith, and Davidson [83] involved stroke patients, who were compared to healthy subjects. Based on task-specific improvements, which were similar for both groups, the authors argued that a partial increase in recollection is possible. They were also able to show some transfer effects on other memory tests. However, because there was no control group of stroke patients, the results of this study are somewhat unclear. In a study by our group, we were able to show that the combination of *repetition lag* and working memory training led to an improvement in an everyday memory test [84]. However, due to the mix of training task types, it remains unclear what the *repetition lag* procedure specifically contributed to the positive effect.

7.4.2 Compensatory, top-down interventions

Compensatory treatment approaches are based on the empirical fact that memory strategies can improve memory performance [85,86]. Using a cognitive strategy to compensate for a deficit is a typical aspect of a top-down approach. This holds for healthy subjects but also for patients. Wilson [87] was one of the first researcher who compared different memory strategies in healthy controls and in patients. She used the strategy of first letter cueing, the method of loci, visual imagery, and story building in both groups and compared immediate and delayed recall performance. It is important to mention that the groups did not apply these strategies by themselves; the experimental make-up guaranteed that both used the strategies in the same way. The results showed that healthy participants profited even more from delayed recall performance from the strategies compared to the patients. However, the patients profited, too, and for both groups, story building showed the largest increase in delayed recall performance.

Many of the memory-impaired patients that Wilson [87] included suffered from nontraumatic hemorrhage, which argues that these results are important for patients with cerebrovascular impairments. Based on her results, Wilson [87] concluded that, if you can teach affected patients effective strategies, this should result in an alleviation of their memory deficit.

Within this group of compensatory approaches, two variations can be distinguished. One approach is to focus on the primarily undamaged functions that are able to compensate for the damaged memory performance. An example of this would be visual imagery, which is a right-hemispheric function. In the case of left hemispheric damage, for example, by a posterior cerebral artery stroke, visuospatial memory is not affected and should take the place of verbal memory. The second approach would be to focus on cognitive processes involved in the processes of encoding, consolidation, and retrieval, and to try to optimize them. This approach integrates top-down and bottom-up aspects for treating the patients.

Kaschel, Sala, Cantagallo, Fahlböck, Laaksonen, and Kazen [88] followed the first approach and taught young TBI patients the method of visual imagery to increase memory performance. The study was an RCT and quite successful. However, it is unclear if this strategy, which presupposes high-level conscious control for executing encoding, can be transferred to older stroke patients. Berg, Koning-haanstra, and Deelman [89] used a combination of story building, deep encoding, and repetition of information to treat young TBI patients. This study was also successful; however, it is not completely clear if it was performed as an RCT, and the strategies which were trained with the patients were rather broad.

Chiaravalloti et al. [90–95] developed the *"modified Story Memory Technique"* (mSMT) with 10 therapy units of 1 hour (for a short overview of the method, compare Table 7.6). In the first four sessions, the formation of mental images is practiced in order to improve memory performance.

TABLE 7.6 The elements of the modified story memorry technique

The 10 x 1 h group sessions are divided into foir parts

- In the first four units, the methodology of visualizing content to support memory performance is practiced.
- The next four units are about the integration of information into semantic units ("story") and their visualization. Example: "dog," "hat," "bite" → "A dog wearing a hat rides a bike."
- The last two sessions practice these methods in different contexts.
- A whole series of high-profile studies have proven the effectiveness of this method in mildly affected patients.

Based on Turgut N., Hildebrandt H. Rehabilitation organisch bedingter gedächtnisstörungen: was, wann, für welche betroffenen?. Neurol Rehabil 2021;27:239–254.

In the next four sessions, more complex facts are linked to semantically connected stories, which are then to be remembered as mental images. In the last 2 hours, the transfer of these methods into everyday life has been trained. The validation of this method was carried out in patients with MS and TBI. There are several RCTs with a high number of cases [91–95]. Both for the wordlist and stories reproduction, the results consistently show improved verbal learning performance. Overall, the effect of this method was very well founded and resulted in a significant increase in verbal learning in MS patients compared to the treatment group and the control group [94]. However, some of the effects were no longer detectable after follow-up. It should also be noted that the study participants tended to suffer from very mild memory impairments. Thus the placebo control group in the study of Chiaravalloti, Moore, Nikelshpur, and DeLuca [94] in the fifth round of the CVLT retrieved more than 10 words. This would be a borderline normal performance, for example, unimpaired German secondary school students. In addition, the study participants were rather young compared to stroke patients.

If one compares the improvements in memory performance in MS patients after the modified story memory technique and after the PC training (as reviewed here [76]), the differences in effects between the two approaches are rather small. The patient using the mSMT improved with five words in total learning performance, whereas the PC training group improved by 3.5 words. When it comes to the question of which therapy should be given, other factors may play a decisive role. The mSMT is performed in groups and requires only 10 hours of therapy. The PC training requires 20 hours of individual training, but the requirement for therapeutic intervention is lower, as the exercises are carried out largely independently by the patients.

In the past, we evaluated the *transfer appropriate processing* strategy in several studies [12,96,97]. This approach is based on various results of memory research to guarantee optimal memory performance, but also integrates training aspects for semantic structuring, which means that it is a combination of top-down and bottom-up approaches. The first aspect concerns the "deep" processing of information: if it is semantically grouped and interpreted, memory performance is normally significantly higher. Corresponding results for patients suffering from memory disorders were published as early as the seventies of the last century [98]. In the meantime, the brain areas that are used for compensatory purposes have also been researched [99–101].

The second aspect concerns the influence of situational context on memory retrieval (*state-dependent memory*). The more the context of the retrieval corresponds to the conditions under which the information was stored, that is, *the encoding* and *retrieval* contexts are similar, the higher the memory performance [102]. Contextual equality can be partially influenced by maximally harmonizing the ordering criteria and the procedure for recording and retrieval. Recent research has shown that the context is an important cue for specific memory performance. Baumel and Trißl (2022) invited participants to study a wordlist. After half an hour, some of the participants recalled some words from the list, but not all. Later, the task was to remember all of the words. The result showed that remembering only aspects of the studied list generalized to all words and had a highly significant impact on total performance.

The third aspect related to results from memory research concerns the fact that the information is better retained if (1) it is actively remembered repeatedly shortly after encoding and (2) is recalled again later at significantly longer intervals (*spaced retrieval*). Schacter, Rich, and Stampp [103] in a seminal series of four patients with memory impairments showed that at least some of the patients were able to learn the strategy of space retrieval, that this was associated with a better response to memory training, and that the memory deficits should be mild to moderate for profiting from such a training. For the individual, the most effective distances of the *spaced retrieval* there seems to be implicit knowledge, which may be related to the amount of left memory performance, as the study of Schacter, Rich, and Stampp [103] showed. Another study on younger and older healthy individuals revealed that the younger ones spontaneously allowed a shorter amount of time to elapse before they remembered, while the older ones spontaneously chose a longer time interval, which was not appropriate for their objective memory performance (Maddox et al., 2011). Therefore the ability to space one's own retrieval should be part of memory rehabilitation, because it is an important and effective strategy to boost the consolidation of information. Based on these results, we developed a short list of actions to improve memory performance, which are repeatedly made known to patients (see Table 7.7).

TABLE 7.7 The three basic rules of transfer appropriate processing.

• "Organize content"
Even at home, you find things best when they have their orderly place!
• "Learning headings"
When remembering, the following applies: first the headings, then comes the corresponding information!
• "Find your own repetition frequency"
As with the Wadden Sea, every piece of information must run over the sand several times to leave traces. The necessary frequency must be learned individually.

Based on Turgut N., Hildebrandt H. Rehabilitation organisch bedingter Gedächtnisstörungen: was, wann, für welche Betroffenen?. Neurol Rehabil 2021;27:239–254.

For the first study on the effectiveness of this treatment, the inclusion criteria were at least two words of free recall after interference in the CVLT, at least seven and not more than nine words in the fifth learning trial, and to focus on moderately impaired patients [97]. Patients were recruited mainly in a postacute stage as inpatients of the local rehabilitation unit and suffered from various etiologies. They were divided into three groups: one with transfer appropriate processing, one with getting different strategies trained similar to the [89] study, and one with low-dosage treatment. For the transfer of appropriate processing treatment, they had to learn either words or figures and were taught how to group them semantically. For realizing the highest similarity between encoding and retrieval, patients were immediately interrupted in their retrieval attempts during the training if they did not proceed in the same steps as for encoding.

They were then asked to first remember the heading of the groups used for semantically organizing the information, and only then the individual items, whereby they should not switch between the semantic groups unsystematically. Subsequently, semantic structuring was practiced as a basic method with different materials, and the patients noticed the advantage of dividing the information into semantic groups over unsorted memorization. The method of *spaced retrievals* was applied during training, starting with inviting the patients to use some seconds for spaced retrieval during the distraction phase. Later, they were asked to perform spaced retrieval without external cueing and to mark doing that on paper, to have a control for the behavior of the patients. They were also instructed to recall the information they had learned between two therapy sessions, that is, retrieve it directly after reaching their rooms and again the next morning before breakfast. Fig. 7.7 based on [96] shows the percentage increase in retrieval performance after therapy in (1) the verum group with a total of 20 hours *transfer appropriate processing* sessions, (2) of an active control group, which also received differentiated strategy training over 20 hours, and in (3) a "low dosage" control group that lasts only 7 hours *transfer appropriate processing* sessions (control).

It becomes clear that, in particular, free recall after distraction (SFR), which is the most ecologically important parameter, is improved by *transfer appropriate processing*. The increase is around 40% in the first study compared to the active control group with low therapy intensity, and by 21% compared to the group with different strategies training getting the same therapy intensity. It is important to mention that the people examined were predominantly stroke patients and were therefore

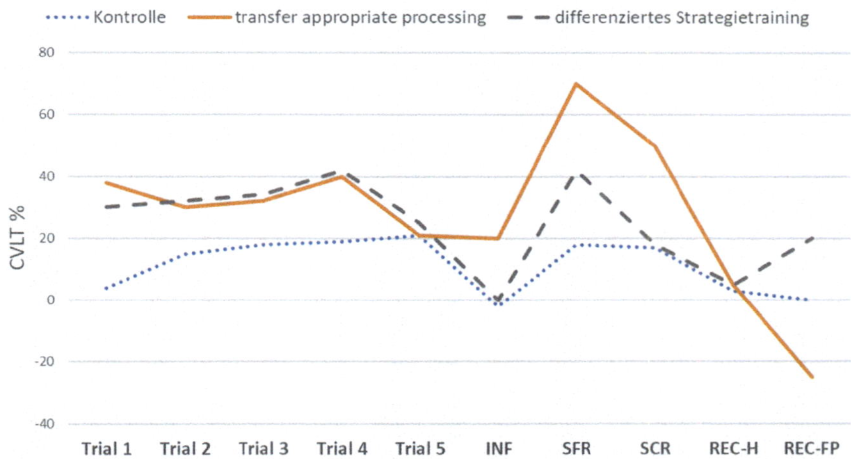

FIGURE 7.7 Improvements in multiple sclerosis patients in California verbal learning test (CVLT) learning performance after 20 sessions with the transfer approbriate processing technique. *Note: INF* interference list, *SFR* short-term free recall, *SCR* short-term cued recall, *REC-H* recognition hits, *REC-FP* recognition false positive. For REC-FEP, a negative percentage is a sign of improvement. *Adapted from "Group therapy for memory impaired patients: A partial remediation is possible." By Hildebrandt et al. (2006).* Journal of Neurology. *https://doi.org/10.1007/s00415-006-0013-6. © 2021 Springer Nature Switzerland AG.*

significantly older and more impaired than the people examined in comparable studies such as [94]. Their learning performance at the time of inclusion was about 25% lower than that of [94]. The results of the replication study [97] are displayed in Fig. 7.8. A comparison with Chiaravalloti, Moore, Nikelshpur, and DeLuca [94] suggests that the patients included in the *transfer appropriate processing* approach could have been a bit more impaired.

Further studies with only elements of the method of *transfer appropriate processing* found that the combination with working memory training and semantic structuring improved prospective memory performance compared to standard training, but not verbal memory performance, which showed a comparable increase as for the active control group with standard memory training [84,104]. Training of working memory and *repetition lag procedure* together leads to improved memory performance in everyday life and an improvement in verbal memory performance comparable to that of memory disorders, compared to standard therapy. Thus in both studies, no improvement in verbal memory performance was achieved. Consequently, the maximum equality of the procedure for

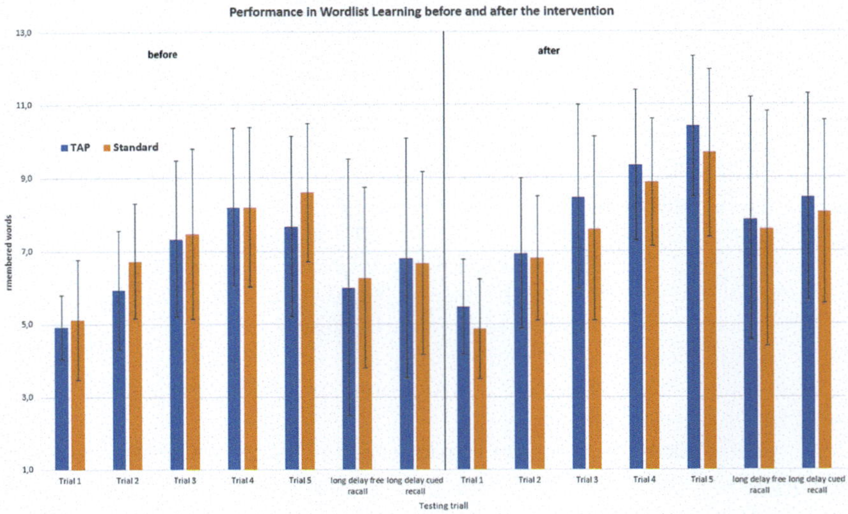

FIGURE 7.8 Improvement of memory performance for wordlist learning by the Transfer Approbriate Processing (TAP) technique in a replication study.

encoding and retrieval of verbal information, as well as the *spaced retrieval*, seems to be of central importance for the significant improvement of verbal memory performance. Training of working memory and semantic structuring or recognition may improve other forms of memory performance, but it is not sufficient to improve verbal memory performance compared to a standard treatment as practised in a neurorehabilitation clinic.

The impact of encoding and retrieval similarity and of spaced retrieval also became evident in a small cross-over study by Ciaramelli, Neri, Marini, and Braghittoni [105] using the PQRST method in memory-impaired patients mainly after rupture of an anterior communicating aneurysm. The patients encoded new texts under three different conditions: the standard condition, requiring reading texts repeatedly, the PQRST-other condition, in which the experimenter formulated questions about the text (Q phase), and the PQRST-self condition, in which patients formulated the relevant questions on their own. In the preview (P) phase, the experimenter read the passage aloud. During the question (Q) phase in the PQRST-other condition, the experimenter read the four (other-generated) questions about the text. In the PQRST-self condition, the patient formulated four questions regarding the text (self-generated questions). In both PQRST conditions, the questions were written on a card that was placed on the desk in front of the participant and remained there throughout the read phase I, in which participants read the material carefully to look for the answers to the questions. In the (S) phase, patients stated the answers, and, if necessary, read the text again. Immediately afterward, the test (T) phase began, in which the experimenter tested memory by (1) asking the same questions that had been embedded in the study phase (i.e., the other-generated questions in the PQRST-other condition, and the self-generated questions in the PQRST-self-condition), (2) asking for free recall of the passage, and (3) asking for delayed free recall of the passage, after 10 min of non-interfering activities. The two experimental conditions therefore entailed similarity of encoding and retrieval guaranteed by the questions and similar to headings on the semantically structured information in the transfer appropriate processing approach. Moreover, there was a kind spaced retrieval attempt by having the questions in front and trying to answer them twice.

The study showed that (1) the patients were able to generate the relevant questions and that they could use them effectively as retrieval cues during immediate and delayed recall (see Fig. 7.9).

Ciaramelli, Neri, Marini, and Braghittoni [105] also analyzed which patients profited most from the PQRST method (compared to the standard condition) and which of the two methods. Patients with weak memory and executive functioning benefited the most from using the PQRST method compared to the standard condition, and patients with more preserved memory and executive functioning achieved similar results in the PQRST-self condition compared to the PQRST-other condition. This argues that strategies should be easy and well-trained to be effective in moderately impaired patients, who often also suffer from additional cognitive impairments.

The *transfer of an appropriate processing* strategy can be taught in a playful way in the group and has the advantage that it is possible to join the group on an ongoing basis, so that groups can take in and discharge participants fluently, which is important for applicability in a rehabilitation clinic. However, the restriction here is that the evaluation of the method is not based on such a high number of cases as in the case of Chiaravalloti, Hillary, Ricker, Christodoulou, Kalnin, Liu, Steffener, and DeLuca [90], Chiaravalloti, Dobryakova, Wylie, and DeLuca [92], Chiaravalloti, Moore, and DeLuca [93]. In addition, it should be borne in mind that those affected by chronic disturbance of memory must be able to retain around seven words in the fifth CVLT learning round and more than two words in free recall for interference.

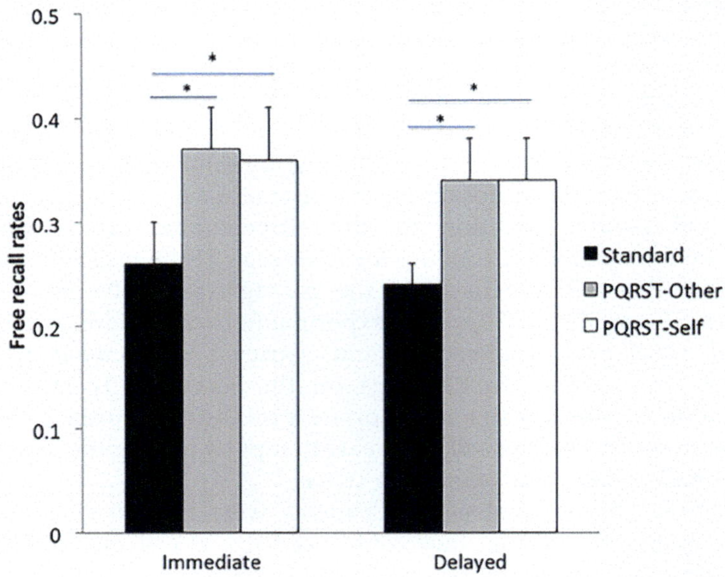

| Free recall rates by encoding condition (Standard, PQRST-Other, PQRST-Self) and test (immediate, delayed). Bars represent the SE of the mean. $^{*}p < 0.05$.

FIGURE 7.9 Effects of the two PQRST memory interventions, compared to an active control group, on immediate and delayed free recall. *From Ciaramelli E., Neri F., Marini L., Braghittoni D. Improving memory following prefrontal cortex damage with the PQRST method. Front Behav Neurosci 2015;9:211.*

7.5 Pharmacological treatment of memory deficits?

A comprehensive discussion on pharmacological treatment of memory deficits is beyond the scope of this chapter. Overall, systematic studies on the treatment of memory deficits after stroke are rare (excluding those on vascular dementia). A clear effect for stroke patients has not been proven [106,107]. The same applies to memory disorders as a result of MS [108,109]. For TBI, the Canadian cognitive rehabilitation guideline states that the acetylcholinesterase inhibitor, donepezil, may be considered for adults with TBI in the chronic stage of recovery, but that methylphenidate and amantadine should not be used to improve memory. An earlier review of Dougall, Poole, and Agrawal [110] was negative. If the field is extended to vascular dementia, some reviews report positive effects of the group of acetylcholinesterase inhibitors on memory performance [107,111] and the use of acetylcholinesterase Inhibitors is approved for vascular dementia in Germany.

7.6 Memory disorder—an effect of increased susceptibility to interference of information consolidation?

Every concrete memory achievement can be broken down into various subaspects, for example, with regard to processes involved at the same time, such as *recollection* and *familiarity*, which together affect memory accuracy. In the previous sections, we implicitly followed a division into encoding, consolidation, and retrieval. Most memory strategies focus on optimizing encoding in the belief that this will also enhance consolidation. Others are purely related to retrieval—such as the use of the SenseCam [112–114]—and a third group targets the relationship between encoding and retrieval, such as the PQRST strategy and transfer appropriate processing.

The consolidation phase, on the other hand, can only be achieved by the method of *spaced retrievals*, based on the idea that consolidation is enhanced by timed intervals of brief recollection. Interestingly, most individuals instinctively select a short delay for the first *spaced retrieval*, which tends to have the strongest effect; subsequent repetitions yield diminishing returns [115]. The choice of a short time for the first spaced retrieval argues that in the first few minutes, the traces of memory are in an unstable state and are highly vulnerable to interference.

How harmful interference immediately after the learning can be for memory performance has also been shown by the early experiments of Cermak, Butters, and Moreines [98], who demonstrated this vulnerability in studies of alcoholics and patients with Korsakoff's syndrome (for similar results [116]). In these experiments, five wordlists were to be learned: the first four with words of the same category, the fifth either with words again from this category or from a semantically different category. During the learning of different words from the same category, an initially steep, then moderate, slump in retrieval performance can be observed. If words from a different category are learned in the fifth learning round, the learning performance immediately returns to the old level of the first learning round with the first category. Interestingly, individuals with severe memory impairment—suffering from a Korsakoff's syndrome—were more susceptible to interference than the control subjects [98]. In other words, not only did they start with fewer words in the first learning round, but their learning performance also decreased even more significantly in the following learning rounds with semantically similar words. In addition, the fifth learning list had to be semantically more clearly different from the previous four lists in order to cancel out the effect of the proactive interference and to restore the original learning performance. These results suggest that people with amnesia displace recently acquired information more easily and quickly, especially when exposed to similar new content. Yet, another interpretation is that information takes a longer time to be stored permanently in memory; however, this does not explain the recovery from proactive interference during the last learning trial with semantically different information.

Dewar, Della Sala, Beschin, and Cowan [117], Dewar, Garcia, Cowan, and Della Sala [118] have investigated what happens when patients with amnesia are given a break (a wakeful rest period) before recall, in which they either have to do nothing or are involved in a relatively simple reaction task. They were able to show that even a simple new task leads to a significant deterioration in memory performance if it is to be carried out immediately after the information has been absorbed. If, on the other hand, there is no additional task for the following 9 minutes and instead the instruction to rest and think a little, then the memory performance increases significantly and reaches not normal, but only slightly impaired levels (see Figs. 7.10 and 7.11). "Protection" from interference during the first few minutes of consolidation seems to be an effective means of significantly improving retention performance.

The results of Dewar, Garcia, Cowan, and Della Sala [118] seem to argue that any distraction rules out consolidation in amnesic patients. According to their interpretation, consolidation is based on active restoration ("replay") of encoded material. If there is not enough time or resources to do so, information will be forgotten. This contradicts the

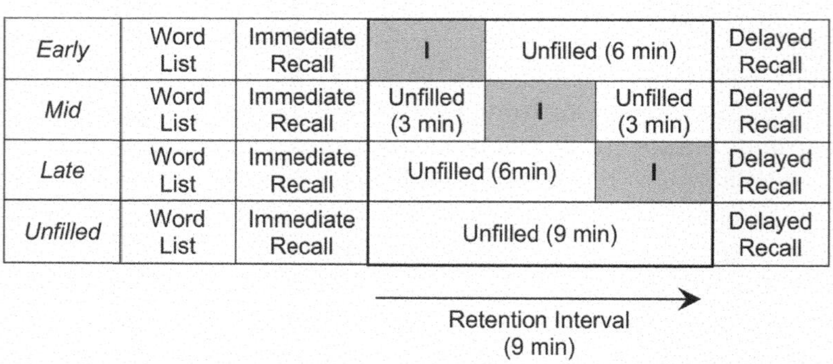

FIGURE 7.10 The four conditions to test the effect of wakeful rest on memory consolidation. *Reproduced from "Delaying interference enhances memory consolidation in amnesic patients " Von Dewar et al. (2009).* Neuropsychology, 23(5), 627–634. *https://doi.org/10.1037/a0015568 © 2009 American Psychological Association.*

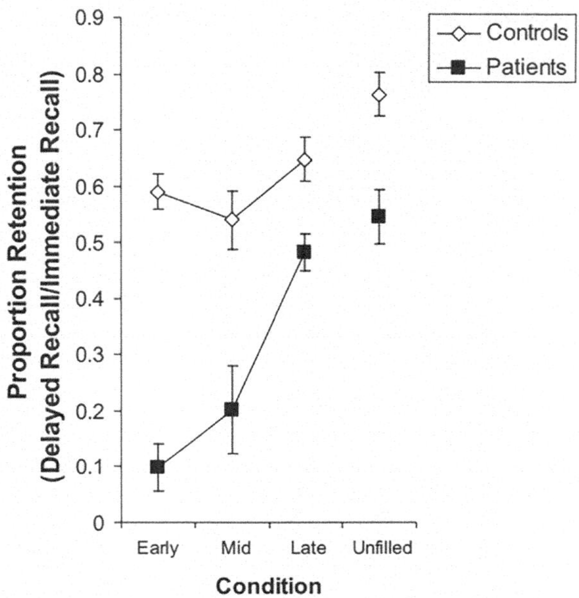

FIGURE 7.11 Effect of interference on delayed recall performance at different time-points during memory consolidation . *Reproduced from "Delaying interference enhances memory consolidation in amnesic patients " Von Dewar et al. (2009).* Neuropsychology, *23(5), 627–634. https://doi.org/10.1037/a0015568 © 2009 American Psychological Association.*

results of Cermak, Butters, and Moreines [98] and [116] on release from proactive interference. The proactive interference effect argues that interference with memory consolidation is caused mainly by the similarity of content and not just by attending to something else.

This is an important question because it also asks *how* interference and its avoidance can be better characterized in order to derive strategies for those affected by memory disorders. It is still unclear what an internal state after encoding and during the wakeful rest phase should look like to optimize consolidation and reduce interference.

Skaggs (1925), who in the first third of the last century dealt intensively with this observation in healthy people, wrote: "(...) it is extremely difficult to secure many 'ideal' rest intervals - ideal in the sense that the subject was mentally passive and indifferent and entirely away from the original learning material (...). Trained subjects are a necessity (...) As subjects become practiced, they are better able to take an indifferent and passive attitude during the rest interval" [119].

However, knowing what kind of internal state is optimal for consolidation is a necessary precondition to use "wakeful rest" for improving the performance of memory-impaired patients. And the results of these studies are highly relevant for clinical practice. On the one hand, they would mean that even people with severe memory disorder retain certain information if they can consolidate it during an unfilled wakeful rest period. This would make it possible to meet the considerable demand for therapeutic help that is implicated using *errorless learning*, which is a very time-consuming training strategy. The results based on Dewar, Della Sala, Beschin, and Cowan [117] argue that any form of interaction with the environment already has an interfering effect during consolidation. Deep non-rapid eye movement (REM) sleep, being a near-perfect interference-free state, further supports this principle [120].

In an experimental pilot study, we tested the effects of different postencoding activities to look for better control on what wakeful rest might be: a distractor task, wakeful rest, or a combination of both in varying order (see Fig. 7.12). Participants included four healthy controls and four patients with mild to moderate memory impairments following right hemisphere MCA stroke. Distractor tasks included a RehaCom attention task, repetitive finger tapping, and progressive muscle relaxation. We hypothesized that repetitive finger tapping, which does not engage the hippocampus, might disrupt consolidation less and that relaxation would promote parasympathetic activity, which enhances consolidation. Indeed, progressive muscle relaxation was the most effective intervention, and patients performed as well as healthy controls using the task during the rest phase (see Fig. 7.13). If replicated in a larger

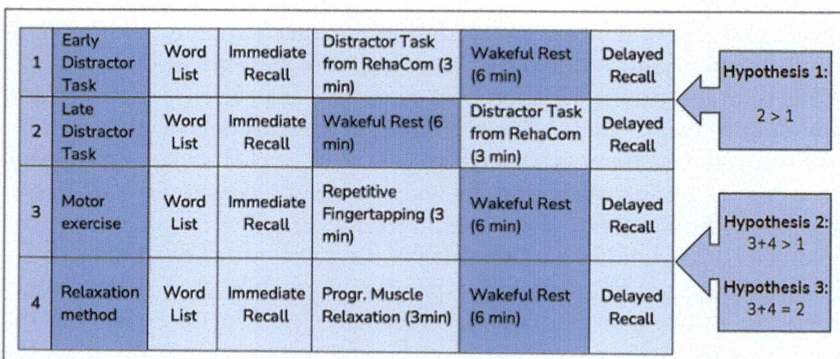

The experimental procedure and the hypotheses. Each row represents one testing session and varies slightly. In parts this design has been adapted from Dewar et al. (2009).

FIGURE 7.12 Design to test the effect of wakeful rest compared to three other conditions on memory performance in stroke patients.

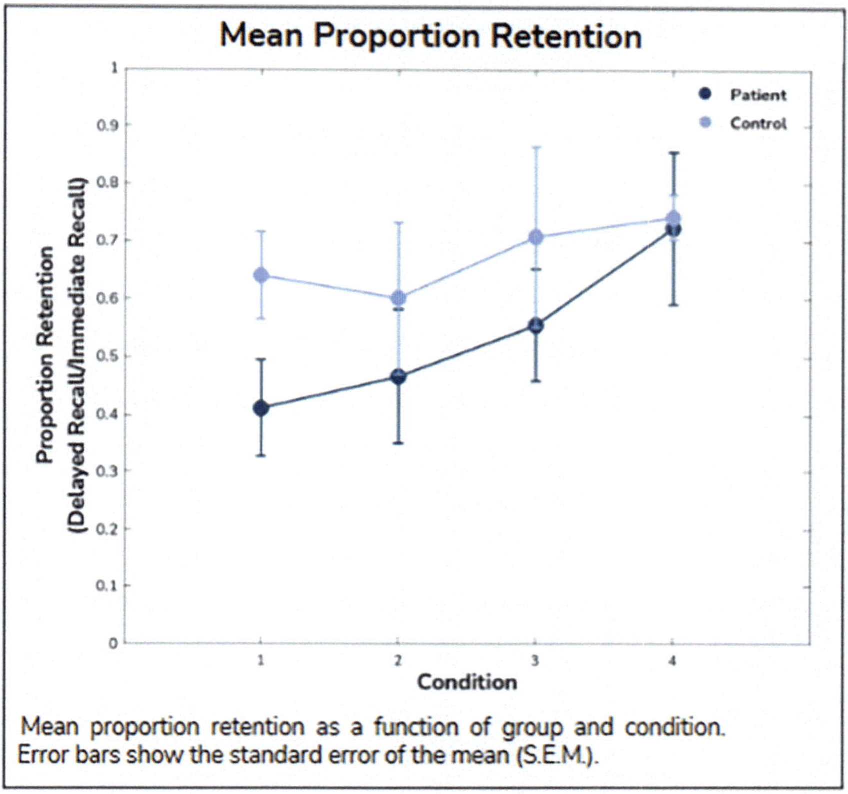

FIGURE 7.13 Results from comparing wakeful rest with three other conditions on memory performance in stroke patients.

study, this would mark a significant step toward incorporating Dewar's findings into everyday clinical practice.

7.7 How to treat mild to moderate memory disorders: a pictorial overview

Fig. 7.14 gives an extensive overview of various strategies to remediate mild to moderate memory disorders, the most important being discussed above. While comprehensive, the figure is quite complex; thus Table 7.5 offers a more confined summary focusing on the key dimensions therapeutic goal, impairment severity, and time since disease onset.

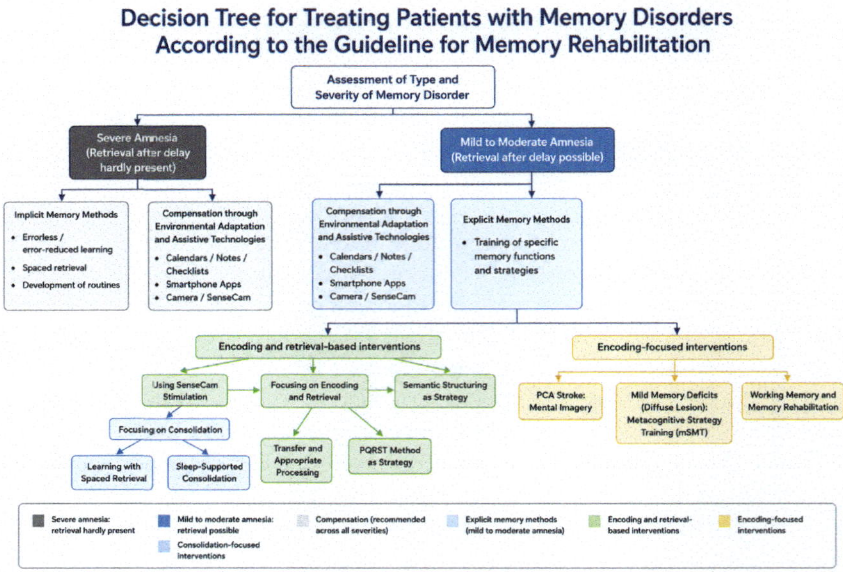

FIGURE 7.14 Decision tree for treating patients with memory disorders according to the guideline for memory rehabilitation.

7.8 Summary

The aim of this chapter was to provide an overview of treatment strategies and methods, as well as to provide a practical decision-making aid on memory rehabilitation (based on the current version of the guideline Thöne-Otto et al., 2020).

We argued that the choice of the neuropsychological treatment should depend on the type and severity of the memory impairment, the stage of recovery, the patient's therapy history, and specific rehabilitation goals. Topics covered included interventions for disorientation, the application of implicit methods such as errorless learning, the selection of appropriate external memory aids, and the availability of cognitive strategies for patients with mild to moderate impairments. Additionally, we emphasized the importance of the recovery phase (early postacute, postacute, and chronic) when choosing treatment approaches. While many studies offer promising directions, many questions remain unanswered to this day. By highlighting these gaps, we hope to encourage future research that will help individuals with memory disorders achieve optimal recovery and independence.

References

[1] Snaphaan L, de Leeuw FE. Poststroke memory function in nondemented patients: a systematic review on frequency and neuroimaging correlates. Stroke 2007;38:198–203.
[2] Chernoff RA, Martin DJ, Schrock DA, Huy MP. Neuropsychological functioning as a predictor of employment activity in a longitudinal study of hiv-infected adults contemplating workforce reentry. J Int Neuropsychol Soc 2010;16:38–48.
[3] Dikmen SS, Machamer JE, Powell JM, Temkin NR. Outcome 3 to 5 years after moderate to severe traumatic brain injury. Arch Phys Med Rehabil 2003;84:1449–57.
[4] Dusankova JB, Kalincik T, Havrdova E, Benedict RH. Cross cultural validation of the minimal assessment of cognitive function in multiple sclerosis (MACFIMS) and the brief international cognitive assessment for multiple sclerosis (BICAMS). Clin Neuropsychol 2012;26:1186–200.
[5] Morrow SA, Drake A, Zivadinov R, Munschauer F, Weinstock-Guttman B, Benedict RH. Predicting loss of employment over three years in multiple sclerosis: clinically meaningful cognitive decline. Clin Neuropsychol 2010;24:1131–45.
[6] de Wall C, Wilson BA, Baddeley AD. The extended rivermead behavioural memory test: a measure of everyday memory performance in normal adults. Memory 1994;2:149–66.
[7] Wilson B, Cockburn J, Baddeley A, Hiorns R. The development and validation of a test battery for detecting and monitoring everyday memory problems. J Clin Exp Neuropsychol 1989;11:855–70.
[8] Ashendorf L, Alosco ML, Bing-Canar H, Chapman KR, Martin B, Chaisson CE, et al. Clinical utility of select neuropsychological assessment battery tests in predicting functional abilities in dementia. Arch Clin Neuropsychol 2018;33:530–40.
[9] Zucchella C, Bartolo M, Bernini S, Picascia M, Malinverni P, Sinforiani E. Modeling alzheimer disease through functional independence and participation. Alzheimer Dis Assoc Disord 2017;31:218–24.
[10] Wilson BA. Memory rehabilitation: integrating theory and practice. New York: Guilford Press; 2009.
[11] Wilson BA, Moffat N. Clinical management of Memory Problems. Rockville, Md.: Aspen Systems Corp; 1984.
[12] Hildebrandt H. Cognitive rehabilitation of memory. Academic Press; 2019. Elsevier.
[13] L.G. Perlman, National Rehabilitation Association. Rehabilitation in the public mind, strategies of marketing: a report on the seventh mary e. Switzer memorial seminar, national rehabilitation association. Alexandria, Va. (633 S. Washington St., Alexandria 22314): The Association; 1983.
[14] A. Thöne-Otto, H. Ackermann, T. Benke, R. Bezold, H. Hildebrandt, C. Meiling, et al. Kurzfassung der s2e-leitlinie „diagnostik und therapie von gedächtnisstörungen bei neurologischen erkrankungen" (awmf-030/124). 2020;31:107-128.
[15] Turgut N, Hildebrandt H. Rehabilitation organisch bedingter gedächtnisstörungen: was, wann, für welche betroffenen? Neurol Rehabil 2021;27:239–54.
[16] Mea M. S1 leitlinie delir und verwirrtheitszustände inklusive alkoholentzugsdelir. DTSCH Ges für Neurologie 2020. Available from https://dgn.org/wp-content/uploads/2020/12/030006_LL_Delir_2020.pdf.
[17] Schenke N, Korabova SD, Thomas, Hildebrandt H. Orientierungsstörungen in der neurologischen rehabilitation. In: Mokrusch T, Gorsler A, Dohle C, Liepert J, Rollnik (Hg.) J, editors. Curriculum neurorehabilitation der Deutschen Gesellschaft für neurorehabilitation e.V. (DGNR). 2023. p. 289–304.
[18] Lipowski ZJ. Delirium (acute confusional states). JAMA 1987;258:1789–92.
[19] O'Keeffe ST, Lavan JN. Clinical significance of delirium subtypes in older people. Age Ageing 1999;28:115–9.

[20] Sandberg O, Gustafson Y, Brannstrom B, Bucht G. Clinical profile of delirium in older patients. J Am Geriatr Soc 1999;47:1300–6.
[21] Balan S, Leibovitz A, Zila SO, Ruth M, Chana W, Yassica B, et al. The relation between the clinical subtypes of delirium and the urinary level of 6-SMT. J Neuropsychiatry Clin Neurosci 2003;15:363–6.
[22] Meagher D, Moran M, Raju B, Leonard M, Donnelly S, Saunders J, et al. A new data-based motor subtype schema for delirium. J Neuropsychiatry Clin Neurosci 2008;20:185–93.
[23] Bellelli G, Morandi A, Davis DH, Mazzola P, Turco R, Gentile S, et al. Validation of the 4at, a new instrument for rapid delirium screening: a study in 234 hospitalised older people. Age Ageing 2014;43:496–502.
[24] Grossmann FF, Hasemann W, Graber A, Bingisser R, Kressig RW, Nickel CH. Screening, detection and management of delirium in the emergency department - a pilot study on the feasibility of a new algorithm for use in older emergency department patients: the Modified Confusion Assessment Method for the Emergency Department (mCAM-ED). Scand J Trauma Resusc Emerg Med 2014;22:19.
[25] Zoremba NCM. Acute confusional states in hospital. Dtsch Arztebl Int 2019;116:101–6.
[26] Farasat S, Dorsch JJ, Pearce AK, Moore AA, Martin JL, Malhotra A, et al. Sleep and delirium in older adults. Curr Sleep Med Rep 2020:1–13.
[27] Fotopoulou A. False selves in neuropsychological rehabilitation: the challenge of confabulation. Neuropsychol Rehabil 2008;18:541–65.
[28] Fotopoulou A. The affective neuropsychology of confabulation and delusion. Cogn Neuropsychiatry 2010;15:38–63.
[29] Fotopoulou A, Conway M, Griffiths P, Birchall D, Tyrer S. Self-enhancing confabulation: revisiting the motivational hypothesis. Neurocase 2007;13:6–15.
[30] Fotopoulou A, Conway MA, Solms M. Confabulation: motivated reality monitoring. Neuropsychologia 2007;45:2180–90.
[31] Lipowski ZJ. Delirium: how its concept has developed. Int Psychogeriatr 1991;3:115–20.
[32] Taskforce DAS, Baron R, Binder A, Biniek R, Braune S, Buerkle H, et al. Evidence and consensus based guideline for the management of delirium, analgesia, and sedation in intensive care medicine. Revision 2015 (das-guideline 2015) - short version. Ger Med Sci 2015;13. Doc19.
[33] Kornfeld DS, Heller SS, Frank KA, Moskowitz R. Personality and psychological factors in postcardiotomy delirium. Arch Gen Psychiatry 1974;31:249–53.
[34] Ren A, Zhang N, Zhu H, Zhou K, Cao Y, Liu J. Effects of preoperative anxiety on postoperative delirium in elderly patients undergoing elective orthopedic surgery: a prospective observational cohort study. Clin Interv Aging 2021;16:549–57.
[35] Jackson TA, Wilson D, Richardson S, Lord JM. Predicting outcome in older hospital patients with delirium: a systematic literature review. Int J Geriatr Psychiatry 2016;31:392–9.
[36] Langan C, Sarode DP, Russ TC, Shenkin SD, Carson A, Maclullich AMJ. Psychiatric symptomatology after delirium: a systematic review. Psychogeriatrics 2017;17:327–35.
[37] Stransky M, Schmidt C, Ganslmeier P, Grossmann E, Haneya A, Moritz S, et al. Hypoactive delirium after cardiac surgery as an independent risk factor for prolonged mechanical ventilation. J Cardiothorac Vasc Anesth 2011;25:968–74.
[38] Seligman ME. Learned helplessness as a model of depression. Comment and integration. J Abnorm Psychol 1978;87:165–79.
[39] Schieveld JNM, Strik JMH. Hypoactive delirium is more appropriately named as "acute apathy syndrome" Crit Care Med 2018;46:1561–2.
[40] Lipowski ZJ. Update on delirium. Psychiatr Clin North Am 1992;15:335–46.

[41] Ferrante LE, Pisani MA, Murphy TE, Gahbauer EA, Leo-Summers LS, Gill TM. Factors associated with functional recovery among older intensive care unit survivors. Am J Respir Crit Care Med 2016;194:299–307.
[42] Inouye SK, Viscoli CM, Horwitz RI, Hurst LD, Tinetti ME. A predictive model for delirium in hospitalized elderly medical patients based on admission characteristics. Ann Intern Med 1993;119:474–81.
[43] Langhorn L, Sorensen JC, Pedersen PU. A critical review of the literature on early rehabilitation of patients with post-traumatic amnesia in acute care. J Clin Nurs 2010;19:2959–69.
[44] De Guise E, Leblanc J, Feyz M, Thomas H, Gosselin N. Effect of an integrated reality orientation programme in acute care on post-traumatic amnesia in patients with traumatic brain injury. Brain Inj 2005;19:263–9.
[45] Langhorn L, Holdgaard D, Worning L, Sorensen JC, Pedersen PU. Testing a reality orientation program in patients with traumatic brain injury in a neurointensive care unit. J Neurosci Nurs 2015;47:E2–10.
[46] Hshieh TT, Yue J, Oh E, Puelle M, Dowal S, Travison T, et al. Effectiveness of multicomponent nonpharmacological delirium interventions: a meta-analysis. JAMA Intern Med 2015;175:512–20.
[47] Francis C, MacCallum F, Pierce S. Interventions for confabulation: a systematic literature review. Clin Neuropsychol 2021:1–24.
[48] Gustafson L, Hagberg B. Recovery in hydrocephalic dementia after shunt operation. J Neurol Neurosurg Psychiatry 1978;41:940–7.
[49] Trivino M, Rodenas E, Lupianez J, Arnedo M. Effectiveness of a neuropsychological treatment for confabulations after brain injury: a clinical trial with theoretical implications. PLoS One 2017;12:e0173166.
[50] Howell S, Griesbach GS. The interplay between neuroendocrine and sleep alterations following traumatic brain injury. NeuroRehabilitation 2018;43:327–45.
[51] Davoudi A, Manini TM, Bihorac A, Rashidi P. Role of wearable accelerometer devices in delirium studies: a systematic review. Crit Care Explor 2019;1:e0027.
[52] Ruan W, Yuan X, Eltzschig HK. Circadian rhythm as a therapeutic target. Nat Rev Drug Discov 2021;20:287–307.
[53] Martinez FE, Ho VW, Brogan G, Pickering C, Leung G, Parrey J, et al. Period-prevalence and risk factors for delirium in a tertiary referral ICU: a prospective cohort study. Acute Med 2021;20:168–73.
[54] Bell KR, Fogelberg D, Barber J, Nakase-Richardson R, Zumsteg JM, Dubiel R, et al. The effect of phototherapy on sleep during acute rehabilitation after traumatic brain injury: a randomized controlled trial. Brain Inj 2021;35:180–8.
[55] West AS, Sennels HP, Simonsen SA, Schonsted M, Zielinski AH, Hansen NC, et al. The effects of naturalistic light on diurnal plasma melatonin and serum cortisol levels in stroke patients during admission for rehabilitation: a randomized controlled trial. Int J Med Sci 2019;16:125–34.
[56] Groves RL. Increasing light exposure for the prevention of delirium: a systematic review. Dimens Crit Care Nurs 2019;38:96–107.
[57] Zhang Y, Su J, Wang J, Tang G, Hu W, Mao J, et al. Cognitive behavioral therapy for insomnia combined with eszopiclone for the treatment of sleep disorder patients transferred out of the intensive care unit: a single-centred retrospective observational study. Med (Baltim) 2018;97:e12383.
[58] Li X, Feng Y, Xia J, Zhou X, Chen N, Chen Z, et al. Effects of cognitive behavioral therapy on pain and sleep in adults with traumatic brain injury: a systematic review and meta-analysis. Neural Plast 2021;2021:6552246.
[59] Pilon L, Frankenmolen N, Bertens D. Treatments for sleep disturbances in individuals with acquired brain injury: a systematic review. Clin Rehabil 2021;35:1518–29.

[60] Smit L, Dijkstra-Kersten SMA, Zaal IJ, van der Jagt M, Slooter AJC. Haloperidol, clonidine and resolution of delirium in critically ill patients: a prospective cohort study. Intensive Care Med 2021;47:316–24.
[61] Benke T, Koylu B, Delazer M, Trinka E, Kemmler G. Cholinergic treatment of amnesia following basal forebrain lesion due to aneurysm rupture–an open-label pilot study. Eur J Neurol 2005;12:791–6.
[62] Wright RA, Boeve BF, Malec JF. Amnesia after basal forebrain damage due to anterior communicating artery aneurysm rupture. J Clin Neurosci 1999;6:511–5.
[63] Keegan LJ, Reed-Berendt R, Neilly E, Morrall MC, Murdoch-Eaton D. Effectiveness of melatonin for sleep impairment post paediatric acquired brain injury: evidence from a systematic review. Dev Neurorehabil 2014;17:355–62.
[64] Lewandowska K, Malkiewicz MA, Sieminski M, Cubala WJ, Winklewski PJ, Medrzycka-Dabrowska WA. The role of melatonin and melatonin receptor agonist in the prevention of sleep disturbances and delirium in intensive care unit - a clinical review. Sleep Med 2020;69:127–34.
[65] Ponsford JL, Ziino C, Parcell DL, Shekleton JA, Roper M, Redman JR, et al. Fatigue and sleep disturbance following traumatic brain injury–their nature, causes, and potential treatments. J Head Trauma Rehabil 2012;27:224–33.
[66] Westermeyer J, Carr TM. Zolpidem-associated consequences: an updated literature review with case reports. J Nerv Ment Dis 2020;208:28–32.
[67] Evans JJ, Emslie H, Wilson BA. External cueing systems in the rehabilitation of executive impairments of action. J Int Neuropsychol Soc 1998;4:399–408.
[68] Wilson BA, Emslie H, Evans JJ, Quirk K, Watson P, Fish J. The neuropage system for children and adolescents with neurological deficits. Dev Neurorehabil 2009;12:421–6.
[69] Wilson BA, Evans JJ, Emslie H, Malinek V. Evaluation of neuropage: a new memory aid. J Neurol Neurosurg Psychiatry 1997;63:113–5.
[70] Wilson BA, Scott H, Evans J, Emslie H. Preliminary report of a neuropage service within a health care system. NeuroRehabilitation 2003;18:3–8.
[71] Sohlberg MM, Mateer CA. Training use of compensatory memory books: a three stage behavioral approach. J Clin Exp Neuropsychol 1989;11:871–91.
[72] Ertas-Spantgar F, Hildebrandt H, Gabel A, Schiering I, Muller SV. Enhancing task performance in adults with intellectual disability through modified goal management training and assistive technology with errorless learning: a randomized controlled trial. Neuropsychol Rehabil 2025;35:982–1003.
[73] Ertas-Spantgar F, Muller SV, Korabova S, Gabel A, Schiering I, Pape AE, et al. Errorless learning and assistive technology did not improve the negative prognosis for severe dressing impairment after stroke if persisting for two weeks: a randomized controlled trial. Appl Neuropsychol Adult 2024;31:939–47.
[74] Roth RH, Ding JB. Cortico-basal ganglia plasticity in motor learning. Neuron 2024;112:2486–502.
[75] Hildebrandt H. Zehn argumente für dialogische interaktion und kognitive modelle als grundlage neuropsychologischer rehabilitation. Z für Neuropsychologie 2021. in Press.
[76] Hildebrandt H. Die rehacom batterie in der behandlung von kognitiven störungen bei patienten mit multipler sklerose. Neurol Rehabil 2016;2:145–50.
[77] Brissart H, Omorou AY, Forthoffer N, Berger E, Moreau T, De Seze J, et al. Memory improvement in multiple sclerosis after an extensive cognitive rehabilitation program in groups with a multicenter double-blind randomized trial. Clin Rehabil 2020;34:754–63.
[78] Fava-Felix PE, Bonome-Vanzelli SRC, Ribeiro FS, Santos FH. Systematic review on post-stroke computerized cognitive training: unveiling the impact of confounding factors. Front Psychol 2022;13:985438.

[79] Gao M, Huang L, Yi J, Zhang T, Zhu G, Zhang Q, et al. The effectiveness of computerized cognitive training in patients with poststroke cognitive impairment: systematic review and meta-analysis. J Med Internet Res 2025;27:e73140.
[80] Jennings JM, Webster LM, Kleykamp BA, Dagenbach D. Recollection training and transfer effects in older adults: successful use of a repetition-lag procedure. Neuropsychol Dev Cogn B Aging Neuropsychol Cogn 2005;12:278–98.
[81] Bailey H, Dagenbach D, Jennings JM. The locus of the benefits of repetition-lag memory training. Neuropsychol Dev Cogn B Aging Neuropsychol Cogn 2011;18:577–93.
[82] Boller B, Jennings JM, Dieudonne B, Verny M, Ergis AM. Recollection training and transfer effects in Alzheimer's disease: effectiveness of the repetition-lag procedure. Brain Cogn 2012;78:169–77.
[83] Stamenova V, Jennings JM, Cook SP, Gao F, Walker LA, Smith AM, et al. Repetition-lag memory training is feasible in patients with chronic stroke, including those with memory problems. Brain Inj 2016:1–11.
[84] Richter KM, Modden C, Eling P, Hildebrandt H. Improving everyday memory performance after acquired brain injury: an RCT on recollection and working memory training. Neuropsychology 2018;32:586–96.
[85] H. Hildebrandt, Cognitive Rehabilitation of Memory. Elsevier: Academic Press, 2019.
[86] Turgut N.H.H. Rehabilitation organisch bedingter gedächtnisstörungen: Was, wann für welche betroffenen? 2022.
[87] Wilson BA. Rehabilitation of Memory. New York: Guilford Press; 1987.
[88] Kaschel R, Sala SD, Cantagallo A, Fahlböck A, Laaksonen R, Kazen M. Imagery mnemonics for the rehabilitation of memory: a randomised group controlled trial. Neuropsychol Rehabil 2002;12:127–53.
[89] Berg IJ, Koning-haanstra M, Deelman BG. Long-term effects of memory rehabilitation: a controlled study. Neuropsychol Rehabil 1991;1:97–111.
[90] Chiaravalloti N, Hillary F, Ricker J, Christodoulou C, Kalnin A, Liu WC, et al. Cerebral activation patterns during working memory performance in multiple sclerosis using fMRI. J Clin Exp Neuropsychol 2005;27:33–54.
[91] Chiaravalloti ND, DeLuca J, Moore NB, Ricker JH. Treating learning impairments improves memory performance in multiple sclerosis: a randomized clinical trial. Mult Scler 2005;11:58–68.
[92] Chiaravalloti ND, Dobryakova E, Wylie GR, DeLuca J. Examining the efficacy of the modified story memory technique (MSMT) in persons with TBI using functional magnetic resonance imaging (fMRI): the TBI-MEM trial. J Head Trauma Rehabil 2015;30:261–9.
[93] Chiaravalloti ND, Moore NB, DeLuca J. The efficacy of the modified story memory technique in progressive MS. Mult Scler 2020;26:354–62.
[94] Chiaravalloti ND, Moore NB, Nikelshpur OM, DeLuca J. An RCT to treat learning impairment in multiple sclerosis: the MEMREHAB trial. Neurology 2013;81:2066–72.
[95] Chiaravalloti ND, Sandry J, Moore NB, DeLuca J. An RCT to treat learning impairment in traumatic brain injury: the TBI-MEM trial. Neurorehabil Neural Repair 2016;30:539–50.
[96] Hildebrandt H, Bussmann-Mork B, Schwendemann G. Group therapy for memory impaired patients: a partial remediation is possible. J Neurol 2006;253:512–9.
[97] Hildebrandt H, Gehrmann A, Modden C, Eling P. Enhancing memory performance after organic brain disease relies on retrieval processes rather than encoding or consolidation. J Clin Exp Neuropsychol 2011;33:257–70.
[98] Cermak LS, Butters N, Moreines J. Some analyses of the verbal encoding deficit of alcoholic korsakoff patients. Brain Lang 1974;1.

[99] Miotto EC. Declarative memory disorders in patients with brain tumors can improve after cognitive training intervention: evidence from functional MRI. J Neurooncol 2012;110:301–2.
[100] Miotto EC, Savage CR, Evans JJ, Wilson BA, Martin MG, Balardin JB, et al. Semantic strategy training increases memory performance and brain activity in patients with prefrontal cortex lesions. Clin Neurol Neurosurg 2013;115:309–16.
[101] Miotto EC, Teixeira MJ. The effects of strategy training on acquisition of new verbal information in patients with acquired brain lesions. Neuro Rehabilitation 2012;31:463–4.
[102] Miller RR. Failures of memory and the fate of forgotten memories. Neurobiol Learn Mem 2021;181:107426.
[103] Schacter DL, Rich SA, Stampp MS. Remediation of memory disorders: experimental evaluation of the spaced-retrieval technique. J Clin Exp Neuropsychol 1985;7:79–96.
[104] Richter KM, Modden C, Eling P, Hildebrandt H. Working memory training and semantic structuring improves remembering future events, not past events. Neurorehabil Neural Repair 2015;29:33–40.
[105] Ciaramelli E, Neri F, Marini L, Braghittoni D. Improving memory following prefrontal cortex damage with the PQRST method. Front Behav Neurosci 2015;9:211.
[106] Farooq MU, Min J, Goshgarian C, Gorelick PB. Pharmacotherapy for vascular cognitive impairment. CNS Drugs 2017;31:759–76.
[107] Kim JO, Lee SJ, Pyo JS. Effect of acetylcholinesterase inhibitors on post-stroke cognitive impairment and vascular dementia: a meta-analysis. PLoS One 2020;15:e0227820.
[108] Bellman S. Pharmacological treatment for memory disorder in multiple sclerosis. Int J Evid Based Healthc 2017;15:186–7.
[109] He D, Zhang Y, Dong S, Wang D, Gao X, Zhou H. Pharmacological treatment for memory disorder in multiple sclerosis. Cochrane Database Syst Rev 2013:CD008876.
[110] Dougall D, Poole N, Agrawal N. Pharmacotherapy for chronic cognitive impairment in traumatic brain injury. Cochrane Database Syst Rev 2015:CD009221.
[111] Baskys A, Hou AC. Vascular dementia: pharmacological treatment approaches and perspectives. Clin Interv Aging 2007;2:327–35.
[112] Silva AR, Pinho MS, Macedo L, Moulin C, Caldeira S, Firmino H. It is not only memory: effects of sensecam on improving well-being in patients with mild alzheimer disease. Int Psychogeriatr 2017;29:741–54.
[113] Silva AR, Pinho S, Macedo LM, Moulin CJ. Benefits of sensecam review on neuropsychological test performance. Am J Prev Med 2013;44:302–7.
[114] Hodges S, Berry E, Wood K. Sensecam: a wearable camera that stimulates and rehabilitates autobiographical memory. Memory 2011;19:685–96.
[115] Maddox GB, Balota DA, Coane JH, Duchek JM. The role of forgetting rate in producing a benefit of expanded over equal spaced retrieval in young and older adults. Psychol Aging 2011;26:661–70.
[116] Warrington EK, Weiskrantz L. Further analysis of the prior learning effect in amnesic patients. Neuropsychologia 1978;16:169–77.
[117] Dewar M, Della Sala S, Beschin N, Cowan N. Profound retroactive interference in anterograde amnesia: what interferes? Neuropsychology 2010;24:357–67.
[118] Dewar M, Garcia YF, Cowan N, Della Sala S. Delaying interference enhances memory consolidation in amnesic patients. Neuropsychology 2009;23:627–34.
[119] Skaggs E. Further studies in retroactive inhibition. Psychol Monogr 1925;34:1–60.
[120] Brodt S, Inostroza M, Niethard N, Born J. Sleep-a brain-state serving systems memory consolidation. Neuron 2023;111:1050–75.

CHAPTER

8

Rehabilitation of disorders of goal-directed behaviour

8.1 Introduction

Executive functions (EFs) are high-level cognitive processes that enable goal-directed behavior, particularly in novel or complex situations [1–6]. They include abilities such as planning, initiation, inhibition, working memory, and cognitive flexibility. Disruptions in these processes affect a patient's ability to initiate tasks, regulate emotions, maintain attention, and adapt to changing demands, ultimately influencing participation in therapy and daily life activities. Recommendations on how to treat executive disorders in the broad sense can be found in the current German guidelines on executive dysfunction [6]. This chapter will focus on disorders in goal-directed behavior, including planning, inhibition, and cognitive flexibility. The reason for focusing on goal-directed behavior is that the more global concept of EFs is rather complex, which leads to ill-defined research results [5]. Another reason is that disorders like increased impulsivity and lack of self-control in social behavior will not be covered, because they most often result from traumatic brain injury (TBI) or other diffuse brain lesions, but not from stroke. Still, most of the following recommendations are derived from clinical practice, as available research is heterogeneous, involves ill-defined patient populations, and is predominantly conducted in chronic phases without distinguishing between different stages of recovery.

Goal-directed behavior relies heavily on the prefrontal cortex (PFC) and its extensive networks [3,4,7]. The PFC is located anterior to the premotor cortex (those regions that start with the premotor sulcus, Chapter 1). The core region of the PFC is the middle frontal gyrus and the inferior frontal gyrus, extending from the sulcus frontalis superior to the ventrolateral orbitofrontal cortex (OFC). The lateral PFC is subdivided into the dorsolateral and the ventrolateral parts by the sulcus arcuatus. The frontal pole (areas 9 and 10 of Brodmann) also belongs to

Applied Neuropsychology of Cerebrovascular Diseases
DOI: https://doi.org/10.1016/B978-0-443-45450-9.00005-9

the PFC as its medial part. The medial PFC, including the anterior cingulate cortex, receives its blood supply primarily from the anterior cerebral artery (ACA). Strokes in this region can lead to motivational deficits, such as apathy and reduced initiation (akinesia and abulia, Chapter 9) [8]. The lateral PFC, particularly on the lateral convexity of the frontal lobe, is mostly supplied by the anterior division of the middle cerebral artery (MCA). The dorsolateral PFC is supplied by the superior anterior branches of the MCA. As a border zone of supply from the MCA and the ACA, it is vulnerable to ischemic events, known as low-flow strokes in watershed areas (Chapter 1) [2,9,10]. Strokes in the OFC, laterally supplied by inferior anterior branches of the MCA and medially by the A1 segment of the ACA, may result in emotional dysregulation and impaired social behavior [11,12]. However, isolated strokes of the OFC are rare events. They occur mainly as a consequence of ruptured aneurysm of the arteria communicans anterior (Chapter 1).

While goal-directed behavior is heavily mediated by the PFC, it also relies on interaction with subcortical structures. The striatum (part of the basal ganglia), thalamus, and limbic structures, for instance, contribute to these processes by forming cortico-subcortical loops. Dysfunction in these loops can result in impairments in goal-directed behavior even if the PFC is not involved [2,10,12,13].

Large studies on stroke patients argue that between 10% and 20% suffer from impairments in EF during the postacute phase of a stroke [14–17]. However, follow-up investigations have shown considerable improvement. On the other hand, they also argue that the risk of persisting cognitive disorders and worse rehabilitative outcomes increases with the existence of such disorders [6,14–17].

There are several excellent books and articles on EFs, associated disorders, and how to use neuropsychological tests for assessing them [1–3,6,7,18,19]. In the following, we will therefore concentrate on disorders of goal-directed behavior and, more specifically, on their treatment.

8.2 Disorders of goal-directed behavior or "Goal Neglect"

Since the PFC is essential for organizing and maintaining goal-directed behavior, neurological damage to the PFC often leads to disorders of planning, learning, and executing complex actions. Patients may understand task rules, or the steps needed to fulfill a plan, but fail to maintain the overarching structure throughout their activity. One influential theory argues that impairment of goal-directed behavior should be termed "goal neglect" [20,21]. This is based on the observation that such patients lose track of task goals over time because they cannot resist distraction or are unable to maintain goal representations in working memory.

However, although goal neglect seems to characterize the behavior of such patients in many respects, it should be mentioned that it may result from different cognitive deficits. First, planning involves the ability to set goals, formulate steps, anticipate outcomes, and monitor execution over time. Key processes for planning encompass the ability to hold subgoals in working memory and to integrate individual steps into one action. Impairment in one of these two functions may result in disorders of goal-directed behavior. Second, while planning is about generating and maintaining a course of action, cognitive flexibility is about changing it when needed. Specifically, cognitive flexibility is the ability to shift mental sets, adapt to changing rules or demands, and adjust behavior based on feedback or environmental contingencies. It becomes essential in novel or dynamic situations where established routines no longer suffice. Deficits in flexibility will also impair goal-directed behavior because contextual adaptation is reduced, which hinders switching between subactions in response to changing task demands.

On a clinical level, disorders of planning become evident as increased distraction, inefficient sequencing of actions, and difficulty anticipating necessary steps, whereas disorders of flexibility primarily result in perseveration and rigidity. Increased distractibility can be observed, for example, when a patient is asked to remember and retrieve specific cards that are placed face down on a table: although they may initially understand the instructions, they quickly lose track of the goal. Instead of methodically searching for the target cards, they may turn over cards at random, become fixated on unrelated details (such as the color or texture of the cards), or stop the task altogether to comment on the table surface. Without continuous external reminders, they often fail to complete the task or may even forget what they were initially asked to do, illustrating a loss of goal maintenance. Perseveration, on the other hand, refers to the inappropriate repetition of a response, thought, or behavior despite changes in task demands or negative feedback for continuing with the behavior. It reflects a breakdown in the ability to disengage from no-longer-relevant cognitive or behavioral sets. On a more abstract level, increased distractibility can be viewed directly as the opposite of perseveration: patients with increased distractibility cope with disinhibited shifting of actions (being mainly controlled by the environment), whereas perseverating patients with impaired flexibility to shift toward the next subaction, remaining mainly controlled by the last dominant internal action presentation.

As far as we know, there is no systematic classification or comparison between different forms of distractibility. Perseveration, however, can be distinguished into *stuck-in-set perseveration*, where individuals persist with an outdated rule or strategy despite negative feedback, *recurrent perseveration*, characterized by the inappropriate intrusion of previously used responses into new tasks, likely due to impaired working memory and deficient task-set reconfiguration; *continuous perseveration*, which refers to the uncontrollable repetition of the same action or movement; and *recurrent perseveration*.

Table 8.1 offers a summary of the most common types of perseverations.

Goal neglect and its clinical presentations seem to differ not only due to involved cognitive processes and association with focal brain lesions, but also related to the stage of recovery. In the early phase following brain injury, planning difficulties are often pronounced and global. Patients may be unable to initiate planning sequences without extensive guidance, abandon tasks due to lapses in goal maintenance, or act without a clear sense of the overarching goal. Poor insight reduces working memory capacity, and impaired attention commonly increases planning failure at this stage [22–25]. One explanation for the high frequency of goal-directed behavior deficits in the early postacute phase is that during this phase, swelling of the brain and global alterations of neurotransmitter availability are common and therefore affect the PFC even without structural lesions. This also aligns with the prevalence rates of executive dysfunction reported above: while 10%–20% of stroke patients in the postacute phase present with such impairments, follow-up data from these large-scale studies suggest partial recovery over time [6,14–17].

In the chronic phase, overt disorganization may lessen, but deficits become more apparent in complex or novel situations. Patients might function relatively well in familiar, routine settings, yet display marked impairments in tasks that require self-initiated planning, prioritization, or adaptation across multiple goals. Now, the remaining structural lesion is of major importance for specific cognitive impairment. Interventions like goal management training (GMT) and the stop-think-check strategies (a simplified form of GMT) become increasingly effective during this stage, particularly as patients regain insight and attentional stamina [26]. Strategies of GMT will be discussed in the next section, arguing that aspects of them can be used already during the early phase of recovery.

8.3 Rehabilitation of goal-directed disorders

8.3.1 Goal-directed disorders according to stage of recovery

Goal-directed disorders differ according to the stage of recovery. In the (early,) severe stages of impairment, patients are often highly distractible

TABLE 8.1 Types of perseverations in neurological rehabilitation—clinical manifestations and neural correlates.

Perseveration type	Stuck-in-set perseveration	Continuous perseveration	Recurrent perseveration	Recurrent utterances	Motor perseverations
Definition	Failure to switch strategies or categories when task demands change failure to shift a mental rule or strategy	Uncontrollable repetition of the same action or movement, even when it is no longer appropriate failing to stop an ongoing behavior	Inappropriate repetition of a previous response during a new activity repeating a past response inappropriately	Verbal perseverations are seen in patients with severe expressive aphasia language-specific subtype common in aphasia	Repetitive, purposeless movements, often directed toward nearby objects, may be exacerbated by environmental triggers or stress movement-based perseveration
Example	Continuing to sort cards by color even after the rule changes to sorting by shape	Repeatedly reaching for an object after the task has ended	Naming an object from a prior trial instead of the current one during a naming task	Persistently naming a previously seen object in a naming task	Repeatedly pulling at bed linens, fiddling with intravenous lines, or feeding tubes
Neural correlates	*Dorso*lateral PFC (DLPFC) (set-shifting and abstract rule maintenance)	Medial frontal cortex and basal ganglia (motor inhibition deficits)	Posterior part of the DLPFC and working memory circuits	Broca's area and anterior cingulate cortex (part of the medial prefrontal cortex)	Diffuse frontal or subcortical pathology, including SMA, premotor cortex, and basal ganglia

Note. This table summarizes the main types of perseveration observed in neurological rehabilitation. SMA = supplementary motor area.

and show great difficulty in following even simple goals due to reduced attentional control. Motor perseveration is frequently observed; for example, patients may react in a stimulus-bound manner to objects such as the bed linens on them, repeatedly grasping or manipulating them without contextual relevance. Continuous perseveration is also common. In brief screening tasks, such as placing an object into a specific shape, patients may continue the action even after being informed that they have (successfully) completed the exercise. Thus at this stage, they require immediate and comprehensive external structuring to reduce cognitive demands, alongside the therapist defining goals, guiding each step, and closely monitoring behavior. The goal here is to begin developing an internal representation of their goals, reduce automatic, perseverative behavior, and enable externally guided attentional control.

As patients progress to more moderate stages, they begin to collaborate with the therapist in defining (sub)goals and gradually assume responsibility for individual steps. The goal here is to strengthen internal goal representation, improve attentional control by slightly increasing environmental distractors, and engage in simple error monitoring techniques. At this stage, the use of external aids (e.g., checklists) is encouraged as well, but still mostly guided by the therapist.

In the mild stages, patients are expected to manage their goals more independently, apply self-monitoring strategies, use external aids, and flexibly adapt their behavior as needed. The therapist's role here is mainly to give feedback, intervene when errors occur that the patient does not recognize or correct themselves, and support the generalization of learned strategies to new settings.

All in all, direct external guidance is progressively replaced by internally supported attention control and, ultimately, by abstract self-regulation. While the overall planning structure remains visible throughout the process, responsibility for its implementation is gradually transferred to the patient.

Table 8.2 below outlines the therapeutic process. Notably, while these aspects should form the foundation of treatment, it is equally important to acknowledge that patients with isolated executive dysfunction are relatively rare. Brain injuries often affect multiple domains, such as additional attention deficits or language impairments. As a result, rehabilitation planning should take into account the broader cognitive profile and adapt interventions accordingly.

8.3.2 Goal management training

One approach for the rehabilitation of goal-directed disorders is goal management, which focuses on goal setting, planning, and plan execution while decreasing automatic, perseverative behavior and susceptibility to distraction. GMT is a metacognitive intervention designed to re-establish top–down attentional control by interrupting automatic responding and fostering intentional, goal-directed behavior [27–30]. While the therapeutic framework (Table 8.2) focuses on the gradual transfer of executive control from therapist to patient, GMT offers a structured method for guiding individual therapeutic tasks *within* that process.

GMT is one of the most widely used and theoretically grounded interventions for executive dysfunction and is recommended by the current German guidelines on neuropsychological rehabilitation, particularly supported in chronic populations Müller and Klein [6]. There are five steps of GMT, namely (1) stop, (2) define, (3) list, (4) learn, and (5) check, which are applied in a cyclical fashion to specific, real-world goals. For example, when preparing a cup of tea, the patient is first prompted to "Stop," pausing to interrupt habitual responding and bring attention to the present moment. They are then asked to "Define" the task goal (e.g., "Make a cup of black tea with sugar and milk"), followed by "Listing" the steps required (e.g., "Boil water," "Place tea bag in cup," "Pour water," "Add sugar and milk," "Stir"). In the "Learn" phase, the patient rehearses or verbalizes this sequence. During the "Check" phase, they are encouraged to monitor their actions (e.g., "Did I remember the sugar?") and evaluate whether the goal was completed as intended.

The following sections outline the rehabilitation of goal-directed disorders across stages of recovery, incorporating GMT as the main intervention and other complementary interventions adapted to the patient's cognitive abilities. All in all, these interventions should support the therapist in guiding their patient to re-engage in goal-directed behavior (Table 8.2).

8.3.3 Rehabilitation of subacute, severe goal-directed disorders

In the severe stages of neurological rehabilitation, patients with goal-directed disorders typically show impaired attentional control, poor impulse regulation, and limited illness insight. For example, during the intake of a patient with right-frontal TBI, she denied experiencing any current difficulties, despite having undergone a craniectomy with visible skull removal on the right side of her head. In our initial interaction, she frequently trailed off mid-sentence and became distracted by objects in the room. When she entered the office for a second session, she immediately began picking up items from the table without any clear purpose. During a simple task such as the line bisection test (used to assess neglect), she stopped midway, changed the subject spontaneously,

TABLE 8.2 The therapeutic process.

Phase	Cognition	Therapist behavior	Patient behavior	Tools	Therapeutic goal
Severe impairment	Poor initiation; high distractibility; highly limited internal goal representation -> severe goal neglect	Provides full external structure (environment, timing, content) to minimize cognitive demands; defines and verbalizes goals; initiates all steps; gives direct commands; disrupts distractive behavior; directs attentional capacities	Passive compliance; follows instructions without initiative; inability to allocate attentional resources -> distractibility; poor illness insight; perseverations	Multimodal "Stop" cues, fixed daily routines, external orientation aids; spaced retrieval; function-specific add-on training to engage in simplified goal management training (GMT) principles	Interrupt automatic, perseverative behavior. Establish a stable routine and external structure. Enable externally guided attentional control sufficient to engage the patient in the simplified GMT protocol
Moderate impairment	Reliable internal goal representation; emerging self-monitoring with partial error awareness; increasing illness insight	Defines (sub)goals together with the patient; models step sequences; facilitates goal rehearsal; teaches and encourages use of external aids (e.g., checklists); monitors behavior and gives support when errors occur. Systematically includes mild to moderate distractions	Recall steps with support; monitors errors inconsistently; needs external prompts; beginning use of external aids	Guided GMT principles; spaced retrieval; guided rehearsal; external aids (e.g., checklists); function-specific add-on training	Strengthen internal goal representation and substeps; improve attention allocation and early monitoring; encourage active external aid use; inhibit moderate distractors
Moderate to mild impairment	Reliable internal representation of multiple goals; initiating and monitoring behavior; mostly independent use of external aids; partial generalization of learned techniques to new tasks; error awareness with minimal reminders	Fades support; intervenes only when errors occur; asks reflective questions to promote self-monitoring; provides feedback; promotes symbolic cue use (e.g., reminders); sets homework	Initiates, plans, and monitors tasks; uses external aids with minimal support; shows error awareness and strategic flexibility	Full goal management training cycle, symbolic cueing, reflective questioning, external aids (e.g., checklists); homework; function-specific add-on training	Self-generated GMT use in activities of daily life; transfer responsibility for planning and monitoring; foster flexible strategy use and goal-directed autonomy

Note. This table represents the overall guiding therapeutic process in the rehabilitation of goal-directed disorders. GMT = goal management training.

or abandoned the task entirely, only continuing when directly prompted. Lastly, during the Trail-Making-Test B (TMT-B), administered to assess cognitive flexibility, she demonstrated perseveration. Having just completed the TMT-A, which required connecting numbers in sequence as fast as possible, she was unable to shift from that strategy. This stuck-in-set perseveration pattern re-emerged in subsequent tasks requiring a change in set. This case illustrates the combination of impaired attentional control, poor task persistence, perseveration, and reduced illness insight.

At this severe stage, the therapist plays an active, directive role. The primary focus is on minimizing cognitive demands by adapting the environment to reduce distractibility and perseveration and by cueing the patient to sustain attentional control toward completing simple, clearly defined goals.

8.3.3.1 *Adaptation of the environment and establishing structured routines*

In terms of minimizing cognitive demands, the therapist first creates a structured and distraction-free environment. This includes keeping the workspace clear of unnecessary items, positioning the patient away from windows or high-traffic areas (e.g., the door), ensuring the door is closed to reduce noise and movement, and sitting directly across from the patient to maintain eye contact and provide a consistent point of focus. In other words, cognitive demands are being lowered to a minimum, supporting the patient to remain engaged with the task at hand [25].

Structured routines are another essential compensatory strategy for the severe phase. While they often build on principles of environmental structuring, they extend further into temporal and behavioral regularity, serving as anchors for attention, orientation, and self-regulation. They restrict executive load via predictability and reduced novelty and allow for greater self-monitoring through repetition [25,31]. Establishing such predictable routines may involve consistent timing, places (the patient's, therapist's, or other rooms), and, when possible, familiar therapeutic staff. In practice, such routines are often difficult to maintain in full due to rotating nursing staff or shifting therapy schedules. However, even small routines, such as beginning the day with the same sequence (e.g., getting out of bed, brushing teeth, getting dressed) or starting each therapy session with the same task, can create a sense of familiarity. When routines change too frequently, the cognitive demands placed on the patient may exceed their current capacity. The overarching goal is to create a reliable framework that patients can orient themselves by.

Nevertheless, while environmental modification may reduce perseverative behavior or distractions, patients may continue to be distracted by internal stimuli, such as intrusive thoughts or emotional concerns, regardless of how well the external environment is controlled. For example, the same patient with right-frontal TBI repeatedly returned to a conversation she had with another person earlier that day. Although there was no apparent external trigger during the session, she was unable to disengage from the topic and redirect her attention. She repeatedly interrupted the exercise she was instructed to complete in order to revisit the conversation and ask further questions about it.

Thus the mere implementation of structured routines and environmental modifications is not sufficient. Patients must be actively supported in understanding and following these routines, using external aids, and practicing them regularly in therapy. Hence such routines do not inherently promote the right usage, flexibility, planning, or problem-solving. Structured routines (as well as environmental modification) do not train the core executive ability to respond flexibly to novel or unpredictable situations. Therefore rehabilitation should also focus on teaching patients generalizable techniques, alongside training their ability to adapt and implement these strategies in new contexts. GMT can serve as an effective framework for this process.

8.3.3.2 *Using goal management training in severe stages*

When implementing GMT in severe stages, the full protocol with all five GMT steps is often not feasible. (Krasny–Pacini et al. [27]). More specifically, holding multiple components in working memory, shifting flexibly between tasks, and continuously monitoring performance overwhelm patients in the severe stage. However, a simplified protocol, focusing on Step 1 ("Stop"), Step 2 ("Define the goal"), and Step 5 ("Check"), can still offer therapeutic value (Table 8.3).

While this simplified three-step GMT protocol reduces cognitive demands, there are still some cognitive prerequisites that need to be met [27]. The patient should be able:

1. …to orient toward and engage with task-relevant stimuli (when externally prompted), maintain focus for short periods, and shift attention between goal and action (when cued) [32]. If this is not possible, sustained attention training should be prioritized, which can include, for instance, computerized continuous performance tasks that require the patient to stay engaged over time [33,34]. Environmental modifications, such as removing visual distractions, as well as the use of salient sensory cues, can further support attentional engagement (see the section above) [32]. Other practical strategies include presenting task materials in high-contrast colors and using verbal (e.g., calling the patient's name), tactile (e.g., gently tapping the table), or

visual cues (e.g., pointing to the task) to redirect attention. This is particularly important for implementing Step 1 ("Stop") of the simplified GMT protocol, which aims to interrupt automatic or disengaged behavior. Effective strategies can include raising a hand while saying "Stop," presenting a red cue card, or gently tapping the patient's hand or arm.

2. …to hold at least one goal in mind (e.g., "I want to prepare a cup of tea") and to verbally repeat the goal throughout the session, indicating sufficient working memory capacity [28,32]. If this is not possible, simple working memory training should be initiated to restore this capacity. The same holds if patients are able to retain task goals (i.e., can engage in the simplified GMT protocol) but struggle in other areas, such as consistency or coordinating multiple task components. Working memory training can include computerized training programs like "RehaCom" or "Cogmed" (e.g., Spikman et al. [33]) as well as strategies during task execution, such as having the patient repeat task goals more frequently or at shorter intervals to support goal maintenance. Furthermore, external memory aids, such as notebooks, written reminders, or visual checklists, can be incorporated to support task understanding and recall.
3. …to recognize when their behavior deviates from the intended goal (when being externally asked to reflect), reflecting basic error awareness and basic cognitive control [32,33]. Some degree of awareness is often considered essential for the independent application of GMT strategies [33]. While limited insight may indeed impede the *independent* use of GMT strategies, it does not necessarily preclude participation in a simplified version. In our clinical experience, even limited engagement in goal-monitoring processes within simplified GMT can facilitate the development of insight over time, serving as a form of awareness training in itself. If engagement is still limited due to insufficient awareness (e.g., the patient attributes mistakes to external factors), other awareness-enhancing techniques may be implemented [30]. These may be immediate error feedback—when the patient makes a mistake during a task (e.g., selecting the wrong item in a cancellation task), the therapist gives a direct prompt such as "Is that what you were supposed to do?"—or prediction–performance comparison—before beginning a task, patients are asked to estimate how well they think they will perform (e.g., "Do you think you'll be able to cross out all the circles in three minutes?")—and task performance will be briefly reviewed after task execution.

Table 8.3 summarizes the simplified GMT protocol, outlining key prerequisites and how to assess them, as well as possible add-on interventions.

TABLE 8.3 Simplified goal management training protocol.

Step	Function/question	External aids	Possible add-ons	Goal
(1) Stop	What am I doing right now? -> Is the patient able to keep one task in mind? *(inhibition, attention)*	– Verbal redirection – Multimodal "stop" cues (e.g., hand tap)	– Inhibition training – Sustained attention tasks – Alertness cueing	– Interrupting automatic/ perseverative behavior – Maintaining task engagement
(2) Define	What is my goal right now? -> Is the patient able to state and recall a goal over a short period of time? *(goal representation and working memory,)*	– Goal cue cards – Therapist modeling – - Checklists	– Working memory training – - Spaced retrieval	– Improving goal clarity and retention of one simple goal over time
(3) Check	"Am I doing what I planned to do?" → Is the patient able to self-monitor and detect deviations? *(error monitoring, insight)*	– Verbal self-check prompts – Structured feedback – Checklists	– Error monitoring strategies – Immediate error feedback	– Supporting externally guided error correction – Increasing awareness of task-related errors

Note. This table outlines the simplified GMT protocol adapted for early rehabilitation, highlighting core cognitive functions, helpful external aids, and possible add-on trainings. The recommendations are based on clinical experience and supported by findings from [27,32–36].

8.3.3.2.1 Case illustration: adapting goal management training for severe executive impairments

A patient with bilateral frontal damage following TBI presented with high distractibility and impulsive, perseverative behavior. He was unable to execute even the simplest tasks independently, becoming easily distracted and reaching for unrelated objects, which he would interact with instead of focusing on the task at hand. However, after modifying the therapeutic environment (e.g., clearing the room of distractions) to reduce distractions and presenting only a basic cancellation task, he was able to repeat back the task instructions, indicating an initial understanding of the goal.

Before initiating the task, we introduced the "Stop" cue (Step 1), as the patient was already reaching for the pen impulsively. This was followed by Step 2: *"What are you supposed to do right now?"*. Steps 3 and 4 (splitting the task and encoding the steps) were externalized by the therapist to reduce cognitive load: *"I am going to give you the pen, and then you are going to cross out all the circles."* In some instances, the patient may repeat these instructions aloud to reinforce task engagement. Externalizing executive steps and scaffolding behavior have also been emphasized in other GMT-adapted programs (e.g., Spikman et al. [33], Novakovic-Agopian et al. [34]).

During task execution, Step 5 ("Check") was applied whenever the patient became distracted, perseverated, or marked the wrong item. A verbal and/or tactile "Stop" cue was introduced, followed by the prompt, *"Are you doing what you are supposed to do?"* In most instances, the patient was able to recognize his error (e.g., marking the wrong item) and correct it—an ability that had not been observed in earlier sessions without this structured approach. As a result, he was able to complete a simple action correctly while effectively ignoring distractors. Although this highly structured and heavily externally guided version of GMT did not lead to independent use of the strategy, it nevertheless appeared to reactivate core executive processes, such as attentional control and error monitoring, within the therapeutic setting. While he remained dependent on external prompts, the patient began to engage in simple performance monitoring.

Ultimately, the goal of the simplified GMT approach is to enable patients to successfully complete simple, structured goals by actively engaging in goal maintenance, performance monitoring, and error correction. Tasks used within the simplified GMT protocol often do not fully reflect real-life complexity, as everyday activities typically involve multiple steps, shifting goals, and unpredictable interruptions. Thus the implementation of ecologically valid tasks is the long-term objective (see e.g., Krasny-Pacini et al. [27]), and once patients are able to carry out the simplified GMT sequence with reduced external support, the full GMT protocol should be introduced.

8.3.4 Rehabilitation of moderate to mild goal-directed disorders

In the moderate stage, patients begin to internally represent goals more reliably, recall step sequences (with or without external aids), and monitor their performance with support. Perseverative behavior is reduced, and the patient only requires minimal interference by the therapist to interrupt perseverations. However, they often still require external prompts and therapist guidance to maintain goal focus and correct errors.

In the mild stage, patients show reliable goal representation, greater planning capacity, and an emerging ability to generalize strategies (i.e., cognitive flexibility) across contexts. The therapist's role becomes more observational and reflective, using symbolic cueing, reflective questioning, and promoting the independent use of external aids to promote autonomy. Patients are increasingly encouraged to take ownership of task planning, problem-solving, and self-monitoring.

8.3.4.1 Environmental adaptation and structured routines

During the moderate impairment stage, a gradual increase in environmental complexity and a corresponding decrease in external control processes become important, and patients should gradually learn to tolerate and manage distractions. For instance, they may be positioned closer to a window or work at a table with some items present. This stepwise reintroduction of distractors supports generalization to everyday situations and helps patients regain some level of attentional control in task execution. Importantly, a gradual increase in distractors does not automatically mean that patients will be able to manage them effectively. The ability to cope with increasing cognitive demands must be supported and trained over time.

When sufficient memory and attentional capacities are present, patients can also be supported in using a structured daily therapy plan. They may be taught to use the timetable to identify which sessions have already taken place (and tick them off), which session is currently ongoing, and which ones are still to come. In this way, rehabilitation progresses from the passive establishment of structured routines to the active involvement of the patient. The patient is encouraged to cognitively engage with the daily structure by understanding what has already happened, what is happening now, and what will happen next.

"Sufficient memory and attentional capacities" refer to the ability to reliably answer basic orientation questions such as: "What is the rough date?," "Where are you?," and "Why are you here?". These orientation markers are crucial to ensure that the patient is anchored in time, place, and situation, which are prerequisites for meaningful engagement with external aids such as a daily timetable (compare Chapter 7 for reorientation and introducing reminders). This is particularly important given that many patients also present with comorbid memory impairments (see Chapter 7 on memory disorders). For example, a patient with right frontal and bilateral temporal lobe damage following TBI exhibited ongoing situational and place disorientation. Firmly believing that his wife was about to pick him up at any moment and continuously asking when his appointment was over, he saw no relevance in consulting the daily schedule. In addition, patients must be able to sustain attention long enough to visually scan the calendar, identify relevant entries, and use it for guidance. Equally important are other basic memory capacities: patients must be able to remember the purpose of the timetable (retrospective memory) and recall consulting it at appropriate moments (prospective memory). Without this foundational level of memory and attention, attempts to foster goal-directed behavior or self-management strategies are likely to be unsuccessful, as the patient may not meaningfully relate to or effectively use the information presented [32].

Once patients can use a basic daily schedule, more complex routines can be introduced and practiced. These may be supported by additional external aids, such as written checklists for morning routines or sequences of therapeutic activities. At this stage, the level of external guidance should be gradually reduced further, encouraging the patient to independently refer to these aids. Table 8.4 informs about environmental structuring and structured routines across recovery stages.

Example: in the case of a patient with right fronto–temporal encephalitis, the patient worked with an occupational therapist to follow a structured morning routine. This involved identifying the current step on a checklist, recalling which steps had already been completed (which had been ticked off last), reading the next step, and carrying it out with support. Although the patient continued to require a high level of guidance (also due to pronounced memory and attentional deficits), he was increasingly able to complete parts of the routine more reliably.

This example also shows that developing and reinforcing such daily routines should ideally be a collaborative effort within the interdisciplinary team, ensuring consistency across therapy sessions, nursing care, and home practice. When well-implemented, structured routines not only compensate for (some) executive dysfunction but also lay the groundwork for habit formation and long-term behavioral stability.

8.3.4.2 Goal management training in moderate to mild stages

In moderate to mild stages of recovery, the full GMT protocol may be employed (Table 8.5). This means that alongside the steps "Stop," "Define," and "Check," the steps "List" and "Learn" are added. "List"

TABLE 8.4 Environmental structuring and structured routines across recovery stages.

Component	Environmental modification	Structured routines
Severe stage	Distraction-free environment; minimal external stimulation; therapist provides full external structuring. *Example:* patient seated away from windows, desk cleared, doors closed, therapist maintains eye contact	Establishing predictability in time, space, and interaction (e.g., same therapist, consistent session start). Routines are therapist-guided. *Example:* starting each session with a visual-scanning task
Moderate to mild stage	Gradual reintroduction of mild distractors; reduced external control; support for generalization to real-world settings. *Example:* patient exposed to mild distractions (e.g., open window, some items on desk)	Expansion to more complex, multistep routines with greater independence. *Example:* morning routine with a checklist and an alarm clock used independently
External aids	Clocks, simple visual calendars, printed daily schedules, and orientation boards	Checklists, alarms, individualized planners, smartphone reminders, and written multistep plans

Note. This table outlines environmental structuring and structured routines across recovery stages, progressing from highly controlled, therapist-guided settings in the severe stage to more complex, independent routines in later stages, supported throughout by external aids.

refers to the process of breaking down the overarching goal into manageable subgoals, while "Learn" involves mentally rehearsing or encoding these substeps to ensure successful execution.

At this stage, patients are expected to engage in more internally driven strategy use, with less reliance on external cueing or therapist guidance. Accordingly, in addition to meeting the cognitive prerequisites for the simplified GMT protocol (see section 3.3), they should also demonstrate the following:

1. **Goal representation**—the ability to independently activate and maintain one or more overarching goals in mind over longer time spans (e.g., "I want to prepare lunch for my children today"), reflecting established goal-directed intention and task orientation across contexts [28].
2. **Goal recall and maintenance**—the capacity to consistently recall and verbally re-state goals throughout multistep tasks, demonstrating functional working memory and the ability to manage interruptions or competing stimuli [7,32].

TABLE 8.5 Structure and all phases of goal management training.

Step	Function/question	External aids	Potential add-on training	Goal
(1) Stop	"Pause and think - what am I doing right now, and is this the task I intended to work on?" → Can the patient accurately identify the current activity, link it to the overarching goal, and inhibit unrelated actions? *(sustained attention, working memory, inhibitory control)*	– Multimodal cues (e.g., verbal "stop" cue) – -Transitional auditory cues (e.g., tone)	– Inhibition training – Attentional control: sustained attention and selective attention tasks, visual scanning – Alertness cueing and training	– Reducing the need for the "Stop" cue – Reducing multimodality of cues – Increasing inhibitory control while increasing distractors
(2) Define	"What is my goal right now?" → Can the patient independently activate, verbalize, and maintain the overarching goal across time and contexts? *(goal representation, maintenance, strategic orientation)*	– Daily schedule or visual day plan – To-do lists	– Working memory training – -Spaced retrieval	– Improving goal clarity – Improving goal retention over time – Using real-life goals, if possible
(3) List	What steps will I need to take to reach my goal, and in what order should I do them? → Can the patient break the goal into logically sequenced, manageable subgoals and anticipate dependencies between them? *(planning, sequencing, problem-solving)*	– Checklists – Step-by-step visual guides	– Problem-solving training (e.g., problem-solving therapy (PST)) – Strategy training – Simplified planning tasks with reduced load	– Enhancing planning skills – Supporting structured sequencing

(*Continued*)

TABLE 8.5 (Continued)

Step	Function/question	External aids	Potential add-on training	Goal
(4) **Learn**	"How will I remember and keep track of these steps while I work? What will I do if I forget one?" → Can the patient mentally rehearse, encode, and plan retrieval of substeps using internal or external strategies? *(prospective memory, rehearsal, contingency planning)*	– Written or visual step lists – Checklists – Prospective memory prompts (e.g., notes, alarms)	– Spaced retrieval – Vanishing cues – Chunking strategies – Working memory training	– Improving recall of steps – Promoting internalization of the plan – Reducing step omissions
(5) **Check**	"Am I following my plan, and if not, what should I change to get back on track?"/"Did the outcome match what I intended, and what would I do differently next time?" → Can the patient monitor progress, detect deviations, and initiate corrective actions with minimal support? *(error monitoring, metacognitive insight, cognitive flexibility)*	– Checklists or tick boxes – Self-check prompts	– Prediction–performance comparison – Problem-solving training (e.g., PST) – Strategy training – Real-time error feedback	– Supporting performance monitoring – Increasing awareness of task-related errors – Promoting strategy adaptation (cognitive flexibility) – Promoting metacognitive reflection

Note. This table outlines the GMT protocol further adapted for moderate to mild rehabilitation of goal-directed disorders. It highlights core cognitive functions, external aids, and possible add-on training. The recommendations are based on clinical experience and supported by findings [32–39].

3. **Task segmentation and planning**—the ability to independently break-down complex goals into subgoals and organize them in a logical, goal-oriented sequence that one is able to follow with little support. This may involve the flexible use of internal strategies or external tools such as written plans or digital reminders, reflecting advanced planning and executive organization skills [28,33].
4. **Performance monitoring and self-correction**—the ability to detect and reflect on errors or inefficiencies during task execution, initiate corrective actions with minimal external prompts, and adjust strategies in response to ongoing task demands. This demonstrates developed self-monitoring, cognitive flexibility, and metacognitive insight [30,33].

Goal representation (Step 2) may be assessed by asking the patient to independently state an overarching goal they intend to pursue, without prior prompting of the content. Goal recall and maintenance (Step 2) may be checked by introducing short delays or mild distractions during a task and then asking the patient to repeat the original goal (i.e., assessing sufficient working memory capacity). In comparison to severe stages of goal-directed disorders, patients should show a more stable ability to repeat the original goal. If performance on this measure is unstable and interferes with subsequent steps of the full GMT protocol, targeted working memory training should be prioritized before progressing to the complete intervention. Regarding task segmentation and planning (Steps 3 and 4), the patient may be asked to outline the steps required to complete a routine task, such as making coffee. In addition, they should be able to correctly identify the step just completed (e.g., "I have now put the coffee in my cup") and the subsequent step, with or without external aids. Finally, performance monitoring (Step 5) can be evaluated by observing whether the patient notices and corrects task errors independently or with subtle prompting (e.g., by asking, "Did that go as planned?") during or after the activity. Possible add-on training options for each individual step in the full protocol, along with examples of external aids, are outlined in Table 8.5.

Additionally, as rehabilitation progresses, the goal is to gradually reduce the intensity and intrusiveness of external cues, fostering greater patient autonomy [34]. To this end, simpler auditory cues, such as a finger tap, a metronome click, or a brief tone, may be introduced to prompt self-initiation of the strategy. These cues can serve as transitional supports that reduce dependency on therapist presence while maintaining engagement with the GMT sequence [38]. Such cues can also later be used in context-independent settings, for instance, when patients want to implement these strategies independently [32].

In parallel, while early recovery phases often require minimizing environmental distractions, controlled reintroduction of distractions may be appropriate in a progressive manner. This gradual increase in environmental complexity can help train inhibitory control (Step 1) [34]. At the same time, gradually increasing distractors is also more similar to real life, thus helping the transition further.

The following training may be added to support greater autonomy in task execution:

1. **Selective attention and visual scanning**—target-detection tasks that require the patient to identify specific stimuli among distractors, implemented through paper-and-pencil (e.g., cancellation tasks) or computerized formats [33,34].
2. **Alertness and responsiveness**—adaptive reaction-time tasks or cued response formats that promote basic orienting and phasic alertness, typically delivered via computerized training programs [39].
3. **Inhibition and flexibility training**—tasks targeting impulsivity and perseveration, such as Go/No-Go or Stroop-like paradigms. These can be integrated into computerized cognitive control training programs [34].

Moreover, tasks may become increasingly complex and self-initiated, requiring patients to apply GMT principles across multiple settings, such as during activities of daily living. The integration of personal goals, such as preparing a meal, managing appointments, or engaging in social interactions, helps anchor the protocol in functionally meaningful behavior, which can enhance motivation and facilitate transfer to everyday life.

Crucially, given that many patients transition to the home environment without continued neuropsychological support, it is essential to prepare them with compensatory strategies (see the section on compensatory strategies) and foster independent self-management. Homework, for instance, can support this by helping patients apply executive strategies in their everyday environment, enhance metacognitive awareness, and foster long-term self-management [29].

Equally important is communication with subsequent care providers or outpatient therapists. Ensuring that these professionals are informed about the strategies and routines already established allows for continuity of care and supports the patient in maintaining and expanding their use of learned strategies. Without such communication, the patient may lose access to interventions that had begun to show effect or may be required to relearn tools already practiced.

8.3.5 Research on goal management training

Importantly, most research on GMT has been done in predominantly chronic acquired brain injury (ABI) populations. Thus research in stroke populations for postacute rehabilitation is limited. Moreover, existing studies are highly heterogeneous and often lack detailed reporting on intervention protocols, making direct comparisons and challenging generalization. Lastly, real-world outcomes are still under-researched and inconsistently reported. Still, the following research is worth noting:

A metaanalysis by Stamenova and Levine [30] demonstrated that GMT is effective as a stand-alone intervention for patients with ABIs, showing small to moderate improvements in EF, such as everyday executive tasks and working memory. The metaanalysis found no statistically significant differences in effectiveness between classic GMT and GMT delivered in combination with other therapeutic approaches (e.g., mindfulness, errorless learning). No significant differences were observed by neurological etiology. The analysis also suggested a dose–response relationship, with longer interventions (often in the range of around 20 hours in standard protocols) associated with stronger effects. Yet, the optimal frequency and spacing of sessions remain unclear, as these parameters were not systematically addressed. The largest effects were found for instrumental activities of daily living (iADL), which were partially sustained at follow-up (often ~5 months), with iADL outcomes remaining improved compared to baseline. However, while most effects were reduced at follow-up but remained statistically significant, subjective ratings of executive functioning by patients or proxies did not maintain statistical significance over time. Moreover, broader real-life outcomes, such as return to work or independent living, were not systematically evaluated in most studies, limiting the evidence for generalizability. Additionally, while time since injury may influence responsiveness to GMT, the metaanalysis noted that the stage of recovery was often either poorly defined or not reported and thus could not be systematically coded or analyzed. Taken together, the evidence supports GMT as a promising intervention, but highlights the need for more rigorous, long-term studies to clarify its most effective components, delivery formats, and real-world impact.

Conversely, Krasny–Pacini et al. [27] systematically examined studies on the effectiveness of GMT across various predominantly chronic ABI populations (mostly TBI or stroke), showing limited evidence for GMT as a stand-alone intervention with regard to ecological outcomes. They rightfully noted that using the same tasks for pretesting and posttesting risks inflating performance gains through practice effects and fails to assess a core feature of executive functioning—the ability to adapt flexibly to novel situations. Gains in everyday functioning were only found when GMT was combined with other components, such as fostering awareness, suggesting that it may be most effective in such contexts. Although the time since injury varied greatly across studies, the review did not examine whether the timing of GMT delivery (e.g., early vs late postinjury) influenced its effectiveness. Additionally, because most studies did not report the severity of dysexecutive functions, no conclusions about the effectiveness of GMT based on severity level can be drawn here either. Only a few studies included a follow-up, with follow-ups not being done later than 6 months. While some reported improvements were maintained, the evidence for long-term efficacy was limited.

Given the structure of GMT-like programs, it appears to be most effective when delivered over multiple sessions, typically at least 5 to 9. Stronger effects have been reported when total training time exceeds 15–20 hours. However, the optimal timing, spacing, and dosing of GMT remain to be systematically investigated. Clinical experience and recommendations support a more flexible, context-sensitive use of GMT, ideally embedded in tasks that closely mirror everyday activities [27]. In an adapted GMT format, Spikman et al. [33] showed that strategy-based interventions tailored to patients' personal goals and supported by therapist feedback resulted in significant improvements not only on trained tasks but also on ecologically valid measures (e.g., Zoo Map Test) of executive functioning. Likewise, Levine et al. [28] demonstrated that patients who completed GMT showed reduced errors and more goal-directed behavior during a meal preparation task, indicating improved real-life executive functioning. These improvements were maintained at 6-month follow-up, highlighting the potential for GMT to produce durable functional gains. However, the broader evidence base, particularly in early rehabilitation and across diverse neurological populations, remains mixed, and these limitations are discussed in later sections. Cantor et al. [37] likewise emphasized the importance of transferring trained skills to daily life in their adaptation of GMT for individuals with chronic EF deficits following TBI (12–14 years postinjury). Their intervention incorporated both homework and the systematic use of external aids, such as to-do lists, workbooks, and daily calendars, to promote strategy generalization beyond the therapy setting.

Given the diversity of patients with impairments in goal-directed behavior, GMT should not be seen as a one-size-fits-all intervention. Potential benefits of add-on training likely depend on the patient's individual profile, including cognitive reserve, stage of recovery, and specific deficits. Thus in clinical practice, add-on modules should be selected thoughtfully and tailored to the patient's needs (see Table 8.5 for specific recommendations). For example, patients who are prone to distraction or stimulus overload may benefit from attentional cueing (e.g., Novakovic–Agopian et al. [34]) or inhibition training, while those with planning difficulties may profit from additional problem-solving interventions (PST; e.g., Miotto et al. [39]) or structured task breakdown exercises.

However, function-specific training should be used as an *additional* intervention; it should not be used as a stand-alone treatment [6]. While improvements of such training may be observed on test-level performance, it is often unclear whether these gains translate into real-world behavior. Therefore ability-specific training is not recommended as a stand-alone intervention, but rather as part of a broader, integrated therapy concept (e.g., GMT).

8.3.6 Pharmacological approaches

According to current clinical guidelines, pharmacological treatment is not considered a first-line intervention for executive dysfunction following ABIs in general [6]. Medication may be considered as a complementary option and only in specific clinical contexts, such as in the presence of comorbid conditions like depression or drive disorders. In such cases, psychostimulants like methylphenidate or dopaminergic agents like amantadine may be used cautiously, though often off-label and based on individual symptom profiles.

8.4 Conclusion

The rehabilitation of goal-directed behavior after stroke requires a stage-sensitive approach that aligns intervention complexity with the patient's cognitive capacities.

In severe stages, intervention should combine externally structured routines, environmental modifications, and errorless learning with highly simplified GMT limited to *stop* (pause before acting), *define* (state the immediate task goal), and *check* (briefly verify progress) elements to foster basic goal maintenance and attentional control.

In moderate stages, a more elaborate but still therapist-guided GMT format can be applied, incorporating spaced retrieval, guided problem-solving, and attentional cueing to strengthen emerging self-monitoring skills. At this stage, partial internalization of key GMT steps, with reduced external prompting and more flexible application across tasks, becomes both a realistic therapeutic goal and an indicator of progress.

In mild stages, standardized GMT protocols embedded in ecologically valid contexts, combined with independent planning and self-monitoring exercises, can help facilitate autonomous goal management. At this stage, patients are able to engage with the complete GMT sequence and apply it flexibly in daily life, marking the entry into the "full GMT" domain where strategies are increasingly self-initiated and generalized across contexts. Add-on methods, such as noninvasive brain stimulation, may provide additional benefits, though the evidence remains preliminary. Future research should clarify optimal combinations, timing, and delivery formats for these approaches, ensuring that structured training leads to durable improvements in everyday goal-directed functioning.

References

[1] Passingham RE. The frontal lobes and voluntary action. New York: Oxford University Press; 1993.
[2] Bonelli RM, Cummings JL. Frontal-subcortical circuitry and behavior. Dialogues Clin Neurosci 2007;9(2):141–51.
[3] Diamond A. Executive functions. Annu Rev Psychol 2013;64:135–68.
[4] Ambrosini E, Arbula S, Rossato C, Pacella V, Vallesi A. Neuro-cognitive architecture of executive functions: a latent variable analysis. Cortex 2019;119:441–56.
[5] Mueller JA, Dollaghan C. A systematic review of assessments for identifying executive function impairment in adults with acquired brain injury. J Speech Lang Hear Res 2013;56(3):1051–64.
[6] Müller S., Klein J., German clinical guidelines on executive function rehabilitation. https://registerawmforg/de/leitlinien/detail/030-125, 2019.
[7] Stuss DT, Alexander MP. Is there a dysexecutive syndrome? Philos Trans R Soc Lond B Biol Sci 2007;362(1481):901–15.
[8] Bush G, Luu P, Posner MI. Cognitive and emotional influences in anterior cingulate cortex. Trends Cogn Sci 2000;4(6):215–22.
[9] Rorden C, Bonilha L, Fridriksson J, Bender B, Karnath HO. Age-specific CT and MRI templates for spatial normalization. Neuroimage 2012;61(4):957–65.
[10] Tekin S, Cummings JL. Frontal-subcortical neuronal circuits and clinical neuropsychiatry: an update. J Psychosom Res 2002;53(2):647–54.
[11] Schoenberg MR, Scott JG. The little black book of neuropsychology: a syndrome-based approach. Springer US; 2016.
[12] Rolls ET, Cheng W, Feng J. The orbitofrontal cortex: reward, emotion and depression. Brain Commun 2020;2(2):fcaa196.
[13] Alexander GE, DeLong MR, Strick PL. Parallel organization of functionally segregated circuits linking basal ganglia and cortex. Annu Rev Neurosci 1986;9:357–81.
[14] Gallucci L, Sperber C, Guggisberg AG, et al. Post-stroke cognitive impairment remains highly prevalent and disabling despite state-of-the-art stroke treatment. Int J Stroke 2024;19(8):888–97.
[15] Lesniak M, Bak T, Czepiel W, Seniow J, Czlonkowska A. Frequency and prognostic value of cognitive disorders in stroke patients. Dement Geriatr Cogn Disord 2008;26(4):356–63.
[16] Nys GM, van Zandvoort MJ, de Kort PL, et al. The prognostic value of domain-specific cognitive abilities in acute first-ever stroke. Neurology 2005;64(5):821–7.
[17] Rasquin SM, Lodder J, Ponds RW, Winkens I, Jolles J, Verhey FR. Cognitive functioning after stroke: a one-year follow-up study. Dement Geriatr Cogn Disord 2004;18(2):138–44.
[18] Kusi-Mensah K, Nuamah ND, Wemakor S, et al. Assessment tools for executive function and adaptive function following brain pathology among children in developing country contexts: a scoping review of current tools. Neuropsychol Rev 2022;32(3):459–82.
[19] Stuss DT, Levine B. Adult clinical neuropsychology: lessons from studies of the frontal lobes. Annu Rev Psychol 2002;53:401–33.

[20] Duncan J, Parr A, Woolgar A, et al. Goal neglect and Spearman's g: competing parts of a complex task. J Exp Psychol Gen 2008;137(1):131–48.
[21] Bhandari A, Duncan J. Goal neglect and knowledge chunking in the construction of novel behaviour. Cognition 2014;130(1):11–30.
[22] Cicerone KD, Goldin Y, Ganci K, et al. Evidence-based cognitive rehabilitation: systematic review of the literature from 2009 through 2014. Arch Phys Med Rehabil 2019;100(8):1515–33.
[23] Cicerone KD, Langenbahn DM, Braden C, et al. Evidence-based cognitive rehabilitation: updated review of the literature from 2003 through 2008. Arch Phys Med Rehabil 2011;92(4):519–30.
[24] Shallice T, Burgess PW. Deficits in strategy application following frontal lobe damage in man. Brain 1991;114(Pt 2):727–41.
[25] Evans JJ. 59 Rehabilitation of executive functioning: an overview. In: Oddy M, Worthington A, Oddy M, Worthington A, editors. Rehabilitation of executive disorders: a guide to theory and practice. Oxford University Press; 2008. p. 0.
[26] Levine B, Stuss DT, Winocur G, et al. Cognitive rehabilitation in the elderly: effects on strategic behavior in relation to goal management. J Int Neuropsychol Soc 2007;13(1):143–52.
[27] Krasny-Pacini A, Chevignard M, Evans J. Goal Management Training for rehabilitation of executive functions: a systematic review of effectiveness in patients with acquired brain injury. Disabil Rehabil 2014;36(2):105–16.
[28] Levine B, Robertson IH, Clare L, et al. Rehabilitation of executive functioning: an experimental-clinical validation of goal management training. J Int Neuropsychol Soc 2000;6(3):299–312.
[29] Levine B, Schweizer TA, O'Connor C, et al. Rehabilitation of executive functioning in patients with frontal lobe brain damage with goal management training. Front Hum Neurosci 2011;5:9.
[30] Stamenova V, Levine B. Effectiveness of goal management training(R) in improving executive functions: a meta-analysis. Neuropsychol Rehabil 2019;29(10):1569–99.
[31] Eslinger PJ, Flaherty-Craig CV, Chakara FM. Rehabilitation and management of executive function disorders. Handb Clin Neurol 2013;110:365–76.
[32] Fish J, Evans JJ, Nimmo M, et al. Rehabilitation of executive dysfunction following brain injury: "content-free" cueing improves everyday prospective memory performance. Neuropsychologia 2007;45(6):1318–30.
[33] Spikman JM, Boelen DH, Lamberts KF, Brouwer WH, Fasotti L. Effects of a multifaceted treatment program for executive dysfunction after acquired brain injury on indications of executive functioning in daily life. J Int Neuropsychol Soc 2010;16(1):118–29.
[34] Novakovic-Agopian T, Chen AJ, Rome S, et al. Rehabilitation of executive functioning with training in attention regulation applied to individually defined goals: a pilot study bridging theory, assessment, and treatment. J Head Trauma Rehabil 2011;26(5):325–38.
[35] Emmanouel A, Kontrafouri E, Nikolaos P, Kessels RPC, Fasotti L. Incorporation of a working memory strategy in GMT to facilitate serial-order behaviour in brain-injured patients. Neuropsychol Rehabil 2020;30(5):888–914.
[36] Chung CS, Pollock A, Campbell T, Durward BR, Hagen S. Cognitive rehabilitation for executive dysfunction in adults with stroke or other adult non-progressive acquired brain damage. Cochrane Database Syst Rev 2013;2013(4):CD008391.
[37] Cantor J, Ashman T, Dams-O'Connor K, et al. Evaluation of the short-term executive plus intervention for executive dysfunction after traumatic brain injury: a randomized controlled trial with minimization. Arch Phys Med Rehabil 2014;95(1):1–9. e3.

[38] Manly T, Hawkins K, Evans J, Woldt K, Robertson IH. Rehabilitation of executive function: facilitation of effective goal management on complex tasks using periodic auditory alerts. Neuropsychologia 2002;40(3):271–81.
[39] Miotto EC, Evans JJ, de Lucia MC, Scaff M. Rehabilitation of executive dysfunction: a controlled trial of an attention and problem solving treatment group. Neuropsychol Rehabil 2009;19(4):517–40.

CHAPTER

9

Rehabilitation of disorders of consciousness

9.1 Introduction

Disorders of consciousness refer to a group of conditions in which patients experience severely restricted abilities to voluntarily interact with their environment due to an acute functional or severe structural brain damage. These disorders have various causes, including stroke, hemorrhage, global hypoxia, traumatic brain injury (TBI), and severe encephalitis. Given the severity of these conditions, patients often require immediate and specialized care through early neurological rehabilitation, as progression to later stages of rehabilitation may not be possible at this stage. This level of care required is typically determined pragmatically using standardized assessment tools such as the Early Rehabilitation Barthel Index (Schonle [1]).

9.2 Diagnostic entities and clinical description

The terminology used to classify syndromes under disorders of consciousness has changed over the past decades (for the following sections, compare: [2–4]). Whereas earlier terms were primarily based on known or suggested causes, such as "post-anoxic coma," the focus has shifted toward describing the most evident symptoms and the essential steps toward recovery. Several disorders of consciousness exist, and they can be viewed as different states through which a patient may progress on the path to full consciousness. However, each disorder can also exist independently, and patients may remain in a particular state permanently.

9.2.1 Comatose state

In a comatose state, the patient is unconscious, with eyes continuously closed and no observable sleep–wake cycle. There is a complete lack of

Applied Neuropsychology of Cerebrovascular Diseases
DOI: https://doi.org/10.1016/B978-0-443-45450-9.00007-2

environmental awareness, evidenced by the absence of responses to visual or auditory stimuli and no ability to communicate or express emotions. The depth of unresponsiveness is such that the patient cannot be awakened by any external means. Vital functions often require support because the brainstem, which regulates essential autonomic processes such as respiration, cardiovascular control, and arousal, is frequently impaired. For instance, breathing may be supported via mechanical ventilation, and other vital functions, such as blood pressure and heart rate, are maintained pharmacologically. If the patient survives this comatose state following brain injury, they may either regain consciousness or transition into unresponsive wakefulness syndrome (UWS).

9.2.2 Unresponsive wakefulness syndrome

Previously referred to as vegetative state or apallic syndrome, UWS is characterized by wakefulness without signs of awareness. In contrast to coma, patients with UWS display a spontaneous sleep–wake cycle, marked by alternating periods of eye opening and closing. Additionally, they typically breathe independently, without the need for mechanical assistance, and display pain-related movements. However, despite this increase in arousal and the return of some spontaneous physiological functions, patients, similar to those in a comatose state, show no purposeful response to environmental stimuli. For instance, despite eye opening, they do not visually fixate on objects, nor do they display goal-directed behavior in response to auditory cues or gentle tactile stimulation. In conclusion, UWS is a state between complete unconsciousness and wakefulness without purposeful interaction.

9.2.2.1 Diagnosing unresponsive wakefulness syndrome

Diagnosing UWS remains challenging, as signs of consciousness are often subtle, inconsistent, or delayed, sometimes emerging only after prolonged or structured stimulation. These signs can easily go unnoticed or be misinterpreted, contributing to a misdiagnosis rate of up to 43% of all cases [5]. In an early study on what was then termed the apallic syndrome (now referred to as UWS), Gerstenbrand [6] and Gerstenbrand [7] identified additional clinical features that could help distinguish UWS from coma, including spasticity, stereotyped motor patterns, and abnormalities in eye movement.

Firstly, patients with UWS typically exhibit generalized, spastic increases in muscle tone, while patients in a coma tend to be hypotonic, meaning they display abnormally low muscle tone. Although these motor patterns appear to offer a useful distinction, they more accurately reflect the duration of the condition rather than the level of consciousness.

Specifically, spasticity in UWS tends to develop gradually over weeks. Consequently, muscle tone abnormalities are unreliable for cross-sectional assessments, particularly in the acute phase following brain injury. Secondly, the presence of disinhibited motor templates, stereotyped, automatic movement patterns not driven by conscious intention, is considered a negative prognostic sign because it reflects a loss of cortical control and the dominance of primitive, subcortical motor patterns, indicating severe disruption of conscious motor regulation. The ability to fixate on or follow objects with the eyes indicates progression toward a minimally conscious state (MCS) (once reliably reproducible, it meets CRS-R criteria for an MCS) [81], as it reflects the emergence of goal-directed behavior; in line with the theoretical framework discussed below, such eye movements are better understood as purposeful actions rather than mere features of motor (dys)function. Thus these distinctions (motor templates and eye movements) are more prognostically relevant than spasticity (due to duration of the state), with motor templates favoring a negative prognosis, and the beginning of eye opening and following indicating a positive development.

Another example of diagnostically significant behavior is the startle response. Many patients with UWS still exhibit a reflexive startle to sudden, intense acoustic stimuli. In healthy individuals, a reduction of the startle response following repeated presentations of sudden acoustic stimuli, known as prepulse inhibition [8,9], reflects normal sensory gating. By definition, patients with UWS should not be able to develop expectations and, thus exhibit habituation. Therefore the emergence of a diminished startle response after repeated stimulation is considered a positive indicator for some recovery. In other words, as soon as a patient's responses begin to change in anticipation of a stimulus, the strict diagnostic criteria for UWS are no longer fulfilled.

Electrophysiology offers a methodological counterpart for the behavioral observation of habituation. In particular, absent cortical somatosensory evoked potentials unexplained by lesions of the lemniscus lateralis are associated with almost 100% negative prognosis concerning reawakening from unresponsive wakefulness [10]. The measurement of the P3 component, a specific brain wave pattern, alternates between frequent and infrequent acoustic stimuli while recording associated electrocortical responses. Two components are of special interest: mismatch negativity (MMN), which consistently arises when an automatic expectation of environmental regularity is violated, and P3, which also responds to deviations from expectation but is more closely linked to conscious attention. Notably, MMN and P3 components have been detected in a subset of patients previously diagnosed with UWS [11–14], which are associated with a better prognosis.

Finally, it is important to note that bilateral brainstem involvement, as can be detected through evoked potential methods, is considered an unfavorable prognostic sign. Conversely, preserved responsiveness of the autonomic nervous system is regarded as a favorable prognostic factor in comatose patients following TBI [15,16].

9.2.3 Minimally conscious state

A minimally conscious state (MCS) is characterized by intermittent but reproducible signs of awareness, distinguishing it from both coma and UWS. These signs may include orienting toward sounds or visual stimuli and recognizing familiar objects. Occasionally, patients may reach for objects upon request, follow simple commands, utter words, or display emotional reactions. However, these responses are typically inconsistent, and due to marked fluctuations in responsiveness, functional communication is not yet possible. A patient is considered to have emerged from the MCS once they can consistently and accurately respond to basic yes/no questions (e.g., "am I clapping my hands right now [clap]?", "Am I touching my nose right now [touch ear]?") or correctly use at least two different familiar objects (e.g., a spoon and a pencil) [81].

MCS is now frequently subcategorized into MCS plus (MCS+) and MCS minus (MCS–), based on the presence or absence of behavioral signs of preserved language functions. This subclassification was initially proposed to have clinical relevance, as patients classified as MCS+, who begin to respond appropriately to questions, demonstrated less functional disability on standardized outcome measures compared to those in MCS–. However, a recent metaanalytic review and a large longitudinal study found no significant differences between the groups [17,18].

As a result, categorizing a patient as being in an MCS– solely based on their inability to respond accurately to verbal questions, may be misleading. This behavior does not reliably reflect the patient's level of consciousness or potential for recovery. For example, failure to respond may stem from profound language impairments (e.g., aphasia) or difficulties initiating speech. When structural damage affects brain regions essential for language processing, an electrophysiological assessment of speech comprehension should be incorporated into the diagnostic process. If impaired comprehension is confirmed, clinical interaction and evaluation should prioritize nonverbal indicators of awareness.

9.2.3.1 Differential diagnosis

MCS is defined both descriptively and as a sequence of evolving stages of recovery. When defined descriptively, it must be carefully distinguished from other syndromes that share similar outward features but are based on different underlying causes. Four syndromes in particular must be differentiated from MCS for this reason: global aphasia, locked-in syndrome, akinetic mutism, and stupor-like drive disorders.

Firstly, global aphasia accompanied by attentional fluctuation can resemble MCS. These patients may appear similar to MCS patients, as they exhibit only basic signs of awareness and are unable to engage in language-based tasks. However, in such cases, their incoherent or absent responses are primarily due to fundamental disorders of language comprehension.

Secondly, locked-in syndrome (see Chapter 2 for a case presentation) is defined by an inability to communicate due to anarthria, meaning (near-) complete paralysis of the muscles required for speech, and tetraplegia. Despite their profound motor impairment, patients with locked-in syndrome are fully conscious and often able to respond using eye movements. Due to sparing of cranial nerves III and IV, basic communication is often possible using vertical eye movements. However, many exhibit fluctuating attention or somnolence, which can complicate diagnosis. A specific subgroup of locked-in patients is additionally unable to respond even with eye movements for communication, a condition termed cognitive motor dissociation syndrome [4,19]. Still, signs of consciousness can be detected using brain-computer interface techniques. Thus it is important to use additional diagnostic tools to avoid overlooking signs of consciousness in patients with severe motor impairments.

The third and fourth syndromes, akinetic mutism and stupor-like drive disorder, will be discussed in the following sections.

9.2.4 Akinetic mutism

Akinetic mutism is a disorder characterized by a severe reduction in the initiation of spontaneous and goal-directed behavior, while motor responses in highly automated contexts remain largely preserved [20,21]. Although patients may process external information to a large extent, they are unable to respond to stimuli intentionally. For instance, they may show automatic head and eye movements toward salient stimuli, and their gaze often conveys a sense of interest in the environment. Additionally, in familiar, highly automated situations, such as grasping for a salient object, they may respond in a seemingly normal and coordinated way. However, when responses require deliberate initiation, this ability is markedly impaired. An example of this is the asymmetry often observed between grasping and releasing movements. While grasping can be triggered reflexively and tends to be preserved, releasing an object demands voluntary control and conscious intent. As a result, patients with akinetic mutism may grasp another person's outstretched hand but are unable to let it go without external prompting. This dissociation between preserved automatic motor execution and impaired volitional control highlights the core deficit of the condition: a breakdown in the initiation of intentional action.

Akinetic mutism has been explained by the existence of two distinct pathways to action [22]. The first pathway is automatic and stimulus-driven. Actions in this pathway are characterized by stereotypy and a fixed coupling to specific environmental features. These connections remain intact in akinetic mutism and account for the patient's automatic responses to specific stimuli. However, since these automatic processes can no longer be inhibited by medial brain areas, actions such as grasping can still be initiated but not voluntarily aborted. Furthermore, intact lateral connections and preserved association areas allow these patients to develop relatively accurate expectations about their environment. Accordingly, a P3 component can often be detected in electrophysiological recordings, although it may be significantly delayed or reduced in latency and amplitude.

The second path to action involves the generation of internal ideas and decisions about target states. This pathway integrates intentions, long-term emotional evaluations (beyond immediate affects), and motivational components. For spontaneous and goal-directed behavior to occur, this second pathway must be intact. It enables the organization of chains of action and flexible shifts in behavior according to overarching goals. This model argues for the existence of a supervisory attentional system, which not only monitors actions but also selects behavioral schemes based on internal goals [23]. In akinetic mutism, it is precisely this latter system that is impaired, resulting in the absence of actions not directly triggered by environmental stimuli. Consequently, patients with akinetic mutism suffer less from a general lack of drive and more from an inability to initiate actions based on internal states (see Table 9.1).

In later, more advanced stages of recovery, patients with akinetic mutism often present with speech comprehension difficulties, working memory impairments, reduced overall memory performance, and a pronounced tendency toward perseveration. These impairments can make tasks such as writing and arithmetic nearly impossible. Additionally, patients frequently display marked distractibility and a tendency to violate rules during structured activities. These symptoms can be attributed to impaired internal control mechanisms: without adequate internal inhibition, environmental stimuli and sometimes internal goals are processed almost directly and impulsively. For example, a patient might name the back of a card they are supposed to memorize because they can no longer recall the actual, covered image, or might move game pieces incorrectly in an impulsive attempt to reach a desired goal.

TABLE 9.1 Disorders of consciousness and their mimics.

Diagnosis	Characteristics	Neuroanatomical cause
Unresponsive wakefulness syndrome (UWS)	• No visible reaction to external stimuli, except possibly to painful stimuli • Sleep-wake cycles preserved • Diagnosis should only be made after verifying the persistence of the condition • Assessment should include observations before and after activating interventions • No habituation and P3 response detectable	Severe cortical damage, especially in the dorsofrontal cortical areas, usually with additional thalamic and/or basal ganglia lesions. Large MCA hemorrhage, hypoxia, or severe traumatic brain injury (TBI)
Akinetic mutism	• Sleep-wake cycles preserved • Environmental events are perceived • No intentional movements, but automatic movements occur in corresponding contexts (e.g., hand closure without hand opening) • No emotional avoidance of stimuli; no emotional aversion toward stimuli; no emotional disengagement from stimuli • P3 response detectable	Lesions in the supplementary motor cortex or premotor cortex, unilateral left-brain lesion is sufficient in principle (e.g., large anterior infarction (left) or nontraumatic SAH as a result of an ACOA aneurysm)
Stupor-like drive disorder	• Sleep-wake cycles preserved • Environmental events are perceived • Intentional movements are rare; automatic movements cannot be triggered significantly more frequently • Emotional withdrawal away from stimulus • P3 response detectable	Lesions in the area of the ventromedial and dorsolateral prefrontal cortex, head of the caudate; usually bilateral lesions, in which case the right hemisphere must be clearly affected (TBI)

Note: unresponsive wakefulness syndrome (UWS), akinetic mutism, stupor-like drive disorder, their characteristics, and neuroanatomical causes. SAH = subarachnoid hemorrhage. ACOA = aneurysm of the anterior communicating artery. TBI = traumatic brain injury. MCA = middle cerebral artery.

9.2.5 Stupor-like drive disorder

A condition that at first glance closely resembles akinetic mutism, but must be carefully distinguished from it, is severe drive disorder (also referred to as "apathy" or "abulia"). In this condition, patients appear mute, immobile, and unresponsive, even though they are capable of initiating actions [24]. The reduction in activity is attributed to a profound loss of drive or motivation due to damage in brain areas responsible for motivational processes, rather than deficits in action initiation. Unlike in akinetic mutism, there is typically no active eye movement toward external stimuli; facial expressions remain rigid, and both facial and bodily gestures clearly signal a lack of interest in the environment.

Patients may either fail to react altogether or actively turn away when addressed, as evidenced by behaviors such as firmer mouth closure and slow, deliberate movements of the head and body. They may also refuse food despite being physically capable of eating and therefore must be fed. Even when they open their mouths for solid food, chewing movements are often minimal, and swallowing may not occur. Importantly, the behavior is not due to physical dysfunction, but rather a breakdown in the association between goal representation and action initiation.

Therefore in purely clinical terms, these patients may resemble individuals in a stupor [25]: a state of extreme unresponsiveness despite wakefulness. In some cases, their presentation even closely mimics catatonic stupor, a subtype of catatonia seen in psychiatric conditions. However, a key distinction lies in motor tone and response to passive movement. While catatonia is often marked by waxy flexibility, where limbs maintain the position in which they are placed, patients with stupor-like drive disorder typically display increased or spastic muscle tone, which Gerstenbrand [6] and Gerstenbrand [7] referred to as rigido-spasticity.

These patients resist passive movement, not due to catatonic features, but due to pathologically elevated muscle tone from underlying neurological damage.

Resistance to passive movement in these patients is therefore a combination of pathologically elevated muscle tone due to underlying neurological damage and negativistic behavior [26]. Patients with stupor-like drive disorder may refuse almost all forms of communication, demonstrating pronounced negativism. This reflects a lack of drive or motivation, rather than the psychomotor and behavioral syndrome typical of catatonia.

Such severe drive disorders can also be accompanied by, or even caused by, depression, particularly in its most severe forms. In this context, the diagnosis of depression should only be made on the basis of observable, objective signs, as a direct psychopathological assessment of subjective experiences is typically not possible.

Stupor-like drive disorder can closely resemble the clinical presentation of patients in a UWS transitioning into an MCS. This similarity places individuals with psychogenic stupor at particular risk of being misdiagnosed as being in a MCS in times before the existence of brain imaging techniques [27,28]. However, patients with stupor-like drive disorder may, in certain situations, demonstrate brief but appropriate verbal responses or engage purposefully in caregiving activities—signs that suggest at least partially preserved information intake and cognitive processing.

The fact that patients with stupor-like drive disorders engage in virtually no behavior that could improve their situation suggests that the association between reward and action is no longer intact. Earlier psychiatric classifications distinguished three forms of stupor-like drive behavior: (1) transient perplexed inhibition, (2) depressive inhibition, and (3) catatonic stupor, with the first being described as fully reversible [25]. Against this background, stupor-like drive disorders may be further differentiated into those with a predominantly depressive or negativistic component and those without direct psychopathological features, in which the generation of goal-directed ideas is impaired. This distinction corresponds to Jasper's [25] classification of depressive inhibition and catatonic stupor.

Patients with stupor-like drive disorder exhibit symptoms similar to what [29,30] described as severe learned helplessness. In his experiments, animals were exposed to uncontrollable electric shocks, meaning the shocks occurred regardless of their behavior. As a result, any behavior became pointless: after an initial phase of intense avoidance activity, the animals eventually ceased all attempts to act. Seligman [29], Seligman et al. [30] observed that the animals had to be physically pulled out of the cages repeatedly in order to relearn that their actions could positively influence their situation—that is, to regain spontaneous activity.

In cognitive terms, the animals lost their understanding of causally effective behaviors. Such understanding is crucial for the formulation of anticipated goals, which must precede and guide goal-directed action. In stupor-like drive disorders, a similar mechanism is proposed: interest in the external environment fades, attention shifts inward, and the ability to represent actions as effective in achieving goals is lost. Two essential cognitive components of stupor-like drive disorders are thus (1) the representation of every action as ineffective for achieving reward and (2) the loss of the ability to mentally represent goal-directed actions.

9.3 Neuroanatomical causes of disorders of consciousness

Disorders of consciousness, such as UWS, akinetic mutism, and stupor-like drive disorders, are characterized by profound disruptions in awareness, responsiveness, or goal-directed behavior. Although these conditions may appear similar in their clinical presentation, they arise from distinct neuroanatomical substrates and pathophysiological

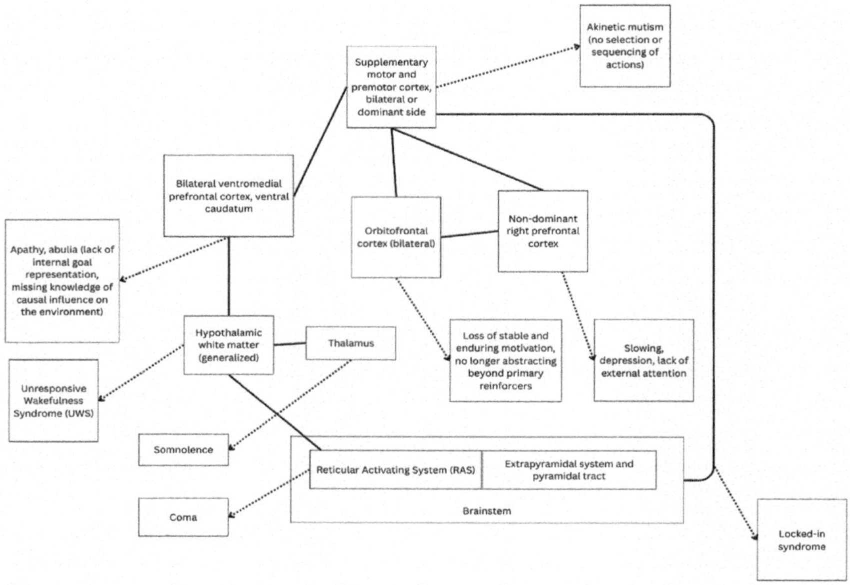

FIGURE 9.1 Diagram of disorders of consciousness and neuroanatomical correlates. *Note.* Correlates of neuropathology with disorders of consciousness. In the diagram, dashed lines represent disorders or symptoms, whereas solid lines represent connections between brain regions [42]. *Source: This figure is originally derived from Hildebrandt H. Neuropsychologische Frührehabilitation: Ein differenzielles Behandlungskonzept für schwerstbeeinträchtigte Patienten. Z für Neuropsychologie 2002;13:91–110.*

mechanisms (see Fig. 9.1). Understanding the underlying brain structures involved is essential for improving diagnostic precision and tailoring therapeutic strategies. Neuroimaging and neuropathological studies have shown that different forms of disorders of consciousness are associated with damage to specific cortical and subcortical regions, including the brainstem, thalamus, and prefrontal networks. The following sections outline the current evidence on the anatomical correlates of UWS, akinetic mutism, and stupor-like drive disorder, highlighting both shared and distinct mechanisms contributing to impaired consciousness and goal-directed behavior.

9.3.1 Unresponsive wakefulness syndrome and minimally conscious state

The definitions of UWS and MCS are based purely on clinical criteria, such as the (non)existence of purposeful behaviors. However, a decoupling of cortical activity from the subcortical arousal system has been discussed as a potential underlying mechanism of UWS. Gerstenbrand

[6,7,31] suggested that decoupling occurs above the hypothalamus at the level of the midbrain, allowing for a spontaneous sleep-wake rhythm, albeit with a reduction in the different sleep stages [32]. Nevertheless, patients with UWS caused by isolated interruption of pathways between the brainstem and cerebral cortex are extremely rare in clinical practice and have been only scarcely described in scientific literature (for an exception, see Chapter 2).

9.3.1.1 *Scientific literature on unresponsive wakefulness syndrome and minimally conscious state*

Most studies investigating the neural correlates of UWS have focused on patients with TBI and anoxic brain injury. However, both conditions result in diffuse rather than focal lesions, making it difficult to identify specific lesions that are both necessary and sufficient to explain the clinical symptoms. In contrast, only about 10%–15% of patients with UWS have suffered a stroke or a nontraumatic subarachnoid hemorrhage. This subgroup offers a valuable opportunity to more precisely identify the brain structures associated with UWS. However, since this subgroup represents only a small proportion of UWS cases, drawing firm conclusions about specific lesion-symptom relationships remains challenging.

In a recent study, Medina Carrion et al. [14] analyzed brain network activity in 99 patients diagnosed with UWS or a MCS using functional magnetic resonance imaging (fMRI)-based measures [33]. They identified distinct functional brain networks (see Fig. 9.2) and assessed which

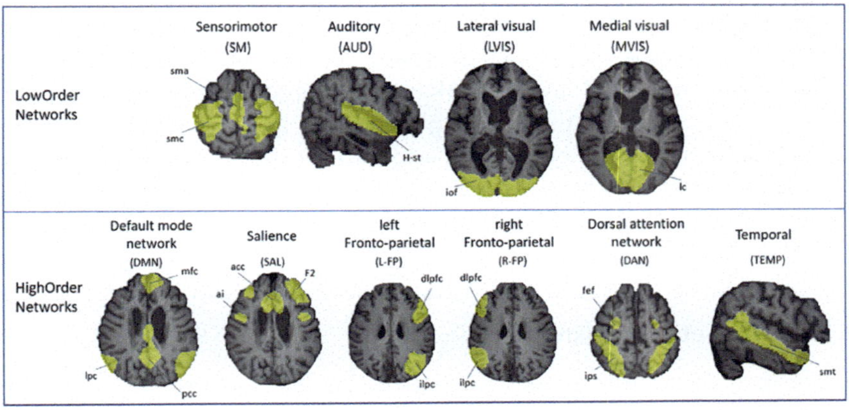

FIGURE 9.2 Templates of low-order and high-order brain networks. *From Medina Carrion J.P., Stanziano M., D'Incerti L., Sattin D., Palermo S., Ferraro S. et al. Disorder of consciousness: structural integrity of brain networks for the clinical assessment. Ann Clin Transl Neurol 2023;10(3):384–396. https://doi.org/10.1002/acn3.51729.*

networks differed between the two patient groups. In TBI and anoxic patients, no significant differences in network activity were found between those with UWS and those in a MCS (although differences were observed compared to a third group of severely impaired but conscious patients). In the TBI and anoxic subgroups, coma recovery scores correlated with lower-order brain networks associated with motor and auditory systems, but not with higher-order cortical systems involved in consciousness.

In contrast, among patients with vascular aetiologies, which encompassed around 30 patients in this study, only two brain networks showed correlations with the coma recovery scale: the auditory network and the salience network. Notably, the salience network also distinguished between UWS and MCS across the entire sample. This network is based on interactions between the anterior insula and the anterior cingulate gyrus and dorsal prefrontal cortices. Thus in patients with vascular lesions, this study demonstrated that bilateral disturbances in premotor, prefrontal, and limbic networks are primarily associated with clinical status and recovery potential. In other words, in patients with focal vascular brain damage, the integrity of higher-order networks, particularly the salience network involved in conscious awareness and goal-directed behavior, is crucial for distinguishing levels of consciousness (UWS vs MCS) and predicting recovery.

It should also be noted that patients with a vascular cause of UWS or MCS tend to have better outcomes compared to patients with anoxic brain injury, and their prognosis is similar to that of TBI patients. Furthermore, age appears to be a major factor influencing recovery, although it does not significantly impact mortality risk [18].

The finding by Medina Carrion et al. [14] is consistent with earlier studies that demonstrated that virtually all patients with UWS show severe brain damage in cortical areas (Gerstenbrand et al. [6,7], [12,31,33,34]). Many of these patients, but not all, also exhibit damage to the thalamus or basal ganglia. In addition, electrophysiological studies have shown that the brainstem can also be affected, despite the presence of a sleep-wake rhythm, [32] particularly in cases where the injuries are due to severe TBI [35].

9.3.2 Akinetic mutism

The neuroanatomical basis of akinetic mutism is typically found in lesions to the dorsomedial areas of the frontal cortex, specifically in the supplementary motor area (SMA) and the presupplementary motor cortex. These areas are involved in the initiation and planning of voluntary movement and internally generated actions. However, rare cases involving bilateral thalamic lesions have also been described [20], particularly when the anterior thalamic nuclei, which are connected to the prefrontal cortex and limbic structures, are affected [36].

Akinetic mutism most commonly occurs following an infarction of the anterior cerebral artery (ACA) or a dorsal watershed infarct involving both the middle cerebral artery (MCA) and the ACA, as these strokes damage parts of the SMA and dorsomedial areas of the premotor cortex. In certain cases, falx meningiomas, tumors arising from the falx cerebri, can also cause akinetic mutism. Unlike vascular lesions, these tumors may develop gradually and can mimic the syndrome by exerting pressure on the SMA or adjacent areas. Finally, unilateral infarctions, especially when affecting the left hemisphere, may cause a more transient form of akinetic mutism.

The SMA and premotor areas are physiologically central to the generation of readiness potentials and the so-called contingent negative variation [37]. Both phenomena are negative shifts in the electroencephalography (EEG) that occur in anticipation of a voluntary, purposeful action [38–40]. In simpler terms, these cortical areas prepare the brain for action; lesions in these regions disrupt the ability to anticipate and initiate voluntary movements.

The medial localization of the affected cortical cells in the frontal lobe is significant, as it reflects particularly strong input from both the visceral centers and the limbic system. This close anatomical and functional connection is illustrated by the cingulate gyrus, a key limbic structure, which lies directly inferior to the SMA. Through this anatomical relationship, the brain is able to integrate information about the current bodily state (factual conditions) with desired goals (target states). This comparison is essential for initiating purposeful action; without it, there is no drive to engage in goal-directed behaviour. Passingham [41] demonstrated this principle experimentally. In animal studies, monkeys were trained to raise their arm spontaneously, that is, without stimulus coupling, to obtain food. Following lesions in the dorsomedial frontal cortex, this behavior almost completely disappeared, although stimulus-coupled behavior (grasping for food visible in the direction of the spontaneous behavior) remained intact. Thus after lesions in this area, information from the environment and the body may still be registered but loses its motivational significance—it no longer triggers spontaneous, goal-directed behavior.

9.3.3 Stupor-like drive disorder

Stupor-like drive disorders can develop directly as a consequence of TBI but may also emerge as residual symptoms in patients recovering from previous UWS [24,42,43]. Functional imaging studies have shown that the anterior prefrontal cortex becomes active when the brain engages in a specific processing mode, namely the generation and maintenance of goals or target states. When this region is bilaterally damaged, patients may lose the ability to generate goals in response to environmental demands. This deficit represents a far more profound limitation than in akinetic mutism, as it reflects a complete breakdown of goal formation itself. Patients are not merely unable to act on internal goals but are incapable of generating purposeful intent in the first place.

If a patient's withdrawal from the environment appears active, accompanied by clinical signs such as negativism or features of depression [43], the orbitofrontal cortex may also be implicated. Rolls [44] and Rolls [45] described centers within the orbitofrontal cortex that are responsible for signaling internal states of need and satiety. Neurons in this region become active when specific physical or social needs arise (e.g., hunger, the need for social attention) and decrease their activity when these needs are satisfied ("satiety"). In this process, the orbitofrontal cortex interacts closely with both the amygdala and anterior prefrontal cortex, forming a network that evaluates the motivational relevance of internal and external stimuli. Corresponding activity in the orbitofrontal cortex has also been demonstrated in humans using functional imaging techniques [46]. Additionally, altered activity in the orbitofrontal cortex and right prefrontal structures has been observed in patients with psychiatric depression [47]. Clinically, loss of appetite and significant weight loss are recognized as one of the physical hallmark symptoms of depression. Taken together, these findings suggest that the active withdrawal from environmental events seen in patients with stupor-like drive disorder could, at least in part, reflect a deficient representation of internal needs resulting from orbitofrontal cortex lesions.

9.4 Treatment of disorders of consciousness

It is no coincidence that improving attention has traditionally been regarded as a core objective in patients with severe disorders of consciousness [24,48–53]. Explicitly or implicitly, the prevailing assumption has been that external stimuli can exceed an internal threshold, thereby triggering recovery from a disorder of consciousness. However, in the following sections, it will be argued that the primary goal of intervention should not be to improve stimulus processing (i.e., attention) but rather to initiate purposeful movements or actions. The core deficit of the various disorders of consciousness (UWS, MCS, akinetic mutism, and severe stupor-like drive disorder [see summary in Table 9.1]) is the absence of goal-oriented, spontaneous behavior, despite the fact that segments of action (i.e., isolated movements) can often be evoked within clearly defined contexts.

In psychiatric terminology, this lack of spontaneous and goal-directed behavior can be classified as a "negative symptom." Negative symptoms are characterized by an extensive reduction in overt behavior, a loss of interest in environmental events, significant learning impairments, and withdrawal from social interactions [54]. This can be observed in various disorders, such as schizophrenia, Alzheimer's disease, and Parkinson's syndrome. Interestingly, many diseases dominated by negative symptoms in their late stages may culminate in a state resembling the apallic syndrome, the earlier term Gerstenbrand [6] and Gerstenbrand [7] used for what is now called UWS.

Unfortunately, it is precisely the spontaneous action aspects of human behavior that have proven to be largely resistant to scientific analysis and therapeutic intervention. Nevertheless, the basic outlines of a theory capable of explaining goal-directed behavior are becoming increasingly clear. In addition to emotional processes, essential components that allow for such behavior include the representation and maintenance of target states (i.e., desired future conditions), the representation of actions with positive or negative consequences for the organism, and the selection and initiation of appropriate actions.

In the following sections, disorders of consciousness will be interpreted as disturbances of this network of emotions, goal representations, and action selection [42]. The primary motivation for this conceptual shift is to design treatment plans for patients with disorders of consciousness. In doing so, new ground will be broken, as established neuropsychological treatment concepts for these conditions do not yet exist. Consequently, the treatment approaches described below are based on clinical experience rather than controlled studies.

9.4.1 Therapy of unresponsive wakefulness syndrome

Therapeutic approaches for patients in UWS aim to support recovery by fostering activation, interaction, and, ultimately, the re-establishment of goal-directed behavior. Historically, treatment has focused on sensory stimulation, which seeks to awaken responsiveness through repeated external input. In theoretical terms, dialogical interaction has gained attention for its emphasis on the patient's emotional and relational context. This section outlines the structure, theoretical foundations, and clinical implications of both approaches, highlighting the importance of personalization, timing, and meaningful engagement in therapy.

9.4.1.1 Two therapeutic approaches: sensory stimulation and dialogical interaction

Historically, the same principles have been formulated for the treatment of patients with UWS as for those in a coma: sensory stimulation [52,55,56] and dialogical interaction [42,49]. Both approaches emphasize frequent and intensive interventions administered several times a day, but with careful attention to dosing and rest periods, to avoid overstimulation. This therapeutic balance, often referred to as sensory regulation, aims to ensure that periods of active input are alternated with phases of minimal external influence to protect the patient's limited cognitive resources.

The principles of sensory stimulation, a widely used intervention for patients with UWS, have been described extensively and are therefore only briefly summarized here (see Table 9.2). Sensory stimulation has been shown to be effective in these patients, although the extent of its effectiveness, especially in the long-term course of rehabilitation, is still unclear (Houston et al. [55], [51–53,56–58]) dialogical interaction, though less commonly employed in this patient group, follows similar principles of intensity, repetition, and rest ([49]; see Table 9.2). Unlike sensory stimulation, which targets specific sensory modalities, dialogical interaction centers around personally meaningful content. It is

TABLE 9.2 Sensory stimulation.

		Sensory stimulation	Dialog development
	Sense channel	Stimuli	Stimuli offers
1	Vestibular, proprioceptive, kinesthetic	Spinning, vibrations, sitting up, moving, rubbing	Hand-supported breathing, rocking, swaying, sitting up, moving, traveling through space
2	Olfactory	Coffee, vanilla, etc.	Aftershave, soap, perfume
3	Gustatory	Sweet-tasting substances	Favorite foods: honey, chocolate
4	Tactile	Touching the hand, arm, shoulder, and face	Stroking, tapping, massaging, rubbing in, hugging, caressing, kissing
5	Auditory	Bell sounds, speaking to, calling, and music	Voices, (heart) sounds, tones, music, calling names, singing, reading aloud, asking questions
6	Visual	Light stimuli, pictures, objects, and faces	Objects (doll, stuffed animal, car), pictures, photos, faces (mirror), gestures, lip-reading

Table derived from Zieger A., Hildebrandt H. Neuropsychologische Frührehabilitation. In: Gauggel S., Kerkhoff G., editors. Fallbuch Neuropsychologie. Göttingen: Hogrefe; 1997. pp. 267–289. Hrsg.

based on a hermeneutic approach, in which the patient's facial expressions, gestures, and behavioral cues are interpreted as potential signs of intentionality or rudimentary interaction. Although such interpretations cannot be objectively verified, given the patient's severely limited ability to communicate, they are grounded in theoretical and ethical assumptions that value the patient as a potentially communicative being [49].

9.4.1.2 Rationale behind sensory stimulation

Two main assumptions underlie the rationale for sensory stimulation: (1) the existence of secondary sensory deprivation and (2) a proposed analogy to sleep physiology.

The first assumption is grounded in the understanding that systematic deprivation of stimuli ("deprivation") can lead to a disintegration and, over time, to a degeneration of neuron assemblies. This secondary deterioration of rehabilitation potential is independent of the primary physiological trauma [59,60]. Animal experiments involving artificially induced brain lesions have documented the positive effects of interaction within an enriched environment and, conversely, the negative effects of sensory deprivation of standard cage living on the reorganization of the brain and functional recovery (see Chapter 3). However, in patients with UWS, self-determined activation and stimulation of the organism are severely impaired due to several factors (e.g., bilateral lesions in frontal regions critical for goal formation and intentional behavior). As a result, their restricted interaction with the environment resembles the sensory deprivation conditions used in experimental control groups in animal experiments [59,60]. This state of deprivation can persist for months and therefore limit the prospect of recovery by missing the critical early-but-not-too-early window for intervention. In purely physical terms, the effects of deprivation are evident in the development of "bed-rest syndrome," in which muscle atrophy occurs due to the absence of stress exposure (cf. Golaszewski et al. [61]). Additional spasticity, due to a lack of movement, may be another consequence of prolonged sensory deprivation.

The second commonly cited rationale for sensory stimulation relates to sleep physiology. It draws an analogy to sleep physiology: intense and repetitive stimuli may elevate the brain's level of attention, reaching a threshold that can interrupt pathological unconsciousness, similar to how sleep can be interrupted by sufficiently intense and repetitive stimuli. Consequently, it is being suggested that various sensory channels should be stimulated systematically and successively, while observing and recording patient reactions (e.g., [50]).

9.4.1.3 The limitations of successive stimulation: a dialogical and neurophysiological perspective

However, from a dialogical perspective, the commonly employed concept of repetitive and successive sensory stimulation is misleading for several reasons. Physiologically, states of consciousness are believed to be associated with the temporal convergence of information from different sensory channels. This convergence (i.e., "binding") leads to the generation of a specific frequency in the electroencephalogram, around 40 Hz in the gamma (γ) band, which has been associated with conscious awareness [62,63]. Accordingly, stimuli from different modalities that coincide in time have a strong arousal value. This is particularly known for the combination of acoustic and visual or tactile and visual stimuli. Neurons in both the midbrain and the cortex become active specifically when they receive convergent input from multiple sensory channels [64]. Subjectively, this process is reflected in the sudden and automatic orientation response we experience when, for example, a sound and a movement occur simultaneously in the same location.

In healthy individuals, this binding mechanism supports rapid orientation and adaptive behavior. In patients with UWS, however, this mechanism appears to be disrupted. Studies of patients with UWS following hypoxia have shown that while stimulus processing reaches the cortex, the neural activity remains in the primary association areas [65]. In other words, neural activity fails to reach higher-order integration networks. Thus effective stimulation does not simply occur due to the crossing of a sensory threshold, but rather through integration of incoming information into a cortically stored pattern of experience.

This has crucial implications for therapeutic strategies. Rather than presenting stimuli in a sequential, repetitive manner (i.e., addressing one modality at a time), interventions may be more effective when they involve simultaneous, convergent stimulation across multiple sensory channels. Simultaneous, convergent stimulation across modalities is likely to be more effective. Such synchronized input is more consistent with the brain's natural processing dynamics and more likely to facilitate arousal and functional connectivity. In contrast, the standard practice of successive stimulation may inadvertently reduce effectiveness by failing to capitalize on the binding mechanisms necessary for conscious awareness.

9.4.1.4 Principles of dialogical interaction: from stimulus to reproducible action

Insights from animal models further emphasize the importance of timing and intensity in rehabilitation, also arguing for a rather dialogical approach instead of sensory stimulation. As discussed in the chapter on stroke rehabilitation in animal models, early-but-not-too-early, intervention is critical. Moreover, such studies have shown that interventions that are too intense can reduce the positive effect of rehabilitation and foster postacute inflammatory processes (see Chapter 3). Thus strengthening a dialogical and empathic form of interaction may be the best strategy to avoid overstimulation and additional stress. At present, there is no biological marker more sensitive to the patient's inner state than the observable effects of dialogical interaction, even in patients with UWS.

From a dialogical perspective, there are also conceptual reasons why drawing analogies between UWS and sleep states (a rationale of sensory stimulation) can be misleading. The primary goal of neuropsychological intervention in patients with UWS is not to achieve wakefulness, as patients in this state already display sleep–wake cycles (i.e., show signs of wakefulness), but rather to facilitate selective and reproducible interaction with the environment. Examples include fixation on stimuli, goal-directed movements, which in the early phase concern the patient's own body, and repetitions of actions without additional stimulation. These early forms of interaction are likely to represent basic components of consciousness. Therapeutically, the focus should therefore not be on simply exceeding a threshold of consciousness, but rather on coupling external stimuli with specific, reproducible reactions. Ultimately, the emphasis should be placed on promoting the patient's independent movement and goal-directed behavior, rather than solely on the processing of stimuli. Moreover, dialogical models also address emotional and trauma-related dimensions of UWS.

9.4.1.5 Trauma, emotional meaning, and the role of familiarity in dialogical interaction

Representatives of the dialogical interaction approach further argue that severe brain injury may induce a global shock reaction in the organism, inhibiting active attention to the environment. In this respect, personally meaningful stimuli, such as familiar voices, faces, or emotionally significant actions, are considered especially important. These stimuli help fulfill the patient's increased need for security and, thereby reduce the stress associated with trauma processing. This assumption is supported by animal studies showing that traumatic experiences can lead to degenerative changes, especially in the limbic system, even when limbic structures are not directly damaged [66,67]. Accordingly, interaction with patients in unresponsive wakefulness should encompass not only sensory stimulation but also emotional engagement to promote recovery.

While these assumptions are supported by theory and observation, biological evidence remains limited. Direct evidence for an additional, nonfocal biological trauma in patients with UWS is not yet available.

However, such evidence should be obtainable in principle, for instance, through the regular measurement of hormone levels (e.g., cortisol, norepinephrine derivatives), which could reveal elevations in peripheral stress indicators. While findings on cortisol levels in humans have so far been inconsistent [68,69], animal studies consistently demonstrate elevated cortisol following brain injury (see Chapter 3), supporting the hypothesis of a systemic stress response.

Clinically, it has been observed that patients with UWS may exhibit a state of withdrawal or inhibited responsiveness, possibly reflecting a trauma-induced global stress reaction. For example, the presence of familiar persons can lead to marked and positive behavioral changes in patients with UWS, including reduced arousal, eye opening, and signs of increased attention. Furthermore, clinical experience has shown that the continuous presence ("rooming-in") of close relatives has a beneficial impact on patient tension levels and the overall course of recovery. Thus the presence of familiar individuals appears to mitigate this withdrawn state, as evidenced by observable behavioral improvements in some patients, supporting the idea that emotionally meaningful interactions retain therapeutic value even in unresponsive conditions.

9.4.1.6 Practical implementations and clinical examples

Building on the theoretical principles outlined above, this section presents practical guidelines for implementing dialogical therapy in patients with UWS. The goal is to move beyond rigid stimulation protocols and instead promote reproducible, meaningful interaction grounded in bodily experience and emotional resonance. Therefore a treatment approach is proposed based on three guiding principles: (1) The principle of primary reinforcement through body-related interaction and involvement of relatives in therapy. This principle aims not only to enhance engagement through physical interaction but also to mitigate the secondary, nonbiological consequences of the injury, meaning the shock and trauma. (2) The principle of temporally closely coupled simultaneous experience of different stimulus qualities with a moderately complex character. Rather than simple, isolated stimuli (e.g., pure sounds or bright lights), more complex stimuli, such as music instead of sounds, or images instead of flashes, should be used. This principle is intended to promote the transgression of neuronal activity within the narrow boundaries of the primary association areas. (3) The principle of passively induced, yet self-initiated stimuli. Stimuli should be designed so that the patient experiences a sense of agency—that is, a perception of being able to influence environmental events, thus reinforcing the possibility of intentional interaction with the environment.

Since the overarching goal of intervention is to achieve reproducible action, therapy should focus on the combination of (initially) passively induced movement and simultaneous visual or acoustic information. In music therapy, for instance, the passive touching of instruments results in an intense coupling of sound and movement—a paradigm example of the principle of temporal convergence of neuronal excitation waves.

The recommendations of the European guideline for the treatment of patients with disorders of consciousness, which suggests mobilizing patients with UWS into a standing position, should be followed wherever possible, provided that the person's bodily expressions do not indicate significant stress. If feasible, passive walking in a therapeutic bath should be considered, as it represents another example of simultaneous stimulation and intensive interaction with the environment, even when performed passively.

Within each therapy session, a summation of stimulation should be achieved, allowing for both periods of activity and periods of rest. Social interactions between the therapist, relatives, and patient are also an essential part of dialogical interaction, focusing on the reproduction of facial and bodily expressions of the patient. The overall progression of dialogical interaction should be guided by the patient's responses: once a reproducible reaction is elicited, the subsequent sequence of interactions should integrate this achievement and offer a next level of complexity, gradually building toward more differentiated and goal-directed behavior.

If patients are stable enough to be mobilized into a wheelchair, the computer can be used as a stimulation instrument. Computers offer the possibility of combining light and acoustic stimuli when touching a keyboard or corresponding switches. The stimulation should take place in a semidarkened room to ensure that the light contrast from the screen reaches a sufficient intensity. We use a "synesthetic piano," where touching specific keys triggers both color changes on the screen and sound changes through the speakers. The patient's hand is either passively guided by the therapist or the therapist activates the keys directly. Throughout the session, attention should be paid to the patient's physical orientation toward the activity. Each stimulation unit typically lasts 5 minutes, followed by a short break during which normal daylight conditions are restored. This change in light and environment also often elicits a noticeable reaction from the patient. Clinically, a maximum of three stimulation units per therapy session has proven effective. After this point, patients usually reach their resilience limit, and a rest phase should be provided.

9.4.1.7 Pharmacological treatment

Pharmacological interventions aimed at improving the condition of patients with UWS are commonly attempted in many rehabilitation facilities, typically using amantadine and L-dopa, based on the assumption that these agents may enhance attentional functioning by modulating neurotransmitter activity. Among these, amantadine currently represents the most evidence-based and widely recommended intervention, particularly for patients with TBI, and it is recommended as a first-line pharmacological option. Studies repeatedly show that transitions from UWS to MCS occur more frequently. However, this advantage diminishes after the medication is discontinued, indicating that the effect may be limited to the period of active treatment. Furthermore, the evidence for nontraumatic causes of UWS remains limited [3].

The scientific evidence supporting L-dopa remains limited, despite its widespread clinical use. To date, only one group study has investigated this approach. Di Rocco et al. [70] found that L-dopa could improve consciousness in comatose patients, but only if the patients had not yet transitioned into a persistent UWS

Furthermore, Zolpidem, a GABA-A receptor agonist primarily used as a hypnotic agent, has been tested off-label. Its exact mechanism remains unclear; however, it has been postulated that through selective inhibition of primarily inhibitory neurons, Zolpidem could lead to an activation of frontal brain regions [71]. While some cases report transient improvements in consciousness, only a small proportion of patients respond (around 5% in reviewed studies; e.g. [72]), and the effects are typically short-lived. Thus in clinical practice, a therapeutic trial with Zolpidem may be considered in order to identify and treat potential responders who have not yet responded to other lines of treatment [3].

More recently, apomorphine has been tested in six patients with prolonged disorders of consciousness, including individuals in a MCS and UWS. Results indicated improvements in behavioral responsiveness, as measured by the CRS-R, and enhancements in brain network function, as evidenced by EEG and positron emission tomography (PET) findings. Notably, four out of six patients in the apomorphine group improved their diagnosis at one year postinjury, compared to one out of seven in the control group. These findings suggest that apomorphine may have a beneficial effect on disorders of consciousness. However, the study had important limitations, including a small sample size, and further controlled studies are needed to confirm its efficacy [73].

Lastly, repetitive transcranial magnetic stimulation (rTMS) may be used for patients with UWS or those in a MCS. rTMS aims to modulate cortical activity and stimulate networks involved in consciousness, with stimulation recommended to target the dorsolateral prefrontal cortex or angular gyrus. While some patients show improvements in behavioral responsiveness after rTMS with indications of a higher benefit in patients with MCS than in UWS (e.g. [74]), the current evidence base is limited and affected by methodological weaknesses, such as small sample sizes, heterogeneous patient groups, and lack of standardized stimulation protocols. Therefore further research is needed to establish its efficacy and define standardized treatment protocols [3].

9.4.2 Therapy of akinetic mutism

The primary therapeutic goal in akinetic mutism is to restore goal-directed behavior, as the core deficit lies not in basic motor function but in the initiation and intentional control of action. Treatment is therefore aimed at gradually shifting patients from passive responsiveness to active engagement. Neuropsychological intervention can typically be structured into four phases:

Phase 1: establishing a stable reaction to a specific communicative situation.
Phase 2: eliciting initial naming and simple goal-directed actions that differ from automatic, stereotyped behaviors.
Phase 3: increasing the time delay between the stimulus and the (speech) response, fostering greater intentional control.
Phase 4: promoting the recovery of spontaneous, self-initiated action.

9.4.2.1 Four phases of recovery

9.4.2.1.1 Phase 1: communication by expression

In the first phase of treatment, communication should be initiated through expressive behavior rather than through verbal content. Expressive behavior arises directly and is controlled primarily by the emotional reactions to environmental stimuli. Despite its simplicity, expressive behavior represents a fundamental form of social interaction, as it provides observable information about the individual's inner states. Neuroanatomically, even the simplest emotional expressions can be triggered subcortically, meaning at a level of neuronal integration that remains intact in patients with frontal lesions.

This foundation of expressive behavior can be therapeutically utilized to establish direct interaction with the patient, aiming to provoke verbal, initially prelinguistic utterances. For example, neuropsychologists can encourage the use of stereotyped or automatic phrases. In one specific case, we achieved the first reproducible vocalizations in a patient who had suffered a ruptured aneurysm of the left anterior communicating artery by introducing a simple "Ey-game" with her. In this exercise, held at the end of each therapy session, the therapist tapped the patient's arm while clearly saying "Ey." This process was repeated several times. Subsequently, it was the patient's turn: her arm had to be guided passively, but at an appropriate speed, to the therapist's arm, as she was not yet capable of such a movement. During this action, the patient was also prompted to vocalize "Ey" when touched.

Although the patient had remained mute for several weeks, it was possible to provoke the first quiet "Ey" within three sessions. Building on this success, we introduced additional automatic language forms, such as "Goodbye," and gradually reconstructed reactive language abilities by prompting sentence completion and picture naming. However, while the patient was able to respond with complete sentences within another 6 weeks, it was not possible for her to spontaneously ask questions or express messages independently.

Another approach to initiating linguistic utterances involves embedding vocalizations into noncommunicative actions. For example, blowing out a candle can be used to elicit an "F" sound. However, our sporadic therapeutic experiences with this method have been less promising. The action of blowing out a candle is already intentional ("blowing out the candle") and therefore harder to trigger automatically. In addition, transferring the isolated sound production into a communicative context presents a generalization problem: even when a vocalization is produced (like when blowing out a candle), it does not inherently carry social or interactive meaning. In other words, the mere ability to produce sounds does not directly translate into the ability to engage in intentional social interaction.

9.4.2.1.2 Phase 2: evoking automatic speech and actions

In the second phase, an overwhelming contextual framework is used to elicit automatic responses. Tasks such as simple naming or sentence completion are effective at this stage, as they offer structure while requiring minimal spontaneous generation of content. Unlike in the first phase, the patient now communicates verbally, and the interaction is linked to specific objects. Initially, patients often find it easier to express themselves through writing rather than speaking. To support this, counting exercises or basic, automated calculations may help provoke written responses.

In terms of speech, fixed and highly overlearned sequences, such as reciting the days of the week or counting, are often effective, as each utterance naturally follows the previous one. These tasks have low communicative demand, as they do not require complex conceptual preparation such as spontaneous speech (see Chapter 6).

For motor actions, tasks with a high degree of automation are particularly helpful. In the early stage of recovery, it is often easier to elicit reactions from the nondominant hand than from the dominant one, since akinetic mutism typically results from a left dorsomedial frontal lesion in right-handed individuals. Automatic responses should gradually be decontextualized and enabled on verbal demand. For instance, a pegboard, a wooden board with vertical slots into which pegs or bars are inserted, can serve as an ideal structured motor task. Its clear spatial layout and repetitive action sequence provide immediate visual and tactile feedback, helping to elicit and reinforce goal-directed movements. Initially, hand-over-hand guidance may be used to initiate the action. As the patient begins to respond more consistently, verbal cues (e.g., "Now take the next peg") or tactile prompts (such as tapping the hand) can facilitate the transition to voluntary execution. The task's simplicity and rhythm make it well-suited for rebuilding motor sequences, and its repetitive structure supports the gradual shift from automatic to intentional movement. Over time, the therapist can increase the level of complexity by prompting verbal initiation or alternating the involved hand to support motor generalization and attentional control.

Basic personal care tasks, such as hygiene routines and food intake, can also be used to provoke initial reactions. The essential goal of this phase is to strip actions of decision-making components and translate them into quasiautomatic action sequences, providing a foundation for further voluntary control.

9.4.2.1.3 Phase 3: delaying automatic speech and actions

The third phase focuses on delaying the patient's response. This delay is intended to prepare the patient for the ability to react spontaneously—that is, without an immediate external trigger. One therapeutic strategy in this phase involves games that require a regulated alternation of activity between two players, such as mill, dice games, or similar. In these games, the end of one player's turn consistently serves as the signal for the other player to become active. Importantly, many simple dice games offer only a limited number of possible moves, thereby avoiding the generation of additional cognitive demands for the patients.

Another therapeutic approach involves the free recall of images or short texts from memory that have been previously presented. However, achieving success in this third phase is accompanied by considerable problems. Patients frequently develop pronounced perseveration during delayed reproduction. Additionally, free retrieval is often accompanied by seemingly nonsensical naming of visible external objects or, not infrequently, by echolalia. These disturbances reflect the dominance of the frontolateral motor system, which remains intact. As a result, the intention to act can still easily fall under the control of the lateral motor system, leading to automatic reactions either to the patient's own previously produced actions or to the environmental stimuli, such as the therapist's verbal cues.

9.4.2.1.4 Phase 4: preparing for prospective speech and actions

The fourth phase is focused on promoting quasispontaneous actions. Prospective actions are agreed upon with the patient and are to be carried out at the appropriate, later moment. Initially, concise external cues, such as the ringing of an alarm clock or a specific action performed by the therapist, are necessary to prompt and help ensure that the agreed-upon action is performed relatively spontaneously within the context. Only in a later phase can these external retrieval cues be gradually phased out, allowing the patient to act more independently and spontaneously.

9.4.2.2 *Pharmacological treatment*

Pharmacological treatment attempts of patients in akinetic mutism have shown improvements following the administration of bromocriptine, a dopamine agonist that stimulates dopamine receptors [75]. Other case reports suggest that tricyclic antidepressants with a high noradrenergic component (e.g., amitriptyline) [76], may also be effective. However, as in the treatment of patients with UWS, controlled studies evaluating the effectiveness of pharmacological interventions are still lacking.

9.4.3 Therapy of stupor-like drive disorder

The primary difficulty for patients with stupor-like drive disorder lies in the initiation and maintenance of cycles of interaction with the environment. This impairment is due to the loss of internal goal representations, reduced environmental attention, or the lack of experience of reward following action (reflecting either depressive or negativistic components). As a therapeutic approach, we therefore propose the following steps:

Phase 1: establishment of continuous, rhythmic movement patterns.
Phase 2: analysis of primary and secondary reinforcers.
Phase 3: establishment of circular reactions.
Phase 4: development of a reproducible interaction system.
Phase 5: expansion of independent actions through a token program or through contingent reinforcement.

9.4.3.1 *Five phases of recovery*

9.4.3.1.1 Phase 1: establishment of passively-induced rhythmic movement patterns

In patients with stupor-like drive disorder, there is a more or less complete decoupling from the environment. Therefore the primary goal of therapeutic intervention is not necessarily the initiation of goal-directed behavior, but at least the maintenance of movement and basic motor activity.

One foundational strategy involves the use of rhythmic movement patterns. These serve both as the basis of many everyday actions and as a starting point for more complex, voluntary behavior due to their repetitive character.

A notable example, also used as a core intervention for patients with stupor-like drive disorders, is passively induced running (if not prohibited by lower body rigid-spasticity). When applied consistently, ideally twice daily over several weeks, this approach has led to surprisingly positive outcomes. During the intervention, one therapist supports the patient's trunk while two others assist with guiding leg movements. Often, the first sign of recovery is the return of trunk stability, followed by the emergence of rhythmic stepping patterns, which are frequently initiated by the passive forward motion of the body. In addition to motor activation, moderate physical exertion and the rhythmic alternation between muscle tension and relaxation appear to have therapeutic benefits, potentially enhancing bodily awareness and facilitating renewed interaction with the environment.

9.4.3.1.2 Phase 2: analysis of primary and secondary reinforcers

The second therapeutic step involves analyzing potential primary and secondary reinforcers, as reinforcing experiences (or internally perceived rewards) are essential for initiating and sustaining actions. Thus an essential prerequisite for effective therapy is the detection of potential reinforcers. These can include primary reinforcers, such as food, physical touch, and verbal attention, as well as secondary reinforcers, most commonly the presence and emotional engagement of close relatives.

Current neuroscientific research suggests that orbitofrontal and limbic structures are organized into compartments that respond to different types of primary and modality-specific reinforcement and are sensitive both to need states and satiety [77,78]. Therefore lesions would need to be very extensive to interrupt all reinforcement pathways, both primary and secondary, which underscores the therapeutic potential even in severely affected patients.

9.4.3.1.3 Phase 3: establishment of circular reactions

The term circular reaction originates from the work of Jean Piaget [79]. It refers to the ability to repeatedly evoke a specific outcome by performing the same movement. In this respect, circular reaction is the starting point of object permanence, working memory loops, and the experience of causality in relation to the environment. In simpler terms, a circular reaction refers to a situation where a person performs a movement, notices the effect it produces, and then repeats the movement to recreate that effect. For example, an infant might accidentally shake a rattle, hear the sound, and then repeat the shaking because they now understand that their action causes a result. This repetition helps form the basis for understanding cause and effect, memory, and intentional action.

In patients with stupor-like drive disorder, therapy aims to restore this causal element of circular reactions as a foundation for re-establishing the sense of environmental control.

To initiate therapeutic dialog, the initial focus is placed on supporting circular reactions. The prerequisite is identifying a body movement that the patient can perform, at least temporarily. Examples include selective spreading of the thumb or repetitive arm movements away from and back toward the body. In the early stages, these movements are fully supported and may need to be passively initiated over a period of several weeks. Any reduction in muscle tone or minimal active participation is immediately reinforced through appropriate physical contact.

The next therapeutic step involves sustaining the initiated movement and ultimately executing it on command, without needing continuous feedback or reinforcement between trials.

Importantly, therapeutic interaction with stupor-like patients should be highly physical. Rolls [44] and Rolls [45] demonstrated that, in addition to food, social tactile touch functions as a primary reinforcer. Corresponding studies in primates revealed that the quality and intensity of tactile stimulation, not the quantity, play a decisive role in emotional and cognitive development, even when other conditions are held constant. Thus touch is more effective than other forms of feedback, such as auditory or visual input, in this therapeutic context.

The achievement of a stable circular reaction is considered a positive prognostic sign, if only because it demonstrates a genuine capacity to act within a specific behavioral domain. This clinical observation aligns with the view of Gerstenbrand [6] and Gerstenbrand [7], who identified the emergence of the so-called "Klüver-Bucy phase" as a critical turning point in patient recovery. From the perspective of action theory, Gerstenbrand's observation can be understood as the occurrence of a first circular reaction. The appearance of spontaneous, sometimes compulsive, movements directed toward the patient's own body or mouth—hallmarks of Klüver-Bucy syndrome—suggests that the previously severe drive disorder is beginning to resolve, making circular reactions possible once again.

9.4.3.1.4 Phase 4: token program

Once a patient has reached a level of participation in everyday activities and therapies, the implementation of a token program can be considered. Positive effects of such programs have been reported in individual cases, particularly among patients with drive disorder or limited cooperation. However, to date, no systematic group studies have been published in this area.

In our own clinical practice, we have observed temporary but significant benefits of token programs. In one case, a patient who demonstrated sufficient cognitive and physical abilities remained highly uncooperative in therapy. It was explained that continuation of his therapy stay on the ward would depend on achieving a minimum number of cooperative therapy sessions per week. Otherwise, transfer to a nursing home would be considered—a realistic consequence, given funding constraints. Daily results were visualized using green and red markers on a pinboard beside the patient's bed and discussed with him regularly. As a result, the patient partially adapted his behavior and became more compliant with therapeutic expectations.

In another case, a patient with severe drive disorder, but without negative symptoms, appeared emotionally euphoric and showed little insight into his condition. Despite his strong slowing in daily activities and refusal to eat without supervision, he expressed a clear interest in woodworking, based on his prior profession. In his case, a token economy was introduced, in which participation in relevant therapy sessions, such as woodworking, was rewarded with tokens that could be exchanged for preferred activities. This system allowed for a degree of behavioral regulation across other therapeutic contexts as well.

When considering a token economy, it is important to first determine whether the core of the disorder lies more in depressive withdrawal or in drive and negativism. In cases where depressive features dominate, the emphasis should be placed on positive reinforcement, rather than confrontation or external pressure.

9.4.3.2 Pharmacological treatment

Some patients with stupor-like drive disorder may benefit from dopaminergic or noradrenergic medication, although typically to a lesser extent than patients with akinetic mutism. This observation is based solely on the individual clinical cases; controlled group studies are currently lacking.

Wroblewski et al. [80] reported successful treatment outcomes using protriptyline (a partially noradrenergic antidepressant) in several patients whose symptoms resembled a stupor-like drive disorder. The patients had right-frontal lesions, mostly commonly following TBI, and generally presented with less severe impairments than the patients described in this chapter.

In our own clinical experience, selective serotonin reuptake inhibitors (SSRIs), prescribed in cases of depression, have not proven effective in treating this disorder. Notably, Wroblewski et al. [80] arrived at the same conclusion following their use of SSRIs in a comparable patient.

9.5 Concluding remarks

This chapter has explored a group of syndromes that, while among the most severe, are nonetheless commonly encountered in neurorehabilitation. We have proposed a unified conceptualization of these conditions as disorders of action, classifying them under "negative symptoms." This classification is supported by consistent, causal involvement of the frontal cortex, long recognized for its central role in action planning, initiation, and evaluation.

The therapeutic approaches outlined here aim to translate this conceptual model into meaningful clinical interventions. While these strategies remain theoretical and largely based on uncontrolled individual observations, they offer a coherent framework that identifies a disruption of the action system as a core deficit in all of these conditions.

By viewing these conditions through the lens of negative symptoms, we can better connect various treatment strategies and move toward more individualized, targeted rehabilitation plans. Whether this approach will prove effective in improving outcomes remains to be determined. The field now stands at a turning point where therapeutic models of dialogical, goal-oriented engagement must be rigorously tested, expanded, and refined. Only through this effort can we hope to transform our current understanding of recovery in disorders of consciousness into effective, individualized clinical practice.

References

[1] Schonle PW. The early rehabilitation Barthel Index-an early rehabilitation-oriented extension of the Barthel Index. Rehabilitation (Stuttg) 1995;34(2):69–73. Available from https://www.ncbi.nlm.nih.gov/pubmed/7624593.

[2] Golden K, Bodien YG, Giacino JT. Disorders of consciousness: classification and taxonomy. Phys Med Rehabil Clin N Am 2024;35(1):15–33. Available from https://doi.org/10.1016/j.pmr.2023.06.011.

[3] Bender A. S3-LL Neurologische Rehabilitation bei Koma und schwerer Bewusstseinsstörung im Erwachsenenalter, 2022.

[4] Kondziella D, Bender A, Diserens K, van Erp W, Estraneo A, Formisano R, et al. European Academy of Neurology guideline on the diagnosis of coma and other disorders of consciousness. Eur J Neurol 2020;27(5):741–56. Available from https://doi.org/10.1111/ene.14151.

[5] Andrews K, Murphy L, Munday R, Littlewood C. Misdiagnosis of the vegetative state: retrospective study in a rehabilitation unit. Br Med J 1996;313(7048):13–6. Available from https://doi.org/10.1136/bmj.313.7048.13.
[6] Gerstenbrand F. Das Apallische Syndrom. Berlin: Springer-Verlag; 1967.
[7] Gerstenbrand F. Das Traumatische Apallische Syndrom, 1967.
[8] Santos-Carrasco D, De la Casa LG. Prepulse inhibition deficit as a transdiagnostic process in neuropsychiatric disorders: a systematic review. BMC Psychol 2023;11(1):226. Available from https://doi.org/10.1186/s40359-023-01253-9.
[9] Zhang J, Wang M, Wei B, Shi J, Yu T. Research progress in the study of startle reflex to disease states. Neuropsychiatr Dis Treat 2022;18:427–35. Available from https://doi.org/10.2147/NDT.S351667.
[10] Arciniegas-Villanueva AV, Fernandez-Diaz EM, Gonzalez-Garcia E, Sancho-Pelluz J, Mansilla-Lozano D, Segura T. Functional and prognostic assessment in comatose patients: a study using somatosensory evoked potentials. Front Hum Neurosci 2022;16:904455. Available from https://doi.org/10.3389/fnhum.2022.904455.
[11] Pruvost-Robieux E, Marchi A, Martinelli I, Bouchereau E, Gavaret M. Evoked and event-related potentials as biomarkers of consciousness state and recovery. J Clin Neurophysiol 2022;39(1):22–31. Available from https://doi.org/10.1097/Wnp.0000000000000762.
[12] Ihalainen R, Annen J, Gosseries O, Cardone P, Panda R, Martial C, et al. Lateral frontoparietal effective connectivity differentiates and predicts state of consciousness in a cohort of patients with traumatic disorders of consciousness. PLoS One 2024;19(7):e0298110. Available from https://doi.org/10.1371/journal.pone.0298110.
[13] Leithner C, Endisch C. Evoked potentials in patients with disorders of consciousness. Handb Clin Neurol 2025;207:147–64. Available from https://doi.org/10.1016/B978-0-443-13408-1.00002-6.
[14] Medina Carrion JP, Stanziano M, D'Incerti L, Sattin D, Palermo S, Ferraro S, et al. Disorder of consciousness: structural integrity of brain networks for the clinical assessment. Ann Clin Transl Neurol 2023;10(3):384–96. Available from https://doi.org/10.1002/acn3.51729.
[15] Hildebrandt H, Zieger A. Unconscious activation of motor responses in a hemiplegic patient with anosognosia and neglect. Eur Arch Psychiatry Clin Neurosci 1995;246(1):53–9. Available from https://doi.org/10.1007/BF02191815.
[16] Hildebrandt H, Zieger A, Engel A, Fritz KW, Bussmann B. Differentiation of autonomic nervous activity in different stages of coma displayed by power spectrum analysis of heart rate variability. Eur Arch Psychiatry Clin Neurosci 1998;248(1):46–52. Available from https://doi.org/10.1007/s004060050016.
[17] Yan D, Simei L, Hongzhao B, Hongyan D, Yuchao D. Prognosis of patients with prolonged disorders of consciousness after brain injury: a longitudinal cohort study. Front Public Health 2024;12:1421779. Available from https://doi.org/10.3389/fpubh.2024.1421779.
[18] Pavlov YG, Spiegelsberger F, Kotchoubey B. Predicting outcome in disorders of consciousness: a mega-analysis. Ann Clin Transl Neurol 2024;11(6):1465–77. Available from https://doi.org/10.1002/acn3.52061.
[19] Golaszewski S, Florea C, Wutzl B, Seidl M, Kunz AB, Schwenker K, et al. The locked-in-plus-syndrome. Eur J Neurol 2016;23:725. <Go to ISI>://WOS:000431634203221.
[20] Ackermann H, Ziegler W. Akinetischer Mutismus – eine Literaturübersicht. Fortschritte der Neurologie und Psychiatrie 1995;63:59–67. Available from https://doi.org/10.1055/s-2007-996603.
[21] Turkstra LS, Bayles KA. Acquired mutism: physiopathy and assessment. Arch Phys Med Rehabil 1992;73(2):138–44. Available from https://www.ncbi.nlm.nih.gov/pubmed/1371915.

[22] Goldberg G, Bloom KK. The alien hand sign. Localization, lateralization and recovery. Am J Phys Med Rehabil 1990;69(5):228–38. Available from https://doi.org/10.1097/00002060-199010000-00002.
[23] Cooper R, Shallice T. Contention scheduling and the control of routine activities. Cogn Neuropsychol 2000;17(4):297–338. Available from https://doi.org/10.1080/026432900380427.
[24] Schoenberg MR, Scott JG. The little black book of neuropsychology: a syndrome-based approach. US: Springer; 2016. Available from https://books.google.de/books?id=C-CJDAEACAAJ.
[25] Jaspers K. Allgemeine psychopathologie (9., univeränderte Aufl. ed.), 1973.
[26] Benegal V, Hingorani S, Khanna S, Channabasavanna SM. Is stupor by itself a catatonic symptom? Psychopathology 1992;25(5):229–31. Available from https://doi.org/10.1159/000284777.
[27] Hintze U, Runge U, Hachenberg T, Wendt M. Dissociative stupor-differential diagnosis of coma following injury. Anasthesiol Intensivmed Notfallmed Schmerzther 1998;33(11):753–5. Available from https://doi.org/10.1055/s-2007-994846.
[28] Oppenheim-Gluckman H, Fermanian J, Derouesne C. Conscient, inconscient, non conscient et comas. Aggressologie 1993;34:147–50. Available from https://www.ncbi.nlm.nih.gov/pubmed/7872467.
[29] Seligman ME. Learned helplessness. Annu Rev Med 1972;23:407–12. Available from https://doi.org/10.1146/annurev.me.23.020172.002203.
[30] Seligman ME, Weiss J, Weinraub M, Schulman A. Coping behavior: learned helplessness, physiological change and learned inactivity. Behav Res Ther 1980;18(5):459–512. Available from https://doi.org/10.1016/0005-7967(80)90011-x.
[31] Kinney HC, Samuels MA. Neuropathology of the persistent vegetative state. A review. J Neuropathol Exp Neurol 1994;53(6):548–58. Available from https://doi.org/10.1097/00005072-199411000-00002.
[32] Golaszewski S, Seidl M, Kunz A, Wipfler P, Kraus J, Nardone R, et al. Functional involvement of cerebral cortex in patients with sleep-wake disturbances after traumatic brain injury: a TMS study. Eur J Neurol 2011;18:57. <Go to ISI>://WOS:000294806600118.
[33] Staquet C, Vanhaudenhuyse A, Kandeepan S, Sanders RD, Ribeiro de Paula D, Brichant JF, et al. Changes in intrinsic connectivity networks topology across levels of dexmedetomidine-induced alteration of consciousness. Anesth Analg 2024;139(4):798–811. Available from https://doi.org/10.1213/ANE.0000000000006799.
[34] Sala A, Gosseries O, Laureys S, Annen J. Advances in neuroimaging in disorders of consciousness. Handb Clin Neurol 2025;207:97–127. Available from https://doi.org/10.1016/B978-0-443-13408-1.00008-7.
[35] Firsching R, Woischneck D, Diedrich M, Klein S, Ruckert A, Wittig H, et al. Early magnetic resonance imaging of brainstem lesions after severe head injury. J Neurosurg 1998;89(5):707–12. Available from https://doi.org/10.3171/jns.1998.89.5.0707.
[36] Jang SH, Byun DH. A review of studies on the role of diffusion tensor magnetic resonance imaging tractography in the evaluation of the fronto-subcortical circuit in patients with akinetic mutism. Med Sci Monit 2022;28:e936251. Available from https://doi.org/10.12659/MSM.936251.
[37] Birbaumer N, Elbert T, Canavan AGM, Rockstroh B. Slow potentials of the cerebral cortex and behavior. Physiol Rev 1990;70:1–40. Available from https://doi.org/10.1152/physrev.1990.70.1.1.
[38] Rockstroh B, Elbert T, Lutzenberger W, Birbaumer N, Roberts LE. Bilateral electrodermal and electrocortical activity in anticipation of sensorimotor tasks. Psychophysiology 1988;25(2):185–92. Available from https://doi.org/10.1111/j.1469-8986.1988.tb00985.x.

[39] Libet B. Subjective antedating of a sensory experience and mind-brain theories: reply to Honderich (1984). J Theor Biol 1985;114(4):563–70. Available from https://doi.org/10.1016/s0022-5193(85)80043-6.
[40] Libet B. Unconscious cerebral initiative and the role of conscious will in voluntary action. Behav Brain Sci 1985;8:529–66.
[41] Passingham RE. The frontal lobes and voluntary action. Oxford: Oxford University Press; 1993. Available from http://www.loc.gov/catdir/enhancements/fy0639/93010270-d.html.
[42] Hildebrandt H. Neuropsychologische Frührehabilitation: Ein differenzielles Behandlungskonzept für schwerstbeeinträchtigte Patienten. Z für Neuropsychologie 2002;13:91–110.
[43] Ludwig L, McWhirter L, Williams S, Derry C, Stone J. Functional coma. Handb Clin Neurol 2016;139:313–27. Available from https://doi.org/10.1016/B978-0-12-801772-2.00028-X.
[44] Rolls ET. The orbitofrontal cortex and reward. Cereb Cortex 2000;10(3):284–94. Available from https://doi.org/10.1093/cercor/10.3.284.
[45] Rolls ET. Memory systems in the brain. Annu Rev Psychol 2000;51:599–630.
[46] Tataranni PA, Gautier JF, Chen KW, Uecker A, Bandy D, Salbe AD, et al. Neuroanatomical correlates of hunger and satiation in humans using positron emission tomography. Proc Natl Acad Sci U S Am 1999;96(8):4569–74. Available from https://doi.org/10.1073/pnas.96.8.4569.
[47] Mayberg HS, Liotti M, Brannan SK, McGinnis S, Mahurin RK, Jerabek PA, et al. Reciprocal limbic-cortical function and negative mood: converging PET findings in depression and normal sadness. Am J Psychiatry 1999;156(5):675–82. Available from https://doi.org/10.1176/ajp.156.5.675.
[48] Schiff ND. Recovery of consciousness after severe brain injury: the role of arousal regulation mechanisms and some speculation on the heart-brain interface. Cleve Clin J Med 2010;77(Suppl 3):S27–33. Available from https://doi.org/10.3949/ccjm.77.s3.05.
[49] Zieger A, Hildebrandt H. Neuropsychologische Frührehabilitation. In: Gauggel S, Kerkhoff G, editors. Fallbuch neuropsychologie. Göttingen: Hogrefe; 1997. p. 267–89. Hrsg.
[50] Gill-Thwaites H, Munday R. The sensory modality assessment and rehabilitation technique (SMART): a comprehensive and integrated assessment and treatment protocol for the vegetative state and minimally responsive patient. Neuropsychol Rehabil 1999;9(3-4):305–20. Available from https://doi.org/10.1080/096020199389392.
[51] Mitchell S, Bradley VA, Welch JL, Britton PG. Coma arousal procedure: a therapeutic intervention in the treatment of head injury. Brain Inj 1990;4(3):273–9. Available from https://doi.org/10.3109/02699059009026177.
[52] Padilla R, Domina A. Effectiveness of sensory stimulation to improve arousal and alertness of people in a coma or persistent vegetative state after traumatic brain injury: a systematic review. Am J Occup Ther 2016;70(3). Available from https://doi.org/10.5014/ajot.2016.021022. 7003180030p7003180031-7003180038.
[53] Pierce JP, Lyle DM, Quine S, Evans NJ, Morris J, Fearnside MR. The effectiveness of coma arousal intervention. Brain Inj 1990;4(2):191–7. Available from https://doi.org/10.3109/02699059009026165.
[54] Brown RG, Pluck G. Negative symptoms: the «pathology» of motivation and goal-directed behaviour. Trends Neurosci 2000;23(9):412–7. Available from https://doi.org/10.1016/s0166-2236(00)01626-x.
[55] Houston AL, Wilson NS, Morrall MC, Lodh R, Oddy JR. Interventions to improve outcomes in children and young people with unresponsive wakefulness syndrome following acquired brain injury: a systematic review. Eur J Paediatr Neurol 2020;25:40–51. Available from https://doi.org/10.1016/j.ejpn.2020.01.015.

[56] Norwood MF, Lakhani A, Watling DP, Marsh CH, Zeeman H. Efficacy of multimodal sensory therapy in adult acquired brain injury: a systematic review. Neuropsychol Rev 2023;33(4):693–713. Available from https://doi.org/10.1007/s11065-022-09560-5.
[57] Rietz S, Hagel K. Specific therapeutic measures in the treatment of waking coma and their efficient application. Aktuelle Neurologie 2000;27(6):252–7. Available from https://doi.org/10.1055/s-2007-1017549.
[58] Mackay LE, Bernstein BA, Chapman PE, Morgan AS, Milazzo LS. Early intervention in severe head injury: long-term benefits of a formalized program. Arch Phys Med Rehabil 1992;73(7):635–41. Available from https://www.ncbi.nlm.nih.gov/pubmed/1622318.
[59] LeWinn EB, Dimancescu MD. Environmental deprivation and enrichment in coma. Lancet 1978;2(8081):156–7. Available from https://doi.org/10.1016/s0140-6736(78)91543-x.
[60] LeWinn EB, Dimancescu MD. Environmental deprivation and enrichment in coma. Lancet 1978;11:156–7.
[61] Golaszewski S, Wutzl B, Florea C, Kunz AB, Seidl M, Schwenker K, et al. Long-term coma-state and the bedrest-syndrome. Eur J Neurol 2016;23:724. <Go to ISI>://WOS:000431634203220.
[62] Steriade M. Arousal: revisiting the reticular activating system. Science 1996;272(5259):225–6. Available from https://doi.org/10.1126/science.272.5259.225.
[63] Tiitinen H, Sinkkonen J, Reinikainen K, Alho K, Lavikainen J, Naatanen R. Selective attention enhances the auditory 40-Hz transient response in humans. Nature 1993;364(6432):59–60. Available from https://doi.org/10.1038/364059a0.
[64] Stein BE, Meredith MA. The merging of the senses. Cambridge, MA, London: Bradford, The MIT Press; 1993.
[65] Laureys S, Faymonville ME, Degueldre C, Fiore GD, Damas P, Lambermont B, et al. Auditory processing in the vegetative state. Brain 2000;123(Pt 8):1589–601. Available from https://doi.org/10.1093/brain/123.8.1589.
[66] Sapolsky RM. Stress, Glucocorticoids, and damage to the nervous system: the current state of confusion. Stress 1996;1(1):1–19. Available from https://doi.org/10.3109/10253899609001092.
[67] Sapolsky RM. Why stress is bad for your brain. Science 1996;273:749–50.
[68] Vogel HP, Kroll M, Fritschka E, Quabbe HJ. Twenty-four-hour profiles of growth hormone, prolactin and cortisol in the chronic vegetative state. Clin Endocrinol (Oxf) 1990;33(5):631–43. Available from https://doi.org/10.1111/j.1365-2265.1990.tb03902.x.
[69] Munno I, Damiani S, Scardapane R, Lacedra G, Megna M, Patimo C, et al. Evaluation of hypothalamic-pituitary-adrenocortical hormones and inflammatory cytokines in patients with persistent vegetative state. Immunopharmacol Immunotoxicol 1998;20(4):519–29. Available from https://doi.org/10.3109/08923979809031513.
[70] Di Rocco C, Maira G, Meglio M, Rossi GF. L-DOPA treatment of comatose states due to cerebral lesions. Preliminary Find J Neurosurg Sci 1974;18(3):169–76. Available from https://www.ncbi.nlm.nih.gov/pubmed/4465415.
[71] Schiff ND. Recovery of consciousness after brain injury: a mesocircuit hypothesis. Trends Neurosci 2010;33(1):1–9. Available from https://doi.org/10.1016/j.tins.2009.11.002.
[72] Whyte J, Myers R. Incidence of clinically significant responses to zolpidem among patients with disorders of consciousness a preliminary placebo controlled trial. Am J Phys Med Rehabil 2009;88(5):410–8. Available from https://doi.org/10.1097/PHM.0b013e3181a0e3a0.
[73] Sanz LRD, Lejeune N, Szymkowicz E, Bonin EAC, Panda R, Sala A, et al. Apomorphine for prolonged disorders of consciousness: a multimodal open-label study.

EClinicalMedicine 2024;78:102925. Available from https://doi.org/10.1016/j.eclinm.2024.102925.

[74] Legostaeva L, Poydasheva A, Iazeva E, Sinitsyn D, Sergeev D, Bakulin I, et al. Stimulation of the angular gyrus improves the level of consciousness. Brain Sci 2019;9(5). Available from https://doi.org/10.3390/brainsci9050103.

[75] Muller U, von Cramon DY. The therapeutic potential of bromocriptine in neuropsychological rehabilitation of patients with acquired brain damage. Prog Neuropsychopharmacol Biol Psychiatry 1994;18(7):1103–20. Available from https://doi.org/10.1016/0278-5846(94)90114-7.

[76] Reinhard DL, Whyte J, Sandel ME. Improved arousal and initiation following tricyclic antidepressant use in severe brain injury. Arch Phys Med Rehabil 1996;77(1):80–3. Available from https://doi.org/10.1016/s0003-9993(96)90225-7.

[77] O'Doherty J, Rolls ET, Francis S, Bowtell R, McGlone F, Kobal G, et al. Sensory-specific satiety-related olfactory activation of the human orbitofrontal cortex. Neuroreport 2000;20:893–7.

[78] O'Doherty J, Rolls ET, Francis S, Bowtell R, McGlone F, Kobal G, et al. Sensory-specific satiety-related olfactory activation of the human orbitofrontal cortex. Neuroreport 2000;11(4):893–7. Available from https://doi.org/10.1097/00001756-200003200-00046.

[79] Piaget J., The construction of reality in he child. New York: Routledge, 1971.

[80] Wroblewski B, Glenn MB, Cornblatt R, Joseph AB, Suduikis S. Protriptyline as an alternative stimulant medication in patients with brain injury: a series of case reports. Protriptyline as an alternative stimulant medication in patients with brain injury: a series of case reports. Brain Inj 1993;7:353–62. Available from https://doi.org/10.3109/02699059309034962.

[81] Giacino Joseph T, Kalmar Kathleen, Whyte John. The JFK Coma Recovery Scale-Revised: measurement characteristics and diagnostic utility. Archives of Physical Medicine and Rehabilitation 2004;85:2020–9. Available from 10.1016/j.apmr.2004.02.033.

CHAPTER

10

Transcranial direct current stimulation of the lesioned brain: evidence and how to use localization of lesions for planning the electrodes' montage

10.1 Introduction

Transcranial direct current stimulation (tDCS) is a noninvasive brain stimulation method that aims to facilitate or inhibit neural activity by means of weak currents (usually 2 mA) applied through scalp electrodes. It changes brain function either by causing the neuron's resting membrane potential to depolarize (excitatory) or hyperpolarize (inhibitory). When anodal (positive) stimulation is used, the current causes a depolarization of the resting membrane potential, which increases neuronal excitability and allows for more spontaneous or experience-triggered (i.e., in response to incoming signals) cell firing. Negative, or cathodal stimulation, causes a hyperpolarization of the resting membrane potential, decreasing neuronal excitability. The specific mechanisms of how tDCS works and descriptions of the physiological mechanisms can be found in Woods, Antal [1].

The number of papers on the use of tDCS in stroke increased during the last 24 years (Fig. 10.1). Still, there are a lot of open questions about its applicability and its effectiveness in stroke rehabilitation. Systematic reviews on motor rehabilitation after stroke are mainly positive, but differ in estimated effect size (trivial to moderate) and evaluation of the methodological quality of studies (low to high quality) [2–14]. A recent large randomized controlled trial (RCT) study on motor rehabilitation in stroke patients, however, showed no effect, which is discouraging after so

Applied Neuropsychology of Cerebrovascular Diseases
DOI: https://doi.org/10.1016/B978-0-443-45450-9.00008-4

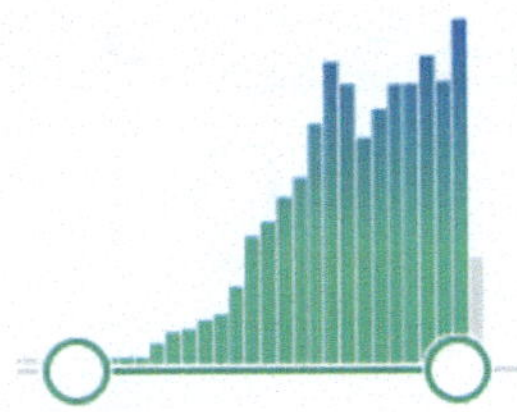

FIGURE 10.1 Development of transcranial Direct Current Stimulation research.

many years of research [15]. In terms of cognitive deficits, recent reviews reveal mixed results (see below). Despite the mixed evidence, there is a broad consensus that tDCS is a safe and cheap intervention without any enduring adverse side effects.

Two major goals of tDCS can be distinguished: (1) to rescue and reintegrate functionally silent but viable neurons (often referred to as "sleeping" neurons that survived the acute phase of a stroke), and (2) to remodel networks to compensate for stroke-related impairments. The effect of tDCS for achieving the first goal depends on the direction of the neuronal cell bodies: the effect is largest if the cells are oriented in the same direction as the current flow and smallest if the current enters the cells in a vertical direction. Activity-dependent excitability of axons plays an important role in achieving the second goal. As argued in Chapter 3, remyelination of axons depends on their specific activity and associated glutamate expression. However, whether tDCS exerts direct effects outside the cell body, that is, at the dendrites and axons, is unclear [16–18]. If the effects are limited to the cell body, tDCS mainly modulates neuronal excitability and firing thresholds; if dendrites and axons are also affected, it could additionally promote synaptic plasticity, axonal remyelination, and long-range network repair. Moreover, the strength of the electrical field decreases subcortically (where the axons are located) due to the resistance of white matter [19]. On the other hand, horizontally running cortico–cortical neurons (e.g., U-fibers) or axons of pyramidal cells in the sulcus area, which initially have a horizontal direction and then make a subcortical bend into the depths, may be suitable for being excited due to directional changes and because these axons are myelinated [19]. Thus any direct modulatory effects of tDCS on axons are likely to be weaker than its effects on cortical cell bodies. In simple terms, these axons are more likely to respond to tDCS because their shape and direction allow the current to flow along them more effectively, making it easier to excite them. Therefore combining training-induced activity with tDCS may help strengthen the neuronal networks underlying cognitive functions and support compensatory reorganization [20,21].

Taken together, while the clinical effectiveness of tDCS in stroke rehabilitation remains somewhat uncertain, its safety profile and low cost continue to support its exploration as a potentially valuable addition to conventional therapies. Therefore we will discuss tDCS for treating (cognitive) deficits in stroke patients in the following sections. While many parts of this chapter remain speculative, such considerations may provide a valuable starting point for new investigations and help to establish a stronger foundation for integrating tDCS into neuropsychological interventions.

10.2 Stage of stroke recovery and related models for transcranial direct current stimulation

The stroke recovery and rehabilitation roundtable [22–24] distinguished between different stages of stroke recovery and argued that these stages may imply different types of intervention (Fig. 10.2). Chapter 3 of this book discusses relevant data from animal studies endorsing stage-specific distinction in stroke recovery, and we followed such a distinction in the chapters on treatment.

Related to tDCS, this differentiation argues for at least two different strategies for stimulation. During the acute phase and the early subacute phase, inflammatory processes prevail and may impact the size and completeness of the remaining lesion (Chapter 3). The major goal during this phase may be to dampen perilesional inflammation by cathodal electrodes. At the same time, starting activity in the contralateral hemisphere plays a role in recovery [22,25,26]. Therefore stimulation of contralesional, unaffected homologous areas may be important.

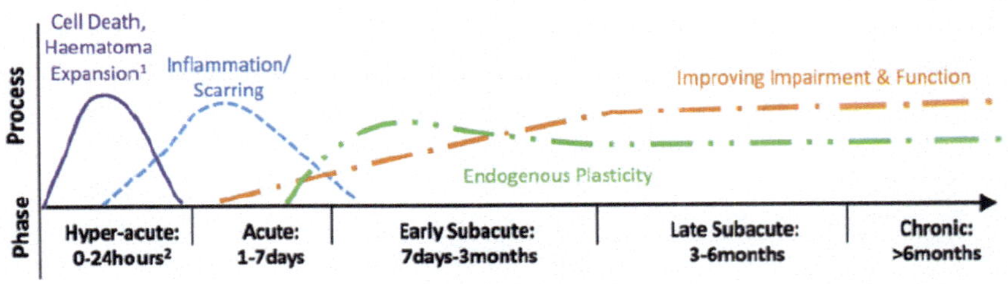

[1] Haemorrhagic stroke specific. [2] Treatments extend to 24 hours to accommodate options for anterior and posterior circulation, as well as basilar occlusion.

FIGURE 10.2 Biological processes related to stroke. *From Bernhardt J., Hayward K.S., Kwakkel G. et al. Agreed definitions and a shared vision for new standards in stroke recovery research: the Stroke Recovery and Rehabilitation Roundtable taskforce. Int J Stroke 2017;12(5):444–450.*

However, after the early subacute stage, recovery is based on improving functions by learning, and effective relearning of functions involves ipsilesional areas of the brain (if still existing). For example, it is well known that neurons of the premotor and sensory parietal cortex have direct access to spinal motor neurons by fibers of the corticospinal tract. Therefore there is a possibility of regaining motor functions by activating these neurons, which might have been redundant before the stroke. Thus in the late postacute and chronic phase, stimulating the perilesional gray matter and functional overlapping ipsilesional structures to increase relearning processes may be the goal of using tDCS.

The assumption here is that relearning skills and functions depend on long-term potentiation, meaning the repeated activation of a synapse leading to a lasting strengthening of the connection between the involved neurons. In this sense, anodal tDCS stimulation might induce such long-term potentiation and therefore speed up the recovery process. However, it should be noted that this assumption could be interpreted in two different ways: either as reactivation of surviving neurons that lost their functional integration or as remodeling of networks necessary for executing the functions. The first of the two interpretations focuses on a direct biological reactivation of neurons inside the perilesional area, whereas the second focuses on learning and networks of learning, which may take place even without activating perilesional areas (for a similar argument [6]).

In this respect, the second interpretation shares some similarity with the inhibition model, which assumes a disturbed network as the cause of the observed deficit. The inhibition model argues that the two hemispheres are connected via the corpus callosum for mutual inhibition [26]. Now, after a stroke, the lesion will lead to a reduced inhibitory effect on the unaffected hemisphere, which increases the activity of the unaffected hemisphere. Such indirect activation may block the functional performance of the affected hemisphere, additionally. In neglect, for instance, insufficient inhibitory control of the intact over the lesioned hemisphere may exacerbate the deficit, pulling attention more strongly to the right side of space (after a right-hemispheric lesion). Cathodal tDCS of the unaffected hemisphere and anodal tDCS of the affected hemisphere might reverse or at least attenuate this additional inhibition of the affected hemisphere. Quite a number of stimulation studies on neglect and aphasia have followed the inhibitory model, and their findings will be discussed below.

The two different goals for tDCS (neuronal reactivation versus remodeling of networks) have consequences for the montage of the electrodes. Neuronal activation tries to optimize the electric field strength in the perilesional areas. However, thinking about networks means that stimulation after stroke should direct current flow along connected areas of the brain. The simplest example then is a bilateral anodal stimulation above the lesion and a cathodal stimulation of the homolog area of the unaffected hemisphere. The combination of activation and inhibition should show a higher effect than only activating or deactivating one hemisphere. And at least one review of electrostimulation after stroke argues that bilateral stimulation for motor rehabilitation has a stronger effect than unilateral stimulation [9]. However, stimulation of networks within *one* hemisphere may also be important and effective. The montage for a parietal lesion, for example, might have an anodal perilesional electrode montage with a cathodal frontal or occipital return electrode, depending on whether the aim is to vary a top-down process or a bottom-up process. An ipsilesional frontoparietal current flow should stimulate top-down processes, whereas a parietooccipital flow supports afferent perceptive functions. However, any unilateral stimulation implicates the risk of inhibiting part of the networks by the activity of the cathode, and therefore bilateral stimulation is safer (see below).

10.3 Safety concerns, basic technical questions, and planning of electrode positions

In Germany, the use of tDCS in hospitals must be legitimized as a healing attempt. Outside of hospitals, applying tDCS does not require legislative certification or education, although some manufacturers require users to attend their own training before using the devices. In any case, stimulation should only be performed using a CE-certified device that meets the requirements of the European Medical Devices Directive 93/42/EEC and the German Medical Devices Act. Further information on the legal basis for using tDCS in the EU and the United States of America, as well as important guidelines, can be found in sections 7.2 and 7.4.1 of Antal, Alekseichuk [27], and we strongly recommend reading these sections thoroughly and following the proposed conduct.

The typical range of current strength for tDCS stimulation in humans lies between 1 and 2 mA, and the duration of the stimulation should not exceed 20 minutes [6]. This is far below stimulations in animal studies, which partly stimulate directly above the brain and not only above the scalp. Still, other safety concerns limit tDCS application in neurorehabilitation even further. Such limitations are any kind of electrical stimulator or pacemaker inside the body, any hint of (prestroke) epilepsy or epilepsy-like patterns in the electroencephalography (EEG), shunt implementation, craniectomy, other openings of the scalp, and metal inside the brain. Even if the question of whether patients who have suffered from convulsions should be excluded in any case is unsettled, for early rehabilitation units with elderly patients, this may lead to about one-third of patients, who cannot be stimulated with tDCS. A clinical neuropsychologist should know these safety concerns and make sure that they are not violated before starting with stimulation. Additionally, using tDCS should be discussed with the respective physician beforehand.

Another methodological problem is that the effects of tDCS cannot be observed directly, because tDCS does not lead to neuronal spiking. This leads to extended observation times to see any effect. Even more problematic is that the localization of electrodes must be estimated and cannot be tested out by piloting. However, this difference from transcranial magnetic stimulation (TMS) depends on the target of stimulation. It may be no coincidence that TMS has been used mainly for motor rehabilitation of hand movements, because the hand knob is located directly below and parallel to the scalp. This allows an easy detection of its localization on clinical images and by provoking finger movements. Higher-order cortical areas do not show such a clear specialization. Their specific performance also depends on their connectivity. The same cortical structure may produce different behavioral effects depending on the task-specific network activation. In this respect, tDCS might even offer enhanced possibilities compared to TMS, which is more localized and does not allow to vary a position of activation and inhibition. Unfortunately, up to now, most of the tDCS studies have investigated the possibility of stimulating networks (except mutually inhibitory ones) but rather focused on stimulating focal regions of interest.

Thirdly, the structural changes in cortical stroke regions during the late postacute and chronic stages must be considered. In those stages, cortical stroke regions fill up with cerebrospinal fluid (CSF) because macrophages (i.e., immune cells of the central nervous system) remove lost neurons, glial cells, and axons. CSF, as a fluid, is a major conductor of current. Therefore a large part of the stimulation will flow into the poststroke CSF-filled lesion cavity and, without specific planning, the remaining current might not be strong enough to elicit any changes at the level of the neurons. Minjoli, Saturnino [28], who simulated the lesions of two stroke patients, found that the average loss of field strength was higher than 30% compared to healthy subjects. Positioning the electrode directly above the stroke lesion reduced the field strength by more than 50%. Such a loss of field strength asks for precise planning of the position of the electrodes. Yoon, Park [29] showed that an adapted positioning of the electrodes to the stroke localization increases the electrical fields of about 20% to 50% compared to the use of standard positions, which is an encouraging result (for similar results [30,31]).

Fourthly, the challenge of predicting current flow across and through the cortex is not limited to the presence of a lesion. CSF and blood vessels are present in the subarachnoid space and in the sulci (Chapter 1). All these structures may redirect the flow of the current. This also argues for an individualized planning of the positions of the electrodes, even if most of the existing clinical tDCS studies worked with nonindividualized standardized positions. Automatized simulation of electric fields and current flow would be feasible after import and normalization of clinical DICOM files, which are the standard digital formats for storing and transmitting medical imaging data. However, access to these files is often not given, and postprocessing takes too long for neuropsychological routine practice. That means that software-based planning of tDCS interventions is only feasible if clinicians can rapidly orient themselves in clinical scans, as introduced in Chapter 2.

In the following, we will first discuss evidence from animal and human studies regarding tDCS in the acute and early postacute stage. Following, human studies on tDCS in the late postacute and chronic stage will be outlined. Afterwards, we will introduce software that can simulate tDCS effects and demonstrate its appropriate use for planning stimulations. It should be emphasized once more that these considerations remain highly speculative, as no comparative studies on different electrode montages across stroke stages are available, and the existing effects of tDCS in treating cognitive and perceptive problems in stroke patients are limited.

10.4 Transcranial direct current stimulation during the acute and the early postacute stage

There are only a few studies including humans that looked at the effect of early tDCS stimulation on recovery. Most studies, at least regarding motor rehabilitation, have been conducted with patients in the chronic stage. Concerning early stimulation, Bahr-Hosseini, Nael [32] and Pruvost-Robieux, Benzakoun [33] applied cathodal tDCS over the affected hemisphere during the acute phase of stroke. Both studies showed that this is feasible and may reduce stroke size. Rossi, Sallustio [34], in contrast, applied *anodal* tDCS above the affected hemisphere. They stimulated during the acute phase (2 days poststroke) and did not observe any significant effect. Considering the animal studies reviewed below, the negative result may be considered plausible. However, Polanowska, Lesniak [35], who initiated anodal stimulation of the affected hemisphere on average 5 days after the stroke, documented an increase in performance on the Jebsen Hand function test (but in none of the other performed motor tests). Bornheim, Croisier [36] similarly reported a significant add-on effect of anodal stimulation during the late postacute phase (one month poststroke). However, patients in this study were treated later and were additionally less impaired compared to the Rossi, Sallustio [34] study, as patients with extensive motor cortex involvement were excluded, and only two patients of the verum group had cortical lesions compared to 7 of the 10 patients of the sham group.

A recent review of Sun, Vecchio [12] concluded that tDCS can support the rehabilitation of gait impairments. No such effect, however, was reported for the rehabilitation of upper limbs. Moreover, the review argued that the effect of tDCS is limited to the subacute phase and tends to diminish once patients reach the chronic phase. Concerning the placement of the electrodes, anodal tDCS of the ipsilesional hemisphere was reported to be more effective than cathodal tDCS of the contralesional hemisphere. Notably, the review defined the subacute phase as up to 6 months poststroke, yet only a few of the studies included assessed patients during the acute or early subacute stage. Thus the review mainly concerned the late subacute and chronic stage, limiting evidence for the early subacute phase. Still, the finding that anodal tDCS appears more effective in the late subacute stage than in the chronic stage is noteworthy, while metaanalytic evaluation of cathodal stimulation of the unaffected hemisphere has yielded inconsistent results [8,12].

Whereas clinical studies mainly concentrate on the late subacute and chronic stages, animal models allow closer examination of the acute and early subacute phases. For instance, Huang, Zhao [37] conducted a metaanalysis of eight studies, each initiating tDCS within the first days poststroke, thereby addressing *the acute or early subacute stage* of recovery. The review reported that cathodal tDCS, rather than anodal tDCS, was effective in improving neurological deficit (assessed by a modified neurological severity score) as well as in reducing the infarct size. A more recent study by Walter, Pikhovych [38] compared the outcomes of tDCS when applied on day 5 versus day 12 following experimental stroke in rodents. It was assessed whether the effect of anodal and cathodal stimulation of the stroke area differed when initiated either in the early subacute or late subacute stage. Walter, Pikhovych [38] found that cathodal tDCS starting on day 5 accelerated functional recovery, increased neurogenesis, as well as decreased microglial activation and inflammatory processes. While anodal tDCS similarly fostered neurogenesis, it did not increase functional recovery when applied in the early stage of recovery. Furthermore, neither cathodal nor anodal stimulation had any impact when applied as late as day 12. Yoon, Oh [39], reported similar results. This study only focused on anodal stimulation above the affected hemisphere and defined early as day 1 and late as day 5 after the stroke. Anodal stimulation on day 5 revealed more improvements when compared to day 1. However, this study did not include a cathodal condition and, since day 5 is still considered the early postacute range, also no late postacute stimulation. Taken together, these findings suggest that cathodal stimulation of the stroke area may be beneficial during the very early phase, whereas anodal stimulation appears to yield stronger effects after some not yet clearly defined number of days. In the chronic phase, however, neither cathodal nor anodal stimulation seems to significantly improve recovery. It should be mentioned that all these studies use tDCS as a single intervention and not as an add-on intervention to functional training. Clinically, however, tDCS is typically applied as an adjunct to rehabilitation, meaning that the findings may not fully represent its potential impact in practice.

Building on this, further experimental work in animal models has explored the neurobiological consequences of tDCS during the early postacute phase. Kaviannejad, Karimian [40] analyzed the effect of tDCS on artificial basilar ischemic strokes in rodents. Again, the stimulation was done during the early postacute phase, that is, day 1 or day 2 after the stroke induction. The neurobiological effect of tDCS was evaluated for the hippocampus. They demonstrated that cathodal, but not anodal, tDCS attenuated the oxidative stress, reduced neuroinflammation, and decreased neuronal death. While reporting benefits on neurobiological mechanisms, they did not present any behavioral data. For instance, they did not assess whether cathodal tDCS also improved memory performance–probably because they decapitated the animals already on day 3 to look for neurophysiological changes. Furthermore, Malinova, Bleuel [41] studied the effect of cathodal and anodal tDCS stimulation in a rodent model after nontraumatic subarachnoid hemorrahge (SAH). The tDCS interventions were initiated on day 3 and day 4 (i.e., early subacute phase) after the induced SAH bleeding. The results showed that cathodal stimulation improved the clinical state of the animals, whereas anodal stimulation worsened it.

Badoiu, Mitran [42] supported previous findings by demonstrating that tDCS reduces inflammatory response, suppresses autophagy, shows antiapoptotic effects and angiogenesis enhancement, attenuates oxidative stress, and influences neurotransmitter metabolism, neurogenesis, and enhances structural neuroplasticity in animal experiments. Rodriguez, Amaya-Pascasio [43] performed a combined systematic review on the effects of TMS and tDCS in animal studies. During the earliest stroke stage, ipsilesional cathodal and contralesional anodal stimulation were more effective than the reverse approaches. They argue that anodal stimulation of the contralesional, nonaffected cortex may play a role in compensating for the deficit (at least in the beginning of the recovery process). However, this is not the only interpretation. It is also plausible that cathodal dampening of neuronal activation in the ipsilesional hemisphere during the acute and early postacute phase exerts a protective effect by reducing additional neuronal loss and neuroinflammation. Concerning the later stages of recovery, Rodriguez, Amaya-Pascasio [43] reported no significant effect of tDCS. All in all, animal literature consistently suggests that tDCS can exert neuroprotective and restorative effects when applied in the acute or early subacute phase, but its benefits diminish once recovery progresses into later stages. However, it should be noted that all animal studies initiated stimulation in the acute or early postacute stage, and none combined tDCS with parallel functional training [44], which is an essential component of human neurorehabilitative studies on tDCS in the late postacute or in the chronic phase. Therefore the nonsignificant results for the later phase of recovery cannot be directly generalized to human stroke patients.

10.5 Evidence on transcranial direct current stimulation in human stroke syndromes

In previous and current clinical studies, tDCS has mainly been applied in three ways. First, as a single anodal stimulation above the lesioned hemisphere, with minimal impact of the return electrode. Second, as single cathodal stimulation above the contralesional hemisphere, and third, as bilateral anodal and cathodal stimulation, following the mutual inhibitory model [6]. As already mentioned, most of the reviews argue for a positive effect on motor rehabilitation after stroke [2–5,7,10,11,13,14,45–47], however a recent large RCT was unable to demonstrate such an effect [15].

Studies using an individualized planning of electrode's position are rare exceptions to this rule, and these studies also included only a small number of patients. One reason for this is that software to simulate the effects of positioning the electrodes has only become available during the last few years. Keeping that in mind, the next sections present a short overview of the results in different domains of cognitive functioning.

10.5.1 Visual field defect

To date, there is no evidence that tDCS or transcranial alternating current stimulation increases the efficacy of training-based treatments in visual field defects due to the lack of high-quality studies. The same holds for combined audiovisual stimulation treatments. Randomized control trials including more than 20 patients are still missing.

Chapter 4 informs about functional training approaches to treat visual field defects.

10.5.2 Neglect

The number of clinical trials investigating tDCS in neglect patients is limited when compared to aphasia and motor rehabilitation. However, a review of studies up to 2017 argues that dual-parietal tDCS might lead to an improvement in visuospatial neglect symptoms [48].

Three more recent controlled trials showed similar results. Turgut, Miranda [49], using a dual approach with right anodal and left cathodal stimulation, documented improved body orientation and clock drawing performance, a common diagnostic tool for neglect. Patients were in a subacute stage and treated with tDCS as well as optokinetic drift. da Silva, de Carvalho Nunes [50] similarly compared anodal right, cathodal left, and sham stimulation. They included outpatients who received physical treatment during the stimulation. Only anodal tDCS (combined with physical therapy) decreased the severity of neglect in neglect tests. Gorsler, Grittner [51] directly compared dual-parietal electrode montage with unilateral anodal stimulation and sham stimulation. Patients were in the subacute stage and trained in visual exploration and saccadic eye movements during the stimulation. The study documented a significant add-on effect only for dual stimulation compared to the sham condition. The difference concerned line bisection but not the cancellation task.

Thus the recent evidence endorses Zebhauser, Vernet [48], an older review that tDCS can contribute to improvements in neglect, particularly on neuropsychological tests and even more particularly in line bisection or body orientation, but not in visual search. However, these effects have not yet translated into clear, observable behavioral changes. Notably, a dual montage with ipsilesional stimulation and contralesional inhibition seems to reveal stronger effects compared to unilateral stimulation or inhibition. These results align with the findings of Sprague [52], which showed that lesioning the contralateral superior colliculus can compensate for the overexcitation of the nonlesioned hemisphere and has been the starting point of many bottom-up treatment approaches for visuospatial neglect (Chapter 5).

In summary, although clinical evidence is still limited, dual-parietal tDCS combining ipsilesional excitation with contralesional inhibition appears to be the most promising approach for alleviating neglect symptoms, particularly in structured neuropsychological tasks, while its translation to everyday functional gains remains uncertain.

Table 10.2 informs about the positioning of electrodes, and Chapter 5 informs about functional training approaches to treat neglect.

10.5.3 Aphasia

The number of studies using tDCS as an add-on intervention in the rehabilitation of aphasia is increasing. A recent metaanalytical study states that the most consistent results are reported for naming measures (i.e., speech production), whereas no effects on speech comprehension have been found yet [53,54]. Another review focusing on long-term effects of tDCS replicated this finding but argued that the effect vanishes over time, becoming insignificant at follow-up [55,56]. However, yet another review [57] argued that tDCS has a significant effect on recovery not only on naming. Still other studies argue that the effect is present in Broca aphasia but not in other types of aphasia [58], which fits the results of Raymer and Johnson [53] that tDCS is effective for naming but not for comprehension.

The stage of recovery is important too. Studies analyzing the effect of tDCS on stroke patients in the subacute state revealed a significant effect for naming performance [56,59]. The effect of tDCS for chronic patients was marginal, but still significant [56].

Concerning the montage of the electrodes, some studies focused on anodal stimulation of premotor areas, and others on the supramarginal or posterior temporal gyrus and the motor cortex. In this respect, anodal left inferior frontal cortex stimulation showed the most promising effects [54]. Right hemisphere cathodal stimulation did not produce consistent effects, which argues against the mutual inhibition model. However, dual stimulation (left anodal with right cathodal stimulation for homologous areas) has not been used in clinical trials.

Whereas most studies applied the same stimulation protocol to all patients, two studies used an individualized stimulation based on stroke localization. Cherney, Babbitt [60] used anodal, cathodal, and sham stimulation of perilesional areas in a small study. Anodal and cathodal stimulation improved performance compared to sham stimulation. There was no difference between the two stimulation polarities, even through both electrodes were placed ipsilesionally. Interestingly, cathodal stimulation resulted in increased areas of cortical activation across both hemispheres, and specifically in perilesional areas (for this counter-intuitive effect, see our simulations below). Stockbridge, Elm [61] performed a single-blinded randomized controlled trial with about 60 patients. On average, recruitment started 2 months after the stroke, which is still in the subacute stage but at the border to the chronic stage. Moreover, stroke severity was only mild to moderate, because more than one-third of the patients showed an anomic pattern (i.e., mainly word-finding difficulties with fluent and grammatically correct speech). Stimulation of gyri was based on the localization of the lesion, however always on the left side. Patients did not improve for the primary outcome variable (picture naming), but there was an effect on the quality of discourse, meaning the overall communication abilities.

Taken together, while tDCS in aphasia rehabilitation shows the most consistent benefits for naming, particularly with anodal stimulation of the left inferior frontal cortex, its broader effects on language recovery remain debated. Individualized, lesion-based approaches may offer additional promise, with results being preliminary.

Table 10.2 informs about the positioning of electrodes, and Chapter 6 informs about functional training approaches to treat aphasia.

10.5.4 Memory and working memory

Essential structures for memory performance are located far medial in the brain (Chapter 1) and are therefore not easily accessible by tDCS. The emitted current will thus not reach the target regions in sufficient quantities. In addition, it is not sufficiently clarified which specific process of memory rehabilitation should be facilitated by tDCS stimulation, which distinguishes it from motor rehabilitation and speech therapy. Another difference is that for aphasia and neglect, inhibition of lesion-induced hyperactivity may play a role, which can be achieved by cathodal stimulation. However, lesion-induced inhibition seems to play no role in memory impairments. One possible reason is that memory function relies on bilateral, distributed networks, whereas aphasia or neglect are strongly lateralized, making them more susceptible to interhemispheric imbalance.

Medvedeva, Materassi [62] investigated the ideal time of tDCS (encoding, consolidation, or retrieval of information) in healthy individuals to achieve an improvement in memory performance and provide an overview of the results of other studies on this topic. It becomes clear that tDCS probably has no effect on consolidation when applied head-on. Frontal stimulation also has no effect on retrieval, but it does have a positive effect on encoding performance. This effect is particularly present for stimulation at F7 of the 10/20 EEG system; results at F3 stimulation are more contradictory (the 10/20 system and the F7/F3 positions are explained below). Positive effects were also demonstrated during encoding by temporoparietal stimulation [63]. It should be emphasized that these results are based on studies in healthy individuals and that they primarily examined recognition performance rather than free recall, which is generally more relevant for neurorehabilitation purposes (after stroke, patients can often still perform reasonably well on recognition because the task provides external cues that guide retrieval). It remains unclear whether the results can be transferred to patients with memory impairment and what role the underlying location of the lesion could play (e.g., in the supply area of the middle cerebral artery compared to the posterior cerebral artery). The Canadian guideline for cognitive impairments in traumatic brain injury patients explicitly states that, up to now, there is no evidence that tDCS has an effect on rehabilitation training [64].

The review of Cruz Gonzalez, Fong [65] on the effectiveness of tDCS in people with mild cognitive impairment documents the problem of a clear assignment of the brain area accessible by tDCS and memory performance. Five RCTs were included, with the left hemisphere being the target of stimulation. All studies showed different electrode positioning—bilateral or unilateral. The results of the review show a significant effect only immediately after stimulation (after-effect of tDCS application), and no study documented a lasting and tDCS-independent effect.

In a recent review, Yan, Zhang [66] analyzed the effect of tDCS on the cognitive performance of patients after stroke. A total of 15 studies with 820 patients were included in the analysis. Compared to the control groups, the verum groups showed a highly significant improvement in the mini-mental state examination and the Montreal cognitive assessment, as well as a significant improvement in attention performance. In contrast, the studies did not show any evidence that tDCS could influence memory performance (see Table 10.1). Attentional performance is based partly on right hemisphere cortical areas, which can be stimulated by tDCS. This may explain why attention performance could be increased by additional tDCS, whereas not for memory performance.

TABLE 10.1 Effect of transcranial direct current stimulation on memory performance.

	anodal tDCS			passive tDCS				Std. Mean Difference
Study or Subgroup	Mean	SD	Total	Mean	SD	Total	Weight	IV, Random, 95% CI
Chen 2019	3.18	1.19	40	2.89	1.25	40	19.0%	0.24 [-0.20, 0.68]
Shaker 2018	8.2	1.36	20	5.8	0.83	20	15.0%	2.09 [1.30, 2.87]
Sun 2016	97	22	26	84	23	27	17.7%	0.57 [0.02, 1.12]
Yun 2015	5	1.2	15	4.9	1.4	15	15.8%	0.07 [-0.64, 0.79]
Zeng 2019	3.36	0.63	14	2.57	0.65	14	14.6%	1.20 [0.38, 2.01]
Zheng 2017	2.99	1.17	27	2.91	1.27	28	18.0%	0.06 [-0.46, 0.59]
Total (95% CI)			142			144	100.0%	0.66 [0.11, 1.20]

Heterogeneity: Tau² = 0.36; Chi² = 23.95, df = 5 (P = 0.0002); I² = 79%
Test for overall effect: Z = 2.35 (P = 0.02)

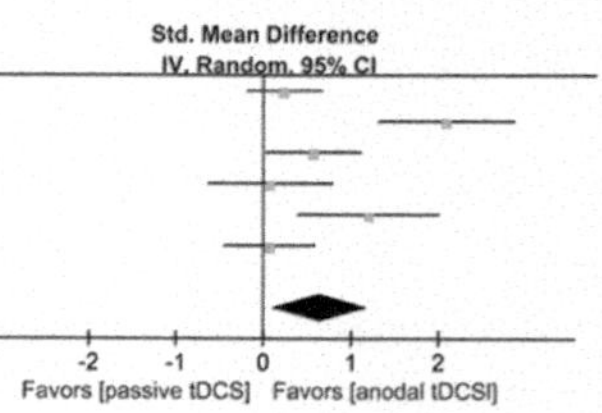

	anodal tDCS			passive tDCS				Std. Mean Difference
Study or Subgroup	Mean	SD	Total	Mean	SD	Total	Weight	IV, Random, 95% CI
Chen 2019	0.647	0.141	40	0.601	0.196	40	35.5%	0.27 [-0.17, 0.71]
Shaker 2018	6.5	1.19	20	4.85	0.81	20	32.3%	1.59 [0.87, 2.31]
Yun 2015	0.6	0.2	15	0.7	0.1	15	32.2%	-0.62 [-1.35, 0.12]
Total (95% CI)			75			75	100.0%	0.41 [-0.67, 1.50]

Heterogeneity: Tau² = 0.81; Chi² = 18.12, df = 2 (P = 0.0001); I² = 89%
Test for overall effect: Z = 0.74 (P = 0.46)

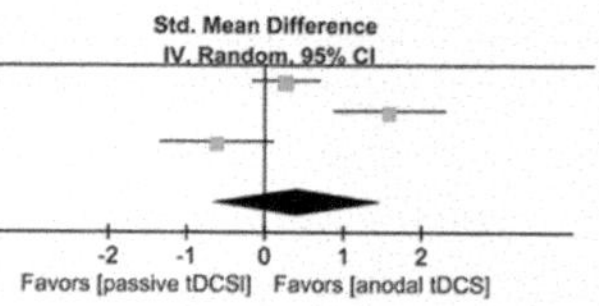

Note: reproduced from 'Effect of transcranial direct-current stimulation on cognitive function in stroke patients: A systematic review and meta-analysis." by Yan, Zhang [66].

A recent review on working memory training combined with tDCS showed significant effects of the training but no additional effects of tDCS [67].

In conclusion, current evidence suggests that while tDCS may transiently enhance encoding, there is no convincing proof that it improves global memory functioning in stroke patients, likely due to the bilateral and deeply located networks underlying memory processes, which remain largely inaccessible to stimulation.

Table 10.2 informs about the positioning of electrodes, and Chapter 7 about functional training approaches to treat memory disorders.

TABLE 10.2 Standard placement of transcranial direct current stimulation electrodes in previous investigations.

	Anode	Cathode
Neglect		
Unilateral	P4	Contralateral supraorbital
Bilateral	P4	P3
Aphasia		
Unilateral	F7	Contralateral supraorbital
Unilateral	F3	Contralateral supraorbital
Unilateral	T5	Contralateral supraorbital
Unilateral	CP5	Contralateral supraorbital
Unilateral	C3	Contralateral supraorbital
Bilateral	F7	F8
Bilateral	T5	T6
Memory disorders		
Unilateral	F3	Contralateral supraorbital
Unilateral	T3 or T5	Contralateral supraorbital
Unilateral	P3 or P4	Contralateral supraorbital
Bilateral	F3	F4
Disorders of consciousness		
Unilateral	F3	Contralateral supraorbital

10.5.5 Goal management training

The current clinical guidelines caution that the evidence base remains limited and further research is warranted [68].

10.5.6 Disorders of consciousness

Evidence for tDCS in the unresponsive wakefulness state (UWS) is inconclusive, and in the minimal consciousness state (MCS) is limited. Some studies report modest improvements in behavioral responsiveness, but these results are often confounded by methodological issues, such as small sample sizes and varying stimulation protocols [69,70]. Thus tDCS cannot yet be considered a standard treatment for UWS. Studies indicate significant improvements in scores on the Coma Recovery Scale-Revised [71–73]. The evidence in MCS is more robust, currently recommending applying anodal tDCS to the left dorsolateral prefrontal cortex, though further research is needed to standardize protocols and confirm long-term benefits [72]. In summary, tDCS appears more effective in MCS than in UWS, but further studies are necessary to establish its clinical utility and optimize treatment parameters [74].

Table 10.2 informs about the positioning of electrodes, and Chapter 9 informs about functional training approaches.

Fig. 10.3 offers information for an understanding of the electrode positions on the scalp according to the EEF 10/20 system.

10.6 Simulating transcranial direct current stimulation interventions

10.6.1 Relation between lesion localization and electrode position for the 10/20 system and starting a first simulation

Previous studies have demonstrated that stroke lesions alter current flow and reduce electric field strength, emphasizing the need for individualized of electrode placement to maximize cognitive rehabilitation effects [6]. To adapt the stimulation to the stroke localization, it is necessary to define a reference system between the scalp and cortical areas. The 10/20 system for the montage of EEG electrodes offers such a reference (for a description on how to use this system and calculate the different electrode position compare Klem, Luders [75]). Fig. 10.3 depicts the various electrode positions of this system and the cortical gyri from four different perspectives. Table 10.3 [76] offers a list of these positions and informs about the targeted cortical areas if using these coordinates for stimulation.

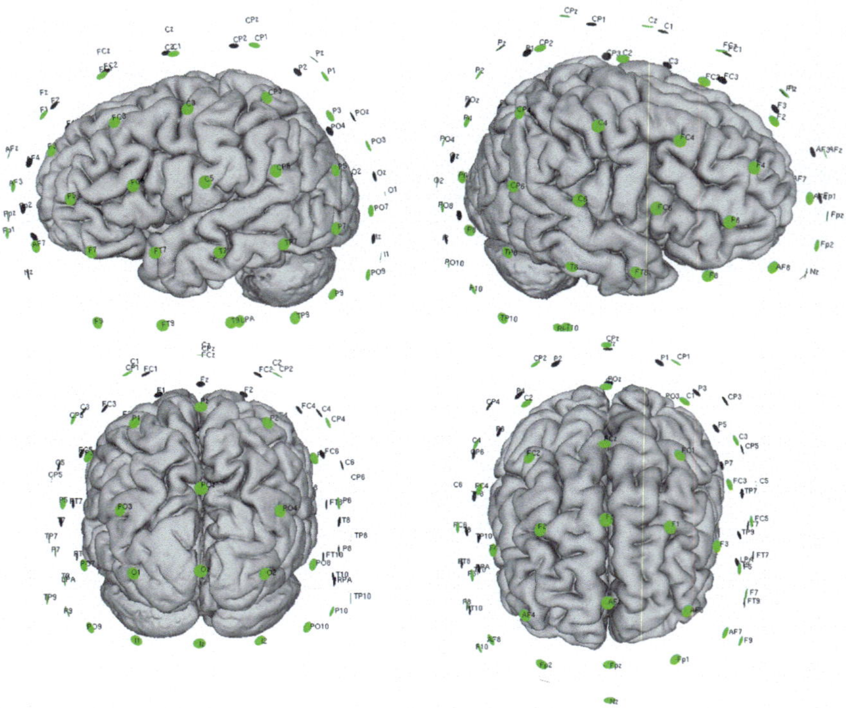

FIGURE 10.3 Electrodes' positions and brain surface visualized by SimNIBS software.

Fig. 10.3 is generated by SimNIBS 4.1.0, a free software to plan and model brain stimulation for TMS and tDCS, and we invite the reader to download this software (https://simnibs.github.io/simnibs/build/html/index.html), since the practical introduction of tDCS will be based on this software. There is a description on how to install the SimNIBS software on the respective website. To see Fig. 10.3, it is necessary (1) to enter the address of the m2m_ernie folder and (2) to activate the gray matter button in the left upper part of the screen (as shown in Fig. 10.4).

To start a simulation, follow the description on the website. In short, go to the lower left part of the software screen and activate the button to add tDCS Poslist. Click "add electrode" and fill in the mA strength (usually between 1 and 2 mA). Click below the position label and choose one of the 10/20 positions by clicking in the field on the left below the position (e.g., C4). Close this window with "okay" and click below the shape. You may use rectangular and circular shapes. Most of the studies use rectangular shapes, but this is only due to material loss when using circular ones. Increasing the shape's extension reduces focal current flow, and reducing the extension increases it. Extensions below 3 cm per

TABLE 10.3 Neuroanatomical structures and related EEG electrodes' positions.

Electrode	Percentage underlying brain regions	Brodmann area
AF3	Frontal pole (100%)	Left BA9
AF4	Frontal pole (100%)	Right BA9
AF7	Frontal pole (100%)	Left BA10
AF8	Frontal pole (100%)	Right BA10
AFZ	Frontal pole (62.5%), superior frontal gyrus (37.5%)	Left BA9
C1	Precentral gyrus (71%), postcentral gyrus (29%)	Left BA4
C2	Precentral gyrus (87.5%), postcentral gyrus (12.5%)	Right BA6
C3	Postcentral gyrus (87.5%), precentral gyrus (12.5%)	Left BA1
C4	Postcentral gyrus (85%), precentral gyrus (15%)	Right BA1
C5	Postcentral gyrus (50%), anterior supramarginal gyrus (44.4%), precentral gyrus (5.6%)	Left BA40
C6	Anterior SMG (72%), postcentral gyrus (28%)	Right BA40
CP1	Superior parietal lobe (SPL) (66.67%), postcentral gyrus (27.78%), superior lateral occipital lobe (5.56%)	Left BA7
CP2	SPL (80%), postcentral gyrus (13%), superior LOC (7%)	Right BA7
CP3	Posterior SMG (47%), SPL (27%), angular gyrus (ANG) (13%), postcentral gyrus (13%)	Left BA40
CP4	ANG (50%), SPL (42%), postcentral gyrus (8%)	Right BA7
CP5	Posterior SMG (61.11%), anterior SMG (16.67%), ANG (11.11%), posterior superior temporal gyrus (STG) (5.56%), superior LOC (5.56%)	Left BA39
CP6	ANG (53%), posterior SMG (40%), superior LOC (7%)	Right BA39
CPZ	Postcentral gyrus (62.5%), precuneus cortex (18.75%), SPL (12.5%), superior LOC (6.25%)	Left BA7
CZ	Precentral gyrus (87%), postcentral gyrus (13%)	Right BA4
F1	SFG (71%), frontal pole (29%)	Left BA6/BA8
F2	SFG (77%), frontal pole (23%)	Right BA6/BA8
F3	Medial frontal gyrus (64%), frontal pole (36%)	Left BA9
F4	Frontal pole (53%), MFG (47%)	Right BA9
F5	MFG (65%), frontal pole (35%)	Left BA9
F6	MFG (50%), frontal pole (50%)	Right BA9
F7	Inferior frontal gyrus (IFG) (pars triangularis) (83%), frontal pole (11%), IFG (pars opercularis) (6%)	Left BA45
F8	IFG (pars triangularis) (66.67%), IFG (pars opercularis) (16.67%), MFG (5.56%), precentral gyrus (5.56%), frontal pole (5.56%)	Right BA45

(Continued)

TABLE 10.3 (Continued)

Electrode	Percentage underlying brain regions	Brodmann area
FC1	SFG (93.75%), MFG (6.25%)	Left BA6
FC2	SFG (82%), precentral gyrus (18%)	Right BA6
FC3	MFG (89%), precentral gyrus (11%)	Left BA6
FC4	MFG (92%), precentral gyrus (8%)	Right BA6
FC5	Precentral gyrus (88%), MFG (6%), IFG (pars opercularis) (6%)	Left BA6
FC6	Precentral gyrus (81%), postcentral gyrus (13%), MFG (6%)	Right BA6
FCZ	Juxtapositional lobule cortex (66.7%), SFG (33.3%)	Left BA6
FP1	Frontal pole (100%)	Left BA10
FP2	Frontal pole (100%)	Right BA10
FPZ	Frontal pole (100%)	Left BA10
FT10	Anterior middle temporal gyrus (MTG) (66.7%), posterior inferior temporal gyrus (11.1%), temporal pole (11.1%), posterior MTG (5.6%), anterior ITG (5.6%)	Right BA21
FT7	Precentral gyrus (64.29%), temporal pole (14.29%), anterior STG (14.29%), IFG (pars opercularis) (7.14%)	Left BA44
FT8	Precentral gyrus (62.5%), anterior STG (25%), central opercular cortex (6.25%), posterior MTG (6.25%)	Right BA6
FT9	Anterior MTG (42%), temporal pole (37%), posterior MTG (16%), anterior ITG (5%)	Left BA38
FZ	SFG (100%)	Left BA6
O1	Occipital pole (100%)	Left BA18
O2	Occipital pole (100%)	Right BA18
OZ	Occipital pole (100%)	Left BA18
P1	Superior LOC (95%), SPL (5%)	Left BA7
P2	Superior LOC (100%) R	Right BA7
P3	Superior LOC (95%), ANG (5%)	Left BA39
P4	Superior LOC (100%)	Right BA39
P5	Superior LOC (89.47%), inferior LOC (5.26%), ANG (5.26%)	Left BA39
P6	Superior LOC (100%) R	Right BA39
P7	Inferior LOC (75%), superior LOC (20%), MTG (temporooccipital part) (5%)	Left BA19
P8	Inferior LOC (85%), superior LOC (10%), ANG (5%)	Right BA19
PO3	Superior LOC (65%), occipital pole (35%)	Left BA19
PO4	Occipital pole (58%), superior LOC (42%)	Right BA19

(Continued)

TABLE 10.3 (Continued)

Electrode	Percentage underlying brain regions	Brodmann area
PO7	Inferior LOC (80%), superior LOC (15%), occipital pole (5%)	Left BA18
PO8	Occipital pole (33.33%), superior LOC (33.33%), inferior LOC (33.33%)	Right BA19
POZ	Cuneal cortex (37.5%), occipital pole (31.3%), superior LOC (25%), precuneus cortex (6.3%)	Left BA19
PZ	Precuneeus cortex (60%), superior LOC (33.33%), SPL (6.66%)	Left BA7
T7	Posterior STG (72.2%), posterior MTG (16.6%), anterior STG (5.6%), anterior SMG (5.6%)	Left BA21
T8	Posterior STG (52.9%), posterior MTG (29.4%), planum temporale (5.9%), anterior SMG (5.9%), central opercular cortex (5.9%)	Right BA22
TP7	MTG (temporooccipital part) (73.7%), posterior SMG (15.8%), posterior MTG (10.5%)	Left BA21
TP8	MTG (temporooccipital part) (75%), ANG (20%), posterior SMG (5%)	Right BA37
TP9	ITG (temporooccipital part) (100%)	Not applicable (cerebellum)
TP10	ITG (temporooccipital part) (89%), MTG (temporooccipital part) (11%)	Not applicable (cerebellum)

From Scrivener C.L., Reader A.T. Variability of EEG electrode positions and their underlying brain regions: visualizing gel artifacts from a simultaneous EEG-fMRI dataset. Brain Behav 2022;12(2e2476.

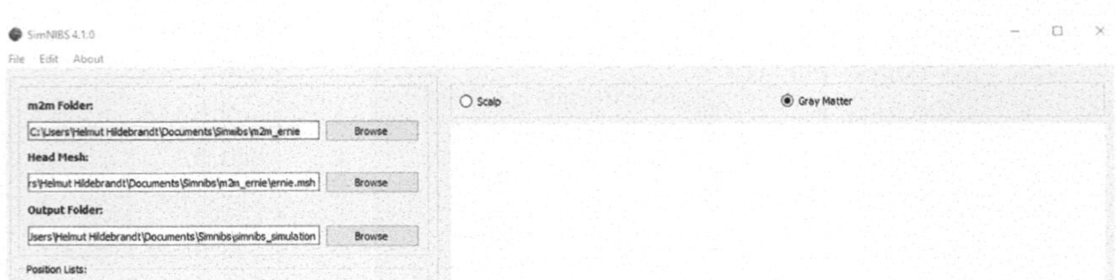

FIGURE 10.4 Screenshot of the SimNIBS software.

dimension increase the risk of feeling skin pain. It is important to compute the current density in the skin underneath the electrode, since there is a threshold of 0.1 mA/cm^2 that should not be exceeded according to the Bundesinstitut für Arzneimittel und Medizinprodukte. For a rectangular electrode of 5 by 7 cm with an area of 35 cm^2, a current of

1 mA would result in a current density of 0.028 mA/cm^2. Now, add a second electrode, define the same level of current but as a negative number, which means that you define the cathodal (return) electrode. For an example based on the mutual inhibitory hemisphere, use C3 as a position. Not using a circular electrode, it is necessary to rotate the second electrode into the correct position. To rotate the electrode, move the cursor to the correct position (vertical below its position), and click twice on the right mouse button. You will see that the virtual electrode moves somewhat. Having done that, you may start your first simulation, which takes some minutes depending on the speed of your PC.

10.6.2 Localization of strokes using the 10/20 EEG system

How to localize stroke areas was the topic of Chapter 2, and we refer to this chapter as relevant background information to understand the following parts of this chapter. In Chapter 2, we defined how to localize the ramus ascendens posterior of the fissure silvii. This ramus defines the 10/20 position "CP" for the electrode, whereas the position "C" for the electrode is related to that of the sulcus centralis (also defined in Chapter 2). The F1 and F2 sites are related to the position of the sulcus frontalis superior, FC5 and FC6 describe a scalp position above Broca's area and its right hemisphere homolog. PO3 and PO4 can be found following the sulcus intraparietalis and are positioned on the scalp related to the angular gyrus. Therefore planning an individualized stimulation of perilesional gray matter or cortical networks involved in stroke lesions presupposes knowledge of where the lesion is localized and which position of the 10/20 system fits that localization.

For a practical example, we focus on case 2 from chapter 2, the images of the fronto–insular stroke. The frontal lesion is clearly visible in row 2, column 1 to 3. The insular lesion is still visible on row 2, column 4. The Heschl's gyrus, described in Chapter 2, can be detected for the right hemisphere in the latter images, for the left hemisphere on row 2, column 3. Cortical areas for transversal sections rostral to this gyrus are mainly part of the frontal lobe (with the exclusion of the first gyrus, which may be the postcentral cortex). The more dorsal pictures show that at least three sulci rostral to Heschl's gyrus are involved in the lesion. This means that the stroke impaired the motor, the premotor cortex, and possibly also the caudal parts of Broca's area. However, more dorsal parts of the frontal cortex are not involved. Projecting that knowledge to Fig. 10.3 showing the 10/20 system, this would mean that one electrode should be placed on the left side of the brain at the site of FC5.

10.6.3 Simulations of electric field strength and current flow by SimNIBS

The simulation of the electric field by SimNIBS ends with its visualization in Gmsh (for an introduction to this software, compare https://www.youtube.com/watch?v=wMCx36EUPwI). You will see the electrodes and the surface (gray matter) of the brain. To focus on other structures, go to *"tools"* in the left upper part of the software window and click on *"visibility."* There are many options available, but one should start with 1, 2, or 3 showing electric field strength in white, gray matter, or CSF, respectively. To focus on the electrical field below the brain's surface, there is a tool menu showing a button called *"clipping,"* which allows dissection of the brain in the three different sagittal, coronal, and transversal directions (for further information on these terms and sectioning the brain in different images, compare Chapter 1). First, decide which direction of the section you want to see, and then from which perspective you want to inspect the sections. We will use transversal sectioning and move through the brain from ventral to dorsal (Fig. 10.5, for the other possibilities). Afterwards, activate *"view one."* Now, clicking into the field of *"D"* in the clipping menu with the left mouse button and moving the mouse from left to right (or vice versa) allows us to inspect the electric field strength at the different levels of the section. It is easy to see that the electric field strengths follow the sulci of the brain, but also reach the subcortical and the white matter of the different gyri. Choosing Volume 9 (blood) in the menu visibility further allows you to visualize the major veins of the brain and their uptake of electricity.

We invite the reader to use the clinical cases of Chapter 2 to simulate different electrode positions related to the lesion localization and to analyze the effect of the cathode position and size on the electric field strength.

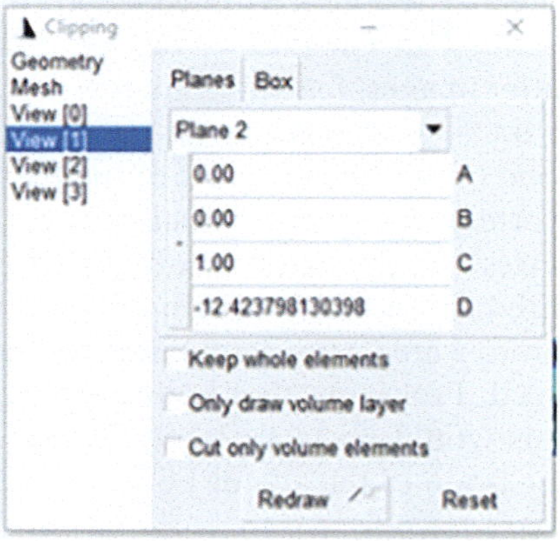

FIGURE 10.5 How to select SimNIBS views of brain regions.

10.7 How to define the electrodes' positions?

10.7.1 The impact of stroke on transcranial direct current stimulation

Table 10.2 lists the standard montages of tDCS for treating different stroke syndromes. As mentioned above, however, there are several arguments that such a standard montage might be suboptimal, because of a limited understanding of the distribution of the resulting electric field and the differences in stroke localization. For instance, placing the anode at P4 for all neglect patients will yield highly variable perilesional fields when the lesion is frontal rather than parietal. Galletta, Cancelli [77] were one of the first to argue against standard montage because of the varying electric field distribution. In two patients with frontal stroke suffering from aphasia, they demonstrated that the position of the cathodal electrode is of major importance for the distribution of the electric field. This contradicts the assumption of the classical montages, where the cathode is mostly attached at a frontopolar position or even outside the head to avoid any inhibition. According to Galletta, Cancelli [77], any placement of the cathode influences the distribution of electric field strength and therefore the amount of current reaching the target region. Or in other words: it is not just the anode, which defines the emitted field strength at a specific area of the brain, but the distance between and the relative positioning of both electrodes. And optimizing the electric field strength at a specific position of the brain is important, because the emitted current which reaches the cortex and subcortical structures, is low.

Galletta, Cancelli [77] further argued that, in the case of Broca's aphasia, the best electrode placement may include a left frontal anode and a right frontal cathode. They propose that this placement allows for the highest field strength at the left frontal Broca's area (because of a smaller distance compared to a contralateral frontopolar position). This is an interesting finding, since bilateral montages seem to have stronger effects. However, following the simulation of Galletta, Cancelli [77], not because of the correctness of the inhibitory model, but simply because of electric field optimization.

Evans, Johnstone [78] simulated the effect of artificial strokes outside the hand knob area for stimulating the hand knob area (i.e., the bulge on the precentral gyrus marking the hand representation of the primary motor cortex) to treat upper extremity motor paresis. From a clinical point of view, this approach is somewhat irritating, since it targets the neuroanatomical substrate of the function to be improved rather than the lesioned tissue itself. Their simulation would act compensatory: increase the function of unimpaired structures to take over the diminished performance.

The study of Evans, Johnstone [78] is highly relevant because they analyzed not only the meaning of the electrode's position, but also the impact of lesion size, lesion distance, and current flow direction. First, lesion size and lesion distance played a major role in the electric field strength in the target area (Fig. 10.6). Large lesions near the target area reduced the field strength considerably. Lesion conductivity also had an effect. If the conductivity is limited (as in the postacute phase without a complete transformation of the center of the stroke area into CSF), the impact on the electric field strength is less than in a situation where scar building is finished, the stroke is completely demarcated and filled with highly conductive CSF (for a similar result [79]).

However, the impact of lesion size and lesion location was also moderated by the direction of current flow. The lesion acted as an attractor: due to the high conductivity, major parts of the emitted current were funnelled into the direction of the lesion. Fig. 10.7 shows the effect of the relative position of the lesion on current flow and electric field strength: if the lesion is located in opposite direction of the intended current flow strengths is decreasing (Part A of Fig. 10.7) and if the lesion is in line with the current flow the strengths might even increase (Part B of Fig. 10.7).

Fig. 10.8 shows the result of the optimal placement of the electrodes depending on the location of the lesion and aiming to increase the field strength at the hand knob of the sulcus centralis. In the case of a lesion on the right of the hand knob area, in an anterior–inferior position (the Fig. 10.8 does not show the third dimension exactly), the anode should be placed at a dorsal parietal position and the cathode contralaterally frontal. In the case of a lesion on the left of the hand knob area, the cathode should be placed much more centrally on the vertex and the anode at the junction of the temporal and occipital lobes.

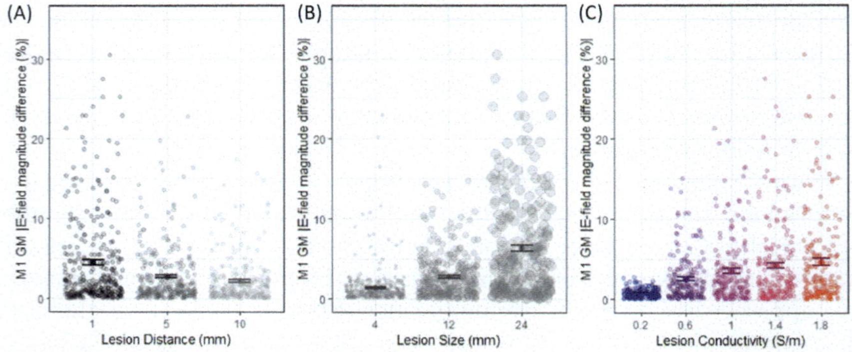

FIGURE 10.6 Impact of lesion characteristics on electrical field magnitude. *From Evans C., Johnstone A., Zich C., Lee J.S.A., Ward N.S., Bestmann S. The impact of brain lesions on tDCS-induced electric fields. Sci Rep 2023;13(119430.*

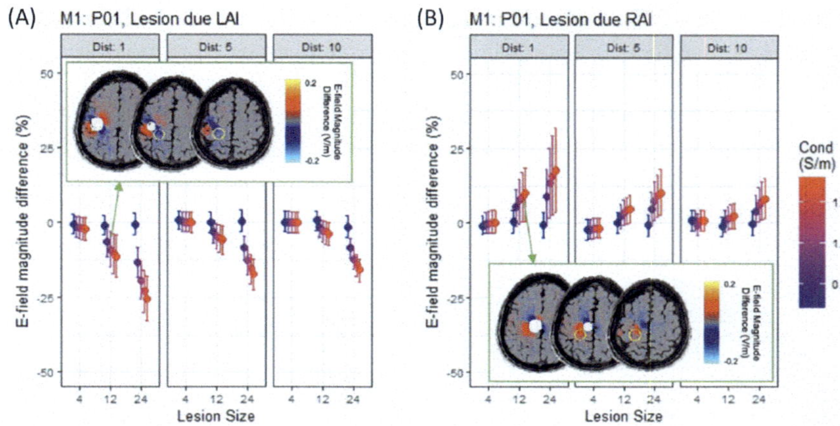

FIGURE 10.7 Impact of lesion size and distance on induced electrical field. *From Evans C., Johnstone A., Zich C., Lee J.S.A., Ward N.S., Bestmann S. The impact of brain lesions on tDCS-induced electric fields. Sci Rep 2023;13(119430.*

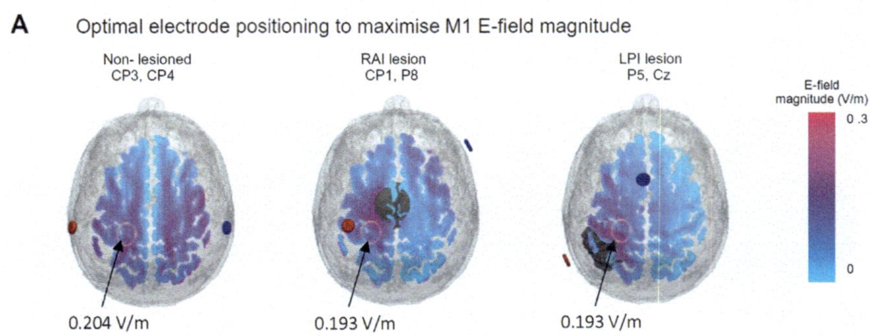

FIGURE 10.8 Effects of electrode positioning. *From Evans C., Johnstone A., Zich C., Lee J.S.A., Ward N.S., Bestmann S. The impact of brain lesions on tDCS-induced electric fields. Sci Rep 2023;13(119430.*

Evans, Johnstone [78] argued that the lesion should be located more inline the position of the two electrodes, to have the highest electric field at the target areas—at least if one does not consider the relative directions of the neurons and the current flow, but only the amount of electrical stimulation.

One question that is not answered by the published simulation studies is whether unilateral stimulation might increase focal electric field strength. A strong argument against unilateral stimulation is that the cathode might inhibit relevant network-related areas located in the same hemisphere. However, technically, it should be possible to moderate this effect by increasing the size of the cathode and therefore reducing its focal impact on specific brain areas. The advantage of unilateral stimulation is that it would reduce the effect of the interhemispheric fissure, which captures electric field strength because the sinus saggitalis superior and its subarachnoid space is filled with CSF and blood, both of which have a large conductivity.

To answer this question, we used SimNIBS to simulate two unilateral montages and increased the size of the cathode. As can be seen in Fig. 10.9,

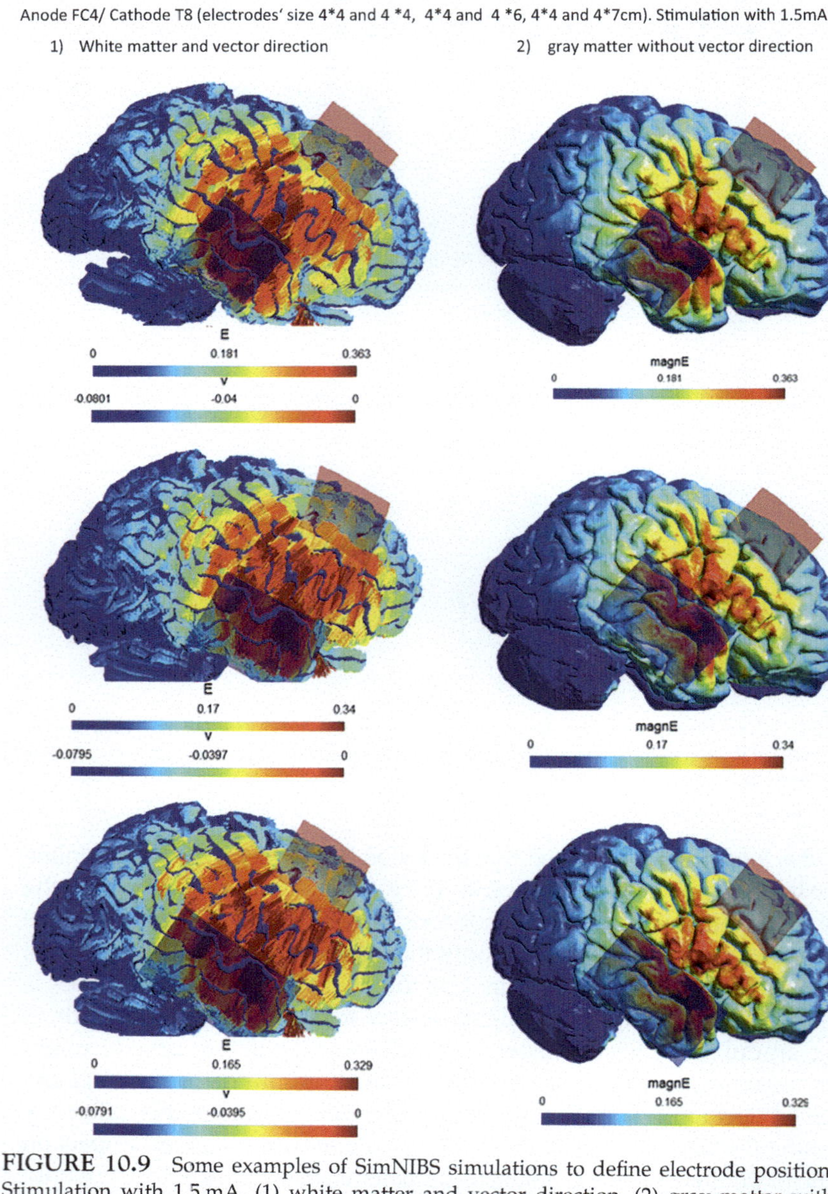

FIGURE 10.9 Some examples of SimNIBS simulations to define electrode positioning. Stimulation with 1.5 mA, (1) white matter and vector direction, (2) gray matter without vector direction, anode FC6/cathode T10 (electrodes' size 4*4 and 4*4, 4*4 and 4*4 and 4*7 cm). Stimulation with 1.5 mA, (1) white matter and vector direction, (2) gray matter without vector direction.

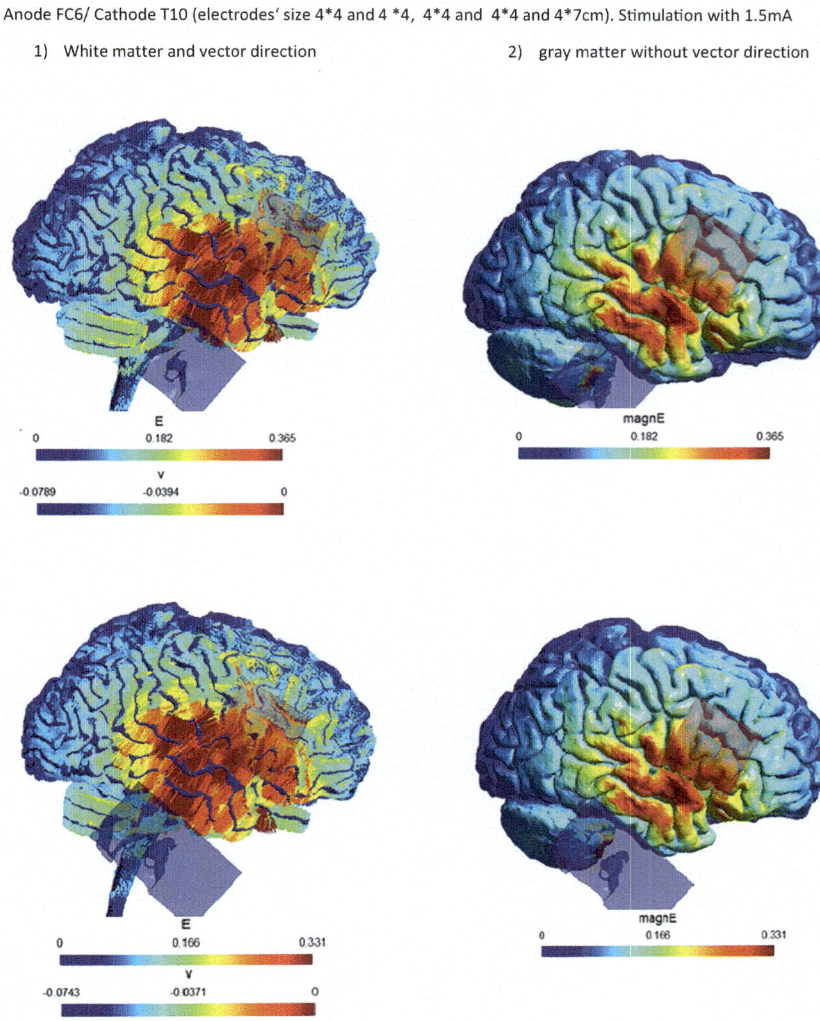

FIGURE 10.9 *(continued)*

the size of the cathode did not play any major role for focal electric field strength (as often assumed). Increasing the size of the cathode from 16 mm^2 to 28 mm^2 reduced the electric field strength by about 10% (comparing the E and magnE of the different simulations). The absolute position of the anode and the cathode similarly did not impact the localization with the highest electrical field significantly. The crossing of the fissure silvii by the direction of the current flow—displayed by the vector field—determined the strength of the electric field. It was always highest on the side of the fissura sylvii of the cathode. Moving the anode nearer to the fissure or increasing the size of the cathode did not change that. Therefore any unilateral stimulation should be explicitly network-guided. The anode should be placed over the target network and the return on the same-hemisphere sites that will not interfere with the targeted function. Moreover, single-anode unilateral montage is often suboptimal; a network-guided setup with a distributed/large return is more likely to confine the field to the target perilesional network and avoid unwanted inhibition.

10.7.2 Speculative suggestions for the montage of transcranial direct current stimulation electrodes

Table 10.4 gives an overview of electrode montages related to stages of stroke recovery.

However, this is not an individualized usage of tDCS. Mathematical modeling of tDCS is out of reach for the near future, because the models still struggle with unsolved problems (e.g., conductivity of the [scattered] lesion,

TABLE 10.4 Speculative relations between post-stroke recovery phase and transcranial Direct Current Stimulation interventions.

Recovery stage	Target area	Possible montage
Acute and early subacute	Perilesional gray matter	Bilateral, cathodal on the affected, anodal on the unaffected hemisphere
Late subacute	Perilesional gray matter	Anodal perilesional stimulation, indifferent cathodal electrode position
Late subacute and chronic	Perilesional gray matter	Anodal perilesional stimulation, indifferent cathodal electrode position
	Inhibition of contralesional hyperactivity	Bilateral stimulation: anodal on the affected, cathodal on the unaffected hemisphere
	Stimulation of networks for the relearning of functions	Bilateral montage along assumed networks (e.g., the dorsal attention system, language areas, etc.). The cathodal position should be in line with the extension of the network, but on the contralesional scalp
	Improving attention by stimulating attentional subsystems	Focal anodal stimulation of attention-relevant brain structures (unclear if unilateral stimulation might be used)

increasing subarachnoid space due to the stroke lesion, available time for treating single patients [80,81], etc.). However, tentatively and based on the simulations reviewed and performed above, a more individualized placement of the electrodes may take into account the following aspects:

1. The distance between the two electrodes should never be too small nor too large.
2. If the cathode activity can be ignored or might even contribute to the intended goal, the size of this electrode should be no larger than that of the anode. Otherwise, the size of the cathode might be increased (however, this reduces the maximal focal electrode strength).
3. If the goal is to stimulate perilesional neurons, both electrodes should be placed in one line before and behind the lesion.
4. Large sulci crossing through the line between anode and cathode should be avoided if possible. They will capture the electric field strength.
5. If the goal is to stimulate a network responsible for the impaired function, both electrodes should be placed in one line before and behind the network. For instance, if the lesion is localized in Broca's area, place the cathode next to but posterior to Broca's area and the anode caudal to Wernicke's area.
6. During the early subacute stage, a cathodal stimulation above the lesion and an anodal contralesional stimulation show the highest effect in animal research.

References

[1] Woods AJ, Antal A, Bikson M, et al. A technical guide to tDCS, and related non-invasive brain stimulation tools. Clin Neurophysiol 2016;127(2):1031–48.

[2] Abdullahi A, Wong TWL, Ng SSM. Effects of home-based neurostimulation on outcomes after stroke: a systematic review and meta-analysis. Neurol Sci 2024;45(11):5157–79.

[3] Chamorro-Hinojosa JA, Molina-Rueda F, Carratala-Tejada M. Transcranial direct current stimulation in the treatment of gait disturbance in post-stroke patients: an overview of systematic reviews. Sens (Basel) 2023;23(23).

[4] Grazia Maggio M, Bonanno M, Filoni S, Ciancarelli I, Quartarone A, Calabro RS. Can non-motor outcomes be improved in chronic stroke? A systematic review on the potential role of non-invasive brain stimulation. Brain Res 2024;1841:149093.

[5] He W, Yaning L, Shaohong Y. Effect of electrical stimulation in the treatment on patients with foot drop after stroke: a systematic review and network meta-analysis. J Stroke Cerebrovasc Dis 2025;34(5):108279.

[6] Hordacre B, McCambridge AB, Ridding MC, Bradnam LV. Can transcranial direct current stimulation enhance poststroke motor recovery? Development of a theoretical patient-tailored model. Neurology 2021;97(4):170–80.

[7] Jiang T, Yan J, Li X, et al. tDCS combined with CIMT for post-stroke upper extremity rehabilitation: a systematic review and meta-analysis. NeuroRehabilitation 2025;56(2):97–112.

[8] Kang N, Weingart A, Cauraugh JH. Transcranial direct current stimulation and suppression of contralesional primary motor cortex post-stroke: a systematic review and meta-analysis. Brain Inj 2018;32(9):1063–70.

[9] Lee S, Yoo Y. A literature review on optimal stimulation parameters of transcranial direct current stimulation for motor recovery after stroke. Brain Neurorehabil 2024;17(3).

[10] Li LL, Wu JJ, Li KP, et al. Comparative efficacy of different noninvasive brain stimulation protocols on upper-extremity motor function and activities of daily living after stroke: a systematic review and network meta-analysis. Neurol Sci 2024;45(8):3641–81.

[11] Rodriguez-Huguet M, Ayala-Martinez C, Vinolo-Gil MJ, Gongora-Rodriguez P, Martin-Valero R, Gongora-Rodriguez J. Transcranial direct current stimulation in physical therapy treatment for adults after stroke: a systematic review. NeuroRehabilitation 2024;54(2):171–83.

[12] Sun Y-Y, Vecchio F, Zheng M-X, et al. Transcranial direct current stimulation for upper and lower limb motor dysfunction after stroke: a systematic review and meta-analysis of randomized controlled trials. Brain Netw Modulation 2025;4(1). 4.

[13] Tang X, Zhang N, Shen Z, et al. Transcranial direct current stimulation for upper extremity motor dysfunction in poststroke patients: a systematic review and meta-analysis. Clin Rehabil 2024;38(6):749–69.

[14] Yu L, Chen H, Chen C, et al. Efficacy of anodal transcranial direct current stimulation for upper extremity function after ischemic stroke: a systematic review of parallel randomized clinical trials. J Stroke Cerebrovasc Dis 2025;34(1):108112.

[15] Schlaug G, Cassarly C, Feld JA, et al. Safety and efficacy of transcranial direct current stimulation in addition to constraint-induced movement therapy for post-stroke motor recovery (TRANSPORT2): a phase 2, multicentre, randomised, sham-controlled triple-blind trial. Lancet Neurol 2025;24(5):400–12.

[16] Nowak LG, Bullier J. Axons, but not cell bodies, are activated by electrical stimulation in cortical gray matter. II. Evidence from selective inactivation of cell bodies and axon initial segments. Exp Brain Res 1998;118(4):489–500.

[17] Nowak LG, Bullier J. Axons, but not cell bodies, are activated by electrical stimulation in cortical gray matter. I. Evidence from chronaxie measurements. Exp Brain Res 1998;118(4):477–88.

[18] Radman T, Ramos RL, Brumberg JC, Bikson M. Role of cortical cell type and morphology in subthreshold and suprathreshold uniform electric field stimulation in vitro. Brain Stimul 2009;2(4):215–28. 28 e1-3.

[19] Siebner HR, Ziemann U. Das TMS-Buch. Handbuch der transkraniellen magnetstimulation. Berlin Heidelberg: Springer-Verlag; 2007.

[20] Boros K, Poreisz C, Munchau A, Paulus W, Nitsche MA. Premotor transcranial direct current stimulation (tDCS) affects primary motor excitability in humans. Eur J Neurosci 2008;27(5):1292–300.

[21] Buch ER, Santarnecchi E, Antal A, et al. Effects of tDCS on motor learning and memory formation: a consensus and critical position paper. Clin Neurophysiol 2017;128(4):589–603.

[22] Bernhardt J, Borschmann K, Boyd L, et al. Moving rehabilitation research forward: developing consensus statements for rehabilitation and recovery research. Neurorehabil Neural Repair 2017;31(8):694–8.

[23] Bernhardt J, Hayward KS, Kwakkel G, et al. Agreed definitions and a shared vision for new standards in stroke recovery research: the Stroke Recovery and Rehabilitation Roundtable taskforce. Neurorehabil Neural Repair 2017;31(9):793–9.

[24] Bernhardt J, Hayward KS, Kwakkel G, et al. Agreed definitions and a shared vision for new standards in stroke recovery research: the Stroke Recovery and Rehabilitation Roundtable taskforce. Int J Stroke 2017;12(5):444–50.

[25] Plow EB, Sankarasubramanian V, Cunningham DA, et al. Models to Tailor brain stimulation therapies in stroke. Neural Plast 2016;2016:4071620.

[26] Brancaccio A, Tabarelli D, Belardinelli P. A new framework to interpret individual inter-hemispheric compensatory communication after stroke. J Pers Med 2022;12(1).

[27] Antal A, Alekseichuk I, Bikson M, et al. Low intensity transcranial electric stimulation: safety, ethical, legal regulatory and application guidelines. Clin Neurophysiol 2017;128(9):1774–809.

[28] Minjoli S, Saturnino GB, Blicher JU, et al. The impact of large structural brain changes in chronic stroke patients on the electric field caused by transcranial brain stimulation. Neuroimage Clin 2017;15:106–17.

[29] Yoon MJ, Park HJ, Yoo YJ, et al. Electric field simulation and appropriate electrode positioning for optimized transcranial direct current stimulation of stroke patients: an in Silico model. Sci Rep 2024;14(1):2850.

[30] Van der Cruijsen J, Dooren RF, Schouten AC, et al. Addressing the inconsistent electric fields of tDCS by using patient-tailored configurations in chronic stroke: implications for treatment. Neuroimage Clin 2022;36:103178.

[31] Dmochowski JP, Datta A, Huang Y, et al. Targeted transcranial direct current stimulation for rehabilitation after stroke. Neuroimage 2013;75:12–9.

[32] Bahr-Hosseini M, Nael K, Unal G, et al. High-definition cathodal direct current stimulation for treatment of acute ischemic stroke: a randomized clinical trial. JAMA Netw Open 2023;6(6):e2319231.

[33] Pruvost-Robieux E, Benzakoun J, Turc G, et al. Cathodal transcranial direct current stimulation in acute ischemic stroke: pilot randomized controlled trial. Stroke 2021;52(6):1951–60.

[34] Rossi C, Sallustio F, Di Legge S, Stanzione P, Koch G. Transcranial direct current stimulation of the affected hemisphere does not accelerate recovery of acute stroke patients. Eur J Neurol 2013;20(1):202–4.

[35] Polanowska KE, Lesniak MM, Seniow JB, Czepiel W, Czlonkowska A. Anodal transcranial direct current stimulation in early rehabilitation of patients with post-stroke non-fluent aphasia: a randomized, double-blind, sham-controlled pilot study. Restor Neurol Neurosci 2013;31(6):761–71.

[36] Bornheim S, Croisier JL, Maquet P, Kaux JF. Transcranial direct current stimulation associated with physical-therapy in acute stroke patients - a randomized, triple blind, sham-controlled study. Brain Stimul 2020;13(2):329–36.

[37] Huang J, Zhao K, Zhao Z, Qu Y. Neuroprotection by transcranial direct current stimulation in rodent models of focal ischemic stroke: a meta-analysis. Front Neurosci 2021;15:761971.

[38] Walter HL, Pikhovych A, Endepols H, et al. Transcranial-direct-current-stimulation accelerates motor recovery after cortical infarction in mice: the interplay of structural cellular responses and functional recovery. Neurorehabil Neural Repair 2022;36(10-11):701–14.

[39] Yoon KJ, Oh BM, Kim DY. Functional improvement and neuroplastic effects of anodal transcranial direct current stimulation (tDCS) delivered 1 day vs. 1 week after cerebral ischemia in rats. Brain Res 2012;1452:61–72.

[40] Kaviannejad R, Karimian SM, Riahi E, Ashabi G. A single immediate use of the cathodal transcranial direct current stimulation induces neuroprotection of hippocampal region against global cerebral ischemia. J Stroke Cerebrovasc Dis 2022;31(3):106241.

[41] Malinova V, Bleuel K, Stadelmann C, et al. The impact of transcranial direct current stimulation on cerebral vasospasm in a rat model of subarachnoid hemorrhage. J Cereb Blood Flow Metab 2021;41(8):2000–9.
[42] Badoiu A, Mitran SI, Catalin B, et al. From molecule to patient rehabilitation: the impact of transcranial direct current stimulation and magnetic stimulation on stroke-a narrative review. Neural Plast 2023;2023:5044065.
[43] Rodriguez A, Amaya-Pascasio L, Gutierrez-Fernandez M, Garcia-Pinteno J, Moreno M, Martinez-Sanchez P. Non-invasive brain stimulation for functional recovery in animal models of stroke: a systematic review. Neurosci Biobehav Rev 2024;156:105485.
[44] Edwards JD, Dominguez-Vargas AU, Rosso C, et al. A translational roadmap for transcranial magnetic and direct current stimulation in stroke rehabilitation: consensus-based core recommendations from the third stroke recovery and rehabilitation roundtable. Neurorehabil Neural Repair 2024;38(1):19–29.
[45] Miranda de Aquino Miranda J, Sousa de Andrade PH, Henrique M, et al. The effect of transcranial direct current stimulation combined with task-specific training on spatiotemporal gait parameters and functional mobility in individuals with stroke: a systematic review and meta-analysis. Top Stroke Rehabil 2025;32(4):438–57.
[46] Qin Y, Xu J, Ng SSM. Effects of transcranial direct current stimulation (tDCS) on motor function among people with stroke: evidence mapping. Syst Rev 2025;14(1):60.
[47] Usman JS, Wong TW, Ng SSM. Effects of treadmill training combined with transcranial direct current stimulation on mobility, motor performance, balance function, and other brain-related outcomes in stroke survivors: a systematic review and meta-analysis. Neurol Sci 2025;46(1):99–111.
[48] Zebhauser PT, Vernet M, Unterburger E, Brem AK. Visuospatial neglect - a theory-informed overview of current and emerging strategies and a systematic review on the therapeutic use of non-invasive brain stimulation. Neuropsychol Rev 2019;29(4):397–420.
[49] Turgut N, Miranda M, Kastrup A, Eling P, Hildebrandt H. tDCS combined with optokinetic drift reduces egocentric neglect in severely impaired post-acute patients. Neuropsychol Rehabil 2018;28(4):515–26.
[50] da Silva TR, de Carvalho Nunes HR, Martins LG, et al. Non-invasive brain stimulation can reduce unilateral spatial neglect after stroke: ELETRON trial. Ann Neurol 2022;92(3):400–10.
[51] Gorsler A, Grittner U, Rackoll T, Kulzow N. Efficacy of unilateral and bilateral parietal transcranial direct current stimulation on right hemispheric stroke patients with neglect symptoms: a proof-of-principle study. Brain Neurorehabil 2022;15(2):e19.
[52] Sprague JM. Interaction of cortex and superior colliculus in mediation of visually guided behavior in the cat. Science 1966;153(3743):1544–7.
[53] Raymer AM, Johnson RK. Effectiveness of transcranial direct current stimulation as an adjuvant to aphasia treatment following stroke: evidence from systematic reviews and meta-analyses. Am J Speech Lang Pathol 2024;33(6S):3431–43.
[54] Elsner B, Kugler J, Mehrholz J. Transcranial direct current stimulation (tDCS) for improving aphasia after stroke: a systematic review with network meta-analysis of randomized controlled trials. J Neuroeng Rehabil 2020;17(1):88.
[55] You Y, Li Y, Zhang Y, Fan H, Gao Q, Wang L. Long-term effects of transcranial direct current stimulation (tDCS) combined with speech language therapy (SLT) on post-stroke aphasia patients: a systematic review and network meta-analysis of randomized controlled trials. NeuroRehabilitation 2023;53(3):285–96.
[56] Chai L, Huang Y, Guo X, Xiong A, Lin B, Huang J. Does SLT combined with NIBS enhance naming recovery in post-stroke aphasia? A meta-analysis and systematic review. NeuroRehabilitation 2024;54(4):543–61.

[57] Han C, Tang J, Tang B, Han T, Pan J, Wang N. The effectiveness and safety of noninvasive brain stimulation technology combined with speech training on aphasia after stroke: a systematic review and meta-analysis. Med (Baltim) 2024;103(2):e36880.

[58] Bonilha L, Rorden C, Roth R, Sen S, George MS, Fridriksson J. Improved naming in patients with Broca's aphasia with tDCS. J Neurol Neurosurg Psychiatry 2024;95(3):273–6.

[59] Rubi-Fessen I, Gerbershagen K, Stenneken P, Willmes K. Early boost of linguistic skills? Individualized non-invasive brain stimulation in early postacute aphasia. Brain Sci 2024;14(8).

[60] Cherney LR, Babbitt EM, Wang X, Pitts LL. Extended fMRI-guided anodal and cathodal transcranial direct current stimulation targeting perilesional areas in post-stroke aphasia: a pilot randomized clinical trial. Brain Sci 2021;11(3).

[61] Stockbridge MD, Elm J, Breining BL, et al. Transcranial direct-current stimulation in subacute aphasia: a randomized controlled trial. Stroke 2023;54(4):912–20.

[62] Medvedeva A, Materassi M, Neacsu V, et al. Effects of anodal transcranial direct current stimulation over the ventrolateral prefrontal cortex on episodic memory formation and retrieval. Cereb Cortex 2019;29(2):657–65.

[63] Antonenko D, Hayek D, Netzband J, Grittner U, Floel A. tDCS-induced episodic memory enhancement and its association with functional network coupling in older adults. Sci Rep 2019;9(1):2273.

[64] Velikonja D, Ponsford J, Janzen S, et al. INCOG 2.0 guidelines for cognitive rehabilitation following traumatic brain injury, part V: memory. J Head Trauma Rehabil 2023;38(1):83–102.

[65] Cruz Gonzalez P, Fong KNK, Chung RCK, Ting KH, Law LLF, Brown T. Can transcranial direct-current stimulation alone or combined with cognitive training be used as a clinical intervention to improve cognitive functioning in persons with mild cognitive impairment and dementia? A systematic review and meta-analysis. Front Hum Neurosci 2018;12:416.

[66] Yan RB, Zhang XL, Li YH, Hou JM, Chen H, Liu HL. Effect of transcranial direct-current stimulation on cognitive function in stroke patients: a systematic review and meta-analysis. PLoS One 2020;15(6):e0233903.

[67] Kazinczi C, Kocsis K, Boross K, et al. The effect of computerized cognitive training and transcranial direct current stimulation on working memory among post-stroke individuals: a systematic review with meta-analysis and meta-regression. BMC Neurol 2024;24(1):314.

[68] Müller S. V., Klein T. et al., Diagnostik und Therapie von exekutiven Dysfunktionen bei neurologischen Erkrankungen, S2e-Leitlinie, 2019, in: Deutsche Gesellschaft für Neurologie (Hrsg.), Leitlinien für Diagnostik und Therapie in der Neurologie. Online: www.dgn.org/leitlinien (abgerufen am TT.MM.JJJJ).

[69] Cavinato M, Genna C, Formaggio E, et al. Behavioural and electrophysiological effects of tDCS to prefrontal cortex in patients with disorders of consciousness. Clin Neurophysiol 2019;130(2):231–8.

[70] Feng Y, Zhang J, Zhou Y, Bai Z, Yin Y. Noninvasive brain stimulation for patients with a disorder of consciousness: a systematic review and meta-analysis. Rev Neurosci 2020.

[71] Angelakis E, Liouta E, Andreadis N, et al. Transcranial direct current stimulation effects in disorders of consciousness. Arch Phys Med Rehabil 2014;95(2):283–9.

[72] Hermann B, Raimondo F, Hirsch L, et al. Combined behavioral and electrophysiological evidence for a direct cortical effect of prefrontal tDCS on disorders of consciousness. Sci Rep 2020;10(1):4323.

[73] Martens G, Lejeune N, O'Brien AT, et al. Randomized controlled trial of home-based 4-week tDCS in chronic minimally conscious state. Brain Stimul 2018;11(5):982–90.

[74] Bender A, S3-LL Neurologische Rehabilitation bei Koma und schwerer Bewusstseinsstörung im Erwachsenenalter,2022.
[75] Klem GH, Luders HO, Jasper HH, Elger C. The ten-twenty electrode system of the International Federation. The International Federation of Clinical Neurophysiology. Electroencephalogr Clin Neurophysiol Suppl 1999;52:3–6.
[76] Scrivener CL, Reader AT. Variability of EEG electrode positions and their underlying brain regions: visualizing gel artifacts from a simultaneous EEG-fMRI dataset. Brain Behav 2022;12(2):e2476.
[77] Galletta EE, Cancelli A, Cottone C, et al. Use of computational modeling to inform tDCS electrode montages for the promotion of language recovery in post-stroke aphasia. Brain Stimul 2015;8(6):1108–15.
[78] Evans C, Johnstone A, Zich C, Lee JSA, Ward NS, Bestmann S. The impact of brain lesions on tDCS-induced electric fields. Sci Rep 2023;13(1):19430.
[79] Manoli Z, Parazzini M, Ravazzani P, Samaras T. The electric field distributions in anatomical head models during transcranial direct current stimulation for post-stroke rehabilitation. Med Phys 2017;44(1):262–71.
[80] Datta A, Baker JM, Bikson M, Fridriksson J. Individualized model predicts brain current flow during transcranial direct-current stimulation treatment in responsive stroke patient. Brain Stimul 2011;4(3):169–74.
[81] McCann H, Pisano G, Beltrachini L. Variation in reported human head tissue electrical conductivity values. Brain Topogr 2019;32(5):825–58.

CHAPTER

11

Dialogical interaction and protective cognitive environments (including virtual reality) as major components of neuropsychological rehabilitation

11.1 How to define neuropsychological rehabilitation?

Decades ago, Barbara Wilson described the task of neuropsychological rehabilitation (NR) as following:

> "NR is concerned with the amelioration of cognitive, emotional, psychosocial, and behavioral deficits caused by an insult to the brain. Major changes in NR have occurred over the past decade or so. NR is now mostly centered on a goal-planning approach in a partnership of survivors of brain injury, their families, and professional staff who negotiate and select goals to be achieved. There is widespread recognition that cognition, emotion, and psychosocial functioning are interlinked, and all should be targeted in rehabilitation. This is the basis of the holistic approach [1]."

This holistic, goal-oriented view [2] is a valuable starting point. It emphasizes the need to integrate cognition, emotion, and psychosocial functioning, and it highlights the importance of involving patients and their families in setting meaningful goals. Yet it also has clear limitations. Wilson's definition primarily addresses patients in the chronic stage, where the task is to manage stable behavioral problems in a relatively constant environment. Acute and postacute phases are omitted, where the central question is whether functional deficits can still be improved or

Applied Neuropsychology of Cerebrovascular Diseases
DOI: https://doi.org/10.1016/B978-0-443-45450-9.00009-6

compensated (the "prognosis"), and where the challenge of gaining awareness of impairments is particularly pressing. The definition also says little about the specific contribution of neuropsychology: the simulation of cognitive environments for diagnosis and therapy. We therefore propose a reframing:

NR is best understood as a dialogical interaction between the patient and the therapists [1]. It is grounded in the neuropsychologist's theoretical assumptions about the patient's disorder, the patient's assumptions about his or her condition, and the concrete results of diagnostic testing carried out against this background. In this sense, NR is also a form of self-enlightenment because the brain cannot monitor its own intactness; impairments become visible only through confrontation with an environment—either real or simulated.

Unawareness is the basic state of patients after brain damage; patients with motor deficits often become aware of them quickly, because failed movements are experienced immediately. Cognitive deficits, however, are typically less obvious, especially in the structured and simplified environments of rehabilitation centers, where severe motor limitations further restrict opportunities for interaction. In addition, patients have a natural tendency to adjust their environment to the complexity of their own abilities for defending the experience of control and agency.

Unawareness can even be rational, as long as personal goals and the rights of others (e.g., family members) are not restricted. Moreover, mere neuropsychological testing because of suffering from brain damage makes little sense, as it has no direct relevance for the somatic treatment and, with a few exceptions (such as driving aptitude diagnostics), it only provides provides limited information about the expected everyday performance of the patients.

Yet for rehabilitation, awareness is essential: without it, motivation and willingness to engage in therapy are limited. Simply reporting deficits is usually insufficient; patients must actively experience their limitations in order to truly understand them. Consequently, before treatment can begin, some degree of insight into the deficits is essential. This is why neuropsychological guidelines—for example, for the treatment of executive dysfunction—emphasize that awareness of deficits is a prerequisite for effective therapy [3].

The central role of simulations based on theoretical models for becoming aware of the extent of the deficit can be illustrated by visual field defects (VFD). Patients typically do not perceive these as a "black hole" in vision; the deficit becomes apparent through interaction with the environment, such as when bumping into objects [4]. Here, cognitive modeling matters. The precise extent and structure of VFD can only be assessed by simulating an appropriate environment—for instance, by requiring patients to keep their gaze fixed while stimuli are presented in the periphery. The choice of stimulus properties (e.g., dark vs bright targets, animated vs static, sudden vs gradual onset) is also not trivial, as different parameters interact with the visual system in different ways. Some VFDs may disappear under certain stimulus conditions (as in the phenomenon of blindsight), while others remain unchanged [5]. Such knowledge has direct therapeutic implications: if a defect is unresponsive to different salience conditions, restorative therapy is unlikely to succeed, and compensation training becomes the only appropriate option [6,7] (compare Chapter 4).

VFDs are sensory deficits; however, the principles of their assessment also hold for cognitive deficits: without keeping certain processes constant (in perimetry, the direction of the eyes' gaze), other processes (in perimetry, the visual field) cannot be systematically investigated. A typical example of this is memory diagnostics. A statement about the impairment of the ability to *consolidate* information presupposes a comparison of learning and retrieval performance achieved under different conditions (i.e., free recall, semantically supported recall, and recognition).

Thus coming back to the definition of Barbara Wilson [1], NR cannot be reduced to pragmatic problem-solving in the chronic stage. It should be conceptualized as a dialogical process between theory, simulated environment, therapist, and patient that:

- Fosters awareness of deficits as a prerequisite for motivation and therapy.
- Uses simulated cognitive environments to diagnose and treat impairments.
- Relies on cognitive models to design tasks that reveal deficits, predict prognosis, and guide the choice between restitution and compensation.

11.2 Cognitive theory of deficit as the basis of intervention

Cognitive models are not only essential for increasing awareness of deficits; they also provide the foundation for designing effective treatments. A good example is the treatment of word-finding problems in aphasic patients. Word-finding problems are a hallmark of almost all forms of aphasia, but they can arise from different underlying causes (Chapter 6).

Traditional theories distinguish between two main mechanisms: a disruption in access to semantic memory or a failure in retrieving the phonological code [8]. Levelt's influential model of language production

[9–11] offers a more fine-grained account, identifying several possible levels at which breakdown can occur:

1. **Conceptual level**—a failure to generate or maintain the conceptual framework of the intended message. This can manifest as losing the communicative thread or mismatching the concept with the chosen word.
2. **Grammatical encoding**—defining the sentence structure for conveying the intended meaning. Impairments may reduce the ability to come up with verbs, adjectives, and relative clauses.
3. **Positioning of lemma**—impaired specification of lemmas, the abstract placeholders for words in a sentence. For example, saying *"furniture"* instead of *"sofa."* This reflects the reduced specificity of semantic search.
4. **Phonological encoding**—problems in retrieving the word's phonological code, leading to blocked or incomplete access.
5. **Phonetic/articulatory level**—breakdown in accessing or programming the articulatory form, as in apraxia of speech (e.g., *"tuh-te-le-sion"* for *"television"*).

Therapy must therefore be tailored to the level of impairment [10]. Depending on the analysis of the disturbance, semantic pathways (by script introduction, by images, pictorial or practical representation of the plot, by sentence completion, etc.) or phonological pathways should be used. In the case of phonological access, other cues such as imitation, phonetic aid, audition, or serial speaking are required. For instance, if a patient struggles to retrieve the word "bicycle" due to a semantic deficit, the therapist might show a picture or say, *"You ride it with two wheels and pedals - what is it?"*. If the problem is in phonological retrieval, phonetic prompts (*"It starts with /bai/..."*), repetition, or auditory modeling may be more effective.

However, even Levelt's model [9] reaches its limit in severe cases such as global aphasia, a common syndrome in the postacute stage. Here, therapy must adopt broader, systematic approaches that combine multiple entry points (see Chapter 6 for details). Still, therapeutic facilitation of speech must be grounded in a cognitive theory of language and communication, which enables the construction of a cognitive environment adapted to the patient's impairment. It is within this environment in which treatment takes place.

11.3 The simulation of a protective cognitive environment has a structural and a dynamical component

Following the example of aphasia treatment above, the essence of neuropsychological therapy can be described as model-guided facilitation or cueing, enabling the patient to perform a cognitive function at the threshold of what is still possible. In abstract terms, this threshold defines a protective cognitive environment created by the therapists.

A protective cognitive environment then has two complementary components:

- A **structural component**, shaped by the design of tasks with appropriate severity and complexity.
- A **dynamic component**, realized through the therapist's targeted interventions and cueing during task performance.

To explain these two components in more detail, two examples will be discussed.

Example 11.1: severe and persistent impairment.

For patients with severe, persistent functional impairments, the method of errorless learning—specifically, backward chaining with vanishing cues—illustrates the principle well. Take the reacquisition of writing one's own name in severe aphasia (see Chapter 7). Training begins with the last letter, which the patient copies. Once successful, the last two letters are practiced, always with therapist guidance to prevent errors. Gradually, the cues are reduced until the patient can complete the entire name. Here, the **structural environment** is the progressively shortened task (letters are removed), while the **dynamic environment** is the therapist's prevention of errors through timely cueing.

Example 11.2: potential for recovery of cognitive ability.

In patients with the possibility of cognitive recovery, environments can be based on a structural analysis of disturbed cognitive components. By structural analysis, we mean breaking down a global function into its elementary cognitive components, identifying which are impaired, and constructing therapeutic environments that specifically target those weaknesses. Visuoconstructive deficits, often neglected in rehabilitation research (for an exception, see [12]), may serve as an example. In the following, it will be postulated that the ability of visual construction is based, among other things, on the following hierarchically organized set of cognitive processes (Table 11.1) [13]: matching (assignment of the same shapes), anticipatory rotation (mental and practical), mirroring (two- and three-dimensional), scaling (recognizing the same shape in different proportions), and segmentation (recognizing shapes in larger structures without being irritated by deviating properties that are additionally present) (see Chapter 5 for some application of this model to treat

TABLE 11.1 Hierarchy of cognitive functions for visuoconstruction and their retraining.

Step	Cognitive environment	Cognitive components involved	Goal/action	Therapeutic approach
1	Initial cognitive environment	Matching, two-dimensional rotation (visuoperceptive and elementary functions).	Create a simple cognitive environment that allows the patient to perform basic functions (e.g., matching shapes).	Minimize difficulty, allow basic performance.
2	Gradual complexity increase	Mirroring (3D rotation), scaling, and segmentation.	Designing the environment to challenge more complex cognitive processes.	Provide external help, reduce complexity progressively.
3	Visible environment offers only relative parameters of objects	Scaling and segmentation.	Segment shapes with visual aids (coordinate system, relative ratios).	Make segmentation tasks easier through scaling and external perceptual aids.
4	Relative parameters more and more limited to size	Segmentation (without external perceptual aid).	Move to more autonomous segmentation tasks.	Reduce external aid while focusing on segmentation ability.
5	Advanced segmentation tasks	Segmentation against visually dominant divisions (verticals and diagonals).	Segment shapes in more complex configurations.	Introduce more complex visual segmentation tasks.

allocentric neglect). Obviously, matching is more of a visuoperceptive function, and two-dimensional rotation is more of an elementary function, because both often succeed even in severely damaged patients. In contrast, mirroring, three-dimensional rotation, scaling, and segmentation are complex functions that are often impaired in patients with larger left and right ACM strokes [13].

Visuoconstructive training begins with identifying which components are impaired and then constructing environments in which performance is just possible (Table 11.1, columns on the right). More complex environments are gradually introduced, with dynamic support from the therapist (e.g., using coordinate systems, scaling aids, or perceptual anchors for segmentation tasks). The ability of segmentation can be treated by initially presenting the relative ratios of the components in a different order of magnitude (segmentation thus becomes a problem of scaling). If patients succeed in doing such tasks safely, the next step is to specify a coordinate system of appropriate size so that the mere length of the elements is an aid (i.e., the segmentation of surfaces is supported by the specification of extent). If this is also possible, then the step can be made to simple segmentation tasks without external help being offered, but the segmentation is still supported by perceptual aspects. After that, one can move on to tasks where segmentation against the visually dominant divisions along the verticals and diagonals has to be done.

A simulated cognitive environment therefore can either be a sequence of situations in which certain movements or actions have to be performed to achieve a goal (e.g., writing one's own name). However, it can also mean a certain level of task complexity at which a certain cognitive function is just about possible through therapeutic intervention (e.g., treating visuoconstructive deficits, whereby the goal is then firstly to transfer this complexity into concrete tasks and secondly to achieve higher degrees of complexity through reduction of cues). In both cases, the role of the therapist is to invent and adapt cues to ensure that so that recovery can proceed step by step within an environment where action remains possible.

11.4 Virtual reality as a protective cognitive environment

11.4.1 Virtual reality - a new tool for neuropsychogical treatments?

Extended reality (XR)—including immersive virtual reality (VR) and augmented/mixed reality—is attracting increasing interest in neuropsychological therapy. Reported advantages include ecological validity, safe and engaging scenarios, systematic task repetition with fine-grained control of task parameters, adaptive difficulty, and the use of gamification to support motivation [14–17].

It is important, however, to situate VR—on which we will focus in the following—within the long tradition of neuropsychological treatment, that is, the design of protective environments for retraining and adaptation [18]. Conventional therapies already build structured protective task environments to observe and train cognitive functions: settings are safe, repeatable, and adaptable to impairment severity. In that sense, VR does not replace core therapeutic principles; it extends them by adding a perceptual simulation layer that may approximate everyday contexts more closely and capture detailed behavioral data.

A distinguished feature of VR is the combination of immersion (the system's technical ability to deliver rich, surrounding sensory input) and embodiment (the patient's subjective sense of "being there" and acting with/through a body in the virtual scene) [14–16]. While conventional therapy occurs in the real world, its effectiveness also depends on how convincingly tasks substitute for real-life challenges. In this broader sense, both VR and traditional therapy face the same problem: creating environments that patients accept as a meaningful substitution for the goal of treatment and/or for everyday contexts. As in classical NR, VR offers patients a simulated protective cognitive environment but adds a virtual perceptive substitution.

11.4.2 Quality criteria for virtual reality applications

Krohn, Tromp [18] proposed a particularly helpful checklist for assessing the quality of VR-based neuropsychological applications, which offers the possibility to compare VR and classical NR as a protective environment more deeply. At the top of their list is "domain specificity," which in the terminology developed here should be anchored in the best available cognitive theory of the targeted cognitive function. In other words, the virtual training environment must reflect the relative autonomy and processing structure of the cognitive system under treatment.

This is not trivial. For example, memory rehabilitation can target encoding, consolidation, and recall, each of which involves different subprocesses that may be selectively impaired (see Chapter 7). A generic "memory game" in VR is unlikely to be effective unless it is clearly aligned with the specific aspect of memory that is compromised. Thus designing VR training requires cognitive models that identify the vulnerable subprocess and build a training environment stressing the relevant mechanisms.

Severity and the recovery stage are also crucial. VR could be particularly well-suited for errorless learning, where endless safe repetitions help patients acquire specific knowledge (e.g., practicing how to use a memory notebook or repeatedly rehearsing the name of a caregiver). Yet in this case, the target is not a basic cognitive process such as encoding, but rather the establishment of specific knowledge. Such timing decisions—when to move from process-oriented training to knowledge acquisition—depend on clinical judgment and cooperation as in classical NR, not on VR itself.

Another principle highlighted by Krohn, Tromp [18] is the ecological relevance. Virtual environments should not only look realistic in their appearance but must also represent the actual cognitive challenges patients face in daily life. Ecological validity, however, is difficult to define. A simulated environment only becomes ecologically valid if it reflects the perceptual and cognitive demands of the real world. Driving simulation illustrates this complexity well, as it has a long tradition in both real-world applications and neuropsychological testing and training. Bruck, Haycock [19] recently reviewed driving simulation and emphasized the importance of integrating detailed knowledge about human senses and human information processing, thus arguing for a cognitive theory for ecological modelling. A recent high-level technical report about a driving simulator still acknowledged the limitations of its own driving scenario, noting that key aspects of driver behavior—such as mirror checking, adjusting speed at intersections, maintaining speed limits, and following traffic rules—should be integrated to improve ecological validity [19,20]. Other fundamental problems, such as providing realistic gravitational feedback while driving through curves or braking, remain unsolved outside highly specialized research settings. The development of driving simulators thus demonstrates how challenging it is to achieve ecological validity, even in a relatively restricted domain like driving. Even more troubling, a recent review concluded that there is no clear evidence that training in driving simulators improves real-world driving performance [21]. This review focuses on healthy young adults, leaving open the question of whether older adults or patients with cognitive impairments might benefit more from such training.

Driving simulation is now supported by highly developed VR software, partly due to advances in the gaming industry and the automotive sector. By contrast, many experimental VR settings in neuropsychology remain far less realistic: for example, presenting shelves with pictures of objects as a "supermarket" (Fig. 11.1). Such a display cannot be considered ecologically valid, though it may serve as a protective cognitive environment designed to optimize memory training. Similarly, Dahdah, Bennett [22] used a VR setup of a living room and a classroom, where patients performed the Stroop task on a screen. This was neither

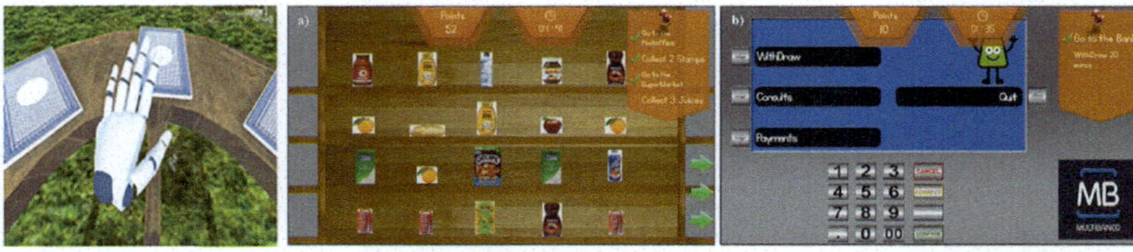

FIGURE 11.1 Are virtual realities ecologically valid? *From Cho D.R., Lee S.H. Effects of virtual reality immersive training with computerized cognitive training on cognitive function and activities of daily living performance in patients with acute stage stroke: a preliminary randomized controlled trial. Med (Baltim) 2019;98(11):e14752; Faria A.L., Andrade A., Soares L. SB IB. Benefits of virtual reality based cognitive rehabilitation through simulated activities of daily living: a randomized controlled trial with stroke patients. J Neuroeng Rehabil 2016;13(1):96.*

more ecologically valid nor more ecologically relevant than performing the same task in a real-world environment. In this respect, what many VR programs really provide is better described as ecological relevance [18], which differs from the often assumed but rarely achieved concept of ecological validity [14,23,24]. However, ecological relevance [18]—alignment with treatment goals and cognitive models—does not distinguish XR from classical NR. Ecological relevance is at the core of it.

Beyond ecological relevance, VR's advantages lie in "Task adaptability," systematic repetition, and "performance quantification" [18]. It allows precise tracking of response times, accuracy, and movements, enabling systematic increases in task difficulty. In this respect, VR shares advantages with traditional computer-based training, offering continuous monitoring and fine-grained adjustments of task complexity. However, as discussed in section 11.6 of this chapter, simply improving task performance (faster responses, fewer errors) does not guarantee recovery of the impaired cognitive function. Effective rehabilitation requires that tasks capture all relevant subfunctions of the impairment, linking VR once again to classical NR as a method of constructing a therapeutically meaningful cognitive environment.

11.4.3 Application domains

From the perspective of offering a protective cognitive environment, VR's role can be differentiated into three prototypical domains:

1. VR can support **knowledge transfer and virtual training**, for example, through principles of errorless learning or spaced retrieval. Here, the focus is not on training a cognitive process itself but on establishing specific pieces of knowledge, such as how to use a memory book or recall the name of a person.

TABLE 11.2 Aspects of virtual reality related to domains of neuropsychological treatments.

	Knowledge transfer	Specific function training	Global cognitive stimulation
Ecological validity	+	++	+/-
Domain specificity	+	++	-
Performance quantification	++	++	+/-
Adaptability	+/-	++	+/-
Automatic cueing	++	+	++
Therapeutic interaction	+/-	+/-	-

2. VR is well-suited for relatively **encapsulated functions** that do not require complex environments. Restorative or blindsight-based training of VFD, as well as treatment of visuospatial neglect, are examples. In these cases, VR offers the ideal combination of high task repetition and precise physiological tracking (e.g., eye, head, and trunk movements) [26–29].
3. VR can target **higher-order cognition**, such as executive functions, problem-solving, or goal management. While adaptability, repetition, and quantification are relatively straightforward in domains (1) and (2), they remain major challenges in (3).

Table 11.2 gives an overview of the strength of VR as a tool for the different contents of NR.

11.4.4 Therapist–patient interaction

Fig. 11.1 illustrates that navigating and task solving in VR often include cues to guide attention and indicate what to do next. In skill learning studies with healthy participants, such cues significantly accelerated learning compared to unguided VR training. Commercial VR systems for healthy people often include automatic cues that anticipate problems of use and prevent breakdowns in performance [30,31]. Sometimes, such a reduction of necessary therapist involvement is also presented as an advantage of VR compared to traditional therapy [4,32,33]. This is misleading. Neuropsychological therapy faces a more difficult challenge: each patient's problems are singular, and effective cueing must be based on the immediate observation of their behavior.

Unfortunately, the therapeutic dimension of therapist–patient interaction and individualized cueing is rarely discussed in VR research. The mere construction of the cognitive environment is not sufficient for therapeutic effectiveness. As argued in Section 11.3 and 11.7, it is the dynamic aspect—the interaction between therapist and patient—that enables functional execution through cues and facilitation.

Recent semiqualitative studies highlight this issue. One study found that therapist–patient collaboration was strongly altered by the introduction of VR: therapists reported a loss of intuitive control over what patients were attending to, and a greater need for verbal instructions during sessions [34]. Another study emphasizes that VR allowed patients to demonstrate their real difficulties, thereby enabling therapists to better understand, discuss, and adapt cueing strategies [35]. Yet, in this study, most therapeutic interventions still occurred outside of the VR environment, which is far from ideal in contexts such as memory rehabilitation. Since the therapist's role is to enable the execution of the impaired function through guided facilitation, VR should allow therapist–patient interaction within the same reality level.

11.4.5 Scientific evidence for virtual reality as treatment tool

Because we advocate the view of neuropsychological treatment as a simulation of a protective cognitive environment, we are convinced that VR will open new windows of opportunity. We expect that VR will become an important tool in NR, yet its integration into therapeutic interaction and its ecological transfer remain unresolved challenges. Table 11.3 summarizes the current landscape: VR shows the most consistent promise in perceptual and attentional domains, but overall, the evidence base is heterogeneous.

VFD—recent randomized controlled trials (RCTs) show that VR-based visual training can modestly expand residual fields. For example, Namgung, Kwon [28] used the Nunap Vision VR-perceptual learning system in hemianopia and found small but significant visual-field gains. A larger double-blind trial reported greater increases in the sensitivity area with VR training versus no treatment [36]. A different approach used an immersive VR supermarket to train visual search in hemianopia/quadrantanopia; this improved scanning, spatial memory, and visuospatial processing [37]. Likewise, Bolognini, Diana [38] showed that a home-based audio-visual VR program improved visual search accuracy, speed, mood, and daily-function scores in chronic hemianopia. Overall, evidence is emerging but still modest; larger RCTs with active controls and standardized outcomes are needed.

TABLE 11.3 Evidence of virtual reality in cognitive neurorehabilitation.

Domain	Systematic review summary (current strength)	Main gaps/notes
Visual field defects	Emerging evidence in multiple trials: virtual reality (VR) perceptual learning and compensatory training can yield small field gains (~1–3 degrees). Stroke-VR reviews report limited cognitive benefits.	Larger randomized controlled trials (RCTs) with active controls are needed. Standardized perimetry outcomes and long-term functional transfer measures are lacking.
Unilateral spatial neglect	Promising but heterogeneous. Many small positive trials, but weak designs and low ecological validity.	Few large RCTs; variable protocols (games vs rehab tasks); usability and therapist facilitation rarely studied.
Aphasia/language	Mixed results. Metaanalyses: small reductions in aphasia severity, no clear effect on functional communication or word-finding.	Mostly small single-center pilots. No evidence that VR improves daily communication. Larger RCTs with functional speech endpoints are needed.
Memory (episodic/prospective)	Limited/mixed. VR-activity of daily living (ADL) studies (e.g., supermarket/apartment tasks) show within-task gains, but inconsistent generalization. No systematic memory-only reviews.	Very few RCTs. Outcome measures vary. Transfer to everyday prospective memory is unclear. Postacute versus chronic differences are underexplored.
Executive function/goal management	Sparse evidence. Gains reported mainly within global cognition reviews.	No dedicated VR executive rehab RCTs. Domain-specific trials with ecologically valid ADL/planning outcomes are needed.
Disorders of consciousness	Very limited. Only case reports/pilots (mostly pediatrics). No systematic reviews.	Extremely scant evidence. Adult feasibility untested. Ethical/safety issues limit trials. Need tolerability studies with electroencephalography (EEG)/functional magnetic resonance imaging (fMRI) outcomes.

(*Continued*)

TABLE 11.3 (Continued)

Domain	Systematic review summary (current strength)	Main gaps/notes
Global cognition	Metaanalyses: modest overall benefits. VR often targets multiple domains, yielding small composite gains.	High heterogeneity and risk of bias. Standardized batteries, active controls, and cost-effectiveness analyses are lacking. Long-term effects unclear.
Usability and implementation	Neglected area. Therapists and patients are rarely studied. Reports highlight barriers (cybersickness, lack of guidelines).	Urgent need for usability/implementation research. How therapists cue in VR, staff training, and workflow integration remains unclear.

Unilateral spatial neglect—reviews highlight VR's promise for neglect but emphasize heterogeneity and methodological weaknesses [39]. For instance, Salatino, Zavattaro [39] found improvements in neglect in most small trials, but few were controlled. Representative trials include Motomura, Amimoto [27], a randomized trial where VR stimulus-response games (with/without moving backgrounds) significantly improved left-sided reaction times compared to control tasks. Shin, Kim [40] reported that an 8-week immersive virtual exploration therapy (VR-VET) led to significant gains in standard neglect tests and daily function versus no-VR training. An earlier RCT by Choi, Shin [26] found that VR-based goal-oriented practice yielded larger improvements in line bisection, neglect perception, and head movement than conventional therapy. Therapist-focused studies (e.g., [41]) note that clinicians see VR's potential (enhancing patient awareness of neglected space) but cite usability issues and the need for clear implementation guidelines. In summary, VR neglect therapy shows benefits in small trials, but larger RCTs and attention to ecological validity and therapist integration are needed.

Aphasia/language—systematic reviews find mixed results. Devane, Behn [42] reviewed VR speech therapy studies (mostly pilots) and reported small gains in impairment scores but no clear improvements in functional communication. Similarly, Cao, Huang [43] metaanalyzed five small trials: they found a borderline significant reduction in overall aphasia severity with VR but no effect on verbal fluency, naming, or repetition. Representative studies include immersive VR conversation tasks or script training. For example, Giachero, Calati [44] used a VR conversational agent and found improved oral comprehension, repetition, and written language in chronic aphasia. However, most trials are small and focus on impairment measures. Thus evidence is limited: VR can reduce aphasia severity in some, but its impact on daily communication remains unproven [42]. Larger controlled trials with real-world speech outcomes are needed.

Memory disorders (episodic/prospective)—few VR trials exist, with mixed results. One RCT Faria, Andrade [25] used an immersive "Reh@City" VR apartment/supermarket training and found significant improvements in memory, attention, and visuospatial tasks versus conventional therapy. Another recent trial with 54 chronic stroke patients showed that a VR cognitive program significantly improved global cognition (MoCA) and memory/reasoning tasks more than conventional training [17]. These suggest VR can enhance trained memory tasks. However, generalization to real-world remembering (e.g., prospective memory) is inconsistent. Systematic evidence is scarce and mixed; any gains often stay within the VR tasks. More RCTs, especially in postacute patients, are needed to assess transfer to daily memory functions.

Executive function/goal management—very few VR trials have targeted executive control alone. A pioneering study [22] had brain-injured patients play an immersive VR Stroop task; participants showed faster reaction times on Stroop conditions and improved inhibitory control after training. In other words, VR training improved specific executive measures (task-switching speed, accuracy under pressure) in a small inpatient sample. Broader reviews of VR cognition note modest positive effects overall [45], but specific "goal-management" programs (e.g., virtual planning tasks) have not been rigorously tested. In sum, VR appears capable of improving some executive outcomes (as in VR-Stroop studies, see [22]), but dedicated trials on realistic planning/ADL tasks are lacking. More domain-specific research and ecologically valid outcome measures (e.g., complex task performance) are required.

Disorders of consciousness (DoC)—the evidence is very limited. No systematic reviews are available. Only isolated case reports and pilot studies exist, mainly in pediatrics. For example, Maggio, Naro [46] described a 17-year-old minimally conscious patient who underwent a tailored VR cognitive program; the patient showed clinically significant behavioral gains and increased EEG connectivity after training. These single-case findings suggest VR multisensory stimuli can transiently boost arousal/awareness. However, there are no controlled trials in adult DoC, and samples are tiny. Overall, VR application to DoC remains experimental: feasibility is noted in case studies, but efficacy is unproven. Larger studies would first need to address safety, stimulation protocols, and integration with EEG/assessment tools.

Global cognition—Metaanalyses and systematic reviews of VR for stroke cognition report only modest overall benefits. For instance, a recent metareview found limited evidence that VR improves poststroke cognition, with most gains in specific domains [45]. No significant effect on global cognition composite scores was found, but the authors noted improved executive, memory, and visuospatial scores with VR. In practice, multidomain VR programs often yield small improvements: for example, Faria, Andrade [25] found VR-ADL training gave larger gains in global cognitive function than conventional rehab, and Chatterjee, Buchanan [47] reported VR cognitive rehab reduced hospital stay and tended to help those with more severe deficits. The new RCT by Maggio, Bonanno [17] showed VR cognitive training significantly raised MoCA and mood versus standard care. In summary, VR may add modest cognitive benefit beyond conventional therapy, but heterogeneity in interventions/outcomes is high. Large multicenter trials with standardized cognition batteries and cost-effectiveness data are still needed.

Usability and implementation—adoption of VR in clinics faces challenges. Few reviews address this; most note a lack of studies on therapist roles, user training, and tech barriers. For example, a therapist survey in VR neglect games found clinicians excited about VR's potential but concerned about usability: they called for better instructions, customization features, and ways to integrate VR with traditional therapy [41]. Other qualitative work highlights issues like VR-induced fatigue/sickness, equipment costs, and the fact that therapists often monitor patients outside the headset (reducing therapist–patient interaction). In short, VR tech can increase patient engagement but introduces new training and workflow hurdles. Future studies should systematically evaluate user experience, ergonomics, and therapist copresence during VR, as well as address cybersickness and infrastructure needs.

Taken together, the current evidence shows that VR is best established for perceptual and attentional impairments, whereas its role in language, memory, and executive dysfunction remains exploratory. Importantly, the neglected aspects of therapist–patient interaction and ecological transfer should be addressed explicitly if VR is to become more than a technological novelty. Still, from the perspective of NR as establishing protective cognitive environments, VR offers, just because of being VR, essential insights.

11.5 Bottom-up treatments—increasingly part of neuropsychological therapy—cannot replace therapeutically guided training in protective cognitive simulations

The effectiveness of strictly bottom-up interventions that function without a protective cognitive environment remains scientifically unproven. An example of a mere bottom-up therapy without a lasting effect beyond placebo conditions is prism adaptation (Chapter 5) for visuospatial neglect. Prism adaptation is used to treat visuospatial neglect and has a significant effect in the short term, that is, during the after-effect phase, on visuomotor coordinates but possibly also on other cognitive functions [48]. The effect of this method is traditionally explained by the fact that there is a functional (unconscious) process of alignment of the visual coordinates shifted from the proprioceptive coordinates. When the prism glasses are doffed again, realignment remains measurable for a certain period. So, if the prism glasses shift the visual world to the right, the motor coordinate system must adapt to it by reaching further to the left compared to the visual world. As a result, after doffing the glasses, the neglect is compensated for by the after-effect. This observation had a great resonance in neglect rehabilitation research, and prism glasses therapy has been proposed as a new, potentially fast and effective bottom-up method of neglect rehabilitation [16,17]. However, despite initial enthusiasm [48,49], three new metaanalyses question its therapeutic value [50–52].

The importance of cognitive theory for bottom-up interventions like prism adaptation can be demonstrated as follows. Research shows that the adaptation process to the glasses is carried out by two processes: a relatively fast cognitive control performance process (recalibration) and a slow motor learning process (realignment). In other words, the faulty motor response is initially compensated for by increased cognitive control, the importance of which recedes later because the motor and visual coordinates are implicitly better matched with each other. The therapeutic consequences for the construction of a protective cognitive environment to be drawn from the fact that at least these two processes exist are quite different: if recalibration is the process that initiates an improvement in neglect (quasi through cognitive compensation and increased insight), then the prism glasses should be put on and taken off more often during a therapy session in order to allow the cognitive error correction to go through as much as possible. However, if realignment is the driving process, then patients should wear the glasses continuously for as long as possible in order to complete the motor adaptation process to the maximum. Up to now, treatment trials have focused almost exclusively on the second assumption.

Word list learning, without appropriate embedding in a cognitive theory and simulation of a cognitive environment, would be another (ineffective) example of a functional bottom-up treatment. Only when guided by a model of memory processes, such training can acquire therapeutic meaning. For example, the repetition lag method [53–55] systematically increases the delay between repeated distractors, forcing patients to rely on conscious recollection rather than familiarity. The procedure also illustrates how theory-based control of task difficulty—here grounded in models of recollection versus familiarity [56]—could be used for designing effective environments (Chapter 7). This distinguishes the repetition lag procedure from mere bottom-up word list learning, even if its efficacy is also under debate.

Brain stimulation interventions—attracting considerable interest—provide another example of bottom-up training. They can be divided into focal nonspecific (e.g., pharmacological acting), focal specific (e.g., transcranial direct current stimulation, Chapter 10), and dynamically linking (e.g., transcranial alternating electrical stimulation). Their general goal is to increase neuroplasticity and, thereby the effect of therapeutic interventions. Metaanalyses suggest small additive benefits in aphasia [57,58] and neglect [59], though effects are less consistent for attention and memory [60] (Chapter 10). However, their use also depends on cognitive modelling: stimulation must target cortical areas known to support recovery, and the excitatory or inhibitory effects. For example, the application of tDCS and TMS should be carried out over the brain regions that play a central role in the recovery of a function. Moreover, due to the spread of currents, tDCS only reaches brain areas adjacent to the skull. It is therefore rather unsuitable for influencing limbic or subcortical processes. In the case of tDCS, the effect of the anode can be distinguished from that of the cathode. Cathodes cause inhibition, so their focal use in the chronic state is only useful if there is a reasonable assumption of dysfunctional cortical inhibition, and therefore it may be restricted to aphasia and neglect. In any case, for both focal and global (e.g., pharmacological) interventions, the parallel implementation of *functional training* is a central component.

These examples converge on a central point: bottom-up procedures cannot bypass the design of protective cognitive environments in NR. Whether using perceptual manipulations, memory paradigms, or brain stimulation, effective treatment requires cognitive models that define the protective environment, guide difficulty progression, and connect interventions to neuroplastic mechanisms.

11.6 No therapy without an understanding of the severity of impairment

Developing and distinguishing between protective cognitive environments always requires a definition of an adequate degree of task difficulty. Only then is dialogic interaction possible: the patient can become aware of their limitations, and the therapist can guide and design the intervention toward the next level of complexity.

Many professional computer training courses vary in task severity and thus simulate a protective cognitive environment. This flexibility and thus the broadening of the treatment spectrum is one of their strengths. However, the criteria by which difficulty levels are adjusted are often arbitrary and rarely grounded in cognitive theory. By contrast, neuropsychological treatment must define severity according to the impaired cognitive function, a model of cognitive complexity, and the patient's actual performance.

The treatment of neglected patients provides a good example (Chapter 5). At first glance, severity might seem determined by how far to the left the target object is positioned from the center. Yet research shows that other factors are just as decisive [61]: the density of distractors, their relative salience, and the symmetry of the search field (e.g., a fixed left-sided border boundary or the existence of a phenomenological gap between left and right stimuli). Protective environments must therefore be structured according to a theory of visual search. A systematic progression might start with parallel search tasks, then expand through reading and more complex conjunction searches. Neglect severity cannot be defined independently of the environment in which patients operate. Its assessment and treatment both depend on theoretical models of attention and visual search, which provide the necessary framework for constructing meaningful protective cognitive environments [61,62].

11.7 Theory-based cueing is a central element of neuropsychological treatment

Above, within the concept of a protective cognitive environment, two essential components were distinguished: a static moment, defined by the task structure (simulated cognitive environment itself), and a dynamic component, which emerges through the therapist's active intervention. Up to this point, the focus has been mainly on the static component. The dynamic element, however, is equally central, and it consists of the facilitation of the desired behavior through theory-based *cueing*.

Neuropsychological treatment is thus fundamentally based on cooperative interaction between patient and therapist. The therapist enables the patient to progress to the next level of difficulty by providing targeted cues at precisely the right time. Cueing is not merely supportive; it is an active means of ensuring that patients remain within their zone of proximal development, avoiding frustration while at the same time stimulating learning.

The importance of cueing was already illustrated in the treatment of severely aphasic patients when relearning how to write one's own name.

Another example is the transfer of an appropriate processing method for improving memory performance (Chapter 7). This approach, grounded in experimental memory research, relies on three key principles [63]:

1. The to-be-learned material should be semantically structured and organized under meaningful headings ("deep encoding").
2. During retrieval, patients are encouraged first to recall the headings (e.g., dairy, vegetables, fruit) before attempting to recall the individual items (e.g., milk, cucumber, oranges). This ensures context-dependent retrieval, since the structure of encoding and retrieval matches.
3. Patients should find an individual rhythm of spaced retrieval, which secures consolidation over time and is adapted to the severity of their impairment.

During the sessions, semantic structuring is initially practiced along easy structured material (such as groceries) and gradually progresses to more complex and abstract content. Responsibility for organizing the material is increasingly shifted from the therapist to the patient. At the same time, retrieval follows the same procedure used during encoding, with close monitoring to ensure adherence to the procedure. As patients gain confidence, they are guided to develop their own rhythm of spaced retrieval.

The therapist's task is to cue these strategic steps, actively preventing unsystematic ordering, random retrieval attempts, and lack of spaced retrieval.

Initially, cueing is frequent and directive; over time, it becomes more contingent on the patients' behavior and performance. Progression to a higher level of difficulty is only recommended once patients can independently follow the defined steps at their current level. This may involve introducing interference tasks during consolidation or increasing the volume of information to be learned.

In this way, cueing not only supports immediate performance but also fosters the development of self-monitoring and self-regulation strategies, which are essential for functional transfer into daily life.

11.8 The goal of neuropsychological therapy is the systematic disappearance of the therapist

The primary goal of neuropsychological therapy is to make the dynamic component of the protective cognitive environment superfluous. Put differently, cueing intervention should gradually "fade out" until patients can perform independently.

A classic example is the case study by Sohlberg and Mateer [64], who trained a severely amnesic patient in the systematic use of a memory book (Chapter 7). Therapy progressed in three stages, each representing a protective cognitive environment: (1) familiarization with the logic of the book, practiced only within sessions; (2) application through structured role plays; and (3) transfer into daily life. In the first stage, only the logic of the memory book was practiced with the patient and only within the treatment sessions. After the patient had gained an overview of the essential components of the memory book and their use, that is, mastered them with a certainty of almost 100%, the direct use of the memory book was practiced (still only during the treatment session). Role plays were used for this purpose. In the third period of therapy, the use within everyday life was practiced. Successful action of patients at a given stage of treatment was initially possible only with the maximum participation of therapists, whose role was then systematically reduced at each stage until the next stage was reached.

A similar principle guided the neglect therapy described by Turgut, Moller [62] (see Chapter 5). For the different degrees of severity of neglect, various protective cognitive environments were defined, which the patients were just able to cope with. At the same time, a hierarchy of dynamic cues was assigned to these levels, which should help to reach the next level of difficulty. Initially, the therapist formed the maximum cue, which safely aligned the patients to the left. For example, in patients with severe neglect, looking into the eyes of the therapist, who was positioned to the left of the patient, was defined as an anchor stimulus. Cueing combined biological, social, and psychological aspects: face recognition as a biologically anchored function with the request for social interaction (attention) and the representation of the presence of another person in the office. In the next step, nonsocial, but nevertheless highly concise stimuli were used for orientation to the left (e.g., movement perception, later on merely based on colors). The therapist's task here was to support the patients in finding and paying attention to the cues. At the same time, the intervention was intended to ensure that the cues remained present in working memory if they were not directly perceived. Working memory performance should increasingly make the dynamic intervention of the therapist superfluous. In the next adaptation of the simulated protective cognitive environment, the conciseness of the cues was further reduced in order to ensure that patients would also remain aware of those that do not provoke a pop-out effect. Over time, responsibility for orienting leftward shifted from external cues to the patient's own working memory, and ultimately toward spontaneous self-generated cues. Importantly, this strategy presupposes sufficient working memory capacity—either preserved or recovering—underlining the central role of cognitive models in therapy design [17,62].

Fading out of therapy ultimately means the transfer into everyday life (where no therapist is permanently present). However, equating the principle of fading out with the demand for "generalization into everyday life" would be too narrow. Patients' everyday lives are not static—they depend on their performance or limitations. In fact, there is no stable everyday life (an ecological niche in which the patient moves) that can be described independently of the cognitive performance of an organism. In this respect, the concept of everyday life refers to the cognitive complexity that is (again) possible for patients in their daily actions or has been chosen by them as a basic structure that can be reproduced in exchange with the environment.

Fading out can occur through different cognitive mechanisms:

- Reducing complexity, for example, simplifying environments.
- Reacquiring routines, supported by methods such as vanishing cues.
- Developing strategies and internal compensation that sustain independence.

A permanent fading-out can only succeed at the maximum level achievable by the patient; a fading-out at a level of cognitive complexity below their potential independence of the patient violates an essential therapeutic goal. It is thus based on a representation of the patient's performance, the simulation of the corresponding cognitive complexity, and the self-representation of the patients with regard to the consequences of the injury and their chosen biography. The primary goal from the point of view of NR is to achieve the greatest possible independence within a cognitively adapted everyday life.

Maximal independence—the primary goal of the treatment—is not always the goal of the patients, who may prefer a reduced everyday life complexity (i.e., make a kind of erroneous compensation through learned nonuse), cannot accept their disability (insist on their right to "unawareness," so to speak) or do not want to stop struggling for full restitution. In this respect, the simulation of a protective cognitive environment remains central: it provides the structured yet adaptable setting in which independence can be safely developed and tested. Therapy must therefore remain dialogical, balancing the patient's goals and lived preferences with a scientifically grounded prognosis that considers lesion characteristics, time since injury, age, insight, and psychosocial resources.

In short, neuropsychological treatment does not aim at endless therapist involvement, but at enabling patients to internalize strategies, self-monitor, and act independently within a cognitively adapted everyday life. The protective cognitive environment is the scaffold for this process—first externally provided by the therapist, and then progressively internalized by the patient until it becomes part of their own everyday functioning. This also implies a professional political obligation of neuropsychological therapy: to a scientifically based prognosis, which includes, for example, the factors of time interval since the event, size and location of the damage, age, insight achieved, and psychosocial resources of the patients.

11.9 Each specific therapy session is based on the most recent update of the patient's performance

Planning of individual treatment sessions and fading out should be based on a specific integration of knowledge based on the models of cognitive performance and the current severity of the patient's impairment. A well-designed therapy session follows a clear cyclic structure: a brief warm-up of easy tasks, a focused middle section presenting challenges at the patient's current upper performance range, and a cool-down of simple tasks. Framing the demanding work between successes preserves the patient's sense of competence and agency while exposing them to the therapeutic difficulty needed for learning.

Textbooks, scientific articles, and guidelines often recommend the adoption of a certain methodology in neuropsychological treatment because evidence-based results have been achieved with its help (e.g. [3,65]). While it is important to use treatment methods with a strong scientific basis and to implement positive research results in therapy as quickly as possible, it is also crucial to recognize that neuropsychological therapy, which involves creating protective cognitive environments without classifying them according to the severity of the patient's impairment, is inadequate. The same applies to sessions based on only one task, which can easily become monotonous. Therefore a combination of different protective cognitive environments in a therapy session seems to be the better choice. Unfortunately, there is currently virtually no systematization of interventions along categorizations of impairment, the specific combination of interventions, and even less about the chronological sequence of different approaches in their distribution over the step-by-step process of compensation.

11.10 Vulnerable periods of the course and the choice of therapeutic priorities

For agreeing on therapeutic goals, the timing of intervention is a major determinant of outcome (or generally the prognosis of impairment, see section 11.9). Across cognitive domains, treatment effects are typically larger when therapy begins earlier in recovery compared to later in the chronic stage (Chapter 3). A recent metaanalysis in the field of aphasia rehabilitation [66], which was able to include so many studies that the course of over a thousand patients could be assessed, shows that the success of treatment is fundamentally influenced by two aspects, patient age and the time elapsed since injury: younger patients and those treated within the subacute window tend to show greater gains. Older patients and those who were in the chronic stage still showed treatment success, but significantly less than younger patients and those in a subacute stage. For the latter, the gain compared to placebo was around 16%, for those whose event occurred more than 6 months ago, only around 4% [66].

Analogous to these results for aphasia treatment, in studies on the effectiveness of working memory training to improve verbal memory performance, we found that when chronic patients were included, it was not effective, that is, not generalized over the narrower range of trained function [67]. In contrast, in studies conducted with subacute patients, working memory training seems to generalize to verbal and prospective memory performance [68,69]. Since all three studies included an active control group, it is reasonable to think that the duration of the functional consequences (still subacute or already chronic) played a decisive role in the different effectiveness.

Accordingly, an interruption of functional, disorder-oriented treatment in a subacute state in the direction of disease management requires an underpinning by other scientific data, such as a lack of therapy progress for several weeks. This means that focusing on the emotional reactions to the consequences of the disease should be postponed (as far as possible) to a state where the cognitive deficits are likely to remain. Accordingly, work should concentrate on the functional consequences in the postacute stage, only later shifting to coping with the consequences of disease in the chronic stage.

11.11 Prognosis is a central element of therapy and thus of a dialogical interaction

Prognosis is not an abstract prediction—it directly shapes therapeutic choices. Clinicians should integrate up-to-date evidence about recovery trajectories with the patient's ongoing response to therapy when deciding whether to pursue restorative versus compensatory goals. In section 11.10, reference was already made to the period of time that has elapsed since the event that led to brain damage. For its precise assessment, etiological considerations are also necessary: for example, recovery after traumatic brain injury is often slower than in the case of a cortical stroke [70], but the period until a chronic condition is reached, in which spontaneous remission can no longer be assumed, is longer and can last longer than a year. In a study of the one-year outcome of early rehabilitation patients with large MCA strokes or intracerebral bleeding in the area of the middle cerebral artery, we found that patients with bleeding initially showed little progress and more often did not reach phase C of neurological rehabilitation [71]. In the further course of the year, however, their recovery was quite comparable to that of patients with MCA strokes. In this respect, the prognosis to be discussed with the patient depends not only on the period since the event, but also on the biological dynamics of brain recovery.

Age is another aspect that influences prognosis. The effect of age on the regression of motor and cognitive deficits is not fully understood, even though the vast majority of stroke studies repeatedly show that the outcome of older patients is worse than that of younger patients. Richter, Modden [72] found that age did not influence improvement in cognitive performance in a phase D rehab clinic for patients under 65 years of age. In the aforementioned study on the course of large MCA strokes and intracerebral bleeding, age also did not play a relevant role, and this group of patients was predominantly older than 60 years. Kolb [73] reports experimentally on the existing learning ability of rats into old age. However, this was not mediated by the same neuroplasticity as in young rats: the latter showed dendritic sprouting, the former did not. Chapter 3 presents other findings from animal studies, arguing that oligodendrocytes differentiate more often in young animals after artificial stroke compared to older animals.

The location of the lesion plays an important role in the prognosis. Functions (like swallowing or walking) that have independent controlling centers at the brainstem level show a significantly better recovery if they are impaired by a cortical or subcortical lesion than those that do not have such brainstem centers [74]. Unfortunately, the latter is the case for most cognitive functions. There is a clear indication that lesions that destroy most or all brain structures specialized for specific functions do not recover or at least very slowly and in a restricted range, whereas those that do not touch essential structures show much better recovery if treated properly (Chapter 3). In short, injuries affecting essential centers and fibre tracts of specific functions more or less completely will show less recovery of function, for example, those of the same size but distributed over different areas.

In addition to the duration of the disease and etiology, the most clinically relevant criterion for the prognosis is probably the duration since no measurable functional change has occurred, and the severity of the damage. Gerafi, Samuelsson [75] found that 10% of all patients still have a lateralized attention deficit 7 years after a stroke, depending on the severity of the specific and global damage at the onset of the disease. In the area of motor skills, it is a golden rule that a complete paralysis of the hand lasting more than 14 days, which cannot be explained by any other circumstances, is likely to persist permanently. Most motor rehabilitation studies therefore focus on patients with mild to moderate paresis, while NR studies often focus on patients with severe and chronic deficits (see, e.g., section 11.1, the quote from [1]). In these cases, the prognosis, as far as the changeability of functional performance is concerned, is rather unfavorable. For example, after severe hypoxia with extensive loss of hippocampal neurons, the prospect for recovery of memory impairments is almost zero.

If, therefore after a certain sequence of intensive therapy (usually after three weeks of intensive and regular training), no measurable progress becomes apparent, then—considering the best knowledge of the duration, etiology, and severity of the disease—the patients must be told that the treatment goal should be changed. The proposed change must be worked out and communicated in dialogue, as it represents an encroachment on the biographical self-definition of the patient, as it means an abandonment of the desire to gain ability in the treated performance. Without having a clear background in evidence-based knowledge, which is communicated in an understandable way, insisting on such a change (wherever it may go) would be authoritarian and not therapeutic. Without the patient's consent to the new treatment content, further therapy is impossible.

The simulation of a cognitive environment relative to the disorder is therefore the starting point of every diagnosis and treatment, and it also accompanies the course. It also represents the point where neuropsychological treatment changes to primary dealing with the psychological consequences of (cerebrovascular) event, because a relative level has been reached for which no significant improvement can be achieved with the current treatment possibilities. Emotionally coping with the consequences of the disease and NR are jointly mediated by the dialogical character of cognitive simulation and the dynamic character of neuropsychological intervention: both aim to help patients overcome the next hurdles arising from brain injury. Acuteness versus chronic state form additional determining components, as well as the insight and motivation achieved through the dialogical character of the intervention.

References

[1] Wilson BA. Neuropsychological rehabilitation. Annu Rev Clin Psychol 2008;4:141–62.
[2] Wilson BA, Gracey F, Evans JJ, Bateman A. Neuropsychological rehabilitation: theory, models, therapy and outcome. Cambridge: Cambridge University Press; 2010.
[3] Müller S-V. Kurzfassung der S2e-Leitlinie Diagnostik und Therapie von exekutiven Dysfunktionen bei neurologischen Erkrankungen (AWMF-030/125). Z für Neuropsychologie 2020;31(3):135–47.

[4] Townend BS, Sturm JW, Petsoglou C, O'Leary B, Whyte S, Crimmins D. Perimetric homonymous visual field loss post-stroke. J Clin Neurosci 2007;14(8):754–6.
[5] Chokron S, Dubourg L, Garric C, Martinelli F, Perez C. Dissociations between perception and awareness in hemianopia. Restor Neurol Neurosci 2020;38(3):189–201.
[6] Kasten E, Poggel DA, Muller-Oehring E, Gothe J, Schulte T, Sabel BA. Restoration of vision II: residual functions and training-induced visual field enlargement in brain-damaged patients. Restor Neurol Neurosci 1999;15(2-3):273–87.
[7] Kasten E, Wuest S, Sabel BA. Residual vision in transition zones in patients with cerebral blindness. J Clin Exp Neuropsychol 1998;20(5):581–98.
[8] Meteyard L, Bose A. What does a cue do? Comparing phonological and semantic cues for picture naming in aphasia. J Speech Lang Hear Res 2018;61(3):658–74.
[9] Levelt WJ. Models of word production. Trends Cogn Sci 1999;3(6):223–32.
[10] Levelt WJ. Spoken word production: a theory of lexical access. Proc Natl Acad Sci U S A 2001;98(23):13464–71.
[11] Levelt WJ, Roelofs A, Meyer AS. A theory of lexical access in speech production. Behav Brain Sci 1999;22(1):1–38. discussion -75.
[12] Kerkhoff G. Rehabilitation of visuospatial cognition and visual exploration in neglect: a cross-over study. Restor Neurol Neurosci 1998;12(1):27–40.
[13] Sander C. Assessment of visuoconstructive abilities, category-specific processing and speech comprehension in patients with inferiorparietal and superiortemporal lesions. Master Thesis Neurocognitive Psychol CvO Univ Oldenbg 2015.
[14] Catania V, Rundo F, Panerai S, Ferri R. Virtual reality for the rehabilitation of acquired cognitive disorders: a narrative review. Bioeng (Basel) 2023;11(1).
[15] Cavedoni S, Cipresso P, Mancuso V, Bruni F, Pedroli E. Virtual reality for the assessment and rehabilitation of neglect: where are we now? A 6-year review update. Virtual Real 2022;26(4):1663–704.
[16] Laver KE, Lange B, George S, et al. Virtual reality for stroke rehabilitation. Cochrane Database Syst Rev 2025;6(6):CD008349.
[17] Maggio MG, Bonanno L, Rizzo A, et al. The role of virtual reality-based cognitive training in enhancing motivation and cognitive functions in individuals with chronic stroke. Sci Rep 2025;15(1):25258.
[18] Krohn S, Tromp J, Quinque EM, et al. Multidimensional evaluation of virtual reality paradigms in clinical neuropsychology: application of the VR-check framework. J Med Internet Res 2020;22(4):e16724.
[19] Bruck L, Haycock B, Emad A. A review of driving simulation technology and applications. IEEE Open J Vehicular Technol 2021;2:1–16.
[20] Taheri SM, Matsushita K, Sasaki M. Virtual reality driving simulation for measuring driver behavior and characteristics. J Transportation Technol 2017;7:123–32.
[21] Krasniuk S, Toxopeus R, Knott M, McKeown M, Crizzle AM. The effectiveness of driving simulator training on driving skills and safety in young novice drivers: a systematic review of interventions. J Saf Res 2024;91:20–37.
[22] Dahdah MN, Bennett M, Prajapati P, Parsons TD, Sullivan E, Driver S. Application of virtual environments in a multi-disciplinary day neurorehabilitation program to improve executive functioning using the Stroop task. NeuroRehabilitation 2017;41(4):721–34.
[23] Cho DR, Lee SH. Effects of virtual reality immersive training with computerized cognitive training on cognitive function and activities of daily living performance in patients with acute stage stroke: a preliminary randomized controlled trial. Med (Baltim) 2019;98(11):e14752.
[24] Rogers JM, Duckworth J, Middleton S, Steenbergen B, Wilson PH. Elements virtual rehabilitation improves motor, cognitive, and functional outcomes in adult stroke: evidence from a randomized controlled pilot study. J Neuroeng Rehabil 2019;16(1):56.

[25] Faria AL, Andrade A, Soares L. SB IB. Benefits of virtual reality based cognitive rehabilitation through simulated activities of daily living: a randomized controlled trial with stroke patients. J Neuroeng Rehabil 2016;13(1):96.
[26] Choi HS, Shin WS, Bang DH. Application of digital practice to improve head movement, visual perception and activities of daily living for subacute stroke patients with unilateral spatial neglect: preliminary results of a single-blinded, randomized controlled trial. Med (Baltim) 2021;100(6):e24637.
[27] Motomura K, Amimoto K, Numao T, Kaneko F. Effects of a stimulus response task using virtual reality on unilateral spatial neglect: a randomized controlled trial. Arch Phys Med Rehabil 2024;105(8):1449–57.
[28] Namgung E, Kwon SU, Han MK, et al. Digital therapeutics using virtual reality-based visual perceptual learning for visual field defects in stroke: a double-blind randomized trial. Brain Behav 2024;14(5):e3525.
[29] Spreij LA, Ten Brink AF, Visser-Meily JMA, Nijboer TCW. Increasing cognitive demand in assessments of visuo-spatial neglect: testing the concepts of static and dynamic tests. J Clin Exp Neuropsychol 2020;42(7):675–89.
[30] Liu R, Xu X, Yang H, Li Z, Huang G. Impacts of cues on learning and attention in immersive 360-degree video: an eye-tracking study. Front Psychol 2021;12:792069.
[31] Muller S, Dekker E, Morris-Binelli K, et al. Attributes of expert anticipation should inform the design of virtual reality simulators to accelerate learning and transfer of skill. Sports Med 2023;53(2):301–9.
[32] Cooper N, Millela F, Cant I, White MD, Meyer G. Transfer of training-virtual reality training with augmented multisensory cues improves user experience during training and task performance in the real world. PLoS One 2021;16(3):e0248225.
[33] Mantovani E, Zucchella C, Bottiroli S, et al. Telemedicine and virtual reality for cognitive rehabilitation: a roadmap for the COVID-19 pandemic. Front Neurol 2020;11:926.
[34] Crowe SE, Shahri B, Piumsomboon T, Hoermann S, Waller A, Modelling patient-therapist collaboration for brain injury rehabilitation in virtual reality, in:UMAP Adjunct '24: Adjunct Proceedings of the 32nd ACM Conference on User Modeling, Adaptation and Personalization, 2024, pp 437-44.
[35] Nunnerley JL, Murphy P, King M, et al. A virtual rehabilitation tool for cognitive rehabilitation after traumatic brain injury. Disabil Rehabil 2025:1–9.
[36] Namgung E, Kim BJ, Kwon JH, et al. Personalized visual perceptual learning digital therapy for visual field defects following stroke: a randomized clinical trial. JAMA Netw Open 2025;8(5):e2511068.
[37] Dehn LB, Piefke M, Toepper M, et al. Cognitive training in an everyday-like virtual reality enhances visual-spatial memory capacities in stroke survivors with visual field defects. Top Stroke Rehabil 2020;27(6):442–52.
[38] Bolognini N, Diana L, Rossetti A, et al. Telerehabilitation for visual field defects with a multisensory training: a feasibility study. J Neuroeng Rehabil 2025;22(1):34.
[39] Salatino A, Zavattaro C, Gammeri R, et al. Virtual reality rehabilitation for unilateral spatial neglect: a systematic review of immersive, semi-immersive and non-immersive techniques. Neurosci Biobehav Rev 2023;152:105248.
[40] Shin JH, Kim M, Lee JY, Kim MY, Jeon YJ, Kim K. Feasibility of hemispatial neglect rehabilitation with virtual reality-based visual exploration therapy among patients with stroke: randomised controlled trial. Front Neurosci 2023;17:1142663.
[41] Bousché E, Bakker MDJ, Holstege MS, Huygelier H, Nijboer TCW. Group KBNS. Virtual and augmented reality gamification of visuospatial neglect treatment: therapists' user experience. BMC Digital Health 2024;2(9):1–11.

[42] Devane N, Behn N, Marshall J, Ramachandran A, Wilson S, Hilari K. The use of virtual reality in the rehabilitation of aphasia: a systematic review. Disabil Rehabil 2023;45(23):3803–22.
[43] Cao Y, Huang X, Zhang B, et al. Effects of virtual reality in post-stroke aphasia: a systematic review and meta-analysis. Neurol Sci 2021;42(12):5249–59.
[44] Giachero A, Calati M, Pia L, et al. Conversational therapy through semi-immersive virtual reality environments for language recovery and psychological well-being in post stroke aphasia. Behav Neurol 2020;2020:2846046.
[45] Khan A, Imam YZ, Muneer M, Al Jerdi S, Gill SK. Virtual reality in stroke recovery: a meta-review of systematic reviews. Bioelectron Med 2024;10(1):23.
[46] Maggio MG, Naro A, La Rosa G, et al. Virtual reality based cognitive rehabilitation in minimally conscious state: a case report with EEG findings and systematic literature review. Brain Sci 2020;10(7).
[47] Chatterjee K, Buchanan A, Cottrell K, Hughes S, Day TW, John NW. Immersive virtual reality for the cognitive rehabilitation of stroke survivors. IEEE Trans Neural Syst Rehabil Eng 2022;30:719–28.
[48] Striemer CL, Danckert JA. Through a prism darkly: re-evaluating prisms and neglect. Trends Cogn Sci 2010;14(7):308–16.
[49] Barrett AM, Goedert KM, Basso JC. Prism adaptation for spatial neglect after stroke: translational practice gaps. Nat Rev Neurol 2012;8(10):567–77.
[50] Longley V, Hazelton C, Heal C, et al. Non-pharmacological interventions for spatial neglect or inattention following stroke and other non-progressive brain injury. Cochrane Database Syst Rev 2021;7(7):CD003586.
[51] Qiu H, Wang J, Yi W, Yin Z, Wang H, Li J. Effects of prism adaptation on unilateral neglect after stroke: an updated meta-analysis of randomized controlled trials. Am J Phys Med Rehabil 2021;100(3):259–65.
[52] Szekely O, Ten Brink AF, Mitchell AG, Bultitude JH, McIntosh RD. No short-term treatment effect of prism adaptation for spatial neglect: an inclusive meta-analysis. Neuropsychologia 2023;189:108566.
[53] Bailey H, Dagenbach D, Jennings JM. The locus of the benefits of repetition-lag memory training. Neuropsychol Dev Cogn B Aging Neuropsychol Cogn 2011;18(5):577–93.
[54] Boller B, Jennings JM, Dieudonne B, Verny M, Ergis AM. Recollection training and transfer effects in Alzheimer's disease: effectiveness of the repetition-lag procedure. Brain Cogn 2012;78(2):169–77.
[55] Stamenova V, Jennings JM, Cook SP, et al. Repetition-lag memory training is feasible in patients with chronic stroke, including those with memory problems. Brain Inj 2017;31(1):57–67.
[56] Yonelinas AP, Aly M, Wang WC, Koen JD. Recollection and familiarity: examining controversial assumptions and new directions. Hippocampus 2010;20(11):1178–94.
[57] Elsner B, Kugler J, Mehrholz J. Transcranial direct current stimulation (tDCS) for improving aphasia after stroke: a systematic review with network meta-analysis of randomized controlled trials. J Neuroeng Rehabil 2020;17(1):88.
[58] Raymer AM, Johnson RK. Effectiveness of transcranial direct current stimulation as an adjuvant to aphasia treatment following stroke: evidence from systematic reviews and meta-analyses. Am J Speech Lang Pathol 2024;33(6S):3431–43.
[59] Gorsler A, Grittner U, Rackoll T, Kulzow N. Efficacy of unilateral and bilateral parietal transcranial direct current stimulation on right hemispheric stroke patients with neglect symptoms: a proof-of-principle study. Brain Neurorehabil 2022;15(2):e19.
[60] Yan RB, Zhang XL, Li YH, Hou JM, Chen H, Liu HL. Effect of transcranial direct-current stimulation on cognitive function in stroke patients: a systematic review and meta-analysis. PLoS One 2020;15(6):e0233903.

[61] Ten Brink AF, Elshout J, Nijboer TCW, Van der Stigchel S. How does the number of targets affect visual search performance in visuospatial neglect? J Clin Exp Neuropsychol 2020;42(10):1010–27.
[62] Turgut N, Møller L, Dengler K, et al. Adaptive cueing treatment of neglect in stroke patients leads to improvements in activities of daily living: a randomized controlled, crossover trial. Neurorehabil Neural Repair 2018;32(11):988–98.
[63] Hildebrandt H. Cognitive Rehabilitation of Memory. Amsterdam: Elsevier; 2019.
[64] Sohlberg MM, Mateer CA. Training use of compensatory memory books: a three stage behavioral approach. J Clin Exp Neuropsychol 1989;11(6):871–91.
[65] Kerkhoff G, Schmidt L. Neglect und assoziierte Störungen. Hogrefe: Göttingen; 2018.
[66] Collaborators R, Brady MC, Ali M, et al. Precision rehabilitation for aphasia by patient age, sex, aphasia severity, and time since stroke? A prespecified, systematic review-based, individual participant data, network, subgroup meta-analysis. Int J Stroke 2022;17(10):1067–77.
[67] Weicker J, Hudl N, Hildebrandt H, et al. The effect of high vs. low intensity neuropsychological treatment on working memory in patients with acquired brain injury. Brain Inj 2020;34(8):1051–60.
[68] Richter KM, Modden C, Eling P, Hildebrandt H. Working memory training and semantic structuring improves remembering future events, not past events. Neurorehabil Neural Repair 2015;29(1):33–40.
[69] Richter KM, Modden C, Eling P, Hildebrandt H. Improving everyday memory performance after acquired brain injury: an RCT on recollection and working memory training. Neuropsychology 2018;32(5):586–96.
[70] Suzuki M, Sugimura Y, Yamada S, Omori Y, Miyamoto M, Yamamoto J. Predicting recovery of cognitive function soon after stroke: differential modeling of logarithmic and linear regression. PLoS One 2013;8(1):e53488.
[71] Dengler K, Fischer J, Kastrup A, Elsner M, Hildebrandt H. Was wird aus Patienten mit Mediainfarkt bzw. -blutung und Behandlung in der Phase B der neurologischen Rehabilitation? Ergebnisse des Einjahres-Follow-ups. Neurol Rehabil 2015;21(1):13–22.
[72] Richter KM, Modden C, Hanken K, Hildebrandt H. Recovery after brain damage: is there any indication for generalization between different cognitive functions? J Clin Exp Neuropsychol 2015;37(6):571–80.
[73] Kolb B. Brain plasticity and behavior. Lawrence Erlbaum; 1995.
[74] Luft AR, Macko RF, Forrester LW, et al. Treadmill exercise activates subcortical neural networks and improves walking after stroke: a randomized controlled trial. Stroke 2008;39(12):3341–50.
[75] Gerafi J, Samuelsson H, Viken JI, Jern C, Blomstrand C, Jood K. The presence and prediction of lateralized inattention 7 years post-stroke. Acta Neurol Scand 2020;141(5):423–30.

APPENDIX

A

Short list of recommendations on the rehabilitation of patients with cerebrovascular lesions

The following recommendations are predominantly derived from our clinical experience. In many respects, they are not evidence-based, since appropriate studies are currently lacking. Therefore the decision regarding the most suitable approach for any given patient remains entirely within the professional judgment and responsibility of the reader.

A.1 Brain arteries and related stroke syndromes for clinical neuropsychologist

Review a cMRT FLAIR and T2 sequence and, in cases of acute stroke, compare it with a diffusion-weighted imaging (DWI) sequence. Otherwise, use cranial computed tomography (cCT) scans.

Decide which cerebral artery on which side suffered an occlusion and look up the possible consequences listed in the four following tables (Tables A.1–A.4). Keep in mind that brain scan images are laterally reversed: the left side of the image corresponds to the patient's right hemisphere, and vice versa. Try to assess which branch(es) may be involved to get a more detailed expectation. Use neuropsychological tests to define severity. Use clinical information to define the recovery stage (early post-acute, late post-acute, and chronic stages). Use clinical impression of the patient to decide on training intensity. Use clinical interviews to find out what the expectations of the patient are and how far the patient has a realistic view for the possibility of recovery.

TABLE A.1 Stroke syndromes related to the middle cerebral artery.

Deficits related to branches of the artery	Left middle cerebral artery	Right middle cerebral artery
Motor (frontal brain)	Distally emphasized paresis on the right. Dysarthria.	Distally emphasized paresis on the left. Dysarthria.
Action (frontal brain)	Apraxia (ideomotor and ideatory) Apraxia of speech	Apraxia for complex posture and visuoconstructional tasks
Sensory (postcentral brain)	Proprioception and tactile perception right	Proprioception and tactile perception left
Language (frontal, parietal, and temporal brain)	Aphasia (Broca, Wernicke, etc.) Central dyslexia, dysgraphia, and dyscalculia	Decreased prosody and decreased understanding of complex messages Mental rotation tasks impaired
Memory (frontal, parietal, and temporal brain)	Verbal learning and working memory reduced	Visuospatial learning and working memory will be reduced. Risk of confabulations.
Attention (frontal, parietal, and temporal brain)	Slowing, disinhibition. Impairment of phonological loop.	Visuospatial neglect, slowing, problems with feature binding
Vision (parietal and temporal brain)	Impaired local visual attention. Quadrantanopia or hemianopia to the right. Optic ataxia (for right half positions).	Impaired global attention. Quadrantanopia or hemianopia to the left.
Emotional regulation (temporal brain)	Depression, lability of affect	Depression, loss of affective empathy

TABLE A.2 Stroke syndromes related to the anterior cerebral artery.

Deficits related to branches of the artery	Left anterior cerebral artery	Right anterior cerebral artery
Motor (paracentral brain)	Monoparesis on the right leg	Monoparesis of the left leg
Action, executive function (pericallosal, callosomarginal brain)	Acting only reactive to environmental changes Severe planning disorder	Severe disorder of discounting and insight. Pathological grasping and alien hand sign.
Language (pericallosal brain)	Akinetic mutism. Dynamic aphasia.	Slowing of speech
Sensory (paracentral, precuneal brain)	Proprioceptive loss of the right leg's sensations	Proprioceptive loss of the left leg's sensations
Vision	None	None
Attention	Slowing, loss of focusing	Contralateral motor neglect, profound slowing
Memory (A1 brain, orbitofrontal brain, perforating brain)	Memory disorder (specifically for verbal information)	Memory disorder (specifically for visuospatial information)
Emotional regulation	Reduced emotional expression. Reduced planning and goal representation.	Reduced emotional expression. Severe apathy. Myopia for the future, inability for discounting.

TABLE A.3 Stroke syndromes related to the posterior cerebral artery.

Possible deficits after posterior cerebral artery strokes	Left posterior cerebral artery	Right posterior cerebral artery
Motor	No paresis (without thalamic involvement)	No paresis (without thalamic involvement)
Somatosensory	Proprioception and tactile perception right (in case of thalamus involvement). Sensitivity for pain increased	Proprioception and tactile perception left (in case of thalamus involvement) Sensitivity for pain increased
Language	Wordfinding problems	No change
Vision	Homonymous hemianopia toward right or quadrantanopia	Homonymous hemianopia toward left or quadrantanopia
Recognizing	Visually associative agnosia, hemianopic reading disorder, pure alexia	Neglect (with thalamus involvement), hemianopic reading disorder, prosopagnosia
Memory	Severe verbal memory impairment	Mild visuospatial impairment
Affective	No change	No change
Acting	No change	No change

TABLE A.4 Stroke syndromes related to the vertebral or basilar artery (brainstem and cerebellum)

Midbrain, Pons		
Choroidal arteries and perforating cerebral posterior arteries	Parinaud syndrome	Vertical eye movement, pupil size adaptation, nystagmus
Core zone		
Arteria basilaris, medial pontine artery	Depression Apathy/somnolence Coma	No response except for painful stimuli, no circadian wake-sleep pattern
Lateral zone		
Arteria basilaris, lateral pontine arteries	Locked-in syndrome Facialis paresis	Complete plegia of all limbs and face except for vertical eye movements. Often drowsiness and somnolence Caused by cortical lesions: without forehead muscles Caused by brain nerve: including forehead muscles
Pons-Medulla		
Arteria basilaris or vertebralis	Cross-symptoms related to ipsilesional brain nerve functions, ipsilesional cerebellar motor control, and contralesional corticospinal tract and lemniscus medialis functions, because these efferences and afferences cross at the basis of the medulla	Some drowsiness and somnolence
Oculomotor paresis		
Arteria basilaris	Oculomotorius paresis Abducens paresis Trochlearis paresis	One eye fixed at temporal position, slightly rotated downward. Increased pupil size. One eye fixed at nasal position and does not follow toward temporal. Head slightly turned downward and laterally. One eye does not move downward.

(*Continued*)

TABLE A.4 (Continued)

Cerebellum		
Superior cerebellar artery Inferior cerebellar artery Anterior inferior cerebellar artery Inferior cerebellar artery	Medial: cerebellar worm Lateral: cerebellar hemispheres	Dizziness, vertigo, nausea, vomiting Limb pronounced ataxia depending on localization of stroke, vertigo Cognitive affective syndrome with executive disorders

A.2 Localizing brain lesions in clinical brain scans

Look for a cMRT FLAIR and T2 sequence and, in cases of acute stroke, compare it with a DWI sequence. Otherwise, use cCT scans. Keep in mind that brain scan images are laterally reversed: the left side of the image corresponds to the patient's right hemisphere, and vice versa.

Look for the ventricles and the midbrain (butterfly-shaped structure located centrally in the scan series). Use Tables A.5 and A.6 to localize the lesion according to the defined subcortical and cortical landmarks.

TABLE A.5 Landmarks of the clinical MRI scan related to the ventricles and cisterns.

Structure	Location in transversal scans	Key characteristics on FLAIR MRI scan
Ventricles		
Lateral ventricles (body)	On dorsal images, located medially	Black parallel structures on dorsal images
Lateral ventricles (cornua or horns)	Frontal horn: in front of plexus choroideus and thalamus Posterior horn: medial border of temporal and parietal lobe Temporal horn: mediobasal position inside temporal lobe	Black paired sickle-like on medial images Black triangles on medial images Black lateral paired sickle-like on inferior images
Plexus choroideus	Inside body part of lateral ventricle and inside third and fourth ventricle	Scattered appearance on images. Starting point for the division between the frontal horn and the body of the lateral ventricles on the most dorsal images
Third ventricle	Midline, below the body of lateral ventricles	Thin/bold black line in anterior–posterior direction
Foramen of Monro	Between frontal horn of lateral ventricle and third ventricle	Tiny paired black lines
Fourth ventricle	Inferior images, between brainstem and cerebellum	Initially a black half-circle, later a curved line on ventral images
Aqueduct	Midline, ventral to third ventricle	Small black dot in posterior part of "butterfly" structure of the midbrain
Basalganglia, motor fibers		
Caudate nucleus (body)	Adjacent to lateral ventricles at centrum semiovale level	Lighter structure next to body of the lateral ventricles on FLAIR
Caudate nucleus (head)	More ventral, adjacent to anterior lateral ventricles	Egg-like lighter structure next to the frontal horn of the lateral ventricle
Tail of the caudate	Laterally adjacent to the temporal horn of lateral ventricle	Not visible on MRI/CT
Nucleus accumbens	Ventral to the caudate head	Not visible on MRI/CT, inside the lighter V-like medial structure below the head of the caudatum
Putamen	Lateral to the internal capsule	Lighter structure lateral and posterior to head of caudate

(Continued)

TABLE A.5 (Continued)

Structure	Location in transversal scans	Key characteristics on FLAIR MRI scan
Globus pallidus	On ventral images medial to putamen	Sometimes not well differentiated from putamen
Internal capsule	Medial to caudate nucleus, putamen and lateral to thalamus	Darker than basal ganglia and thalamus, contains corticospinal fibers
Limbic system		
Hippocampus	Medially adjacent to the temporal horn of lateral ventricle	Forms medial/posterior border of temporal horn
Amygdala	Anterior/inferior to the temporal horn	Lighter structure but not touching the midbrain
Fornix	Below plexus choroideus, runs medially	Part of the Papez circuit, involved in memory
Columnae fornicis	Anterior of the thalamus, inside frontal horn of lateral ventricle.	On the two inferior images lateral to the third ventricle
Thalamus	Borders third ventricle	On FLAIR scans lighter than the capsula interna
Anterior nucleus (thalamus)	Dorsal imaging showing the thalamus	Inside the stroke visible on Figure 2.5 (Chapter 2) line 2, column 5
Hypothalamus	Borders ventral tip of third ventricle	Small liplike structure anterior of the "butterfly" structure of the midbrain
Mammillary bodies	Posterior to ventral tip of third ventricle	Posterior border of the lip-like structure anterior of the "butterfly" structure of the midbrain
Visual system		
Lateral geniculate nucleus (thalamus)	Borders anterior part of posterior horn of lateral ventricle	Part of visual pathway
Optic radiation	Posterior of lateral geniculate nucleus. Splits into two parts.	Dorsal part: remains medial and curves somewhat dorsal and posterior to reach the medial occipital lobe. Ventral part (Meyer's loop): turns anteriorly and somewhat laterally to get in a lateral position of the posterior horn of the lateral ventricle to reach the medial occipital lobe

(*Continued*)

TABLE A.5 (Continued)

Structure	Location in transversal scans	Key characteristics on FLAIR MRI scan
Pulvinar (thalamus)	Posterior thalamus, adjacent to cisterna quadrigemina	Visible posterior to the stroke on Figure 2.5 (Chapter 2) line 3, column 1
Dorsal core structures		
Corpus callosum (genu and splenium)	Anterior (genu) and posterior (splenium) to lateral ventricles	Because connecting the hemispheres the corpus callosum is visible as homogenous structure without interruption by the fissura longitudinalis
Cingulate gyrus	Surrounding the corpus callosum	Either anterior or posterior or directly superior to the corpus callosum

TABLE A.6 Localization of the cortical sulci and gyri based on landmarks on clinical brain scans.

Structure	Location in transversal scans	Key characteristics on FLAIR MRI scans
Temporal lobe		
Sylvian fissure (fissura sylvii)	Between frontal and temporal lobes	Visible from ventral to dorsal; wedge-shaped lateral border; transforms into medial sulcus dorsally
Ramus ascendens anterior	Branching from Sylvian fissure, anteriorly	Surrounded by Broca's area; appears as dorsally running sulcus
Broca's area	Left inferior frontal gyrus	Located around ramus ascendens anterior; visible as a pattern of three parallel sulci lateral to the anterior insula
Heschl's gyrus	Within lateral sulcus	Finger-like gyrus starting directly posterior to the dorsal insular cortex
Wernicke's area	Posterior to Heschl's gyrus	Located in superior and medial temporal gyri; posterior and/or ventral to the ramus ascendens posterior
Ramus ascendens posterior	Dorsal extension of Sylvian fissure	A dorsally oriented sulcus visible on different images at the same position coarsely above the Heschl's gyrus

(Continued)

TABLE A.6 (Continued)

Structure	Location in transversal scans	Key characteristics on FLAIR MRI scans
Gyrus supramarginalis	Anterior and posterior the ramus ascendens posterior	Extends dorsally beyond the ramus ascendens
Parietal lobe		
Sulcus parieto-occipitalis	Medial sulcus running from parietal cortex toward the ventral splenium	Visible first as two parallel then horizontal sulci moving more and more anterior on more ventral images
Cuneus	Posterior to sulcus parieto-occipitalis	On images superior to the sulcus calcarinus
Sulcus calcarinus	Starts ventral to splenium	Scrumbled structure of sulci located medially in the occipital lobe
Gyrus fusiformis	Lateral to cerebellar vermis	Below the sulcus calcarinus first inside the posterior temporal lobe, more ventrally as its medial oriented surface
Sulcus collateralis	Sulcus inside the posterior temporal lobe	The orientation is first anterior-posterior, more ventral medial to lateral
Sulcus intraparietalis	Two parallel sulci starting in the posterior parietal cortex	Runs anteriorly then splits and shows anterior and lateral direction
Gyrus angularis	Lateral to sulcus intraparietalis	Starting on images directly above the cingulate cortex, but posteriorly in the parietal lobe
Frontal lobe		
Sulcus centralis	Between precentral and postcentral sulci	Identified by three parallel sulci, hand knob and the most posterior extension of the sulcus frontalis superior
Hand knob	Central sulcus, dorsal levels	Half-circle shape; corresponds to hand motor representation
Sulcus frontalis superior	Anterior to sulcus precentralis	Starting at the dorsal frontal images and running on several images in a posterior direction
Supplementary motor area	Most dorsal medial anterior cerebral artery territory	Medially and dorsal to the sulcus frontalis superior
Orbitofrontal cortex	Ventral of anterior commissure	Anterior to the hypothalamus, posterior and medial to two eyes
Prefrontal cortex	Dorsal of anterior commissure	Anterior to the precentral gyrus

A.3 How to perform neurorehabilitation: answers based on artificial middle cerebral artery strokes in animals

Remember the information of Table A.7 for all further decisions about treatment.

TABLE A.7 Fundamental aspects of neurorehabilitation based on stage of recovery and lesion localization.

1	Brain plasticity and the effects of neurorehabilitation vary related to the different phases of organic recovery and appear to follow an inverted U-shape with the greatest potential observed in the post-acute phase. Therefore, rehabilitation during the late post-acute phase should focus primarily on restoration and internal compensatory mechanisms while other aspects, such as emotional challenges due to the condition, may be deferred to later stage.
2	Interventions initiated too early may have a detrimental effect by increasing inflammatory processes and stress response. Therefore, interventions during this state should be avoided or restricted to passive stimulation.
3	Strokes (and other brain lesions) may lead to secondary passivity behavior, and guiding the patients into functional treatment is necessary to increase their motivation and self-confidence. However, distinguishing between primary (neurological) and secondary (psychological) passivity is a clinical decision, which relies on the interaction with the patient.
4	Functionally relevant brain plasticity is greater after only partial damage to specialized brain areas but markedly reduced when specialized areas or their connections are fully destroyed.
5	Interventions for restitution should be discontinued if key areas subserving core functions have been irreversibly destroyed and, once the patient is able to accept it, (often external) compensation is the only realistic goal.
6	Motivated organisms in complex settings like enriched environments (EE) may develop adaptive solutions to cope with the consequences of brain lesions. However, these adaptations do not necessarily restore the precision of coordination of behavior. Such a refinement requires targeted training interventions, which, however, do not guarantee a broader generalization of adaptation.

A.4 Rehabilitation of visual field deficits

Determine the stage of recovery, lesion localization, and severity of impairment. Use Table A.8 to decide on the correct treatment. If the patient is in an early acute stage, passive stimulation should be prioritized. If the patient is in subacute or chronic stage and still shows exploratory deficits, top-down compensatory treatment should be initiated. If the patient is able to compensate for the visual field defect in everyday life and shows a transition zone with residual visual abilities, one may use restorative treatment. If the patient does not recover from the exploratory impairment and/or shows no progress in restorative training, audio-visual stimulation in the blind field may be used.

TABLE A.8 Treatment of visual field defects according to stage of recovery.

Stage of recovery	Top-down (compensatory therapy)	Bottom-up (restorative computerized training)
Approach		
(Early) post-acute visual field defect		Passive visual stimulation of the blind field with acoustic cuing (spatial synchronized tone position)
Post-acute severe to moderate visual field defect	Training of large saccades inside the impaired visual field, learning of a systematic search strategy. Increased checking behavior in fast changing and unknown environments, which should be avoided if possible.	Training of letter and word recognition which move in the direction of the visual field loss. Intensive training of target detection at the border of the field defect if amblyopic transition zone is present.
Chronic visual field defect	Transfer of compensatory strategies to different situations, which are important for the patient. Advice concerning environmental re-arrangement if necessary.	Intensive training of target detection at the border of the field defect if amblyopic transition zone is present. Audio-visual stimulation of the blind field (spatial synchronized position).

A.5 Rehabilitation of unilateral visuospatial deficits ("neglect")

Use clinical information to determine the recovery stage of the patient. If the patients show rather intact visuospatial working memory, follow the top-down approach of Tables A.9 and A.10. If the dorsal parietal lobe is included in the lesion, bottom-up approach is probably less effective. Determine the severity of the deficit (and the stage of recovery). Both approaches may be combined; however, it should be clear what the main interventional goal and strategy is.

TABLE A.9 Two Approaches in Neglect Rehabilitation.

	Approach for Neglect Rehabilitation	
Stage of Recovery	**Top-Down (via cognition)**	**Bottom-Up (via stimulation)**
(Early) Post-Acute Severe Neglect	Eye fixation training Guided movement of the right hand toward the midline Single word reading with leftward cueing and eye contact prompts	Acoustic cueing (right-left moving tones) Passive optokinetic stimulation
Post-Acute Severe to Moderate Neglect	Index finger cueing on the left Flickering stimuli on the left of critical objects/words	Active following of optokinetic stimuli Neck stimulation Gamified prism adaptation Acoustic cueing
Moderate Neglect	Guided search for the first letter of a word at the beginning of a text line Use of elongated objects with salient endpoints for searching toward the left	Active optokinetic tracking with tasks on the left Neck stimulation, Gamified prism adaptation
Moderate to Mild Neglect	Frequent spontaneous reminders to attend to the left side	Active optokinetic tracking with tasks on the left Neck stimulation Any form of prism adaptation
Mild Neglect	Reactive reminders during search tasks↓	Active optokinetic tracking with tasks on the left Neck stimulation Any form of prism adaptation
Very Mild Neglect	Search tasks with adaptive attentional load using rehabilitation software	

TABLE A.10 Hierarchical steps for neglect intervention across domains.

Stages of recovery	Sensory cueing	Working memory	Reading	Searching
1	Ask: "Where are my eyes?"	Move the right hand to midline, remove it, and ask for repositioning	Single words of increasing length	Large pop-out target search
2	Guide gaze orientation toward other spatial position via hand movements	Sit on the left and ask the patient to pass objects	Words with ambiguous beginnings	Small nonpop-out target search
3	Use elongated, well-structured objects to guide attention leftward	Ask for repeated leftward eye movements	Multi-digit numerical strings	Search for highly salient features among increasing distractors
4	Use pop-out, visual anchors (e.g., colored lines)	Ask for repeated fixation just left of the middle	Narrow paragraphs in large fonts	Feature conjunction search with increasing distractors
5	Use the patient's left hand as an attentional anchor	Copy the right-sided patterns on the left	Wide paragraphs in small fonts	Compare objects for salient features
6	Provide occasional verbal reminders to focus on the left	Observe and reinforce balanced eye movements	Scattered paragraph layouts	Compare patterns for non-salient features

Note. The hierarchy presents structured interventions across sensory cueing, working memory, reading, and search domains. Each step builds on the previous, allowing task complexity and cueing demands to be adapted to the patient's current level of neglect severity and cognitive capacity.

A.6 Rehabilitation of language disorders

Determine the major deficits and symptoms of the patients to distinguish between the different subgroups of aphasia. Determine the severity of the aphasic disorder. Follow Tables A.11 and A.12 depending on the diagnosis.

TABLE A.11 Treating impairments in production of speech according to stage of recovery

	Motor aphasia	
Stage of recovery	**Conceptual preparation**	**Phonological preparation**
Massive motor aphasia (speaking any words)	Speaking in series: prescribing the numbers when naming loudly, reading aloud (twice with a delay per number the second time), starting the third time, waiting for the initiative of the patients, speaking along quietly when the patient starts. Working through a hierarchical sequence of cueing from showing, semantic cues to initiate speaking of the word "hand".	Read numbers 1 to 9, use of first letter cueing, imitation mouth movement Choir shadowing with decrease loudness If reasonably confident counting, transition to simple object naming Use writing down, phonological first letter cueing or mouth movement imitation to achieve work speaking
Moderate motor aphasia (individual words can be cleared safely, but rather as a series of words or after a combination of different cues)	Conceptual preparation for simple but changing meanings Semantic: different body parts or distinguished pictures from similar categories Search for single number between distractors that must be found and named. Facilitation by counting starting two numbers before	Read written body parts, use of first letter cueing, imitation mouth movement, choir intonation use of first letter cueing, if necessary
Mild motor aphasia, amnestic aphasia (in interaction about simple facts, the telegram style and a word-finding disorder dominate)	Formulate a sentence to describe actions on pictures (i.e. "x is doing y"). Sentences as cues (read aloud and then passively complete).	Writing down the sentence. Use agent as cue for verb produced by the patient. Sentence Completion Tasks (shadow reading of the patient, pronounce phonological cues)

(*Continued*)

TABLE A.11 (Continued)

Motor aphasia		
Stage of recovery	**Conceptual preparation**	**Phonological preparation**
	Words first with, then without visible images from memory with increasing delay, using visuospatial cues ("which picture was here and which here?")	
Amnestic aphasia (The word-finding disorder occurs in the context of sentences that have been started)	Formulate stories displayed on 4 to 6 action pictures. Position of the individual images as cue for keeping track of the story Cover picture to formulate from working memory with a growing delay from last seeing. Introduce distraction between picture viewing and storytelling. Repetition of fictitious, recurring everyday situations	Write down a word with the most important information for the single picture and point to that word in the case of hesitating speech.

TABLE A.12 Treating impairment in comprehension of speech according to stage of recovery.

Sensory aphasia		
Stage of recovery	**Conceptual preparation**	**Phonological preparation**
Severe speech comprehension disorder without excessive speech production (patient understands max. simplest prompts)	Sorting objects by semantic categories (excluding visual agnosia!) Assigning semantically different, frequent and well-known images/objects to written words. Expand this training to infrequent and more similar objects.	Read the words for the patients. Encourage the patient to repeat the word phonologically (if possible) or to copy the word.
Moderate sensory aphasia or speech comprehension disorder without excessive speech production (simple tasks are understood situationally, without situational context little language understanding)	Ask for of labels for images or words for semantic relationships between objects. Selection of action statements or descriptions for action representations Introduce delay and distraction before naming. Play the game that everybody gets a mix of images and should take turns requesting	Propose written exemplars of labels or for semantic relationships, which should be read aloud and chosen afterwards. Introduce synonyms for same objects

(*Continued*)

TABLE A.12 (Continued)

Sensory aphasia		
Stage of recovery	**Conceptual preparation**	**Phonological preparation**
	without using the direct name of the picture	
Mild speech comprehension disorder (understanding becomes difficult when the situation or context does not guide understanding or when the facts become complex or abstract)	Sentence completion tasks: **1.** Use the same conceptual space for consecutive sentences **2.** Use more and more changing conceptual space for different sentences **3.** Increase sentence length and grammatical complexity Ask for term definitions and headings for different abstract terms Deducing the meaning of words from complex stories	Write down underlying word forms components and ask to sort them in the necessary order for noncanonical sentences or sentences with relative clauses. Use anagrams as games to find semantical meaning words.
Mild comprehension deficit (speech comprehension fails with somewhat longer sentences)	Responding to requests of increasing complexity Relative clauses, such as "Give me the small square that lies next to the rectangle"	Addition problems with two then three terms, alternation of addition and subtraction at three terms. Keeping results and further calculating others.
Wernicke's"Aphasia	Conceptual preparation	Phonological preparation
Sensory aphasia with excessive speech production that is not intelligible.	Introduce Stop Signal Gaining insight into the incomprehensibility of speech production Gain insight into the cause of the malfunction Plus, the same therapy as for simple speech comprehension disorder	Individual words instead of sentences For stopping speech showing of hands. Record patient's speech and play it back. Introduce timer to decrease speech production.

A.7 Rehabilitation of disorientation and memory deficits

Use clinical information to determine the recovery stage of the patient. If the stage is early subacute and concerns orientation, analyze main problems and follow Table A.13.

TABLE A.13 Treatment of early sub-acute disorientation disorders.

Functional treatment of orientation disorders							
Cognition				**Emotion**			
Memory		**Perception and attention**		**hyperactive**		**hypoactive**	
Design of the hospital ward, external memory aids, orientation training	Source Memory Training CSF relief puncture or shunt implantation?	Sleep hygien-e, physical strain, daylight lighting	Sensory training, passive relaxati-on	passive relaxation, music therapy, physical exertion, calming conversations	Positive Biographical Cues, Conversations, Music Therapy, Aromatherapy	Passively guided forced use, gait trainer, positive reinforcement	Passive relaxation

If the stage is late subacute versus chronic, the memory disorder is severe (almost no retention after distraction of 2 min) and the lesion shows a complete interruption of the Papez circuit at some point; follow Table A.14, as far as the patients already accept external memory aids as primary perspective.

If the stage is late subacute versus chronic, the lesion shows no complete interruptions of the Papez circuit at some point, and the memory disorder is either light or moderate; follow Table A.15.

TABLE A.14 Interventions for severe memory disorders depending on recovery stage.

Stage of recovery	Goals	Specific interventional approaches
Early post-acute	Reducing orientation disorder and managing affective stress	Reestablishing wake-sleep pattern Supportive interactions and providing relevant information
Post-acute	Focus on external memory aids if the prognosis argues for enduring severe deficits Source memory training for the treatment of confabulation	Spaced retrieval of orientation-relevant information Errorless learning, depending on whether the error stems from impaired memory consolidation or a storage-related deficit
Chronic state	Establishment of external memory aids: Depending on the additional cognitive disorders, exercise in external memory aids or use of a memory aid for a specific purpose	Self-preservation therapy (external memory aid for maintaining a certain self-identity)

TABLE A.15 Rehabilitation of post-acute and chronic moderate to mild memory disorders.

Stage of recovery	Compensatory interventions	Restorative interventions
Post-acute	Mild impairment: modified story memory technique Moderate impairment: transfer appropriate processing	Mild impairment: combined PC training for attentional and memory functions. The repetition lag procedure is a theoretically sound method for restitutive training; however, the existing evidence is rather limited with only training specific improvement.
Chronic	Mild impairment: modified story memory technique Mild to moderate impairment: transfer appropriate processing. If the major problem is remembering reading text, the PQRST method should be introduced	Mild impairment: combined PC training for attentional and memory functions

A.8 Rehabilitation of goal directed behavior deficits

8.1 Rehabilitation of disorders of consciousness

Use Table A.16 to establish the correct diagnosis.
Use Tables A.17–A.19 for treatment.
Compare the chapter for additional interventions and treatment possibilities.

TABLE A.16 Syndromes of disorders of consciousness.

Diagnosis	Characteristics	Neuroanatomical cause
Unresponsive wakefulness syndrome (UWS)	No visible reaction to external stimuli, except possibly to painful stimuli Sleep-wake cycles preserved Diagnosis should only be made after verifying persistence of the condition Evaluate the patient's responses before and after an activating intervention (typically no change) No habituation and P3 response detectable	Severe cortical damage, especially in the dorsofrontal cortical areas, usually with additional thalamic and/or basal ganglia lesions Large intracerebral hemorrhage of MCA, hypoxia, or severe TBI
Akinetic mutism	Sleep-wake cycles preserved Environmental events are perceived No intentional movements, but automatic movements occur in corresponding contexts (e.g., hand closure without hand opening) No affective avoidance of stimuli; no emotional aversion toward stimuli; no emotional disengagement from stimuli P3 response detectable	Lesion in the supplementary motor cortex (SMA) or premotor cortex, unilateral left-brain lesion is sufficient in principle (e.g., large anterior infarction (left) or nontraumatic SAH as a result of an ACOA aneurysm)
Stupor-like drive disorder	Sleep-wake cycles preserved Environmental events are perceived Intentional movements are rare; automatic movements cannot be triggered significantly more frequently Emotional turning away from stimulus P3 response detectable	Lesion in the area of the ventromedial and dorsolateral prefrontal cortex, head of the caudatum; usually bilateral lesion, in which case the right hemisphere must be clearly affected (TBI)

Note: Unresponsive wakefulness syndrome (UWS), akinetic mutism, stupor-like drive disorder, their characteristics, and neuroanatomical causes. *ACM*, Anterior cerebral artery; *SAH*, subarachnoid hemorrhage; *ACOA*, aneurysm of the anterior communicating artery; *TBI*, traumatic brain injury.

TABLE A.17 Functional treatment of patients in unresponsive wakefulness state.

	Sensory stimulation		**Dialog development**
	Sense channel	Stimuli	Stimuli offers
1	Vestibular, proprioceptive, kinesthetic	Spinning, vibrations, sitting up, moving, rubbing	Hand-supported breathing, rocking, swaying; sitting up, moving, traveling through space
2	Olfactory	Coffee, vanilla, etc.	Aftershave, soap, perfume
3	Gustatory	Sweet-tasting substances	Favorite foods: honey, chocolate
4	Tactile	Touching the hand, arm, shoulder, and face	Stroking, tapping, massaging, rubbing in, hugging, caressing, kissing
5	Auditory	Bell sounds, speaking to, calling, and music	Voices, (heart) sounds, tones, music, calling names, singing, reading aloud, asking questions
6	Visual	Light stimuli, pictures, objects, and faces	Objects (doll, stuffed animal, car), pictures, photos, faces (mirror), gestures, lip-reading

TABLE A.18 Treatment phases for patients with akinetic mutism.

Stage of recovery	**Interventions**
Phase 1	Establishing a stable reaction to a specific communicative situation.
Phase 2	Eliciting initial naming and simple goal-directed actions that differ from automatic, stereotyped behaviors.
Phase 3	Increasing the time delay between the stimulus and the (speech) response, fostering greater intentional control.
Phase 4	Promoting the recovery of spontaneous, self-initiated action.

TABLE A.19 Treatment phases for patients with stupor-like drive disorder.

Stage of recovery	**Interventions**
Phase 1	Establishment of continuous, rhythmic movement patterns.
Phase 2	Analysis of primary and secondary reinforcers.
Phase 3	Establishment of circular reactions.
Phase 4	Development of a reproducible interaction system.
Phase 5	Expansion of independent actions through a token program or through contingent reinforcement.

A.9 Direct current stimulation of the lesioned brain: evidence and how to use localization of lesions for planning the electrodes' montage

Read section 3 of the chapter for safety concerns using tDCS and follow them.

Look for a cMRT FLAIR and T2 sequence and, in acute stroke, compare it with a DWI sequence. Otherwise use cCT scans. Use information of Chapter 1 to localize the stroke lesion.

Use the figures of the chapter to determine the electrodes' position according to the EEG 10–20 system. Use clinical information to determine the recovery stage of the patient. If the stage is not early subacute, define the specific goal of the stimulation (compensatory learning by preserved networks or activation of "sleeping" perilesional neurons). Follow the table below for a nonindividualized montage. Follow the comments below the table for a more individualized approach (Tables A.20–A.21).

TABLE A.20 Standard positions for tDCS depending on stage of recovery.

Stage of recovery	Target area	Possible montage
Acute and early subacute	Perilesional gray matter	Bilateral, cathodal on affected, anodal on unaffected hemisphere
Late subacute	Perilesional gray matter	Anodal perilesional stimulation, indifferent cathodal electrode position
Late subacute and chronic	Perilesional gray matter	Anodal perilesional stimulation, indifferent cathodal electrode position
	Inhibition of contralesional hyperactivity	Bilateral stimulation: anodal on affected, cathodal on unaffected hemisphere
	Stimulation of networks for relearning of functions	Bilateral montage along assumed networks (e.g., dorsal attention system, language areas, etc.). The cathodal position should be in line with the extension of the network but on the contralesional scalp
	Improving attention by stimulating attentional subsystems	Focal anodal stimulation of attention relevant brain structures (unclear if unilateral stimulation might be used)

TABLE A.21 Aspects for individualizing tDCS according to stroke localization.

1	The distance between the two electrodes should be not too small and not too large.
2	If the cathode activity can be ignored or might even contribute to the intended goal, the size of this electrode should be no larger than that of the anode. Otherwise, the size of the cathode might be increased (however, this reduces the maximal focal electrode strength).
3	If the goal is to stimulate perilesional neurons both electrodes should be placed in one line before and behind the lesion.
4	Large sulci crossing through the line between anode and cathode should be avoided if possible. They will capture electric field strength.
5	If the goal is to stimulate a network responsible for the impaired function both electrodes should be placed in one line before and behind the network. For example, if the lesion is localized in Broca's area, place the cathode next to but posterior to the Broca's area and the anode caudal to the Wernicke's area.
6	During the early subacute stage, a cathodal stimulation above the lesion and an anodal contralesional stimulation show the highest effect in animal research.

A.10 Dialogical interaction and protective cognitive environments (including virtual reality) as major components of neuropsychological rehabilitation

A more individualized placement of the electrodes may consider aspects of Tables 22 and 23.

TABLE A.22 Rehabilitation of visuoconstructive disorders according to stage of recovery.

Stage of recovery	Cognitive environment	Cognitive components involved	Goal/action	Therapeutic approach
1	Initial cognitive environment	Matching, two-dimensional rotation (visuoperceptive and elementary functions)	Create a simple cognitive environment that allows the patient to perform basic functions (e.g., matching shapes)	Minimize difficulty, allow basic performance.
2	Gradual complexity increase	Mirroring (3D rotation), scaling, segmentation	Designing the environment to challenge more complex cognitive processes	Provide external help, reduce complexity progressively.
3	Visible environment offers only relative parameters of objects	Scaling and segmentation	Segment shapes with visual aids (coordinate system, relative ratios)	Make segmentation tasks easier through scaling and external perceptual aids.
4	Relative parameters more and more limited to size	Segmentation (without external perceptual aid)	Move to more autonomous segmentation tasks	Reduce external aid while focusing on segmentation ability.
5	Advanced segmentation tasks	Segmentation against visually dominant divisions (verticals and diagonals)	Segment shapes in more complex configurations	Introduce more complex visual segmentation tasks.

TABLE A.23 Evidence for the use of virtual reality across domains of neuropsychological rehabilitation.

Domain	Systematic review summary (current strength)
Visual field defects (VFD)	Emerging evidence in multiple trials: VR perceptual learning and compensatory training can yield small field gains (~1–3°). Stroke-VR reviews report limited cognitive benefits.
Unilateral spatial neglect	Promising but heterogeneous. Many small positive trials, but weak designs and low ecological validity.
Aphasia/Language	Mixed results. Meta-analyses: small reductions in aphasia severity, no clear effect on functional communication or word-finding.
Memory (episodic/ prospective)	Limited/mixed. VR-ADL studies (e.g., supermarket/ apartment tasks) show within-task gains, but inconsistent generalization. No systematic memory-only reviews.
Executive function/goal management	Sparse evidence. Gains reported mainly within global cognition reviews.
Disorders of consciousness (DoC)	Very limited. Only case reports/pilots (mostly pediatrics). No systematic reviews.
Global cognition	Meta-analyses: modest overall benefits. VR often targets multiple domains, yielding small composite gains.
Usability and implementation	Neglected area. Therapists and patients rarely studied. Reports highlight barriers (cybersickness, lack of guidelines).

Index

Note: Page numbers followed by "*f*" and "*t*" refer to figures and tables, respectively.

R

S

Printed and bound by CPI Group (UK) Ltd, Croydon, CR0 4YY
21/09/2026
02219915-0004